oul

Differential Diagnosis in Physical Therapy

D1319928

LEEDS BECKETT UNIVERSITY LIBRARY

DISC

Leeds Metropolitan University

17 0103411 3

ISBN 0-7216-5267-0

heart, lungs, intestines, kidneys/bladder, and liver, with specialty areas of study including cardiology, pulmonary medicine, hematology, gastroenterology, urology/nephrology, hepatic/biliary problems, endocrinology, oncology, and immunology.

Hematology, endocrinology, immunology, and oncology sections are included because the physical therapist may treat a client with musculoskeletal problems who also has a disease involving one of these specialties. The information presented in these sections may assist the physical therapist in planning a treatment program that takes into consideration the client's overall compromised health, especially when exercise may precipitate or aggravate one of these conditions.

With the continual expansion of physical therapy skills, physical therapy protocols are being developed for people with diagnoses such as acquired immunodeficiency syndrome (AIDS), diabetes, allergies, asthma, and various cancers. The material in this text provides the physical therapist with an overview of these disease entities.

PHYSICIAN REFERRAL

The hallmark of professionalism in any health care practitioner is the ability to understand the limits of his or her professional knowledge. The physical therapist, either on reaching the limit of his or her knowledge or on reaching the limits prescribed by the client's condition, should refer the patient to the physician (APTA, 1990). Each physical therapist must work within the scope of his or her level of skill, knowledge, and practical experience.

Guidelines for appropriate referral to a physician (or other health care practitioner) have been outlined in the APTA Code of Ethics, Guide for Professional Conduct and Standards for Physical Therapy Services and Physical Therapy Practitioners (APTA, 1990):

If symptoms are present for which physical therapy is contraindicated or which are indicative of conditions for which treatment is outside the scope of his knowledge, the physical therapist must refer [clients] *to a licensed practitioner of medicine.*

In the event that a medical diagnosis is required and has not been established prior to treatment, then the physical therapist must refer to a licensed practitioner of medicine, dentistry, or podiatry.

Knowing how to refer the client or how to notify the physician of important findings is not always clear. It is ultimately the client's responsibility to act on the information provided by the physical therapist, whether this information is about a home program or involves a recommendation to seek additional medical care.

In the case of a client referred to physical therapy by a physician or dentist, a summary of findings is recommended, whether it is filed in the client's chart in the hospital or sent in a letter to the outpatient's physician or dentist. (For a sample letter, see Fig. 1–3.)

When the client has come to physical therapy without a medical referral (i.e., self-referred) and the physical therapist recommends medical follow-up, the client should be referred to the primary care physician. Occasionally, the client indicates that he or she has not contacted a physician or was treated by a physician (whose name cannot be recalled) a long time ago, or that he or she has just moved to the area and does not have a physician. In these situations, the client can be provided with a list of recommended physicians. It is not necessary to list every physician in the area, but the physical therapist should provide several appropriate choices. Whether or not the client makes an appointment with a medical practitioner, the physical therapist is urged to document subjective and objective findings carefully, as well as the recommendation made for medical follow-up. The client should make these physical therapy records available to the consulting physician.

PHYSICIAN REFERRAL

IMMEDIATE MEDICAL ATTENTION

- Client with anginal pain not relieved in 20 minutes
- Client with angina who has nausea, vomiting, profuse sweating
- Diabetic client demonstrating signs of confusion, lethargy, or changes in mental alertness and function
- Client with bowel/bladder incontinence and/or saddle anesthesia secondary to cauda equina lesion
- Client in anaphylactic shock (see Chapter 11)

MEDICAL ATTENTION NECESSARY

General Systemic

- Unknown cause
- Lack of significant objective neuromusculoskeletal signs and symptoms
- Lack of expected progress with physical therapy treatment
- Development of constitutional symptoms or associated signs and symptoms over the course of treatment
- Discovery of significant past medical history (PMH) unknown to physician
- Changes in health status that persist 7 to 10 days beyond expected time period
- Client who is jaundiced and has not been diagnosed or treated
- Changes in size, shape, tenderness, and consistency of lymph nodes in more than one area, which persist more than 4 weeks; *painless,* enlarged lymph nodes

For Women

- Low back, hip, pelvic, groin, or sacroiliac symptoms without known etiology and in the presence of constitutional symptoms
- Symptoms correlated with menses
- Any spontaneous uterine bleeding after menopause
- For pregnant women:

    Vaginal bleeding
    Elevated blood pressure
    Increased Braxton-Hicks contractions during exercise

Vital Signs (Report these findings)

- Persistent rise or fall of blood pressure
- Blood pressure evaluation in any woman taking birth control pills (should be closely monitored by her physician)

- Pulse amplitude that fades with inspiration and strengthens with expiration
- Pulse increase over 20 BPM lasting more than 3 minutes after rest or changing position
- Difference between systolic and diastolic measurements of more than 40 mm Hg in pulse pressure
- Persistent low-grade (or higher) fever, especially associated with constitutional symptoms, most commonly sweats

Cardiac

- Angina at rest
- Anginal pain not relieved in 20 minutes
- More than three sublingual nitroglycerin tablets required to gain relief
- Nitroglycerin does not relieve anginal pain
- Rest does not relieve angina
- Angina continues to increase in intensity after stimulus (e.g., cold, stress, exertion) has been eliminated
- Changes in pattern of angina
- Abnormally severe chest pain
- Client has nausea, vomiting
- Anginal pain radiates to jaw/left arm
- Upper back feels abnormally cool, sweaty, or moist to touch
- Patient has any doubts about his or her condition

Cancer

- Early warning sign(s) of cancer:

    Seven early warning signs plus two additional signs pertinent to the physical therapy examination: proximal muscle weakness and change in deep tendon reflexes
- All soft tissue lumps that persist or grow, whether painful or painless
- Any woman presenting with chest, breast, axillary, or shoulder pain of unknown etiology, especially in the presence of a positive medical history (self or family) of cancer
- Bone pain, especially on weight-bearing, that persists more than 1 week and is worse at night

Pulmonary

- Shoulder pain that is aggravated by supine positioning
- Shoulder, chest (thorax) pain that subsides with autosplinting (lying on the painful side)
- (For the client with asthma): Signs of asthma or bronchial activity during exercise

Genitourinary

- Abnormal urinary constituents—e.g., change in color, odor, amount, flow of urine
- Any amount of blood in urine

Musculoskeletal

- Symptoms that seem out of proportion to the injury, or symptoms persisting beyond the expected time for the nature of the injury
- Severe or chronic back pain accompanied by constitutional symptoms, especially fever

PRECAUTIONS/CONTRAINDICATIONS TO THERAPY

- Uncontrolled chronic heart failure or pulmonary edema
- Active myocarditis
- Resting heart rate >120 or 130 BPM*
- Resting systolic rate >180 to 200 BPM*
- Resting diastolic rate >105 to 110 BPM*
- Moderate dizziness, near-syncope
- Marked dyspnea
- Unusual fatigue
- Unsteadiness
- Loss of palpable pulse
- Postoperative posterior calf pain
- (For the client with diabetes): Chronically unstable blood sugar levels must be stabilized (normal: 80 to 120 mg/dl; "safe": 100 to 250 mg/dl)

---

* Unexplained or poorly tolerated by client.

Summary

This text is designed to help physical therapists in any practice or clinical setting to screen for medical disease when it is appropriate to do so. In this chapter, four parameters are introduced for use throughout the text in this decision-making process:

1. Client history
2. Pain patterns/pain types
3. Systems review
4. Signs and symptoms of systemic diseases

"The Problem of Pain." Pain is often the primary symptom we face in many physical therapy practices. Recognizing pain patterns characteristic of systemic disease is an important step, so this first chapter includes a detailed overview of pain patterns that can be used as a foundation for all the organ systems presented.

Physical therapists are often called upon to wear many different hats representing a multitude of trades and professions. Although we would like to think that our clients have access to all the services necessary for recovery or rehabilitation from their injury or medical condition, the fact is that we are often their counselor, friend, support person, priest, rabbi, and so on. For this reason, a new section has been

Referral. A 32-year-old female university student was referred for physical therapy through the health service 2 weeks ago. The physician's referral reads: "Possible right oblique abdominis tear/possible right iliopsoas tear." This woman was screened initially by a faculty member, and the diagnosis was confirmed as being a right oblique abdominal strain.

History. Two months ago, while the patient was running her third mile, she felt "severe pain" in the right side of her stomach, which caused her to double over. She felt immediate nausea and had abdominal distention. She couldn't change the position of her leg to relieve the pain at the time. Currently, she still cannot run without pain.

Presenting Symptoms. Pain increases during situps, walking fast, reaching, turning, and bending. Pain is eased by heat and is reduced by activity. Pain in the morning versus evening depends on body position. Once the pain starts, it is intermittent and aches. The patient describes the pain as being severe, depending on her body position. She is currently taking aspirin when necessary.

SAMPLE LETTER

Date

John Smith, M.D.
University of Montana Health Service
Eddy Street
Missoula, MT 59812

Re: Jane Doe

Dear Dr. Smith,
Your patient, Jane Doe, was evaluated in our clinic on 5/2/93 with the following pertinent findings:

Subjective. The patient has severe pain in the right lower abdominal quadrant associated with nausea and abdominal distention. Although the patient notes that the onset of symptoms started while she was running, she denies any precipitating trauma. She describes the course of symptoms as having begun 2 months ago with temporary resolution and now with exacerbation of earlier symptoms. Additionally, she has chronic fatigue and frequent night sweats.

Objective. Presenting pain is reproduced by resisted hip or trunk flexion with accompanying tenderness/tightness on palpation of the right iliopsoas muscle (compared with the left iliopsoas muscle). There are no implicating neurologic signs or symptoms.

Assessment. A musculoskeletal screening examination is consistent with your diagnosis of a possible iliopsoas or abdominal oblique tear. Jane appears to present with a combination of musculoskeletal and systemic symptoms, such as those outlined earlier. Of particular concern are the symptoms of fatigue, night sweats, abdominal distention, nausea, repeated episodes of exacerbation and remission, and severe quality of pain and location (right lower abdominal quadrant). These symptoms appear to be of a systemic nature rather than caused by a musculoskeletal lesion.

Recommendations. I suggest that the client return to you for further medical follow-up to rule out any systemic involvement before the initiation of physical therapy services. I am concerned that my proposed treatment plan of ultrasound, soft tissue mobilization, and stretching may aggravate an underlying disease process.

I will contact you directly by telephone by the end of the week to discuss these findings and to answer any questions that you may have. Thank you for this interesting referral.

Sincerely,

Catherine C. Goodman, M.B.A., P.T.

Result. This client returned to the physician, who then ordered laboratory tests. After an acute recurrence of the symptoms described earlier, she had exploratory surgery. A diagnosis of a ruptured appendix and peritonitis was determined at surgery. In retrospect, the proposed treatment of ultrasound and soft tissue mobilization would have been contraindicated in this situation.

Figure 1–3
Sample letter of the physical therapist's findings that is sent to the referring physician.

added that addresses the psychologic factors associated with pain.

This inclusion does not endorse physical therapists' practicing outside the scope of our expertise and experience. It merely recognizes that in treating the whole client, not only the physical but also the psychologic, emotional, and spiritual needs of that person will be represented in his or her magnitude of symptoms, length of recovery time, response to pain, and responsibility for recovery.

Finally, not every situation can be anticipated, but this text attempts to provide a basic outline for decision making as it relates to medical referral. The bottom line is: *If the client or the physical therapist is in doubt, communication with the physician, dentist, referral source, or family member is indicated.*

References

American Physical Therapy Association: House of Delegates Policies. Alexandria, Virginia, 1984, p. 19.

American Physical Therapy Association: Competencies in Physical Therapy—An Analysis of Practice. Alexandria, Virginia, March 1985.

American Physical Therapy Association: Direct Access to Physical Therapy—Information Packet. Alexandria, Virginia, Government Affairs Department, 1990.

Bauwens, D.B., and Paine, R.: Thoracic pain. *In* Blacklow, R.S. (ed.): MacBryde's Signs and Symptoms, 6th ed. Philadelphia, J.B. Lippincott, 1983, pp. 139–164.

Black, J.L., and Martin, M.J.: Musculoskeletal symptoms and anxiety disorders. Journal of Musculoskeletal Medicine 5(9):67–84, September 1988.

Blacklow, R.S. (ed.): MacBryde's Signs and Symptoms, 6th ed. Philadelphia, J.B. Lippincott, 1983.

Bonica, J.J.: The Management of Pain. Philadelphia, Lea & Febiger, 1953.

Cyriax, J.: Textbook of Orthopaedic Medicine, 8th ed. Vol. 1. London, Baillière Tindall, 1982.

Delitto, A., Tcibulka, M., Erhard, R., Bowling, R.W., and Tenhula, J.A.: Evidence for use of an extension-mobilization category in acute low back syndrome: A prescriptive validation pilot study. Physical Therapy 73(4):216–226, April 1993.

Engel, G.L.: Pain. *In* Blacklow, R.S. (ed.): MacBryde's Signs and Symptoms, 6th ed. Philadelphia, J.B. Lippincott, 1983, pp. 41–60.

Hendrix, M.L.: Understanding Panic Disorder. Washington, D.C., National Institutes of Health, 1993.

Hertling, D., and Kessler, R.M.: Management of Common Musculoskeletal Disorders, 2nd ed. Philadelphia, J.B. Lippincott, 1990.

Ignatavicius, D.D., and Bayne, M.V.: Problems of protection: Management of clients with disruptions of the integumentary system. *In* Ignatavicius, D.D., and Bayne, M.V. (eds.): Medical-Surgical Nursing. Philadelphia, W.B. Saunders, 1993, pp. 1148–1151.

Jacox, A.: Pain: A Source Book for Nurses and Other Health Professionals. Boston, Little, Brown, 1977.

Kirkaldy-Willis, W.H. (ed.): Managing Low Back Pain. New York, Churchill Livingstone, 1983.

Koop, C.E.: Incidence of anxiety-based medical problems. Personal communication, 1992.

Kozol, J.: Illiterate America. New York, Doubleday, 1985.

Magistro, C., et al.: Diagnosis in physical therapy: A roundtable discussion. P.T. Magazine 1(6):58–65, June 1993.

Matassarin-Jacobs, E.: Pain assessment and intervention. *In* Black, J.M., and Matassarin-Jacobs, E. (eds.): Luckmann and Sorensen's Medical-Surgical Nursing, 4th ed. Philadelphia, W.B. Saunders, 1993, pp. 311–358.

Matheson, L.N.: Work capacity evaluation: Systematic approach to industrial rehabilitation. Anaheim, California, Employment and Rehabilitation Institute of California, 1986.

Matheson, L.N.: Symptom magnification casebook. Anaheim, California, Employment and Rehabilitation Institute of California, 1987.

Matheson, L.N.: Symptom magnification syndrome structured interview: Rationale and procedure. Journal of Occupational Rehabilitation 1(1):43–56, 1991.

McKenzie, R.: The Lumbar Spine: Mechanical Diagnosis and Therapy. New Zealand, Spinal Publications, 1981.

Melzack, R.: The McGill Pain Questionnaire: Major properties and scoring methods. Pain 1:277, 1975.

Mennell, J.M.: Joint Pain: Diagnosis and Treatment Using Manipulative Techniques. Boston, Little, Brown, 1964.

Merskey, H., et al. (eds.): Classification of chronic pain: Descriptions of chronic pain syndromes and definitions of pain terms. Pain (Suppl. 3, 1986), reprinted 1991, p. S5.

O'Toole, M.: Miller-Keane Encyclopedia and Dictionary of Medicine, Nursing, and Allied Health, 5th ed. Philadelphia, W.B. Saunders, 1992.

Ridge, J.A., and Way, L.W.: Abdominal pain. *In* Sleisenger, M.H., and Fordtran, J.S. (eds.): Gastrointestinal Disease, 5th ed. Philadelphia, W.B. Saunders, 1993, pp. 150–161.

Rose, S.J.: Physical therapy diagnosis: Role and function. Physical Therapy 69:535–537, 1989.

Rothstein, J.M.: Patient classification. Physical Therapy 73(4): 214–215, April 1993.

Sahrmann, S.A.: Diagnosis by the physical therapist—a prerequisite for treatment. A special communication. Physical Therapy 68:1703–1706, 1988.

Sternbach, R.A.: Pain Patients: Traits and Treatment. New York, Academic Press, 1974.

Travell, J.G., and Simons, D.G.: Myofascial Pain and Dysfunction: The Trigger Point Manual, Vol. 1. Baltimore, Williams & Wilkins, 1983.

Travell, J.G., and Simons, D.G.: Myofascial Pain and Dysfunction, Vol. 2. Baltimore, Williams & Wilkins, 1992.

Waddell, G., Bircher, M., Finlayson, D., and Main, C.: Symptoms and signs: Physical disease or illness behavior? British Medical Journal 289:739–741, 1984.

Wolf, G.A., Jr.: Collecting Data from Patients. Baltimore, University Park Press, 1977.

Zohn, D.A., and Mennell, J.: Musculoskeletal Pain: Diagnosis and Physical Treatment, 2nd ed. Boston, Little, Brown, 1988.

Bibliography

Eddy, L.: Physical Therapy Pharmacology. St. Louis, C.V. Mosby, 1992.

Guccione, A.A.: Physical therapy diagnosis and the relationship between impairments and function. Physical Therapy 71:499–504, 1991.

Jette, A.M.: Diagnosis and classification by physical therapists: Special communication. Physical Therapy 69:967–969, 1989.

Rose, S.J.: Musing on diagnosis: Editorial. Physical Therapy 68(11):1665, November 1988.

2

Introduction to the Interviewing Process

Clinical Signs and Symptoms of:

Menopause

You are interviewing a client for the first time and she tells you, "The pain in my hip started 12 years ago when I was a waitress standing on my feet 10 hours a day. It seems to bother me most when I am having premenstrual symptoms. My left leg is longer than my right leg, and my hip hurts when the scars from my bunionectomy ache. This pain occurs with any changes in the weather. I have a bleeding ulcer that bothers me, and the pain keeps me awake at night. I dislocated my shoulder 2 years ago, but I can lift weights now without any problems." She continues her monologue, and you feel out of control and unsure of how to proceed. This scenario was taken directly from a clinical experience and represents what we in the medical profession term "an organ recital." In this situation, the client provides detailed information regarding all previously experienced illnesses and symptoms that may or may not be related to the current problem.

Interviewing is an important skill for the clinician to learn. It is generally agreed that 80 per cent of the information needed to clarify the cause of symptoms is contained within the subjective assessment. This chapter is designed to provide the physical therapist with interviewing guidelines and important questions to ask the client. The materials presented are not intended to teach the therapist how to interview a client. Other more appropriate texts that emphasize interviewing for the health care professional are available (see the Bibliography).

Medical practitioners (including nurses, physicians, and therapists) begin the interview by determining the client's chief complaint. The chief complaint is usually a symptomatic description by the client (i.e., subjective sensations reported, such as fatigue, dizziness, night sweats, fever).

The subjective examination may also reveal any contraindications to physical therapy treatment or indications for the kind of treatment that is most likely to be effective. Questioning the client may also assist the physical therapist in determining whether an injury is in the acute, subacute, or chronic stage. This information guides the clinician in providing symptomatic relief for the acute injury, more aggressive treatment for the chronic problem, and a combination of both methods of treatment for the subacute lesion.

The interviewing techniques, interviewing tools, core interview, and review of the inpatient hospital chart in this chapter will help the therapist determine the location and potential significance of any symptom (including pain).

The interview format provides detailed information regarding the frequency, duration, intensity, length, breadth, depth, and anatomic location as these relate to the client's chief complaint. The physical therapist will later correlate this information with objective findings from the examination to rule out possible systemic origin of symptoms. The information obtained from the interview guides the physical therapist in either referring the client to a physician or in planning physical therapy treatment.

INTERVIEWING TECHNIQUES

An organized interview format assists the physical therapist in obtaining a complete and accurate data base. Using the same outline with each client ensures that all pertinent information related to previous medical history and current medical problem(s) is included. This information is especially important when correlating the subjective data with objective findings from the physical examination.

Many interviewing techniques can be used by the skilled interviewer (Bates,

1990; Coulehan and Block, 1992; Greenberger and Hinthorn, 1992). For the physical therapist, several techniques are essential building blocks that can be expanded upon with experience. The most basic skills required for a physical therapy interview include

- Open-ended questions
- Closed-ended questions
- Funnel sequence or technique
- Paraphrasing technique

Open-Ended and Closed-Ended Questions

Beginning an interview with an *open-ended question* (i.e., questions that elicit more than a one-word response) is advised even though this gives the client opportunity to control and direct the interview. Initiating an interview with the open-ended directive, "Tell me why you are here" can potentially elicit more information in a relatively short (5 to 15 minute) period than a steady stream of *closed-ended questions* requiring a "yes" or "no" type of answer (Table 2–1).

Table 2–1
INTERVIEWING TECHNIQUES

Open-Ended Questions	Closed-Ended Questions
1. How does bed rest affect your back pain?	1. Do you have any pain after lying in bed all night?
2. Tell me how you cope with stress and what kinds of stressors you encounter on a daily basis.	2. Are you under any stress?
3. What makes the pain (better) worse?	3. Is the pain relieved by food?
4. How did you sleep last night?	4. Did you sleep well last night?

A client who takes control of the interview by telling the therapist about every ache and pain of every friend and neighbor can be rechanneled effectively by interrupting the client with a polite statement such as, "I'm beginning to get an idea of the nature of your problem. Now I would like to obtain some more specific information" (Hertling and Kessler, 1990). At this point, the interviewer may begin to use closed-ended questions (i.e., questions requiring the answer to be "yes" or "no") in order to characterize the symptoms more clearly. Moving from the open-ended line of questions to the closed-ended questions is referred to as the *funnel technique* or *funnel sequence.*

Each question format has advantages and limitations. The use of open-ended questions to initiate the interview may allow the client to control the interview but can also prevent a false-positive or false-negative response that would otherwise be elicited by starting with closed-ended (yes or no) questions. False responses elicited by closed-ended questions may develop from the client's attempt to please the health care provider or to comply with what the client believes is the correct response or expectation.

Closed-ended questions tend to be more impersonal and may set an impersonal tone for the relationship between the client and the physical therapist. These questions are limited by the restrictive nature of the information received so that the client may respond only to the category in question and may omit vital, but seemingly unrelated, information.

Use of the funnel sequence to obtain as much information as possible through the open-ended format first (before moving on to the more restrictive but clarifying "yes" or "no" type of questions at the end) can establish an effective forum for trust between the client and physical therapist.

Follow-up Questions (FUPs)

The funnel sequence is aided by the use of *follow-up* questions, referred to as *FUPs*

in the text. Beginning with one or two open-ended questions in each section, the interviewer may follow up with a series of closed-ended questions, which are listed in the core interview presented later in this chapter. For example: How does rest affect the pain or symptoms?

- Are your symptoms aggravated or relieved by any activities?
    - If yes, what?
- How has this problem affected your daily life at work or at home?
- How has it affected your ability to care for yourself without assistance (e.g., dress, bathe, cook, drive)?

Paraphrasing Technique

A useful interviewing skill that can assist in synthesizing and integrating the information obtained during questioning is the paraphrasing technique. When using this technique, the interviewer repeats information presented by the client. This technique can assist in fostering effective, accurate communication between the health care recipient and the health care provider.

For example, once a client has responded to the question, "What makes you feel better?," the physical therapist can paraphrase the reply by saying, "You've told me that the pain is relieved by such and such, is that right? What other activities or treatment brings you relief from your pain or symptoms?" If you cannot paraphrase what the client has said, or you are unclear about the meaning of the client's response, ask for clarification by requesting an example of what the person is talking about.

INTERVIEWING TOOLS

With the changing requirements of hospital accreditation and payment sources, physical therapists are required more and more to identify problems, to quantify symptoms (e.g., pain), and to demonstrate the effectiveness of treatment. The use of interviewing tools such as the *McGill Pain*

Questionnaire (Melzack, 1975; Wolf, 1985) can also assist physical therapists in documenting a client's progress and in justifying services provided. This can be accomplished by utilizing information about the client to establish objective and measurable goals against which progress can be measured.

No single instrument or method of pain measurement can be considered to be the best under all circumstances. However, for the clinician who is interested in quantifying pain as part of a goal-writing procedure and in order to measure improvement by using pain as a guide, some form of assessment is necessary.

The McGill questionnaire is presented in this chapter in a form adapted for use by physical therapists. This particular questionnaire is included because it assesses overall pain experience and is not limited to a single disease, injury, or body part. It provides a good baseline for assessing pain. Other forms of pain indices are available, including assessment scales designed specifically for back pain and back disability (see the Bibliography).

McGill Pain Questionnaire

Classes of Word Descriptors

The McGill Pain Questionnaire, which was designed by Melzack (1975), consists of three major classes of word descriptors —sensory, affective, and evaluative—that are used by clients to describe subjective pain experience (Fig. 2–1). *Sensory* words (Groups 1 to 10) describe pain in terms of time, space, pressure, heat, and other properties. *Affective* qualities (Groups 11 to 15) include aspects of tension, fear, and autonomic properties that are a part of the pain experience. *Evaluative* words (Group 16) describe the overall intensity of the pain phenomenon by using subjective labels (Jacox, 1977; Wolf, 1985).

The remaining groups (17 to 20) are considered to be a miscellaneous category. Each word selected in the miscellaneous category should be evaluated for possible etiology (e.g., radiating may be more neurogenic, whereas torturing is more descriptive of an affective quality). Words within each subgroup (1 to 20) were determined by Melzack and Torgerson (1971) to be ranked according to intensity of pain. For example, pounding pain is considered worse than pulsing pain, and stabbing implies more pain than boring which, in turn, represents more pain than pricking (Jacox, 1977).

Questionnaire Administration

The questionnaire was designed to provide quantitative measures of clinical pain that can be treated statistically. Proper questionnaire administration requires that the client select only one word from each category and describe only the present pain. The questionnaire should be administered by the physical therapist or by trained ancillary staff.* The client should be instructed to check only words listed that best describe the pain. Any categories that do not describe the client's pain should remain blank.

The anatomic figure should be explained and presented at the same time. The physical therapist will note additional indicators between the two anatomical figures in the questionnaire (see Fig. 2–1) to outline areas of numbness, moderate or severe pain, or shooting pain. These descriptors were not part of the original questionnaire but have been added as a modification for use by physical therapists. These additional notations can be drawn in by the physical therapist while the client is being interviewed about the description of pain sensation.

---

* Any clinician who decides to use the interview tools presented here is advised to read the original articles describing the research and intentions for use of these pain scales.

UNIVERSITY OF MONTANA
PHYSICAL THERAPY CLINIC

CLIENT'S NAME _____

DATE _____

DIRECTIONS: There are many words that describe pain. Some of these words are grouped below. Check (✔) one word in each category that best describes your pain. Any category that does not describe your pain should remain blank.

1 Flickering
Quivering
Pulsing
Throbbing
Beating
Pounding

2 Jumping
Flashing
Shooting

3 Pricking
Boring
Drilling
Stabbing
Lancinating

4 Sharp
Cutting
Lacerating

5 Pinching
Pressing
Gnawing
Cramping
Crushing

6 Tugging
Pulling
Wrenching

7 Hot
Burning
Scalding
Searing

8 Tingling
Itchy
Smarting
Stinging

9 Dull
Sore
Hurting
Aching
Heavy

10 Tender
Taut
Rasping
Splitting

11 Tiring
Exhausting

12 Sickening
Suffocating

13 Fearful
Frightful
Terrifying

14 Punishing
Gruelling
Cruel
Vicious
Killing

15 Wretched
Blinding

16 Annoying
Troublesome
Miserable
Intense
Unbearable

17 Spreading
Radiating
Penetrating
Piercing

18 Tight
Numb
Drawing
Squeezing
Tearing

19 Cool
Cold
Freezing

20 Nagging
Nauseating
Agonizing
Dreadful
Torturing

||||| Numbness

⚫ Severe pain

〰 Moderate pain

↓ Shooting pain

ACCOMPANYING SYMPTOMS:
Nausea
Headache
Dizziness
Drowsiness
Constipation
Diarrhea

COMMENTS:

SLEEP:
Good
Fitful
Can't sleep

COMMENTS:

ACTIVITY:
Good
Some
Little
None

FOOD INTAKE:
Good
Some
Little
None

COMMENTS:

COMMENTS:

A form of the McGill Pain Questionnaire.

KEY:
Group 1   suggests vascular disorder
Groups 2-8   suggests neurogenic disorder
Group 9   suggests musculoskeletal disorder
Groups 10-20 suggests emotional lability

SCORING: Add up total number of checks. Patients who mark
4-8 = Within normal limits (WNL)
≥ 6 = may be getting a "little into pain"
≥ 10 = may be helped more by a clinical psychologist than by physical therapy
≥ 16 = unlikely to respond to therapy procedures

Figure 2–1

A form of the McGill Pain Questionnaire. The key and scoring information at the bottom are for the therapist's use only to determine the type of disorder and how to handle the disorder. (Adapted from Wolf, S.L.: Clinical decision making in physical therapy. *In* Paris, S. [ed.]: Clinical Decision Making: Orthopedic Physical Therapy. Philadelphia, F.A. Davis, 1985.)

Questionnaire Scoring

The score is determined by adding the total number of checks in Groups 1 to 20. This total is then compared with the key provided (see Fig. 2–1). The results allow physical therapists to determine the degree of emotional involvement experienced by the person. By reviewing the score and the categories selected by the client to describe pain, the physical therapist may be able to recognize a potential need for psychologic counseling in place of, or as an adjunct to, physical therapy procedures (Melzack, 1975; Wolf, 1985).

Categories selected may also serve as a screen for symptoms of possible vascular, neurogenic (nervous system), or musculoskeletal involvement. For example, Group 1 suggests a vascular disorder, Groups 2 to 8 suggest a neurogenic disorder, and Group 9 suggests a musculoskeletal lesion. Accompanying (or associated) symptoms are more indicative of possible systemic involvement.

Physical therapists may choose to modify the standardized questionnaire procedure in order to assess previous and present pain patterns. This modification provides better understanding of the client's history. If the test is not administered according to the standardization, then the scoring cannot be considered valid as described.

When used as intended, the McGill Pain Questionnaire also should be administered after treatment to assess changes in pain. Although it was designed to be readministered after each treatment, individual physical therapists may determine a schedule of less frequent use depending on the type of facility, the type of client, and time factors.*

---

* We have found that the McGill Pain Questionnaire is most useful in the case of people with chronic pain or pain of unknown etiology. The major disadvantage of this tool is the use of uncommon words, such as lancinating, rasping, and lacerating.

When the questionnaire is given after treatment, it is important to determine whether the client tends to choose the same word descriptors on successive presentations of the questionnaire. Variations in the quality and intensity of pain, as well as changes in mood and other psychologic variables such as personality, would produce some variation in word choices on successive questionnaires. Clients who have a particular pain syndrome would be expected to show a considerable degree of consistency by choosing subclasses that characterize the pain syndrome (Melzack, 1975).

SUBJECTIVE EXAMINATION

The core interview is the primary substance of the subjective examination and is intended to provide a database that can be expanded to add information. Information obtained is extremely important in determining immediate treatment referral, and it must be conducted in a complete and organized manner. An example of a core interview follows. The complete subjective examination consists of several major components, each of which is discussed further in this chapter. These components include

- Family/Personal History
  - Age
  - Past medical history
  - Medical testing/previous surgery
  - General health
  - Special questions for women and men
  - Work environment
  - Vital signs

- Core Interview
  - History of present illness
  - Assessment of pain and symptoms
  - Medical treatment and medications
  - Current level of fitness
  - Sleep-related history
  - Psychogenic considerations

Family/Personal History

It is unnecessary and probably impossible to complete the entire subjective examination on the first day. Most clinics or health care facilities use what is called an initial intake form before the client's first visit with the physical therapist. The *Family/Personal History* form is an example of an initial intake form.

This component of the subjective examination can elicit valuable data regarding the client's family history of disease and personal life style, including working environment and health habits. Once the client has completed the Family/Personal History intake form, the clinician can then follow up with appropriate questions based on any "Yes" selections made by the client.

For example, a client who circles "Yes" on the Family/Personal History form indicating a history of ulcers or stomach problems now presents a chief complaint of back pain during the History of Present Illness. Obtaining further information at the first appointment with the client by using *Special Questions to Ask* from Chapter 6 is necessary so that a decision regarding treatment or referral can be made immediately.

This treatment-versus-referral decision is further clarified as the interview and other objective evaluation procedures continue. Thus, if further questioning fails to show any association of back pain with gastrointestinal symptoms and the objective findings from the back evaluation point to a true musculoskeletal lesion, medical referral is unnecessary and treatment with physical therapy can begin.

Each clinical situation requires slight adaptations or alterations to the interview. These modifications, in turn, affect the depth and range of questioning. For example, a client who has pain associated with an anterior shoulder dislocation and who has no history of other disease is unlikely to require in-depth questioning to rule out systemic origins of pain. Conversely, a woman with no history of trauma with

previous history of breast cancer who is self-referred to the physical therapist without a previous medical examination and who complains of shoulder pain should be interviewed more thoroughly. The simple question "How will the answers to the questions I am asking permit me to help the client?" can serve as a guide to you (Wolf, 1977).

Continued questioning may occur both during the objective examination and during treatment. In fact, the physical therapist is encouraged to carry on a continuous dialogue during the objective examination, both as an educational tool (i.e., for the client's education) and as a method of reducing any apprehension on the part of the client. This open communication may bring to light other important information (Swisher and Enelow, 1985).

The client may wonder about the extensiveness of the interview, thinking, for example, "Why is the therapist asking questions about bowel function when my primary concern relates to back pain?" The physical therapist may need to make a qualifying statement to the client regarding the need for such detailed information. For example, questions about bowel function to rule out gallbladder involvement (which can refer pain to the back) may seem to be unrelated to the client but make sense when the physical therapist explains the possible connection between back pain and systemic disease.

Throughout the questioning, record both positive and negative findings in the subjective and objective reports in order to correlate information when making an initial assessment of the client's problem. Efforts should be made to quantify all information by frequency, intensity, duration, and exact location (including length, breadth, depth, and anatomic location).

This Family/Personal History form may be set up in a variety of ways. One type is outlined in the sample on page 31. More detailed information and follow-up questions can be found in subsequent chapters under each system heading.

FAMILY/PERSONAL HISTORY

DATE: _____

CLIENT'S NAME _____ DOB _____ AGE _____

DIAGNOSIS _____ DATE OF ONSET _____

PHYSICIAN _____ THERAPIST _____ PRECAUTIONS _____

Past Medical History

Have you or any immediate family member ever been told you have:

Circle one:

(Do **NOT** complete) **For the therapist:**

			Relation to Client	Date of Onset	Current Status
■ Cancer	Yes	No			
■ Diabetes	Yes	No			
■ Hypoglycemia	Yes	No			
■ Hypertension or high blood pressure	Yes	No			
■ Heart disease	Yes	No			
■ Angina or chest pain	Yes	No			
■ Shortness of breath	Yes	No			
■ Stroke	Yes	No			
■ Kidney disease/stones	Yes	No			
■ Urinary tract infection	Yes	No			
■ Allergies	Yes	No			
■ Asthma, hay fever	Yes	No			
■ Rheumatic/scarlet fever	Yes	No			
■ Hepatitis/jaundice	Yes	No			
■ Cirrhosis/liver disease	Yes	No			
■ Polio	Yes	No			
■ Chronic bronchitis	Yes	No			
■ Pneumonia	Yes	No			
■ Emphysema	Yes	No			
■ Migraine headaches	Yes	No			
■ Anemia	Yes	No			
■ Ulcers/stomach problems	Yes	No			

Therapists: Use this space to record baseline information. This is important in case something changes in the client's status. You are advised to record the date and initial this form for documentation and liability purposes, indicating that you have reviewed this form with the client.

Continued on following page

Circle one:

<table>
<tr><td></td><td></td><td></td><td colspan="3">(Do NOT complete) For the therapist:</td></tr>
<tr><td></td><td></td><td></td><td>Relation to Client</td><td>Date of Onset</td><td>Current Status</td></tr>
<tr><td>■ Arthritis/gout</td><td>Yes</td><td>No</td><td></td><td></td><td></td></tr>
<tr><td>■ AIDS/HIV-positive</td><td>Yes</td><td>No</td><td></td><td></td><td></td></tr>
<tr><td>■ Hemophilia/slow healing</td><td>Yes</td><td>No</td><td></td><td></td><td></td></tr>
<tr><td>■ Guillain-Barré syndrome</td><td>Yes</td><td>No</td><td></td><td></td><td></td></tr>
<tr><td>■ Epilepsy</td><td>Yes</td><td>No</td><td></td><td></td><td></td></tr>
<tr><td>■ Thyroid problems</td><td>Yes</td><td>No</td><td></td><td></td><td></td></tr>
<tr><td>■ Multiple sclerosis</td><td>Yes</td><td>No</td><td></td><td></td><td></td></tr>
<tr><td>■ Tuberculosis</td><td>Yes</td><td>No</td><td></td><td></td><td></td></tr>
<tr><td>■ Fibromyalgia/myofascial pain syndrome</td><td>Yes</td><td>No</td><td></td><td></td><td></td></tr>
<tr><td>■ Other (please describe)</td><td>Yes</td><td>No</td><td></td><td></td><td></td></tr>
</table>

Work Environment

1. Occupation:

2. Does your job involve: [　] prolonged sitting (e.g., desk, computer, driving)
   [　] prolonged standing (e.g., equipment operator, sales clerk)
   [　] prolonged walking (e.g., mill worker, delivery service)
   [　] use of large or small equipment (e.g., telephone, fork lift, typewriter, drill press, cash register)
   [　] lifting, bending, twisting, climbing, turning
   [　] exposure to chemicals, pesticides, toxins, or gases
   [　] other: please describe

3. Do you use any special supports:
   [　] back cushion, neck cushion
   [　] back brace, corset
   [　] other kind of brace or support for any body part

4. History of falls:　[　] I have had no falls
   [　] I have just started to lose my balance/fall
   [　] I fall occasionally
   [　] Certain factors make me cautious (e.g., curbs, ice, stairs, getting in and out of the tub)

For the physical therapist:

Vital Signs

Resting pulse rate

Oral temperature

Blood pressure: 1st reading _____ 2nd reading _____

　　　　　　　　Position:　　　　　　　　　　　　Extremity:

Medical Testing

1. Are you taking any prescription or over-the-counter medications?

   Yes   No

If yes, please list:

2. Have you have any x-rays, sonograms, computed tomography (CT) scans, or magnetic resonance imaging (MRI) done recently?

   Yes   No

If yes, when?   Where?   Results?

3. Have you had any laboratory work done recently (urinalysis or blood tests)?

   Yes   No

If yes, when?   Where?   Results (if known)?

4. Please list any operations that you have ever had and the date(s):

Operation   Date

General Health

1. Have you had any illnesses within the last 3 weeks (e.g., colds, influenza, bladder or kidney infection)?

   Yes   No

2. Have you noticed any lumps or thickening of skin or muscle anywhere on your body?

   Yes   No

3. Do you have any sores that have not healed or any changes in size, shape, or color of a wart or mole?

   Yes   No

4. Have you had any unexplained weight gain or loss in the last month?

   Yes   No

5. Do you smoke or chew tobacco?

   Yes   No

If yes, how many packs/day? _____ For how many months or years?

_____

6. How much alcohol do you drink in the course of a week? _____

7. Do you use recreational drugs? If yes, what, how much, how often? _____

_____

8. How much caffeine do you consume daily (including soft drinks, coffee, tea, or chocolate)?

9. Are you on any special diet prescribed by a physician?

10. Do you have a pacemaker, transplanted organ, or metal implants?

    Yes   No

Physical therapists may modify the information required depending on individual differences in client base and specialty areas served. For example, an orthopedic-based facility or a sports medicine center may want to include questions on the intake form concerning current level of fitness and orthopedic devices used, such as orthotics, splints, or braces. Physical therapists working with the geriatric population may want more information regarding levels of independence in activities of daily living. ■

Age and Aging (Resnick, 1993)

The age of a client is an important variable to consider when evaluating the underlying neuromusculoskeletal pathology and when screening for medical disease. Table 2–2 provides some of the age-related systemic and neuromusculoskeletal pathologies. (Table 10–3 also lists common malignant tumors by age.)

Of all the people who have ever lived to age 65 years, more than half are currently alive. Although the implications of this

Table 2–2

SOME AGE-RELATED MEDICAL CONDITIONS

Diagnosis	Sex	Age (Years)
Neuromusculoskeletal		
Guillain-Barré syndrome		Any age; hx of infection/alcoholism
Multiple sclerosis		15–50
Rotator cuff degeneration		30+
Spinal stenosis	Men > women	60+
Tietze's syndrome		Before 40, including children
Costochondritis	Women > men	40+
Neurogenic claudication		40–60+
Systemic		
AIDS/HIV	Men > women	20–49
Buerger's disease	Men > women	20–40 (smokers)
Abdominal aortic aneurysm	(Hypertensive) Men > women	40–70
Cancer		See Table 10–3
Breast cancer	Women > men	45–70 (peak incidence)
Hodgkin's disease	Men > women	20–40; 50–60
Osteoid osteoma (benign)	Men > women	10–20
Pancreatic carcinoma	Men > women	50–70
Skin cancer	Men = women	Rarely before puberty
Gallstones	Women > men	40+
Gout	Men > women	40–59
Gynecologic conditions	Women	20–45 (peak incidence)
Prostatitis	Men	40+
Primary biliary cirrhosis	Women > men	40–60
Reiter's syndrome	Men > women	20–40
Renal tuberculosis	Men > women	20–40
Rheumatic fever	Girls > boys	4–9; 18–30
Shingles		60+
Spontaneous pneumothorax		20–40
Systemic backache		45+
Thyroiditis	Women > men	30–50
Vascular claudication		40–60+

startling statistic are usually viewed in demographic and economic terms, the impact of age on medical care is also substantial and requires significant alterations in the approach to the older client.

Human aging is best characterized as the progressive constriction of each organ system's homeostatic reserve. This decline (Table 2–3), often referred to as "homeostenosis," begins in the third decade and is gradual, linear, and variable among individuals. Each organ system's decline is independent of changes in other organ systems and is influenced by diet, environment, and personal habits.

An abrupt change or sudden decline in any system or function is always due to disease and not to "normal aging." In the absence of disease, the decline in homeostatic reserve should cause no symptoms and impose no restrictions on activities of daily living regardless of age. In short, "old people are sick because they are sick, not because they are old."

The onset of a new disease in elderly people generally affects the most vulnerable organ system, which often is different from the newly diseased organ system and explains why disease presentation is so atypical in this population. For example, less than one fourth of older clients with hyperthyroidism present with the classic triad of goiter, tremor, and exophthalmos; more likely symptoms are atrial fibrillation, confusion, depression, syncope, and weakness.

Because the "weakest link" is so often the brain, lower urinary tract, or cardiovasular or musculoskeletal system, a limited number of presenting symptoms predominate no matter what the underlying disease. These include

■ acute confusion

■ depression

■ falling

■ incontinence

■ syncope

The corollary is equally important: The organ system usually associated with a particular symptom is less likely to be the cause of that symptom in older individuals than in younger ones. For example, acute confusion in older patients is less often due to a new brain lesion, incontinence is less often due to a bladder disorder, falling to a neuropathy, or syncope to heart disease.

Questions to assess balance and function of elderly persons are included on the Family/Personal History form. Well elderly people have no falling patterns but may have a fear of falling in specific instances (e.g., getting out of the bath or shower; walking on ice, curbs, or uneven terrain). Elderly clients who have just started to fall or who fall frequently may be fearful of losing their independence by revealing this information even to a physical therapist. Even though the client indicates no difficulty with falling, the therapist is encouraged to review this part of the form carefully with the client.

For women, gender-linked protection against coronary artery disease ends with menopause. At age 45 years, one in nine women develops heart disease. By age 65 years, this statistic changes to one in three women. Women who have heart attacks are twice as likely as men to die within the first 2 weeks. Whether this is due to discriminatory medicine, natural physiologic differences between men and women, or some other factor is unknown at this time (Diethrich and Cohen, 1992).

Past Medical History

The initial Family/Personal History form also provides the physical therapist with some idea of the client's previous medical history, medical testing, and current general health status. It is important to take time with these questions and to ensure that the client understands what is being asked. As stated earlier, the interviewer may follow up on any "Yes" response on

Table 2–3

SELECTED AGE-RELATED CHANGES AND THEIR CONSEQUENCES

Organ/System	Age-Related Physiologic Change*	Consequence of Age-Related Physiologic Change	Disease, Not Age
General	↑ Body fat	↑ Volume of distribution for fat-soluble drugs	Obesity
	↓ Total body water	↓ Volume of distribution for water-soluble drugs	Anorexia
Eyes/Ears	Presbyopia Lens opacification ↓ High-frequency acuity	↓ Accommodation ↑ Susceptibility to glare Difficulty discriminating words if background noise is present	Blindness Deafness
Endocrine	Impaired glucose tolerance	↑ Glucose level in response to acute illness	Diabetes mellitus
	↓ Thyroxine clearance (and production)	↓ T_4 dose required in hypothyroidism	Thyroid dysfunction
	↑ ADH, ↓ renin, and ↓ aldosterone	—	↓ Na^+, ↑ K^+
	↓ Testosterone	—	Impotence
	↓ Vitamin D absorption and activation	Osteopenia	Osteoporosis Osteomalacia
Respiratory	↓ Lung elasticity and ↑ chest wall stiffness	Ventilation/perfusion mismatch and ↓ pO_2	Dyspnea Hypoxia
Cardiovascular	↓ Arterial compliance and ↑ systolic BP → LVH	Hypotensive response to ↑ HR, volume depletion, or loss of atrial contraction	Syncope
	↓ β-adrenergic responsiveness	↓ Cardiac output and HR response to stress	Heart failure
	↓ Baroreceptor sensitivity and ↓ SA node automaticity	Impaired blood pressure response to standing, volume depletion	Heart block

the intake form. For example, a "Yes" response to questions on this form directed toward *allergies, asthma,* and *hay fever* should be followed up by asking the client to list the allergies and to list the symptoms that may indicate a manifestation of allergies, asthma, or hay fever. The physical therapist can then be alert for any signs of respiratory distress or allergic reactions during exercise or with the use of topical agents.

Likewise, clients may indicate the presence of *shortness of breath* with only mild exertion or without exertion, possibly even after waking at night. This condition of breathlessness can be associated with one of many conditions, including heart disease, bronchitis, asthma, obesity, emphysema, dietary deficiencies, pneumonia, and lung cancer. A "Yes" response to any question in this section would require further questioning, correlation to objective findings, and consideration of referral to the client's physician.

Medical Testing

Tests contributing information to the physical therapy assessment may include radiography (x-rays, sonograms), computed tomography (CT) scans, magnetic resonance imaging (MRI), lumbar puncture analysis, urinalysis, and blood tests. The client's medical records may contain information regarding which tests have been performed and the results of the test. It

Table 2-3
SELECTED AGE-RELATED CHANGES AND THEIR CONSEQUENCES *Continued*

Organ/System	Age-Related Physiologic Change*	Consequence of Age-Related Physiologic Change	Disease, Not Age
Gastrointestinal	↓ Hepatic function	Delayed metabolism of some drugs	Cirrhosis
	↓ Gastric acidity	↓ Ca^+ absorption on empty stomach	Osteoporosis B_{12} deficiency
	↓ Colonic motility	Constipation	Fecal impaction
	↓ Anorectal function	—	Fecal incontinence
Hematologic/ Immune System	↓ Bone marrow reserve (?)	—	Anemia
	↓ T-cell function	False-negative PPD response	—
	↑ Autoantibodies	False-positive rheumatoid factor, antinuclear antibody	Autoimmune disease
Renal	↓ Glomerular filtration rate	Impaired excretion of some drugs	↑ Serum creatinine
	↓ Urine concentration/dilution (see also *Endocrine*)	Delayed response to salt or fluid restriction/overload; nocturia	⇅ Na^+
Genitourinary	Vaginal/urethral mucosal atrophy	Dyspareunia Bacteriuria	Symptomatic urinary tract infection
	Prostate enlargement	↑ Residual urine volume	Urinary incontinence Urinary retention
Musculoskeletal	↓ Lean body mass, muscle	—	Functional impairment
	↓ Bone density	Osteopenia	Hip fracture
Nervous System	Brain atrophy	Benign senescent forgetfulness	Dementia Delirium
	↓ Brain catechol synthesis	—	Depression
	↓ Brain dopaminergic synthesis	Stiffer gait	Parkinson's disease
	↓ Righting reflexes	↑ Body sway	Falls
	↓ Stage 4 sleep	Early wakening, insomnia	Sleep apnea

* Changes generally observed in healthy elderly subjects free of symptoms and detectable disease in the organ system studied. The changes are usually important only when the system is stressed or other factors are added (e.g., drugs, disease, or environmental challenge); they rarely result in symptoms otherwise.

The table displays selected changes that occur normally with age and their physiologic consequences. Changes due to disease rather than to age are listed in the last column. ADH = antidiuretic hormone, BP = blood pressure, HR = heart rate, LVH = left ventricular hypertrophy, PPD = purified protein derivative, T_4 = thyroxine.

From Resnick, N.M.: Geriatric Medicine. *In* Harrison's Principles of Internal Medicine. New York, McGraw-Hill, 1994.

may be helpful to question the client directly by asking

■ What medical test have you had for this condition?

After giving the client time to respond, you may need to probe further by asking

■ Have you had any x-ray films, sonograms, CT scans, or MRIs in the last 2 years?

■ Do you recall having any blood tests or urinalyses done?

If yes, the physical therapist will want to know when and where these tests were performed and the results (if known to the client). Knowledge of where the test took place provides the therapist with access to the results (with the client's written permission for disclosure).

As often as possible, the physical therapist will want to examine the available test results either with a radiologist or with the client's physician or assistant. Familiarity with the results of these tests, combined with an understanding of the clinical presentation, can assist physical therapists in knowing what to look for clinically with future clients and to offer some guidelines for knowing when to suggest or recommend additional testing for clients who have not had a radiologic work-up or other potentially appropriate medical testing.

For a current and informative comparison of each of these test procedures, including expected results, risk factors, advantages, and disadvantages, the reader and client are referred to *The Patient's Guide to Medical Tests* (Pickney and Pickney, 1986) or *Laboratory Tests and Diagnostic Procedures* (Chernecky et al., 1993). Laboratory values of interest to physical therapists are displayed on the inside covers of this book.

Previous Surgery

Previous surgery or surgery related to the client's current symptoms may be indicated on the Family/Personal History form. Whenever treating a client postoperatively, the physical therapist should try to read the surgical report and should look for notes on complications, blood transfusions, and the position of the client during the surgery and the length of time in that position.

Clients in an early postoperative stage (within 3 weeks of surgery) may have stiffness, aching, and musculoskeletal pain unrelated to the diagnosis, which may be attributed to position during the surgery. Postoperative infections can lie dormant for months. Accompanying constitutional symptoms may be minimal with no sweats, fever, or chills until the infection progresses with worsening of symptoms or significant change in symptoms.

Specific follow-up questions differ from one client to another depending on the type of surgery, age of client, accompanying medical history, and so forth, but it is always helpful to assess how quickly the

client recovered from surgery in order to determine an appropriate pace for a therapy treatment program.

General Health

Recent Infections. Recent infections such as mononucleosis, hepatitis, or upper respiratory infections may precede the onset of Guillain-Barré syndrome. Recent colds, influenza, or upper respiratory infections may also be an extension of a chronic health pattern of systemic illness. Further questioning may reveal recurrent influenza-like symptoms associated with headaches and musculoskeletal complaints. These complaints could originate with medical problems, such as endocarditis (a bacterial infection of the heart) or pleuropulmonary disorders, which should be ruled out by a physician.

Knowing that the client has had a recent bladder, vaginal, uterine, or kidney infection, or that the client is likely to have such infections, may help explain back pain in the absence of any musculoskeletal findings. The client may or may not confirm previous back pain associated with previous infections. If there is any doubt, a medical referral is recommended. On the other hand, chest or sacroiliac pain may be caused by repeated coughing after a recent upper respiratory infection.

Screening for Cancer. Any responses in the affirmative to early screening questions for cancer (General Health questions 2, 3, and 4) must be followed up by a physician. Changes in appetite and unexplained weight loss can be associated with cancer, onset of diabetes, hyperthyroidism, depression, or pathologic anorexia (loss of appetite). Weight loss significant for neoplasm would be a 10 per cent loss of total body weight over a 4-week period not related to any intentional diet or fasting.

A significant, unexplained weight gain can be caused by congestive heart failure, hypothyroidism, or cancer. Weight gain/ loss does not always correlate with appetite. For example, weight gain associated with neoplasm may be accompanied by appetite loss, whereas weight gain associated with hyperthyroidism may be accompanied by increased appetite.

Substance Abuse. "Substance" refers to all mood-affecting chemicals. Among the substances most commonly used that cause druglike reactions but are not usually thought of as drugs are

- alcohol
- tobacco
- coffee
- black tea
- caffeinated carbonated beverages

Other substances commonly abused include *depressants* such as barbiturates (barbs, downers, pink ladies, rainbows, reds, yellows, sleeping pills), *stimulants* such as amphetamines and cocaine (crack, coke, snow, white, lady, blow, rock), *opiates* (heroin), *cannabis derivatives* (marijuana, hashish), and *hallucinogens* (LSD or acid, mescaline, magic mushroom, PCP, angel dust) (Kneisl, 1993).

Physiologic Effects. Behavioral and physiologic responses to any of these substances depend on the characteristics of the chemical itself, the route of administration, and the adequacy of the client's circulatory system. A brief description of the physiologic effects is included in each section below. A few general findings are reported here.

Separate from disturbances of cardiac rhythm, heart palpitations may result from effort, excitement, infection, tobacco, alcohol, or caffeine. Heavy smoking is commonly associated with chronic alcohol abuse (Matsuo et al., 1987), and both addictions have a negative influence on bone formation, probably a result of defective osteoblastosis (de Vernejoul et al., 1983). The combination of coffee ingestion and smoking raises the blood pressure of hypertensive clients about 15/33 mm Hg for as long as 2 hours (Freestone and Ramsay, 1982).

Questions designed to screen for the presence of chemical substance abuse need to become part of assessment whenever clients are seen by health professionals (Kneisl, 1993). After asking questions about use of alcohol, tobacco, caffeine, and recreational drugs, conclude with

- Are there any drugs or substances you take that you haven't told me about yet?

Tobacco. Tobacco is considered a "gateway" drug. People who smoke are more likely to drink alcohol, eat poorly, and abuse other drugs. Cigarette smoking and the use of other tobacco products constitutes the single most devastating preventable cause of death in the United States today. Smoking contributes substantially to hundreds of thousands of deaths each year from heart attacks and strokes; tens of thousands of deaths from lung, bladder, and other cancers; and immeasurable suffering and disability from chronic bronchitis and emphysema, angina pectoris, nonfatal strokes, and other tobacco-induced diseases (Quick and Quick, 1984).

Tobacco contains nicotine, which acts on the heart, blood vessels, digestive tract, kidneys, and nervous system. The effects of tobacco use (whether in the form of chewing tobacco or pipe or cigarette smoking) on the heart and lungs are well documented. For the client with respiratory or cardiac problems, tobacco stimulates the already compensated heart to beat faster, narrows the blood vessels, reduces the supply of oxygen to the heart, and increases the client's chances of developing blood clots (Wong, 1981). These effects have a direct impact on the client's ability to exercise and must be considered when starting a treatment program.

Smoking markedly increases the need for vitamin C, which is poorly stored in the body. One cigarette can consume 25 mg of vitamin C (one pack would consume 500 mg/day) (Bresler, 1979). The capillary fragility associated with low ascorbic acid levels greatly increases the tendency for tissue bleeding, especially at injection sites

(Travell and Simons, 1983). The detrimental effects of cigarette smoking on wound healing and peripheral circulation are well known (Riefkohl et al., 1986; Sherwin and Gastwirth, 1990; Webster et al., 1986; Yaffe et al., 1984).

Several studies have linked smoking with acute lumbar and cervical intervertebral disc herniation (Frymoyer et al., 1983; Heliövaara et al., 1987; Holm and Nachemson, 1988). It is unclear why smoking aggravates these conditions, but it is hypothesized that the decreased blood circulation limits nutrients to the disc. Another study by Rimoldi (1993) found that tobacco has a direct adverse effect on bone remodeling.

Alcohol. The National Institute on Alcohol Abuse and Alcoholism reports that 2 to 10 per cent of individuals aged 65 years or older are alcoholics. That percentage translates into about three million older Americans and is likely a gross underestimate. As the graying of America continues, this figure may escalate, especially as "baby boomers" (people born between 1945 and 1960), having grown up in an age of alcohol and substance abuse, carry that into old age.

Alcohol is a toxic drug that is harmful to all body tissues. It has both vasodilatory (capable of opening blood vessels) and depressant effects that may produce fatigue and mental depression or alter the client's perception of pain or symptoms. Alcohol raises systolic blood pressure, so that ingestion of alcohol may intensify already existing throbbing pain associated with the cardiovascular system.

Besides deleterious effects on the gastrointestinal, hepatic, cardiovascular, hematopoietic, genitourinary, and neuromuscular systems, prolonged used of excessive alcohol may affect bone metabolism, resulting in reduced bone formation, disruption of the balance between bone formation and resorption, and incomplete mineralization (Lalor et al., 1986; Schapira, 1990). Alcoholics are often malnourished, which exacerbates the direct effects of alcohol on bones. Alcohol-induced osteoporosis may progress for years without any obvious symptoms.

Osteoporosis, osteomalacia, or both are histologic manifestations of deficient bone metabolism in chronic alcoholism, in which vitamin D deficiency plays a major role (Lalor et al., 1986; Long et al., 1978; Verbanck et al., 1977). Osteoporosis is the predominant bone condition in most people with cirrhosis (Matloff et al., 1982; Mobarhan et al., 1984).

Regular consumption of alcohol may indirectly perpetuate trigger points through reduced serum and tissue folate levels. Ingestion of alcohol reduces the absorption of folic acid while increasing the body's need for it (Travell and Simons, 1983). Of additional interest to physical therapists, alcohol diminishes the accumulation of neutrophils necessary for "clean-up" of all foreign material present in inflamed areas. This phenomenon results in delayed wound healing and recovery from inflammatory processes involving tendons, bursae, and joint structures.

Alcohol may interact with prescribed medications to produce various effects, including death. Unless the client has a chemical dependency on alcohol, appropriate education may be sufficient for the client experiencing negative effects of alcohol use during physical therapy treatment. For example, when interviewing the client, you may want to say

■ Alcohol, tobacco, and caffeine often increase our perception of pain and may mask or even increase other symptoms. I would like to ask you to limit as much as possible your use of any of these stimulants. At the very least, it would be better if you didn't drink alcohol before our therapy sessions, so I can accurately assess your symptoms and progress and move along quickly through our treatment plan.

If the client's breath smells of alcohol, you may want to say more directly

■ I can smell alcohol on your breath right

now. How many drinks have you had today?

Clients who depend on alcohol and/or recreational drugs require in-depth medical treatment and follow-up. Because of the controversial nature of interviewing the alcohol- or drug-dependent client, the following is only a suggested guideline of follow-up questions that may be considered. Specific screening tools for assessing alcohol abuse are available (see the Bibliography).

- Do you ever drink alcoholic beverages (or use drugs recreationally)?
  - If yes, estimate how many drinks you have on an average day.
- (Alternative question) How many drinks have you had today?

Caffeine. Caffeine is a stimulant drug, but its exact mechanism remains unclear. Some researchers believe that caffeine stimulates the adrenal glands to release hormones that stimulate activity of cells in the brain, heart, skeletal muscles, and kidneys (Silverman et al., 1992). In moderation (50 to 200 mg a day), it *seems* relatively harmless for *most* people (Weinhouse et al., 1991), although the study of Silverman and associates indicates that even small amounts can produce disruptive symptoms. Caffeine is known to constrict cerebral arteries, so it has been used in treating headaches (Gilman and Goodman, 1975).

Two hundred milligrams is a little more than two cups of coffee. Caffeine ingested in toxic amounts (more than 250 mg/day, or three cups of caffeinated coffee) has many effects, including nervousness, irritability, agitation, sensory disturbances, tachypnea (rapid breathing), heart palpitations (strong, fast, or irregular heart beat), nausea, urinary frequency, diarrhea, and fatigue. People who drink 8 to 15 cups of coffee a day have been known to have problems with sleep, dizziness, restlessness, headaches, muscle tension, and intestinal disorders (Blacklow, 1983; Work, 1991). Caffeine may enhance the client's

perception of pain. Pain levels can be reduced dramatically by reducing the daily intake of caffeine.

In large doses, caffeine is a stressor, but the withdrawal from caffeine can be equally stressful. Withdrawal from caffeine induces a withdrawal syndrome of headaches, lethargy, fatigue, poor concentration, nausea, impaired psychomotor performance, and emotional instability, which begins within 12 to 24 hours and lasts about 1 week (Hughes et al., 1992; Work, 1991). Other sources of caffeine are

- tea (black and green)
- cocoa
- chocolate
- caffeinated carbonated beverages
- some drugs, many over-the-counter medications

Cocaine and Amphetamines. Cocaine and amphetamines affect the cardiovascular system in the same manner as does stress (Majid et al., 1992). The drugs stimulate the sympathetic nervous system to increase its production of adrenaline. Surging adrenaline causes severe constriction of the arteries, a sharp rise in blood pressure, rapid and irregular heart beats, and seizures (Christan et al., 1990). Heart rate can accelerate by as much as 60 to 70 beats per minute. In otherwise healthy, fit people, this overload can cause death in minutes, even to first-time cocaine users. In addition, cocaine can cause the aorta to rupture, the lungs to fill with fluid, the heart muscle and its lining to become inflamed, blood clots to form in the veins, and strokes to occur as a result of cerebral hemorrhage. Although life-threatening complications are not common, they are unpredictable and appear to have no correlation to dose, length of use, or method of administration (Diethrich and Cohen, 1992).

Special Questions for Women

Gynecologic disorders can refer pain to the low back, hip, pelvis, groin, or sacroiliac (SI) joint. Any woman presenting with pain or symptoms in any one or more of these areas should be screened for a possible systemic origin. The need to screen for systemic disease is essential when there is no known cause of the symptoms/pain. In addition to the questions included in the Family/Personal History form, specific questions for women who have pain in these areas are included here (see Screening for Medical Disease: Special Questions for Women). Any woman with a positive personal/family history of cancer should be screened for medical disease even if the current symptoms can be attributed to a known neuromusculoskeletal etiology.

General Health. All women should be encouraged to have a Pap test annually. Any woman over the age of 40 years with a positive family history for breast cancer should have a mammogram annually. Breast self-examination should be performed monthly; instructions in techniques are readily available through the American Cancer Society or in any nursing or medical physical examination text. The best time to conduct breast self-examination is right after the menstrual period, or the

---

SCREENING FOR MEDICAL DISEASE: SPECIAL QUESTIONS FOR WOMEN

GENERAL HEALTH

- Date of last Pap smear:
- Date of last breast examination:
- Do you perform a monthly breast self-examination?
- Where are you in your menstrual cycle (pre/mid/postmenstrual):
- Are you taking birth control pills?
- For the menopausal woman: Are you taking estrogen replacement therapy (ERT)?
- Have you experienced any of the following (constitutional) symptoms associated with your current problem(s):
  - (night) sweats
  - low-grade fever
  - nausea
  - diarrhea/constipation
  - dizziness
  - fainting
  - fatigue

PAST MEDICAL HISTORY

- Have you had vaginal surgery or a hysterectomy? **(Hysterectomy: joint pain and myalgias may occur; vaginal surgery: incontinence)**
- Have you ever had (or do you now have) pelvic inflammatory disease or any sexually transmitted disease (STD)?
- How many pregnancies have you had?
- How many live births have you had?
- Do you have "brittle bones" (osteoporosis)?
- Have you ever had a compression fracture of your back?

LEEDS METROPOLITAN UNIVERSITY LIBRARY

fourth through seventh day of the menstrual cycle, when the breasts are the smallest and least congested. The pregnant or menopausal woman who is not having menstrual periods should select a date to examine her breasts each month.

The use of estrogen-containing oral contraceptive pills remains the most common cause of secondary hypertension. Subsequent stroke can occur, although recent studies have shown that, with the exception of subarachnoid hemorrhage, there is no increase in risk of stroke among smokers who use oral contraceptives. Older age and obesity are the only known predisposing factors to pill-induced hypertension (Kaplan, 1990). Most women demonstrate a slight elevation in blood pressure with their use, and approximately 5 per cent develop hypertension that persists after discontinuation of the pill (Crane et al., 1971; Weir, 1978; Dennison and Black, 1993). Careful screening of premonitory symptoms, especially headaches, is important (Henderson et al., 1991).

The relative risk of venous thrombosis for current users is an estimated five times that for nonusers. Venous thrombosis and pulmonary embolism are related to the pill's estrogenic component, whereas other cardiovascular complications relate primarily to the progesterone component (Henderson et al., 1991).

The introduction and use of oral contraceptives in the United States have occurred at the same time that breast cancer rates have risen. The effect, if any, of oral contraceptives on breast cancer is under investigation (Henderson et al., 1991). All contraceptives cause breast cancer to the extent that delaying a woman's first pregnancy (and probably reducing her total number of pregnancies) increases her risk of breast cancer (Layde et al., 1989).

It is biologically plausible that exogenously administered steroidal hormones such as those in the pill could have an effect on breast carcinogenesis. Estrogen causes proliferation of breast tissue and would be expected to increase the risk of breast cancer by stimulating growth of stem cells and intermediate cells (Thomas, 1984).

The epidemiology of breast cancer suggests that hormone-related events during puberty, during fertile years, around menopause, and after menopause can independently or synergistically influence breast cancer. By way of education, women should be alerted that hormone exposure information must be collected by the physician throughout a majority of a woman's adult years, and the consequences of exposure must be monitored (Henderson et al., 1991).

Menopause. Like menarche, menopause (cessation of menstruation) is an important developmental event in a woman's life. Menopause is not a disease but rather a complex sequence of biologic aging events during which the body makes the transition from fertility to a nonreproductive status. The usual age for menopause is between 48 and 54 years, although it may occur as early as age 35 years (Clark et al., 1993), and early undetected physiologic changes have often begun in women's mid-30s (Cutler and Garcia, 1992; Dranov, 1993).

The pattern of menstrual cessation varies. It may be abrupt but more often occurs over 1 to 2 years. Periodic menstrual flow gradually occurs less frequently, becoming irregular and less in amount. Occasional episodes of profuse bleeding may be interspersed with episodes of scant bleeding. Menopause is said to have occurred when there have been no menstrual periods for 12 consecutive months (Clark et al., 1993). *Any spontaneous uterine bleeding after this time is abnormal and requires medical evaluation.*

Estrogen provides a natural protective defense against heart disease by blocking the formation of plaque on the intimal lining of the blood vessels. This gender-linked protection from cardiac incidents ends with menopause. Levels of LDL cholesterol (the "bad" cholesterol) increase in women for 10 to 15 years following the cessation of the menstrual cycle. Estrogen replacement therapy decreases LDL ("bad") cholesterol levels and raises HDL ("good") cholesterol levels.

Within the past decade, removal of the uterus (hysterectomy) has become a common major surgery in the United States. In fact, more than one third of the women in the United States have hysterectomies. The majority of these women have this operation between the ages of 25 and 44 years. Removal of the uterus and cervix, even without removal of the ovaries, usually brings on an early menopause, within 2 years of the operation. Oophorectomy (removal of the ovaries) brings on menopause immediately, regardless of the age of the woman, and early surgical removal of the ovaries (before 30 years of age) doubles the risk of osteoporosis.

Clinical Signs and Symptoms of Menopause

- Fatigue and malaise
- Depression, mood swings
- Headache
- Altered sleep pattern (insomnia)
- Hot flashes
- Irregular menses, cessation of menses
- Vaginal dryness, pain during intercourse
- Atrophy of breasts and vaginal tissue
- Pelvic floor relaxation (cystocele/rectocele)
- Urge incontinence

Diagnosis and Treatment. A blood test to measure the levels of luteinizing hormone (LH), estrogen hormone, and follicle-stimulating hormone (FSH)* is a reliable means of determining the state of menopause. High FSH and LH levels in the pres-

* The reader is referred to Table 9–2 for detailed information about these hormones.

ence of low estrogen is indicative of menopause.

Menopause is a natural process that may be left unaltered to complete its course. It will lower a woman's exposure to hormones and reduce the risk of breast cancer. If a woman chooses to pursue medical treatment, hormone replacement therapy (HRT) is one method of treatment. Pros and cons of HRT are listed in Appendix A at the end of this chapter, but each individual client must discuss this with her physician in the context of her own health history.

Estrogen replacement with an agent such as Premarin (estrogen made from pregnant mares' urine) provides only one quarter of the estrogen that a fertile ovary would produce but carries a known increase in the risk of cancer of the endometrium (mucous membrane lining the uterus that is sloughed during menstrual periods). Synthetic progesterone (progestin) is prescribed along with the estrogen to protect against that risk.

One study (Prince et al., 1991) on prevention of postmenopausal osteoporosis reported that an exercise program plus calcium supplements slowed or stopped bone loss. The best results were obtained when estrogen was combined with exercise; bone mass was increased and symptoms such as hot flashes and sleeplessness improved.

Past Medical History. Detailed questions about past labors and methods of delivery, past surgical procedures, incontinence, history of sexually transmitted or pelvic inflammatory disease(s), and history of osteoporosis and/or compression fractures are important for women. For example, pregnancy and birth history are important because the hormone relaxin, secreted by the corpus luteum, is elevated in a woman's system during pregnancy and 7 to 10 days before menstruation begins. Women who have had multiple pregnancies or births may have sacroiliac or low back pain associated with poor abdominal tone and ligamentous laxity. Relaxin increases elongation of ligaments by placing ligaments at the end-range and has a relaxation effect on joints, therefore increasing the chances for injury (Maitland, 1986). The symptomatic sacroiliac problem may be aggravated by intercourse in the supine position. Change in position can alter painful intercourse when the cause of pain is musculoskeletal. Additionally, the risk of developing chronic postpartum back pain may be doubled among women who received epidural anesthesia during labor (Pauls, 1993).

Incontinence. As with any medical problem, some women are more at risk for urinary incontinence than others. Though it can affect women of any age, it is estimated that 37 per cent of adult women 60 years and older are affected by urinary incontinence (Fantl et al., 1991). Women with a history of pelvic floor trauma during delivery and women who have undergone vaginal surgery are more prone to develop incontinence problems. Other medical conditions that may contribute to this problem include repeated infection, chronic urinary problems, and the loss of sufficient muscle strength that occurs with the postmenopausal stage of life.

Physician Referral. Women who have a history of hip, sacroiliac, pelvic, groin, or low back pain without traumatic etiology should be referred for a gynecologic evaluation if there is a history of fever or night sweats or an indication of correlation between menses and symptoms. Any woman with a positive family or personal history of breast cancer who has chest or shoulder pain of unknown etiology should make an appointment with her physician. Any woman whose blood pressure is elevated and who is currently taking birth control pills should be monitored closely by her physician. Any spontaneous uterine bleeding after menopause is abnormal and requires medical evaluation (see Screening for Medical Disease: Special Questions for Women, Special Questions for Women Experiencing Back, Groin, Pelvic, Hip, or Sacroiliac [SI] Pain, and Special Questions for Women Experiencing Shoulder Pain/Dysfunction).

SPECIAL QUESTIONS FOR WOMEN EXPERIENCING BACK, GROIN, PELVIC, HIP, OR SACROILIAC (SI) PAIN

- Since your back/SI (or other) pain/symptoms started, have you seen a gynecologist to rule out any gynecologic cause of this problem?

- Have you ever been told that you have

  - Retroversion of the uterus (tipped back)
  - Ovarian cysts
  - Fibroids or tumors
  - Endometriosis
  - Cystocele (sagging bladder)
  - Rectocele (sagging rectum)

- Have you ever had pelvic inflammatory disease?

- Do you have any known sexually transmitted diseases? **(Cause of PID)**

- Do you have any premenstrual symptoms (e.g., water retention, mood changes including depression, headaches, food cravings, painful or tender breasts)? Have you noticed any pattern between your back/SI (or other) symptoms and PMS?

- Do you have an intrauterine coil or loop (IUCD)? **(PID and ectopic pregnancy can occur)**

- Have you (recently) had a baby? **(Birth trauma)**

  If yes:

Continued on following page

- Did you have an epidural (anesthesia)? **(Postpartum back pain)**
- Did you have any significant medical problems during your pregnancy or delivery?
- Have you ever had a tubal or ectopic pregnancy? Is it possible you may be pregnant now?
- Have you had any spontaneous or induced abortions? **(Weakness secondary to blood loss, infection, scarring; blood in peritoneum irritating diaphragm)**

    If yes, how many, and when was onset of symptoms in relation to incident?

- Do you ever leak urine with coughing, laughing, lifting, exercising, or sneezing? **(Stress incontinence; tension myalgia of pelvic floor)**
- Do you ever feel a "falling-out" feeling or pelvic heaviness after standing for a long time? **(Incontinence; prolapse; pelvic floor weakness)**
    - If yes to incontinence, ask several additional questions to determine the frequency, the amount of protection needed, as measured by the number and type of pads used daily, and how much this problem interferes with daily activities and lifestyle.
- Recent history of bladder or kidney infections? **(Referred back pain)**
- Presence of vaginal discharge? **(Referred back pain)**

    If yes:

    - Do you know what is causing this discharge?
    - How long have you had this problem?
    - Is there any connection between when the discharge started and when you first noticed your back/SI (or other) symptoms?
- Is there any connection between your (back, hip, SI) pain/symptoms and your menstrual cycle (related to either ovulation, mid-cycle, or menses)?
- Where were you in your menstrual cycle when your injury or illness occurred?
- Have you ever been told you have endometriosis?

SPECIAL QUESTIONS FOR WOMEN EXPERIENCING SHOULDER PAIN/DYSFUNCTION

- Have you had any recent kidney infections, tumors, or kidney stones? **(Pressure from kidney on diaphragm referred to shoulder)**
- Have you ever had a breast implant or mastectomy? **(Altered lymph drainage, scar tissue)**
- Have you ever had a tubal or ectopic pregnancy?
- Have you had any spontaneous or induced abortions recently? **(Blood in peritoneum irritating diaphragm)**
- Have you recently had a baby? **(Excessive muscle tension during birth)**

    If yes:

    - Are you breast feeding with the infant supported on pillows?
    - Do you have a breast discharge or have you had mastitis?

Special Questions for Men

Men describing symptoms related to the groin, low back, hip, or sacroiliac joint may have some urologic involvement. The screening questions presented on the intake form assess the need for further medical follow-up.

A positive response to any or all of these questions may be evaluated further following the format provided. Additional *Special Questions to Ask* may assist the physical therapist in making an appropriate referral for a possible urologic evaluation (see Special Questions for Men Experiencing Back, Hip, Groin, or Sacroiliac Pain).

Work Environment

Questions related to the client's daily work activities and work environment are included in the Family/Personal History to assist the physical therapist in planning a program of client education consistent with the objective findings and proposed treatment plan. For example, the physical therapist is alerted to the need for follow-up with a client complaining of back pain who sits for prolonged periods without a back support or cushion. Likewise, a worker involved in bending and twisting who complains of lateral thoracic pain may be describing a muscular strain from repetitive overuse. These work-related questions may help the client report significant data contributing to symptoms that may otherwise have been undetected.

Questions related to occupation and exposure to toxins such as chemicals or gases are included because well-defined physical (e.g., cumulative trauma disorder) and health problems occur in people engaging in specific occupations. For example, seven diseases (asthma, laryngitis, chronic bronchitis, emphysema, and three eye ailments) have been identified by the Department of Veterans Affairs for compensation as a result of soldiers' exposure to toxic chemicals during World War II (P.T. Bulletin, 1993a). Survivors of the Vietnam war who have been exposed to the defoliant Agent Orange are at risk for the development of soft tissue sarcoma, non-Hodgkin's lymphoma, Hodgkin's disease, and a skin-blistering disease, chloracne (Dalager et al., 1991; P.T. Bulletin, 1993b; Uzych, 1991).

Other examples include pesticide exposure among agricultural workers, lung disease in miners, and silicosis in those who must work near silica. Each geographic area has its own specific environmental/occupational concerns.

Vital Signs

Assessment of baseline vital signs, including resting pulse, blood pressure, and

---

SPECIAL QUESTIONS FOR MEN EXPERIENCING BACK, HIP, GROIN, OR SACROILIAC PAIN

- Do you ever have difficulty with urination (e.g., difficulty starting or continuing flow or a very slow flow of urination)?
- Do you ever have blood in your urine?
- Do you ever have pain, burning or discomfort on urination?
- Do you urinate often, especially during the night?
- Does it feel like your bladder is not emptying completely?
- Have you ever been treated for prostate problems (prostate cancer, prostatitis)?
- Have you recently had kidney stones, bladder or kidney infections?
- Have you ever been told that you have a hernia, or do you think you have a hernia?

temperature should be a part of the initial data collected so that correlations and comparisons with the baseline are available when necessary. Ancillary staff can be trained to perform these simple tests. Normal ranges of values for the vital signs are provided for your convenience. However, these ranges can be exceeded by a client and still represent normality for that person. It is the unusual vital sign in combination with other signs and symptoms, medications, and medical status that gives clinical meaning to the pulse rate, blood pressure, and temperature.

Pulse Rate. A resting pulse rate (normal range: 60 to 100 beats/min), taken at the carotid artery or radial artery pulse point, should be available for comparison with the pulse rate taken during treatment or after exercise. A rate above 100 beats per minute indicates tachycardia; below 60 beats per minute indicates bradycardia.

Pulse amplitude (weak or bounding quality of the pulse) that fades with inspiration and strengthens with expiration is *paradoxic* and should be reported to the physician (Keene, 1993). A pulse increase of over 20 beats per minute lasting for more than 3 minutes after rest or changing position should also be reported. The resting pulse may be higher than normal with fever, anemia, infections, some medications, hyperthyroidism, or pain.

Blood Pressure. Blood pressure is the measurement of pressure in an artery at the peak of systole (contraction of the left ventricle) and during diastole (when the heart is at rest after closure of the aortic valve, which prevents blood from flowing back to the heart chambers) (O'Toole, 1992). The measurement (in mm Hg) is listed as systolic (contraction phase)/diastolic (relaxation phase).

The normal range varies slightly with age and varies greatly among individuals. Normal systolic pressure ranges from 100 to 140 mm Hg, and diastolic pressure ranges from 60 to 90 mm Hg. It is more accurate to evaluate consecutive blood pressure readings over time rather than make an isolated measurement for reporting blood pressure abnormalities. Blood pressure also should be correlated with any related diet or medication.

The blood pressure should be taken in the same arm and in the same position (supine or sitting) each time the blood pressure is measured (see Appendix B at the end of the chapter). This information should be recorded with the initial reading (see Family/Personal History form). Blood pressure depends on many factors, including age, vessel size, blood viscosity, force of contraction, current medications, diet, time of last meal (systolic), amount of caffeine ingested, and presence or perceived degree of pain.

Hypotension is a systolic pressure below 95 mm Hg or a diastolic pressure below 60 mm Hg. *Hypertension* is a systolic pressure above 140 mm Hg or a diastolic pressure above 90 mm Hg. The difference between the systolic and diastolic pressure readings is called pulse pressure. A difference of more than 40 mm Hg is abnormal and should be reported (Keene, 1993). The overall goal of treating clients with hypertension is to prevent morbidity and mortality associated with high blood pressure. The specific objective is to achieve and maintain arterial blood pressure below 140/90 mm Hg, if possible (Dennison and Black, 1993).

Postural hypotension is defined as a blood pressure fall of more than 10 to 15 mm Hg of the systolic pressure or more than 10 mm Hg of the diastolic pressure *and* a 10 to 20 per cent increase in heart rate; changes must be noted in both the blood pressure and the heart rate (Braunwald, 1992).

Gravitational effects on the circulatory system can cause a 10 mm Hg drop in systolic blood pressure when a person changes position from supine to sitting to standing. This drop usually occurs without symptoms as the body quickly compensates to ensure no reduction in cardiac output. In clients on prolonged bed rest or on antihypertensive drug therapy, there may be either no reflexive increase in heart rate or a sluggish vasomotor response. These clients may experience larger drops in blood pressure and often experience lightheadedness (Cohen and Michel, 1988).

A difference of 10 mm Hg in either systolic or diastolic measurements from one extremity to the other may be an indication of vascular problems (look for associated symptoms). With a change in position (supine to sitting), the normal fluctuation of blood pressure and heart rate increases slightly (about 5 mm Hg for systolic and diastolic pressures and 5 to 10 beats per minute in heart rate). After changing the postural position of the client, a time delay of 1 to 3 minutes should be permitted before auscultating blood pressure and palpating the radial pulse (Ignatavicius and Bayne, 1993).

A slightly elevated blood pressure may be considered a normal finding in the elderly as a protective mechanism to maintain adequate blood flow to the brain and essential organs (Libow and Butler, 1981; Smith, 1988). Blood pressure values greater than 180 mm Hg (systolic) and 100 mm Hg (diastolic) are treated in elderly clients toward a target value of 160/90 mm Hg (Ciccone, 1993; Potter and Haigh, 1990).

Systolic pressure increases with age and with exertion in a linear progression. If systolic pressure does not rise as work load increases, or if this pressure falls, it may be an indication that the functional reserve capacity of the heart has been exceeded. For any person, exercise or activity should be reduced or stopped if the systolic pressure exceeds 225 mm Hg. Diastolic blood pressure increases during upper extremity exercise or isometric exercise involving any muscle group. Activity or exercise should be decreased or halted if the diastolic pressure exceeds 130 mm Hg (Hillegass and Sadowsky, 1993).

Before reporting abnormal blood pressure readings, measure both sides for comparison, remeasure both sides, have another health professional check the readings, correlate blood pressure measurements with other vital signs, and screen for associated signs and symptoms such as pallor, fatigue, perspiration, and/or palpitations. A persistent rise or fall in blood pressure requires medical attention and possible intervention.

Temperature. Normal body temperature is not a specific number but a range of values that depends on factors such as the time of day, age, medical status, or presence of infection. Oral body temperature ranges from 36° to 37.5° C (96.8° to 99.5° F), with an average of 37° C (98.6° F). Temperatures above the normal range are *hyperthermic,* those below are *hypothermic* (Keene, 1993). There is a tendency among the aging population to develop an increase in temperature on hospital admission or in response to any change in homeostasis.

Any client who has back, shoulder, hip, sacroiliac, or groin pain of unknown cause must have a temperature reading taken. Temperature should also be assessed for any client who has constitutional symptoms, especially night sweats (gradual increase followed by a sudden drop in body temperature), pain, or symptoms of unknown etiology, and for clients who have not been medically screened by a physician. When measuring body temperature, the physical therapist should ask if the person's normal temperature differs from 37° C (98.6° F).

The therapist should use discretionary caution with any client who has a fever. Exercise with a fever stresses the cardiopulmonary system, which may be further complicated by dehydration. It is important to ask whether the client has taken aspirin to reduce the fever, which might mask an underlying problem.

Core Interview

History of Present Illness

The history of present illness (often referred to as the chief complaint) may best

Text continued on page 54

THE CORE INTERVIEW

HISTORY OF PRESENT ILLNESS

Chief Complaint (Onset)

■ Tell me why you are here today.

■ Tell me about your injury.
   Alternative question: What do you think is causing your problem/pain?

   FUPs: How did this injury or illness begin?

   Was your injury or illness associated with a fall, trauma, assault, or repetitive activity (e.g., painting, cleaning, gardening, filing papers, driving)?

   When did the present problem arise and did it occur gradually or suddenly?

   Systemic disease: Gradual onset without known cause.

   Have you ever had anything like this before? If yes, when did it occur? Describe the situation and the circumstances.

   How many times has this illness occurred? Tell me about each occasion.

   Is there any difference this time from the last episode?

   How much time elapses between episodes?

   Do these episodes occur more or less often than at first?

   Systemic disease: May present in a gradual, progressive, cyclical onset: worse, better, worse.

PAIN/SYMPTOM ASSESSMENT

■ Do you have any pain associated with your injury or illness? If yes, tell me about it.

Location

■ Show me exactly where your pain is located.

   FUPs: Do you have this same pain anywhere else?

   Do you have any other pain or symptoms anywhere else?

   If yes, what causes the pain or symptoms to occur in this other area?

Description

■ What does it feel like?

   FUPs: Has the pain changed in quality, intensity, frequency, or duration (how long it lasts) since it first began?

Pattern

■ Tell me about the pattern of your pain or symptoms.
   Alternative question: How does your pain or symptoms change with time?

FUPs: Have you ever experienced anything like this before?

If yes, do these episodes occur more or less often than at first?

When does your back/shoulder/(name body part) hurt?

Describe your pain/symptoms to me from first waking up in the morning to going to bed at night. (See the special "sleep-related" questions that follow.)

Are your symptoms worse in the morning or in the evening?

Frequency

■ How often does the pain/symptoms occur?

FUPs: Is your pain constant or does it come and go (intermittent)?

Are you having this pain now?

Did you notice these symptoms this morning immediately after awakening?

Duration

■ How long does the pain/symptom(s) last?

Systemic disease: Constant.

Intensity

■ On a scale from 0 to 10 with 0 being no pain and 10 being the worst pain you have experienced with this condition, what level of pain do you have right now?
Alternative question: How strong is your pain?
1 = mild
2 = moderate
3 = severe

FUPs: Which word describes your pain right now? _____

Which word describes the pain at its worst? _____

Which word describes the least amount of pain? _____

Systemic disease: Pain tends to be intense.

Associated Symptoms

■ What other symptoms have you had that you can associate with this problem?

FUPs: Have you experienced any

Burning
Difficulty in breathing
Difficulty in swallowing
Dizziness
Heart palpitations

Hoarseness
Nausea
Night sweats
Numbness

Problems with vision
Tingling
Vomiting
Weakness

Systemic disease: Presence of symptoms bilaterally (e.g., edema, nail bed changes, bilateral weakness, paresthesia, tingling, burning). Determine the frequency, duration, intensity, and pattern of symptoms. Blurred vision, double vision, scotomas (black spots before the eyes), or temporary blindness may indicate early symptoms of multiple sclerosis (MS), cerebral vascular accident (CVA), or other neurologic disorders.

Continued on following page

Aggravating Factors

■ What kinds of things affect the pain?

> **FUPs:** What makes your pain/symptoms worse (e.g., eating, exercise, rest, specific positions, excitement, stress)?

Relieving Factors

■ What makes it better?

> **Systemic disease:** Unrelieved by change in position or by rest.

■ How does rest affect the pain/symptoms?

> **FUPs:** Are your symptoms aggravated or relieved by any activities? If yes, what?
>
> How has this problem affected your daily life at work or at home?
>
> How has it affected your ability to care for yourself without assistance (e.g., dress, bathe, cook, drive)?

MEDICAL TREATMENT AND MEDICATIONS

Treatment

■ What medical treatment have you had for this condition?

> **FUPs:** Have you been treated by a physical therapist for this condition before? If yes,
>
> When?
>
> Where?
>
> How long?
>
> What helped?
>
> What didn't help?
>
> Was there any treatment that made your symptoms worse? If yes, please elaborate.

Medications

■ Are you taking any prescription or over-the-counter medications?

> **FUPs:** If no, you may have to probe further regarding use of laxatives, aspirin, acetaminophen (Tylenol), and so forth. If yes,
>
> What medication do you take?
>
> How often?
>
> What dose do you take?
>
> What are you taking these medications for?
>
> When was the last time that you took these medications? Have you taken these drugs today?
>
> Do the medications relieve your pain or symptoms?
>
> If yes, how soon after you take the medications do you notice an improvement?

If prescription drugs, who prescribed them for you?

How long have you been taking these medications?

When did your physician last review these medications?

CURRENT LEVEL OF FITNESS

■ What is your present exercise level?

FUPs: What type of exercise or sports do you participate in?

How many times do you participate each week (frequency)?

When did you start this exercise program (duration)?

How many minutes do you exercise during each session (intensity)?

Are there any activities that you could do before your injury or illness that you cannot do now? If yes, please describe.

Dyspnea: Do you ever experience any shortness of breath (SOB) or lack of air during any activities (e.g., walking, climbing stairs)?

FUPs: Are you ever short of breath without exercising?

If yes, how often?

When does this occur?

Do you ever wake up at night and feel breathless?

If yes, how often?

When does this occur?

SLEEP-RELATED

■ Can you get to sleep at night? If no, try to determine whether the reason is due to the sudden decrease in activity and quiet, which causes you to focus on your symptoms.

■ Are you able to lie or sleep on the painful side? If yes, the condition may be considered to be chronic, and treatment would be more vigorous than if no, indicating a more acute condition requiring more conservative treatment.

■ Are you ever wakened from a deep sleep by pain?

FUPs: If yes, do you awaken because you have rolled onto that side? Yes may indicate a subacute condition requiring a combination of treatment approaches depending on objective findings.

Can you get back to sleep?

FUPs: If yes, what do you have to do (if anything) to get back to sleep? (The answer may provide clues for treatment.)

■ Have you had any unexplained fevers, night sweats, or unexplained perspiration?
Systemic disease: Fevers and night sweats are characteristic signs of systemic disease.

Continued on following page

STRESS

- What major life changes or stresses have you encountered that you would associate with your injury/illness?
  Alternative question: What situations in your life are "stressors" for you?

- On a scale from 0 to 10, with 0 being no stress and 10 being the most extreme stress you have ever experienced, in general, what number rating would you give to your stress at this time in your life?

- What number would you assign to your level of stress today?

- Do you ever get short of breath or dizzy, or lose coordination with fatigue (anxiety-produced hyperventilation)?

FINAL QUESTIONS

- Do you wish to tell me anything else about your injury, your health, or your present symptoms that we have not discussed yet?

- Is there anything else you think is important about your condition that I haven't asked yet?

---

be obtained through the use of open-ended questions. This section of the interview is designed to gather information related to the client's reason(s) for seeking clinical treatment.

The following statements may be appropriate to start an interview.

- Tell me why you are here today.
- Tell me about your injury.
- (Alternatively) What do you think is causing your problem or pain?

During this initial phase of the interview, allow the client to carefully describe his or her current situation. Follow-up questions (FUPs) and paraphrasing can now be used in conjunction with the primary, open-ended questions (see The Core Interview).

Insidious Onset. When the client describes an insidious onset or unknown cause, it is important to ask further questions. Did the symptoms develop after a fall, trauma (including assault), or some repetitive activity (such as painting, cleaning, gardening, filing, or driving long distances)? The alert therapist may recognize causative factors requiring medical screening.

Likewise, the client may wrongly attribute onset of symptoms to a particular activity that is really unrelated to the current symptoms. When the symptoms seem out of proportion to the injury, or when the symptoms persist beyond the expected time for that condition, a red flag should be raised in the therapist's mind.

Twenty-five per cent of clients with primary malignant tumors of the musculoskeletal system report a prior traumatic episode. Often the trauma or injury brings attention to a preexisting malignant or benign tumor. Whenever a fracture occurs with minimal trauma or involves a transverse fracture line, the physician considers the possibility of a tumor. The presence of night pain or lack of change with activity or position is a red flag. A growing mass, whether painless or painful, is a tumor unless diagnosed otherwise by a physician. A hematoma should decrease in size over time, not increase (Lane, 1990).

Finally, extrinsic trauma from a motor vehicle accident, assault, fall, or known accident or injury may result in intrinsic trauma to another part of the musculoskeletal system or other organ system. Such intrinsic trauma may be masked by the more critical injury and may become more symptomatic as the primary injury resolves.

Assessment of Pain and Symptoms

Characteristics of Pain. It is very important to be able to identify how the client's description of pain as a symptom relates to sources and types of pain discussed in Chapter 1. Many characteristics of pain can be elicited from the client during the core interview to help define the source or type of pain in question. These characteristics include

- Location
- Description of sensation
- Pattern
- Frequency
- Intensity or duration

Other additional components are related to factors that aggravate the pain, factors that relieve the pain, and other symptoms that may occur that are associated with the pain. Specific questions are included for each descriptive component. Keep in mind that a gradual increase in frequency, intensity, or duration of symptoms over time can indicate systemic disease.

Location of Pain. Questions related to the location of pain focus the client's description as precisely as possible. An opening statement might be

- Show me exactly where your pain is located.

Follow-up questions may include:

- Do you have any other pain or symptoms anywhere else?
  - If yes, what causes the pain or symptoms to occur in this other area?

If the client points to a small, localized area and pain does not spread, the cause is more likely to be a superficial lesion and is probably not severe. If the client points to a small, localized area but the pain does spread, this is more likely to be a diffuse, segmental, referred pain that may originate in the viscera or deep somatic structure (Hertling and Kessler, 1990).

Description of the Sensation of Pain. To assist the physical therapist in obtaining a clear description of pain sensation, pose the question

- What does it feel like?

Allow the client some choices in potential descriptors. Some common words might include

knifelike	dull
boring	burning
throbbing	prickly
deep aching	sharp

An assessment tool such as the McGill Pain Questionnaire may assist in providing additional descriptors. Follow-up questions may include

- Has the pain changed in quality since it first began?
- Changed in intensity?
- Changed in duration (how long it lasts)?

When a client describes the pain as knifelike, boring, colicky, coming in waves, or a deep aching feeling, this description should be a signal to the physical therapist to consider the possibility of a systemic origin of symptoms. Dull, somatic pain of an aching nature can be differentiated from the aching pain of a muscular lesion by squeezing or by pressing the muscle overlying the area of pain. This reproduces aching of muscular origin with no connection to deep somatic aching.

Pattern of Pain. In determining the pattern of the pain, the client should be asked to describe how the symptoms of pain change with time. Some choices may include the following (Melzack, 1975):

A	B	C
Continuous	Brief	Rhythmic
Steady	Momentary	Intermittent
Constant	Transient	Periodic

Follow-up questions may include

- Have you ever had anything like this before?
  - If yes, do these episodes occur more or less often than at first?
- When does your back/shoulder (name the body part) hurt?
- Describe your pain/symptoms to me from when you wake up in the morning to when you go to bed at night.

(See the special questions regarding Sleep, pp. 53 and 62.)

The pattern of pain associated with systemic disease is often a progressive pattern with a cyclical onset (i.e., the client describes symptoms as being alternately worse, better, and worse over a period of months). This pattern differs from the sudden sequestration of a discogenic lesion that presents with a pattern of increasingly worse symptoms followed by a sudden cessation of all symptoms. Such involvement of the disc occurs without the cyclical return of symptoms weeks or months later, which is more typical of a systemic disorder.

If the client appears to be unsure of the pattern of symptoms or has "avoided paying any attention" to this component of pain description, it may be useful to keep a record at home assisting the client to take note of the symptoms for 24 hours. A chart such as the McGill Home Recording Card (Melzack, 1975) (Fig. 2–2) may help the client outline the existing pattern of the pain and can be used later in treatment to assist the therapist in detecting any change in symptoms or function.

A client frequently will comment that the pain or symptoms have not changed despite 2 or 3 weeks of treatment with physical therapy. This information can be discouraging to both client and therapist; however, when the symptoms are reviewed, in fact a decrease in pain, increase in function, reduced need for medications, or other significant improvement in the pattern of symptoms may be seen. The improvement has been gradual and is best documented through the use of a baseline of pain activity established at an early stage in treatment by using a record such as the Home Recording Card.

However, if no improvement in symptoms or function can be demonstrated, the therapist must again consider a systemic origin of symptoms. Repeating screening questions for medical disease is encouraged throughout the treatment process even if such questions were included in the intake interview. Because of the progressive nature of systemic involvement, the client may not have noticed any constitutional symptoms at the start of physical therapy treatment that may now be present. Constitutional symptoms affect the whole body and are characteristic of systemic disease or illness.

Some constitutional symptoms are

- Fever
- Diaphoresis (unexplained perspiration)
- Night sweats (can occur during the day)
- Nausea
- Vomiting
- Diarrhea
- Pallor
- Dizziness/syncope (fainting)
- Fatigue
- Weight loss

Frequency and Duration. The frequency of occurrence is related closely to the pattern of the pain, and the client should be asked how often the symptoms occur and whether the pain is constant or intermittent. Duration of pain is a part of this description.

- How long do the symptoms last?

For example, pain related to systemic disease has been shown to be a *constant* rather than an *intermittent* type of pain experience. Clients who indicate that the pain is constant should be asked

---

McGill Home Recording Card

NAME: _____   DATE STARTED: _____

Please record:

	Morning	Noon	Dinner	Bedtime
M				
Tu				
W				
Th				
F				
Sa				
Su				

1. Pain intensity #:
   0 = no pain
   1 = mild
   2 = discomforting
   3 = distressing
   4 = horrible
   5 = excruciating
2. # analgesics taken
3. Note any unusual pain, symptoms or activities on back of card.
4. Record # hours slept in morning column.

Please note: If the client previously rated the pain on a scale from 0–10, substitute the 0–10 scale in place of the 0–5 scale used to describe pain intensity.

Figure 2–2
McGill Home Recording Card. (From Melzack, R.: The McGill Pain Questionnaire: Major properties and scoring methods. Pain *1:*298, 1975.)

- Do you have this pain right now?
- Did you notice these symptoms this morning immediately when you woke up?

Further responses may reveal that the pain is perceived as being constant but in fact is not actually present hourly and/or can be reduced with rest or position change, which is more characteristic of musculoskeletal origin.

Intensity. The level or intensity of the pain is an extremely important, but difficult, component to assess in the overall pain profile. Assist the client with this evaluation by providing a rating scale. For example, the physical therapist might ask the client to rate the pain on a scale from 0 (no pain) to 10 (worst pain experienced with this condition).

An alternative method provides a scale of 1 to 5 with word descriptions for each number (Melzack, 1975) and asks

- How strong is your pain?

   1 = mild

   2 = discomforting

3 = distressing

4 = horrible

5 = excruciating

As with the Home Recording Card, this scale for measuring the intensity of pain can be used to establish a baseline measure of pain for future reference. A client who describes the pain as "excruciating" (or a 5 on the scale) during the initial interview may question the value of therapy when several weeks later there is no subjective report of improvement. A quick check of intensity by using this scale often reveals a decrease in the number assigned to pain levels. This can be compared with the initial rating, providing the client with assurance and encouragement in the rehabilitation process. A quick assessment can be made by asking

■ How strong is your pain?

1 = mild

2 = moderate

3 = severe

The description of intensity is highly subjective. What might be described as "mild" for one person could be "horrible" for another person. Careful assessment of the person's nonverbal behavior (e.g., ease of movement, facial grimacing, guarding movements) and correlation of the person's personality with his or her perception of the pain may help clarify the description of the intensity of the pain. Pain of an intense, unrelenting (constant) nature is often associated with systemic disease.

Associated Symptoms. These symptoms may occur alone or in conjunction with the pain of systemic disease. The client may or may not associate these additional symptoms with the chief complaint. The physical therapist may ask

■ What other symptoms have you had that you can associate with this problem?

If the client denies any additional symptoms, follow up this question with a series of possibilities such as

Burning

Difficulty in breathing

Difficulty in swallowing

Dizziness

Heart palpitations

Hoarseness

Nausea

Night sweats

Numbness

Problems with vision

Tingling

Vomiting

Weakness

Whenever the client says "Yes" to such associated symptoms, check for the presence of these symptoms bilaterally. Also, bilateral weakness either proximally or distally should serve as an indicator of more than a musculoskeletal lesion.

Blurred vision, double vision, scotomas (black spots before the eyes), or temporary blindness may indicate early symptoms of MS or may possibly be warning signs of an impending CVA. The presence of any associated symptoms, such as those mentioned here, would require contact with the physician to confirm the physician's knowledge of these symptoms.

Aggravating/Relieving Factors. Finally, a series of questions addressing aggravating and relieving factors must be included. The McGill Pain Questionnaire provides a chart, shown in Figure 2–3, that may be useful in determining the presence of relieving or aggravating factors (Melzack, 1975). A question related to aggravating factors could be

■ What kinds of things make your pain or symptoms worse (e.g., eating, exercise, rest, specific positions, excitement, stress)?

To assess relieving factors, ask

	Indicate a plus (+) for aggravating factors or a minus (−) for relieving factors.		
	Liquor		Sleep/rest
	Stimulants (e.g., caffeine)		Lying down
	Eating		Distraction (e.g., television)
	Heat		Urination/defecation
	Cold		Tension, stress
	Weather changes		Loud noises
	Massage		Going to work
	Pressure		Intercourse
	No movement		Mild exercise
	Movement		Fatigue
	Sitting		Standing

Figure 2–3

Factors aggravating and relieving pain. (From Melzack, R.: The McGill Pain Questionnaire: Major properties and scoring methods. Pain *1*:277, 1975.)

■ What makes the pain better?

Follow-up questions include

■ How does rest affect the pain/symptoms?

■ Are your symptoms aggravated or relieved by any activities?
  ■ If yes, what?

■ How has this problem affected your daily life at work or at home?

■ How has this problem affected your ability to care for yourself without assistance (e.g., dress, bathe, cook, drive)?

Systemic pain tends to be relieved minimally, relieved only temporarily, or unrelieved by change in position or by rest. However, musculoskeletal pain is *often* relieved both by a change of position and by rest.

In summary, careful, sensitive, and thorough questioning regarding the multifaceted experience of pain can elicit essential information necessary when making a decision regarding treatment or referral. The use of pain assessment tools may facilitate clear and accurate descriptions of this critical symptom.

Medical Treatment and Medications

Medical Treatment. Medical treatment includes any intervention performed by a physician (family practitioner or specialist), dentist, physician's assistant, nurse,

nurse practitioner, physical therapist, or occupational therapist. The client may also include chiropractic treatment when answering the question

- What medical treatment have you had for this condition?

In addition to eliciting information regarding specific treatment performed by the medical community, follow-up questions relate to previous physical therapy treatment:

- Have you been treated by a physical therapist for this condition before?
  - If yes, when, where, and for how long?
- What helped and what didn't help?
- Was there any treatment that made your symptoms worse? If yes, please elaborate.

Knowing the client's response to previous types of treatment techniques may assist the therapist in determining an appropriate treatment protocol for the current chief complaint. For example, previously successful treatment techniques described may provide a basis for initial treatment until the therapist can fully assess the objective data and consider all potential types of treatments.

Medications. Medications (either prescription or over-the-counter) may or may not be listed on the Family/Personal History form. Often, it is necessary to probe further regarding the use of aspirin, acetaminophen (Tylenol), laxatives, or other drugs that can alter the client's symptoms.

Seventy-five per cent of all elderly clients take over-the-counter (OTC) medications that may cause confusion, cause or contribute to additional symptoms, and interact with other medications. Sometimes the client is receiving the same drug under different brand names, increasing the likelihood of drug-induced confusion. Because many older people do not consider these "drugs" worth mentioning, it is important to ask specifically about OTC drug use. Additionally, drug abuse and alcoholism are more common in elderly people than is generally recognized, especially in depressed clients (Resnick, 1993).

Medications can mask signs and symptoms or produce signs and symptoms that are seemingly unrelated to the client's current medical problem. For example, long-term use of steroids resulting in side effects such as proximal muscle weakness, tissue edema, and increased pain threshold may alter objective findings during the examination of the client (Hertling and Kessler, 1990). A detailed description of gastrointestinal (GI) disturbances caused by nonsteroidal antiinflammatory drugs (NSAIDs) resulting in back, shoulder, or scapular pain is presented in Chapter 6.

In the aging population, drug side effects can occur even with low doses that usually produce no side effects in younger populations. Older people are two or three times more likely than young to middle-aged adults to have adverse drug reactions, for a number of reasons. Drug clearance is often markedly reduced owing to a decrease in renal plasma flow and glomerular filtration rate, as well as reduced hepatic clearance. The volume of the drug distributed is also affected, because elderly people have a decrease in total body water and a relative increase in body fat (Resnick, 1993).

Many people who take prescribed medications cannot recall the name of the drug or tell you why they are taking it. It is essential to know whether the client has taken OTC or prescription medication before the physical therapy examination or treatment, because the symptomatic relief or possible side effects may alter the objective findings. Similarly, when appropriate, treatment can be scheduled to correspond with the time of day when clients obtain maximal relief from their medications.

For every client, the therapist is strongly encouraged to take the time to look up indications for use and possible side effects of prescribed medications. The *Nursing Drug Handbook, The Complete Drug Reference* (available in hospital libraries or pharmacies), and *Drug Use–Education Tip (Du-et)** are easy-to-use reference guides. Pharmacists are invaluable sources of easy-access information. Other references are included in the Bibliography.

Distinguishing drug-related signs and symptoms from disease-related symptoms may require careful observation and consultation with family members or other health professionals to see whether these signs tend to increase following each dose (Ciccone, 1993).

The physical therapist is often in the role of educator and may find it necessary to reeducate the client regarding the importance of taking medications as prescribed, whether on a daily or other regular basis. In the case of hypertension medication, the therapist should ask whether the client has taken the medication today as prescribed. It is not unusual to hear a client report, "I take my blood pressure pills when I feel my heart starting to pound." The same situation may occur with clients taking antiinflammatory drugs, antibiotics, or any other medications that must be taken consistently for a specified period to be effective.

Appropriate FUPs include the following:

- Why are you taking these medications?

- When was the last time that you took these medications?

- Have you taken these drugs today?

- Do the medications relieve your pain or symptoms?
  - If yes, how soon after you take the medications do you notice an improvement?

- If prescription drugs, who prescribed this medication for you?

- How long have you been taking these medications?

- When did your physician last review these medications?

---

* Available from the American Academy of Family Physicians, Kansas City, Missouri. Telephone: 1-(800)-274-2237.

Current Level of Fitness

An assessment of current physical activity and level of fitness (or level just before the onset of the current problem) can provide additional necessary information relating to the origin of the client's symptomatology. The level of fitness can be a valuable indicator of potential response to treatment based on the client's motivation (i.e., those who are more physically active and healthy seem to be more motivated to return to that level of fitness through disciplined self-rehabilitation).

It is important to know what type of exercise or sports activity the client participates in, the number of times per week (frequency) that this activity is performed, the length (duration) of each exercise or sports session, as well as how long the client has been exercising (weeks, months, years), and the level of difficulty of each exercise session (intensity). It is very important to ask

- Since the onset of symptoms, are there any activities that you can no longer accomplish?

The client should give a detailed description concerning these activities, including how physical activities have been affected by the symptoms.

Follow-up questions include

- Do you ever experience shortness of breath or lack of air during any activities (e.g., walking, climbing stairs)?

- Are you ever short of breath without exercising?

- Are you ever awakened at night breathless?
  - If yes, how often and when does this occur?

If the Family/Personal History form is not completed, it may be helpful to ask some of the questions under "Work Environment." For example, assessing the history of falls with elderly people is essential. One third of community-dwelling and a higher proportion of institutionalized elderly people fall annually. Aside from the serious injuries that may result, a debilitating "fear of falling" may cause many elderly people to reduce their activity level and restrict their social life. This is one area that is often treatable and even preventable with physical therapy.

Elderly persons who are in bed for prolonged periods of time are at risk for secondary complications, including pressure ulcers, urinary tract infections, pulmonary infections and/or infarcts, congestive heart failure, osteoporosis, and compression fractures.

Sleep-Related History

Sleep patterns are valuable indicators of underlying physiologic and psychologic disease processes. The primary function of sleep is believed to be the restoration of body function. When the quality of this restorative sleep is decreased, the body and mind cannot perform at optimal levels. Physical problems that result in pain, increased urination, shortness of breath, changes in body temperature, perspiration, or side effects of medications are just a few causes of sleep disruption. Any factor precipitating sleep deprivation can contribute to an increase in the frequency, intensity, or duration of a client's symptoms.

For example, fevers and night sweats are characteristic signs of systemic disease. Night sweats occur as a result of a gradual increase followed by a sudden drop in body temperature. This change in body temperature can be related to pathologic changes in immunologic, neurologic, and endocrine function. Certain neurologic lesions may produce local changes in sweating associated with nerve distribution. For example, a client with a spinal cord tumor may report changes in skin temperature above and below the level of the tumor. Any client presenting with a history of either night sweats or fevers should be referred to the primary physician. This is es-

pecially true for clients with back pain or multiple joint pain without traumatic origin.

Pain is usually perceived as being more intense during the night owing to the lack of outside distraction when the person lies quietly without activity. The sudden quiet surroundings and lack of external activity create an increased perception of pain that is a major disruptor of sleep. It is very important to ask the client about pain during the night. Is the person able to get to sleep? If not, the pain may be a primary focus and may become continuously intense so that falling asleep is a problem.

■ Does a change in body position affect the level of pain?

If a change in position can increase or decrease the level of pain, it is more likely to be a musculoskeletal problem. If, however, the client is awakened from a deep sleep by pain in any location that is unrelated to physical trauma and is unaffected by a change in position, then it may be an ominous sign of serious systemic disease, particularly cancer. FUPs include

■ If you wake up because of pain, is it because you rolled onto that side?

■ Can you get back to sleep?
  ■ If yes, what do you have to do (if anything) to get back to sleep? (This answer may provide clues for treatment.)

Many other factors (primarily environmental and psychologic) are associated with sleep disturbance, but a good, basic assessment of the main characteristics of physically related disturbances in sleep pattern can provide valuable information related to treatment or referral decisions.

Psychogenic Considerations

(See also Psychologic Factors in Pain Assessment, Chapter 1.)

By using the interviewing tools and techniques described in this chapter, the physical therapist can communicate a willingness to consider all aspects of illness,

---

INTERVIEWING DOs AND DON'Ts

DOs

Do use a sequence of questions that begins with open-ended questions.

Do leave closed-ended questions for the end as clarifying questions.

Do select a private location where confidentiality can be maintained.

Do listen attentively and show it both in your body language and by occasionally making reassuring verbal prompts, such as "I see" or "Go on."

Do ask one question at a time and allow the client to answer the question completely before continuing with the next question.

Do encourage the client to ask questions throughout the interview.

Do listen with the intention of assessing the client's current level of understanding and knowledge of his or her current medical condition.

Do eliminate unnecessary information and speak to the client at his or her level of understanding.

Do correlate signs and symptoms with medical history and objective findings to rule out systemic disease.

Do provide several choices or selections to questions that require a descriptive response.

DON'Ts

Don't jump to premature conclusions based on the answers to one or two questions. (Correlate all subjective and objective information before consulting with a physician.)

Don't interrupt or take over the conversation when the client is speaking.

Don't destroy helpful open-ended questions with closed-ended follow-up questions before the person has a chance to respond (e.g., How do you feel this morning? Has your pain gone?).

Don't use professional or medical jargon when it is possible to use common language (e.g., don't use the term myocardial infarct instead of heart attack).

Don't overreact to information presented. Common overreactions include raised eyebrows, puzzled facial expressions, gasps, or other verbal exclamations such as "Oh, really?" or "Wow!" Less dramatic reactions may include facial expressions or gestures that indicate approval or disapproval, surprise, or sudden interest. These responses may influence what the client does or does not tell you.

Don't use leading questions. Pain is difficult to describe, and it may be easier for the client to agree with a partially correct statement than to attempt to clarify points of discrepancy between your statement and his or her pain experience (Jacox, 1977).

Leading Questions	Better Presentation of the Same Questions
Where is your pain?	Do you have any pain associated with your injury? If yes, tell me about it.
Does it hurt when you first get out of bed?	When does your back hurt?
Does the pain radiate down your leg?	Do you have this pain anywhere else?
Do you have pain in your lower back?	Point to the exact location of your pain.

whether biologic or psychologic. Client self-disclosure is unlikely if there is no trust in the health professional, if there is fear of a lack of confidentiality, or a sense of disinterest.

Stress. Most symptoms (pain included) are aggravated by unresolved emotional stress. Prolonged stress may lead gradually to physiologic changes.

Stress may result in depression, anxiety disorders, and behavioral consequences such as smoking, alcohol and substance abuse, and accident proneness (Mitchell and Larson, 1987).

The effects of emotional stress may be increased by physiologic changes brought on by the use of medications or poor diet and health habits (e.g., cigarette smoking or ingestion of caffeine in any form). Finally, the client's ability to remember secondary to the use of medications, age, depression, anxiety, or other factors may limit information given.

As part of the core interview, the physical therapist may asses the client's subjective report of stress by asking

■ What major life changes or stresses have you encountered that you would associate with your injury/illness?

or

■ What situations in your life are "stressors" for you?

It may be helpful to quantify the stress by asking the client

■ On a scale from 0 to 10, with 0 being no stress and 10 being the most extreme stress you have ever experienced, what number rating would you give your stress in general at this time in your life?

Emotions such as fear and anxiety are common reactions to illness and treatment and may increase the client's awareness of pain and symptoms. These emotions may cause autonomic (branch of nervous system not subject to voluntary control) distress manifested in such symptoms as pallor, restlessness, muscular tension, per-

spiration, stomach pain, diarrhea or constipation, or headaches.

It may be helpful to screen for anxiety-provoked hyperventilation by asking

■ Do you ever get short of breath or dizzy or lose coordination when you are fatigued?

After the objective evaluation has been completed, the physical therapist can often provide immediate relief of emotionally based symptoms by explaining the cause of pain, by outlining a treatment plan, and by providing a realistic prognosis for improvement. This may not be possible if the client demonstrates signs of hysterical symptoms or conversion symptoms.

Whether the client's symptoms are systemic or caused by an emotional/psychologic overlay, if the client does not respond to treatment it may be necessary to notify the physician that you are unable to find a satisfactory explanation for the client's complaints. Further medical evaluation may be indicated.

HOSPITAL INPATIENT INFORMATION

Medical Chart

The core interview presented in this chapter can provide the physical therapist with the basic information required for beginning to assess the patient's* condition. Treatment of hospital or nursing home inpatients requires a slightly different interview (or information gathering) format. Reviewing the patient's chart thoroughly for information (see Hospital Inpatient Information) will assist the physical therapist in developing a safe and effective treatment plan. It is important for the physical therapist to be aware of this vital information before beginning treatment. Important information to look for might include

---

* Clients are still more likely to be referred to as "patients" in a hospital setting.

- Age
- Diagnosis
- Surgery
- Physician's report
- Associated or additional problems relevant to physical therapy
- Medications
- Restrictions
- Laboratory results
- Vital signs

An evaluation of the patient's medical status in conjunction with age and diagnosis can provide valuable guidelines for treatment. The neurophysiologic and behavioral implications of the aging process are well documented and should be considered on an individual basis (Jackson, 1987).

If the patient has had recent surgery, the physician's report should be scanned for preoperative and postoperative orders. For example, was the patient treated preoperatively with physical therapy for gait, strength, range of motion, or other objective assessments?

For the postoperative patient, how was the patient positioned during the procedure? Prolonged time in the lithotomy position (supine, legs flexed on thighs, thighs flexed on abdomen and abducted) for men undergoing prostate surgery often results in residual musculoskeletal complaints. This surgical position for men and for women during laparoscopy (examination of the peritoneal cavity) may place patients at increased risk for thrombophlebitis because of the decreased blood flow to the legs during surgery.

Other valuable information that may be contained in the physician's report may include

- What are the current short-term and long-term medical treatment plans?
- Are there any known or listed contraindications to physical therapy treatment?
- Does the patient have any weight-bearing limitations?

Associated or additional problems to the primary diagnosis may be found within the chart contents (e.g., diabetes, heart disease, peripheral vascular disease, or respiratory involvement). The physical therapist should look for any of these conditions in order to modify exercise accordingly and to watch for any related signs and symptoms that might affect the exercise program:

- Are there complaints of any kind that may affect exercise (e.g., shortness of breath [dyspnea], heart palpitations, rapid heart rate [tachycardia], fatigue, fever, or anemia)?

If the patient is diabetic, the therapist should ask

- What are the current blood glucose levels?
- When is insulin administered?

Avoiding peak insulin levels in planning exercise schedules is discussed more completely in Chapter 9. Other questions related to medications can follow the core interview outline with appropriate follow-up questions:

- Is the patient receiving oxygen or receiving fluids/medications through an intravenous line?
  - If the patient is receiving oxygen, will he or she need increased oxygen levels prior to, during, or following physical therapy? What level(s)?
- Are there any dietary or fluid restrictions?
  - If so, check with the nursing staff to determine the full limitations. For example:
    - Are ice chips or wet washcloths permissible?
    - How many ounces or milliliters of fluid are allowed during therapy?
    - Where should this amount be recorded?

Laboratory values and vital signs should be reviewed. For example:

- Is the patient anemic?
- Is the patient's blood pressure stable?

Anemic patients may demonstrate an increased normal resting pulse rate that should be monitored during exercise. Patients with unstable blood pressure may require initial standing with a tilt table or monitoring of the blood pressure before, during, and after treatment. Check the nursing record for pulse rate at rest and blood pressure to use as a guide when taking vital signs in the clinic or at the patient's bedside.

Nursing Assessment

After reading the patient's chart, check with the nursing staff to determine the nursing assessment of the individual patient. The essential components of the nursing assessment that are of value to the physical therapist may include

- Medical status
- Pain
- Physical status
- Patient orientation
- Discharge plans

The nursing staff are usually intimately aware of the patient's current medical and physical status. If pain is a factor

- What is the nursing assessment of this patient's pain level and pain tolerance?

Pain tolerance is relative to the medications received by the patient, the number of days after surgery or after injury, fatigue, and the patient's personality.

To assess the patient's physical status, ask the nursing staff

- Has the patient been up at all yet?
- If yes, how long has the patient been sitting, standing, or walking?
- How far has the patient walked?

- How much assistance does the patient require?

Ask about the patient's orientation:

- Is the patient oriented to time, place, and person?

In other words, does the patient know the date and the approximate time, where he or she is, and who he or she is? Treatment plans may be altered by the patient's awareness; for example, a home program may be impossible without family compliance.

- Are there any known or expected discharge plans?
- If yes, what are these plans and when is the target date for discharge?

Cooperation between nurses and the physical therapist is an important part of the multidisciplinary approach to planning the patient's treatment. The aforementioned questions to present and factors to consider provide the physical therapist with the basic hospital or nursing home–related information necessary to carry out an objective examination and to plan a treatment protocol. Each individual patient's situation may require that the physical therapist obtain additional pertinent information.

PHYSICIAN REFERRAL

The physical therapist may be able to determine detailed and specific information regarding symptoms of possible systemic origin by using the questions presented in this chapter to interview the client. Then, by correlating the client's answers with family/personal history, vital signs, and objective findings from the physical examination, the therapist can screen for medical disease and decide whether a referral to the physician is indicated (see Systemic Signs and Symptoms Requiring Physician Referral).

This information is not designed to be used to provide the client with a medical diagnosis, but rather to accurately assess

Medical Chart

- **Patient age**
- **Diagnosis**
- **Surgery:** Did the patient have surgery?
  FUPs: See Surgery on pages 33 and 38 in this chapter.
- Physician's report
  FUPs: Check the physician's preoperative and postoperative orders. (Was the patient treated preoperatively by a physical therapist for gait, strength, or range of motion evaluation?)
  - What are the short-term and long-term medical treatment plans?
  - Are there contraindications for treatment?
  - Are there weight-bearing limitations?
- **Associated or additional problems,** such as diabetes, heart disease, peripheral vascular disease, respiratory involvement
  FUPs: Are there complaints of any kind that may affect exercise?
  - If diabetic, what are the current blood glucose levels (normal range: 70 to 120 mg/dl)?
  - When is insulin administered? (Use this to avoid the peak insulin levels in planning an exercise schedule.)
- **Medications** (what, when received, what for, potential side effects)
  FUPs: Is the patient receiving oxygen or receiving fluids/medications through an intravenous line?
- **Restrictions:** Are there any dietary or fluid restrictions?
  FUPs: If yes, check with the nursing staff to determine the patient's full limitation.
  - Are ice chips or a wet washcloth permissible?
  - How many ounces or cubic centimeters of fluid are allowed during therapy?
- **Laboratory values:** Hematocrit/hemoglobin level (see Chapter 3 for normal values and significance of these tests); exercise tolerance test results if available for cardiac patients; pulmonary function test (PFT) to determine severity of pulmonary problem; arterial blood gas (ABG) levels to determine the need for supplemental oxygen during exercise
- **Vital signs:** Is the blood pressure stable?
  FUPs: If no, consider initiating standing with a tilt table or monitoring the blood pressure before, during, and after treatment.

Nursing Assessment

- **Medical status:** What is the patient's current medical status?
- **Pain:** What is the nursing assessment of this patient's pain level and pain tolerance?
- **Physical status:** Has the patient been up at all yet?
  FUPs: If yes, is the patient sitting, standing, or walking? How long and (if walking) what distance, and how much assistance is required?
- **Patient orientation:** Is the patient oriented to time, place, and person? (Does the patient know the date and the approximate time, where he or she is, and who he or she is?)
- **Discharge plans:** Are there any known or expected discharge plans?
  FUPs: If yes, what are these plans and when will the patient be discharged?
- **Final question:** Is there anything else that I should know before exercising the patient?

Table 2–4
SYSTEMIC SIGNS AND SYMPTOMS REQUIRING PHYSICIAN REFERRAL

Constitutional Symptoms	Pattern of Symptoms	Associated S&S
Fever	Constant pain/night pain	Pain on urination
Diaphoresis	Cyclic pattern	Blood in urine
Night sweats	Pain description:	Tachycardia
Nausea	boring	Bradycardia
Vomiting	knifelike	Difficulty in swallowing
Diarrhea	deep ache	Dyspnea
Pallor	colicky	Vision changes
Dizziness/syncope	Bilateral symptoms:	Hoarseness
Fatigue	edema	Heart palpitations
Weight loss	clubbing	
	numbness	
	tingling	
	nail bed changes	
	skin pigmentation changes	
	skin rash	
	Unusual menstrual history	
	Association between menses and symptoms	
	Temporary relief/no relief with rest or change in position	

pain and systemic symptoms that may mimic or occur simultaneously with a musculoskeletal problem.

Some of the specific indications for physician referral mentioned in this chapter include the following:

■ Spontaneous postmenopausal bleeding

■ A growing mass, whether painful or painless

■ Persistent rise or fall in blood pressure

■ Hip, sacroiliac, pelvic, groin, or low back pain in a woman without traumatic etiology who reports fever, night sweats, or an association between menses and symptoms

■ A positive family/personal history of breast cancer in a woman with chest, back, or shoulder pain of unknown etiology

■ Elevated blood pressure in any woman taking birth control pills; this should be closely monitored by her physician

Table 2–4 lists systemic signs and symptoms that were evaluated as part of the client's subjective examination. In each chapter, a list of possible signs or symptoms is provided for your consideration when making an evaluation and referral. As always, correlate *history* with *patterns of pain* and any *unusual findings* that may indicate *systemic disease.*

Key Points to Remember

■ Most of the information needed to determine the cause of symptoms is contained within the subjective assessment (interview process).

■ The Family/Personal History form can be used as the first tool to screen clients for medicinal disease. Any "Yes" responses should be followed up with appropriate questions. The therapist is strongly encouraged to review the form with the client, entering the date and his or her own initials. The form can be used as a document of baseline information.

■ Medical screening examinations (interview and vital signs) should be completed for any person experiencing back, shoulder, scapular, hip, groin, or sacroiliac symptoms of unknown cause. The presence of constitutional symptoms will almost always warrant a physician's referral but *definitely* requires further follow-up questions in making that determination.

■ It may be necessary to explain the need to ask such detailed questions about organ systems seemingly unrelated to the musculoskeletal symptoms.

■ With the older client, a limited number of presenting symptoms predominate no matter what the underlying disease is, including acute confusion, depression, falling, incontinence, and syncope.

■ A recent history of any infection (bladder, uterine, kidney, vaginal, upper respiratory), mononucleosis, influenza, or colds may be an extension of a chronic health pattern of systemic illness.

■ Special Questions for Women and Special Questions for Men are provided to screen for gynecologic or urologic involvement for any woman or man presenting with back, shoulder, hip, groin, or sacroiliac symptoms of unknown origin.

■ Other red flags: symptoms that seem out of proportion to the injury, symptoms that persist beyond the expected time for that condition, presence of night pain, or no change in symptoms with change in activity or position.

CASE STUDY*

REFERRAL

Your latest referral is a 28-year-old white man who has had a diagnosed progressive idiopathic Raynaud's syndrome of the bilateral upper extremities for the last 4 years. The client has been examined by numerous physicians and by an orthopedist. He has complete numbness and cyanosis of the right second, third, fourth, and fifth digits upon contact with even a mild decrease in temperature. He says that his symptoms have progressed to the extent that they appear within seconds if he picks up a glass of cold water.

He works almost entirely outside, often in cold weather, and uses saws and other power equipment. The numbness has created a very unsafe job situation.

The client received a gunshot wound in a hunting accident 6 years ago. The bullet entered the posterior left thoracic region, lateral to the lateral border of the scapula, and came out through the anterior, lateral, superior chest wall. He says that he feels as if his shoulders are constantly rolled forward. He reports no cervical, shoulder, or elbow pain or injury.

PHYSICAL THERAPY INTERVIEW

Please note that not all of these questions would necessarily be presented to the client, because his answers may determine the next question and may eliminate some questions.

Tell me why you are here today. (Open-ended question)

---

* This case study was adapted and used with permission from the primary physical therapist.

■ ■ ■ ■ ■   ■ ■ ■ ■ ■ ■

Pain

Do you have any pain associated with your past gunshot wound? If yes, describe your pain.

> **FUPs:** Give the client a chance to answer and prompt only if necessary with suggested adjectives such as "Is your pain sharp, dull, boring, or burning?" or "Show me on your body where you have pain."
>
> To pursue this line of questioning, if appropriate:
>
> **FUPs:** What makes your pain better or worse?
> What is your pain like when you first get up in the morning, during the day, and in the evening?
> Is your pain constant or does it come and go?
> On a scale from 0 to 10 with zero being no pain and ten being the worst pain you have ever experienced with this problem, what level of pain would you say that you have *right now?*
> Do you have any other pain or symptoms that are not related to your old injury?
> If yes, pursue as above to find out about the onset of pain, etc.

You indicated that you have numbness in your right hand. How long does this last?

> **FUPs:** Besides picking up a glass of cold water, what else brings it on?
> How long have you had this problem?
> You indicated that this numbness has progressed over time. How quickly has this progression occurred?
> Do you ever have similar symptoms in your left hand?

Associated Symptoms

Even though this person has been seen by numerous physicians, it is important to ask appropriate questions to rule out a systemic origin of current symptoms, especially if there has been a recent change in the symptoms or presentation of symptoms bilaterally. For example:

What other symptoms have you had that you can associate with this problem?

In addition to the numbness, have you had any

- tingling
- burning
- weakness
- vomiting
- hoarseness
- difficulty with breathing
- nausea

- dizziness
- difficulty with swallowing
- heart palpitations or fluttering
- unexplained sweating or night sweats
- problems with your vision

How well do you sleep at night? (Open-ended question)

Do you have trouble sleeping at night? (Closed-ended question)

■ ■ ■ ■ ■ ■ ■ ■ ■ ■ ■ ■

Does the pain awaken you out of a sound sleep? Can you sleep on either side comfortably?

Medications

Are you taking any medications? If yes, and the person doesn't volunteer the information, probe further:

> What medications?
> What are you taking this medication for?
> When did you last take the medication?
> Do you think the medication is easing the symptoms or helping in any way?
> Have you noticed any side effects? If yes, what are these effects?

Previous Medical Treatment

Have you had any recent x-ray examinations? If yes, find out where and when the radiographs were taken and also what parts of the body were x-rayed.

Tell me about your gunshot wound. Were you treated immediately?

Did you have any surgery at that time or since then? If yes, pursue details with regard to what type of surgery and where and when it occurred.

Did you have physical therapy treatment at any time after your accident? If yes, relate when, for how long, with whom, what was done, did it help?

Have you had any other kind of treatment for this injury (e.g., acupuncture, chiropractic, osteopathic, naturopathic, and so on)?

Activities of Daily Living (ADLs)

Are you right handed?

How do your symptoms affect your ability to do your job or work around the house?

How do your symptoms affect caring for yourself (showering, shaving, other activities of daily living such as eating or writing)?

Final Question

Is there anything else you feel that I should know concerning your injury, such as your health or your present symptoms, that I have not asked about?

Note: If this client had been a woman, the interview would have included questions about breast pain, the date when she was last screened for cancer with a physician (cervical and breast), and whether she does monthly self-examination of her breasts.

References

Barnhardt, E.R. (ed.): Physicians' Desk Reference, 47th ed. Oradell, New Jersey, Medical Economics Company, 1993.

Bates, B.: Guide To Physical Exam and History Taking, 5th ed. Philadelphia, J.B. Lippincott, 1990.

Blacklow, R.S. (ed.): MacBryde's Signs and Symptoms, 6th ed. Philadelphia, J.B. Lippincott, 1983.

Braunwald, E. (ed.): Heart Disease: A Textbook of Cardiovascular Medicine, 4th ed. Philadelphia, W.B. Saunders, 1992.

Bresler, D.: Free Yourself from Pain. New York, Simon and Schuster, 1979.

Chernecky, C., Krech, R., and Berger, B.: Laboratory Tests and Diagnostic Procedures. Philadelphia, W.B. Saunders, 1993.

Christan, T., Turnbull, T., and Cline, D.: Cardiopulmonary abnormalities after smoking cocaine. Southern Medical Journal 83(3):335–338, 1990.

Ciccone, C.D.: Geriatric pharmacology. In Guccione, A.A. (ed.): Geriatric Physical Therapy. St. Louis, C.V. Mosby, 1993, pp. 171–197.

Clark, A.J., Matassarin-Jacobs, E., and Carpenter, L.C.: Structure and function of the female and male reproductive systems. In Black, J.M., and Matassarin-Jacobs, E. (eds.): Luckmann and Sorensen's Medical-Surgical Nursing, 4th ed. Philadelphia, W.B. Saunders, 1993, pp. 2037–2052.

Cohen, M., and Michel, T.H.: Cardiopulmonary symptoms in physical therapy practice. New York, Churchill Livingstone, 1988.

Coulehan, J.L., and Block, M.R.: The Medical Interview: A Primer For Students of the Art, 2nd ed. Philadelphia, F.A. Davis, 1992.

Crane, M.G., Harris, J.J., and Winsor, W., III: Hypertension, oral contraceptive agents and conjugated estrogens. Annals of Medicine 74:13, 1971.

Cutler, W.B., and Garcia, C.-R.: Menopause: A Guide for Women and the Men Who Love Them, 2nd ed. New York, W.W. Norton Company, 1992, p. 63.

Dalager, N.A., Kang, H.K., Burt, V.L., and Weatherbee, L.: Non-Hodgkin's lymphoma among Vietnam veterans. Journal of Occupational Medicine 33(7):774–779, 1991.

Dennison, P.D., and Black, J.M.: Nursing care of clients with peripheral vascular disorders. In Black, J.M., and Matassarin-Jacobs, E. (eds.): Luckmann and Sorensen's Medical-Surgical Nursing, 4th ed. Philadelphia, W.B. Saunders, 1993, pp. 1253–1314.

de Vernejoul, M.C., Bielakoff, J., Herve, M., et al.: Evidence for defective osteoblastic function. A role of alcohol and tobacco consumption in osteoporosis in middle-aged men. Clinical Orthopaedics and Related Research 179:107–115, 1983.

Diethrich, E.B., and Cohen, C.: Women and Heart Disease. New York, Times Books, Random House, 1992.

Dranov, P.: Estrogen: Is it right for you? New York, Simon and Schuster, 1993.

Drug Use–Education Tip (Du-Et). Rockville, Md., Pharmaceutics Manufacturers Association, 1988.

Fantl, J.A., Wyman, J.F., and McClish, D.K., et al.: Efficacy of bladder training in older women with urinary incontinence. Journal of the American Medical Association 265:609–613, 1991.

Freestone, S., and Ramsay, L.E.: Effect of coffee and cigarette smoking on the blood pressure of untreated and diuretic-treated hypertensive patients. American Journal of Medicine 73(3):348–353, 1982.

Frymoyer, J.W., Pope, M.H., Clements, J.H., et al.: Risk factors in low back pain. Journal of Bone and Joint Surgery 65-A:213–218, 1983.

Gilman, A., and Goodman, L.S. (eds.): The Pharmacological Basis of Therapeutics, 5th ed. New York, Macmillan, 1975.

Greenberger, N.J., and Hinthorn, D.R.: History Taking and Examination. St. Louis, Mosby–Year Book, 1992.

Heliövaara, M., Knekt, P., and Aromaa, A.: Incidence and risk factors of herniated lumbar intervertebral disc or sciatica leading to hospitalization. Journal of Chronic Diseases 40:251–258, 1987.

Henderson, M.M., Dorflinger, L.J., Fishman, J., et al.: Oral Contraceptives and Breast Cancer. Washington, D.C., National Academy Press, 1991.

Hertling, D., and Kessler, R.M.: Management of Common Musculoskeletal Disorders, 2nd ed. Philadelphia, J.B. Lippincott, 1990.

Hillegass, E., and Sandowsky, H.S.: The Essentials of Cardiopulmonary Physical Therapy. Philadelphia, W.B. Saunders, 1993.

Holm, S., and Nachemson, A.: Nutrition of the intervertebral disc: Acute effects of cigarette smoking. An experimental animal study. Upsala Journal of Medical Science 83:91–98, 1988.

Hughes, J.R., Oliveto, A.H., Helzer, J.E. et al.: Should caffeine abuse, dependence, or withdrawal be added to DSM-IV and ICD-10? American Journal of Psychiatry 149(1):33–40, 1992.

Ignatavicius, D.D., and Bayne, M.V.: Assessment of the cardiovascular system. In Ignatavicius, D.D., and Bayne, M.V. (eds.): Medical-Surgical Nursing. Philadelphia, W.B. Saunders, 1993, pp. 2067–2114.

Jackson, O.L. (ed.): Therapeutic Considerations for the Elderly. New York, Churchill Livingstone, 1987.

Jacox, A.: Pain: A Source Book for Nurses and Other Health Professionals. Boston, Little, Brown, 1977.

Kaplan, N.M.: Clinical Hypertension, 5th ed. Baltimore, Williams and Wilkins, 1990.

Keene, A.: Physical examination. In Black, J.M., and Matassarin-Jacobs, E. (eds.): Luckmann and Sorensen's Medical-Surgical Nursing, 4th ed. Philadelphia, W.B. Saunders, 1993, pp. 215–246.

Kneisl, C.R.: Nursing care of clients with substance abuse. In Black, J.M. and Matassarin-Jacobs, E. (eds.): Luckmann and Sorensen's Medical-Surgical Nursing, 4th ed. Philadelphia, W.B. Saunders, 1993, pp. 2199–2216.

Lalor, B.C., Franco, M.V., and Powell, D.: Bone and mineral metabolism and chronic alcohol abuse. Quarterly Journal of Medicine *59*:497–511, 1986.

Lane, J.M.: When to consider malignant tumor in the differential diagnosis after athletic trauma. Editorial comment. Journal of Musculoskeletal Medicine *7*(5):16, 1990.

Layde, P.M., Webster, L.A., Baughman, A.L., et al.: The independent associations of parity, age at first full term pregnancy and duration of breastfeeding with the risk of breast cancer. Journal of Clinical Epidemiology *42*:963–973, 1989.

Libow, L.S., and Butler, R.N.: Treating mild diastolic hypertension in the elderly: Uncertain benefits and possible dangers. Geriatrics *36*:55–62, 1981.

Long, R.G., Meinhard, E., and Skinner, R.K.: Clinical, biochemical and histological studies of osteomalacia, osteoporosis and parathyroid function in chronic liver disease. Gut *19*:85–90, 1978.

Maitland, G.D.: Vertebral Manipulation, 5th ed. Boston, Butterworth-Heinemann, 1986.

Majid, P.A., Cheirif, J.B., Rokey, R., et al.: Does cocaine cause coronary vasospasm in chronic cocaine abusers? A study of coronary and systemic hemodynamics. Clinical Cardiology *15*(4):253–258, 1992.

Matloff, D.S., Kaplan, M.M., and Neer, R.M.: Osteoporosis in primary biliary cirrhosis: Effects of 25-hydroxyvitamin D treatment. Gastroenterology *83*:97–102, 1982.

Matsuo, K.M., Mirohata, T., and Sugioka, Y.: Influence of alcohol intake, cigarette smoking and occupational status on idiopathic osteonecrosis of the femoral head. Clinical Orthopaedics and Related Research *234*:115–123, 1987.

Melzack, R.: The McGill Pain Questionnaire: Major properties and scoring methods. Pain *1*:277, 1975.

Melzack, R., and Torgerson, W.S.: On the language of pain. Anesthesiology *34*:50, 1971.

O'Toole, M. (ed.): Miller-Keane Encyclopedia and Dictionary of Medicine, Nursing, and Allied Health, 5th ed. Philadelphia, W.B. Saunders, 1992.

Mitchell, T.R., and Larson, J.R.: People in Organizations: An Introduction to Organizational Behavior, 3rd ed. New York, McGraw-Hill, 1987.

Mobarhan, S.A., Russell, R.M., Recker, R.R., et al.: Metabolic bone disease in alcoholic cirrhosis: A comparison of the effect of vitamin D_2, 23-hydroxyvitamin D_3, or supportive treatment. Hepatology *4*:266–273, 1984.

Nursing Drug Handbook '93: Springhouse, Pennsylvania, Springhouse Corporation, 1993.

Pauls, J.: Physical therapy for women. P.T. Magazine of Physical Therapy *1*(2): 64–67, 1993.

Pickney, C., and Pickney, E.R.: The Patient's Guide to Medical Tests, 3rd ed. New York, Facts on File, 1986.

Potter, J.F., and Haigh, R.A.: Benefits of antihypertensive therapy in the elderly. British Medical Bulletin *46*:77–93, 1990.

Prince, R.L., Smith, M., Dick, I.M., et al.: Prevention of postmenopausal osteoporosis. New England Journal of Medicine *325*(17):1189–1195, 1991.

P.T. Bulletin: VA may see more ailments caused by toxins. January 20, 1993a.

P.T. Bulletin: Two diseases added to list attributed to Agent Orange. August 11, 1993b.

Quick, J.C., and Quick, J.D.: Organizational Stress and Preventive Management. New York, McGraw-Hill, 1984.

Resnick, N.M.: Geriatric medicine and the elderly patient. *In* Tierney, L.M., McPhee, S.J., Papadakis, M.A., and Schroeder, S.A.: Current Medical Diagnosis and Treatment. Norwalk, Connecticut, Appleton and Lange, 1993, pp. 21–39.

Riefkohl, R., Wolfe, J.A., Cox, E.B., and McCarty, K.S.: Association between cutaneous occlusive vascular disease, cigarette smoking and skin slough after rhytidectomy. Plastic Reconstructive Surgery *77*(4):592–595, 1986.

Rimoldi, R.: Unpublished paper presented at the 60th Annual Meeting of the American Academy of Orthopaedic Surgeons, San Francisco, February, 1993.

Schapira, D.: Alcohol abuse and osteoporosis. Seminars in Arthritis and Rheumatism *19*(6):371–376, 1990.

Sherwin, M.A., and Gastwirth, C.M.: Detrimental effects of cigarette smoking on lower extremity wound healing. Journal of Foot Surgery *29*(1):84–87, 1990.

Silverman, K., Evans, S.M., Strain, E.C., and Griffiths, R.: Withdrawal syndrome after the double-blind cessation of caffeine consumption. New England Journal of Medicine *327*(16):1109–1114, 1992.

Smith, W.F.: Epidemiology of hypertension in older patients. American Journal of Medicine *85*(Suppl 3b):2–6, 1988.

Swisher, S.N., and Enelow, A.J.: Interviewing and Patient Care, 3rd ed. London, Oxford University Press, 1985.

The Complete Drug Reference. Yonkers, New York, 1992.

Thomas, D.B.: Do hormones cause breast cancer? Cancer 53:595–604, 1984.

Travell, J.G., and Simons, D.G.: Myofascial Pain and Dysfunction: The Trigger Point Manual. Baltimore, Williams and Wilkins, 1983.

Uzych, L.: Agent Orange, the Vietnam war, and lasting health effects. Environmental Health Perspectives *95*:211, 1991.

Verbanck, M., Verbanck, J., and Brauman, J.: Bone histology and 25-OH vitamin D plasma levels in alcoholics without cirrhosis. Calcified Tissue Research *22*:538–541, 1977.

Webster, R.C., Kazda, G., Hamdan, U.S., et al.: Cigarette smoking and face lift: Conservative versus wide undermining. Plastic Reconstructive Surgery *77*(4): 596–604, 1986.

Weinhouse, S., et al.: Nutrition and Cancer: American Cancer Society Guidelines on Diet, Nutrition and Cancer. A Cancer Journal for Clinicians *41*(6):337, 1991.

Weir, R.J.: When the pill causes a rise in blood pressure. Drugs *16*(6):522–527, 1978.

Wolf, G.A., Jr.: Collecting Data from Patients. Baltimore, University Park Press, 1977.

Wolf, S.L.: Clinical decision making in physical therapy. *In* Paris, S.: Clinical Decision Making: Orthopedic Physical Therapy. Philadelphia, F.A. Davis, 1985.

Wong, C.: Learning to Live with Angina. New York, MIPI Publications, 1981.

Work, J.A.: Are java junkies poor sports? The Physician and Sportsmedicine *19*(1):83–88, 1991.

Yaffe, B., Cushin, B.J., and Strauch, B.: Effect of cigarette smoking on experimental microvascular anastomoses. Microsurgery *5*(2):70–72, 1984.

Bibliography

Advice for the Patient, Vol 2, 7th ed. United States Pharmacopeial Dispensing Information (USPDI), Rockville, Maryland, 1987.

Barnhardt, E.R. (ed.): Consumer's Guide to Nonprescription Drugs, 11th ed. Oradell, New Jersey, Medical Economics Company, 1990.

Barnhardt, E.R. (ed.): Physicians' Desk Reference: Drug Interactions and Side Effects Index, 44th ed. Oradell, New Jersey, Medical Economics Company, 1990.

Bergner, M., Bobbitt, R.A., and Kressel, S.: The sickness impact profile: Conceptual formulation and methodology for the development of a health status measure. International Journal of Health Services *6*:393, 1976.

Bernstein, L., and Bernstein, R.: Interviewing: A Guide for Health Professionals. Norwalk, Connecticut, Appleton-Century-Crofts, 1985.

Cash, W.B., Jr., and Stewart, C.I.: Interviewing: Principles and Practices. Dubuque, Iowa, W.C. Brown, 1985.

Ciccone, C.D.: Pharmacology in Rehabilitation. Philadelphia, F.A. Davis, 1990.

Cohen-Cole, S.A.: The Medical Interview: The Three Function Approach. St. Louis, Mosby–Year Book, 1990.

Dirckx, J.H.: History and Physical: The Nonphysicians Guide to the Medical History and Physical Examination. Modesto, California, Health Professions Institute, 1991.

Fairbanks, J.C.T., Couper, J., Davies, J.B., and O'Brien, J.P.: The Oswestry Low Back Pain Disability Questionnaire. Physiotherapy *66*:271, 1980.

Malone, T. (ed.): Physical and Occupational Therapy: Drug Implications for Practice. Philadelphia, J.B. Lippincott, 1989.

McKenzie, R.A.: The Lumbar Spine: Mechanical Diagnosis and Therapy. Wakanae, New Zealand, Spinal Publications, 1981.

Million, R., Hall, W., and Haavik, R.D.: Assessment of the progress of the back-pain patient. Spine *7*:204, 1982.

Roland, M., and Morris, R.: A study of the natural history of back pain. Part I: Development of a reliable and sensitive measure of disability in low-back pain. Spine *2*:141, 1983.

Rose, S.J., Shulman, A.D., and Strube, M.J.: Functional assessment of patients with low back syndrome. Topics in Geriatric Rehabilitation *1*:9, 1986.

Selzer, M.L., et al.: A self-administered Short Michigan Alcoholism Screening Test. Journal of Studies on Alcohol *36*(117), 1975.

Tamburro, C.H.: Chronic liver injury in phenoxy herbicide-exposed Vietnam veterans. Environmental Research *59*(1):175–188, 1992.

United States Pharmacopeial Dispensing Information (USPDI). Rockville, Maryland, 1993.

Waddell, G., and Main, C.J.: Assessment of severity of low-back disorders. Spine *9*:204, 1984.

What are the signs of alcoholism? New York, National Council on Alcoholism, 1990.

Appendix A

Advantages and Disadvantages of Hormone Replacement Therapy (HRT)

RISKS

Continued menstruation

Possible increase in risk of breast cancer with prolonged use

Possible increase in risk of uterine cancer

Breast swelling or tenderness

Premenstrual syndrome with use of progesterone

Administration of estrogen by transdermal patch delivers higher levels of hormone, increasing the risk of breast cancer

BENEFITS

Provides natural protection against coronary artery disease

Prevents osteoporosis

Eliminates hot flashes

May improve memory and concentration

Improves mood and sense of well-being

Reduces fatigue and restores energy

Appendix *B*
Guidelines for Blood Pressure Measurement

■ Select the proper cuff size:

Pediatric cuff size is 8 to 10 cm wide and 26 cm long.

Adult cuff size is 12 to 14 cm wide and 30 cm long.

Larger adult cuff size is 18 to 20 cm wide.

■ Make sure that equipment is properly assembled and calibrated:

Cuff bladder should be intact inside the cuff.

Sphygmomanometer should be calibrated to 0 mm Hg every few months to ensure reliability.

Cuff must be placed above the area to be auscultated (e.g., the left arm is recommended for more distinct sounds; the cuff is placed above the brachial artery).

■ Follow these steps to measure and record blood pressure accurately:

1. Palpate the brachial or radial pulse.
2. Inflate the cuff 30 mm Hg above the level at which those pulses disappear. As soon as the blood begins to flow through the artery again, Korotkoff's sounds are heard. The first sounds are tapping sounds that gradually increase in intensity.
3. The initial tapping sound that is heard for at least two consecutive beats is recorded as *systolic* blood pressure.

The first phase of sound may be followed by a momentary disappearance of sounds that can last from 30 to 40 mm Hg as the needle descends. Following this temporary absence of sound, there are murmuring or swishing sounds. As deflation of the cuff continues, the sounds become sharper and louder. These sounds represent phase 3. During phase 4, the sounds become muffled rather abruptly and then are followed by silence, which represents phase 5. Phase 5, or the point at which sounds disappear, is most often used as the *diastolic* blood pressure.

■ Measurements should be recorded on both arms to assess for thoracic outlet (cardiovascular component), vascular obstruction, and errors in measurement. Subsequent measurements should be done on the extremity with the highest pressure.

■ If arms are inaccessible (e.g., after amputation or mastectomy), pressures can be obtained using an appropriately sized cuff on the client's thigh or calf. The popliteal artery or posterior tibial artery is auscultated.

■ The position of the client and the site used to obtain the blood pressure are recorded. Any signs or symptoms of distress should be observed and recorded.

■ Always measure the blood pressure twice. No rest or pause between readings is necessary.

Adapted from Ignatavicius, D.D., and Bayne, M.V.: Assessment of the cardiovascular system. *In* Ignatavicius, D.D., and Bayne, M.V. (eds.): Medical-Surgical Nursing. Philadelphia, W.B. Saunders, 1993, p. 2093.

Overview of Cardiovascular Signs and Symptoms

■ ■ ■ ■ ■ ■ ■ ■ ■ ■ ■

Clinical Signs and Symptoms of:

Myocardial Ischemia
Angina Pectoris
Heartburn
Myocardial Infarction
Pericarditis
Left-Sided Heart Failure
Right-Sided Heart Failure Aneurysm
Ruptured Aneurysm
Cardiac Valvular Disease
Rheumatic Fever
Endocarditis
Mitral Valve Prolapse
Fibrillation
Tachycardia
Sinus Bradycardia
Arterial Disease

Arteriosclerosis Obliterans
Buerger's Disease
Raynaud's Phenomenon and Disease
Superficial Venous Thrombosis
Deep Venous Thrombosis
Lymphedema
Hypertension
Transient Ischemic Attack
Orthostatic Hypotension
Herpes Zoster (Shingles)
Dorsal Nerve Root Irritation
Thoracic Outlet Syndrome
Gastrointestinal Disorders
Breast Pathology
Chest Pain Due to Anxiety

The trouble with heart disease is that the first symptom is often hard to deal with: sudden death.

MICHAEL PHELPS, M.D.

Heart disease remains the leading cause of death in industrialized nations. In the United States alone, cardiovascular disease (CVD) is responsible for approximately one million deaths each year. More than one in four Americans has some form of cardiovascular disease. The American Heart Association reports that about half of all deaths from heart disease are sudden and unexpected.

Fortunately, during the last two decades, cardiovascular research has greatly increased our understanding of the structure and function of the cardiovascular system in health and disease. Despite the formidable statistics regarding the prevalence of CVD, during the last 15 years a steady decline in mortality from cardiovascular disorders has been witnessed. Effective application of the increased knowledge regarding CVD and its risk factors will assist health care professionals to educate clients in achieving and maintaining cardiovascular health (Abraham and Kavanaugh, 1991).

CARDIOVASCULAR STRUCTURE AND FUNCTION (Abraham and Kavanaugh, 1991; Ott, 1993a)

The cardiovascular system consists of the heart, arteries, capillaries, veins, and lymphatics. The functions of the heart are to pump oxygenated blood into the arterial system, which carries it to the cells, and to collect deoxygenated blood from the venous system and deliver it to the lungs for reoxygenation (Fig. 3–1).

The function of the arteries, capillaries, veins, and lymphatics is to carry blood to and from tissues and cells throughout the body.

Heart

The heart is a relatively small organ located in the middle of the mediastinum, where the lungs partially overlap it. This pulsatile, four-chambered pump beats approximately 72 times per minute and

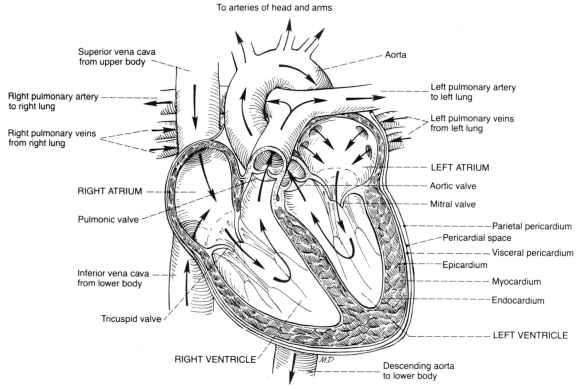

Figure 3–1

Structure and circulation of the heart. Blood entering the left atrium from the right and left pulmonary veins flows into the left ventricle. The left ventricle pumps blood into the systemic circulation through the aorta. From the systemic circulation, blood returns to the heart through the superior and inferior venae cavae. From there, the right ventricle pumps blood into the lungs through the right and left pulmonary arteries. (From Black, J.M., and Matassarin-Jacobs, E. [eds.]: Luckmann and Sorenson's Medical-Surgical Nursing, 4th ed. Philadelphia, W.B. Saunders, 1993, p. 1093.)

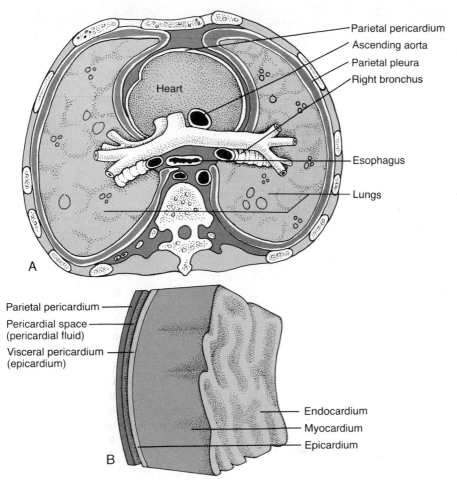

Figure 3–2

The heart and associated layers of membranes. *A,* Cross-section through the thorax just above the heart, emphasizing the lining of the cavity that contains the lungs (parietal pleura) and the lining of the cavity that contains the heart (parietal pericardium). *B,* Sagittal view of the layers of the heart.

pumps more than 5 liters of blood each minute, or about 2000 gallons per day. It continually propels oxygenated blood into the arterial system and receives poorly oxygenated blood from the venous system. The heart muscle rests on the diaphragm and is tilted forward and to the left such that the apex of the heart is rotated anteriorly.

Pericardium. The heart is enclosed by the pericardium, which consists of two layers, one sac inside another (Fig. 3–2):

■ Visceral pericardium (the inner layer)
■ Parietal pericardium (the outer layer)

The two pericardial surfaces are separated by a pericardial space that normally contains approximately 10 to 20 ml of thin, clear pericardial fluid. This lubricating fluid moistens the contacting surfaces of the pericardial layers. It serves to reduce the friction produced by the pumping action of the heart and cushions the heart against external trauma. The visceral pericardium actually encases the heart and extends several centimeters onto each of the great vessels. The parietal pericardium, the tough, fibrous outer membrane, is attached anteriorly to the manubrium and xiphoid process of the sternum, posteriorly to the thoracic vertebrae, and inferiorly to the diaphragm.

There are three layers of cardiac tissue:

■ Epicardium (outer layer of the heart, which has the same structure as the visceral pericardium)

■ Myocardium (middle layer of the heart, composed of striated muscle fibers; the actual contracting muscle of the heart)

■ Endocardium (inner layer, consisting of endothelial tissue that lines the inside of the heart's chambers and covers the heart valves)

Coronary Arteries

The blood circulating through the heart does not supply the heart muscle itself with oxygen and nutrients. The blood vessels that nourish the heart muscle are called the *coronary arteries*. These arteries lie on the surface of the heart and arise from the aorta (just behind the cusps of the aortic valve) in an area known as the sinuses of Valsalva.

Two main coronary arteries (right and left) branch off the aorta just above the aortic valve, encircle the heart, and supply blood to the myocardium. Unlike the case with other arteries, 75 per cent of the coronary artery blood flow occurs during diastole, when the heart is relaxed (Ahrens and Taylor, 1992).

For adequate blood flow through the coronary arteries, the diastolic blood pressure must be at least 60 mm Hg. Coronary blood flow increases with increased activity (e.g., exercise) and increased stimulation of the sympathetic nervous system. Coronary blood supply to the myocardium can be limited by several conditions, including coronary artery disease, spasm, and myocardial infarction (Cohen and Michel, 1988).

Despite scientific advances in the field of cardiology, coronary artery disease and its complications are still the leading cause of death in the United States.

Valves

The four cardiac valves are delicate, flap-like structures that function to maintain unidirectional (forward) blood flow through the heart chambers. These valves open and close in response to changes in pressure and volume within the heart chambers. The cardiac valves can be classified into two types: the atrioventricular (AV) valves, which separate the atria from the ventricles; and the semilunar valves, which separate the pulmonary artery and the aorta from their respective ventricles.

Atrioventricular

The AV valves include

■ The tricuspid valve (located between the right atrium and the right ventricle)

■ The bicuspid (mitral) valve (located between the left atrium and left ventricle)

The tricuspid valve contains three leaflets held in place by fibrous cords called the chordae tendineae. The mitral valve on the left side of the heart is a bicuspid valve with two valve cusps or leaflets. It is also attached by the chordae tendineae, which are extremely important because of the support they give to the AV valves during ventricular systole to prevent valvular prolapse (falling downward) into the atrium. There is also a degree of leaflet overlapping during closure of the AV valves, which helps prevent the backward flow of blood.

Semilunar

The semilunar valves include

■ The aortic valves

■ The pulmonic valves

The structural design of the semilunar valves consists of three cuplike cusps. The valves lie between each ventricle and the great vessel into which it empties. These valves are open during ventricular systole (contraction) to permit blood flow into the aorta and pulmonary artery. They are closed during diastole (relaxation) to prevent retrograde (backward) flow from the aorta and pulmonary artery back into the ventricle when it is relaxed.

Cardiac Nervous System
(Ott, 1993a)

The cardiac conduction system consists of modified cardiac muscle cells characterized by their ability to conduct electrical impulses very rapidly. The conduction system acts to spread the action potential, initiated in one area of the myocardium, rapidly through the whole heart. Spread of the action potential stimulates synchronized contraction of the atria and ventricles. The conduction system consists of the sinoatrial node (SA node), the atrioventricular node (AV node), the bundle of His, and Purkinje's fibers.

Both the sympathetic and parasympathetic nervous systems innervate the heart. Sympathetic nervous system (SNS) efferent fibers originate in the thoracolumbar region, travel through the superior, middle, and inferior cervical ganglia, and are received in the atria and ventricles (Cohen and Michel, 1988).

The catecholamines epinephrine, norepinephrine, and dopamine are the neurotransmitters for the sympathetic nervous system. The parasympathetic nervous system (PNS) efferent fibers traverse the vagus nerve and supply the atria and the SA and AV nodes. Acetylcholine is the primary neurotransmitter for the PNS. Both the PNS and the SNS have afferent fibers that send impulses from the heart and great vessels to higher centers in the brain (Cohen and Michel, 1988).

Although the heart rate is controlled primarily by the autonomic nervous system, excitability is influenced by hormones, electrolytes, nutrition, oxygen supply, medications, body temperatures, infection, and nerve characteristics. Impulses from the cerebral cortex also can have a significant effect on the heart rate. For example, pain, fear, anger, and excitement all can cause a substantial increase in the heart rate.

The *sinoatrial node,* or pacemaker, is located at the junction of the superior vena cava and right atrium. Under normal circumstances, the SA node initiates each heart beat. This node consists of two types of specialized cells within a network of dense fibers. P cells in the center of the node initiate electrical impulses approximately 60 to 100 times per minute. T cells on the circumference transmit these impulses to surrounding atrial muscle.

The sympathetic and parasympathetic nervous systems control the SA node. Any myocardial tissue in the atria, AV bundle, or ventricles has the capability of taking over the role of pacemaker if that tissue generates impulses at a higher rate than that of the SA node.

The *atrioventricular node,* or AV junction, is located in the lower aspect of the atrial septum. The AV node receives electrical impulses from the SA node. Within the AV node, the impulse is delayed while the atria contract. This delay enables atrial contraction to be completed before the ventricles are stimulated and contract.

The *bundle of His* (AV bundle) fuses with the AV node to form another pacemaker site. If the SA node fails, the bundle of His can initiate and sustain a heart rate of 40 to 60 beats per minute (BPM). The bundle of His branches into two segments, right and left, which terminate in Purkinje's fibers.

Purkinje's fibers are a diffuse network of conducting strands on the endocardial surface, penetrating the myocardium of both ventricles. They rapidly spread the wave of depolarization (rapid reversal of the resting membrane potential to generate an electrical current) through the ventricles. Activation of the ventricles begins in the septum and then moves from the apex of the heart upward.

Within the ventricular walls, depolarization is initiated by an impulse from the SA node. The impulse first spreads through the right atrium and then activates the left atrium. Shortly after the impulse reaches the left atrium, it also activates the region at the junction and subsequently the AV node. The impulse continues to activate the ventricular muscle from the apex toward the base of the heart to complete the process. Repolarization is a passive event that occurs in each cell and does not involve the conduction system.

CARDIAC PATHOPHYSIOLOGY

Three components of cardiac disease are discussed (Table 3–1):

Diseases affecting the heart muscle

Diseases affecting heart valves

Defects of the cardiac nervous system

Within these categories, there are diseases that are not mentioned here, either because they are rare or because they do not mimic musculoskeletal symptoms.

Degenerative Heart Disease
(Arizona Heart Institute, 1991; Reigle and Ringel, 1993)

Degenerative heart disease refers to the changes in the heart and blood supply to the heart and major blood vessels that occur with aging. As the population ages, degenerative heart disease becomes the most prevalent form of cardiovascular disease. Degenerative heart disease is also called *atherosclerotic cardiovascular disease, arteriosclerotic cardiovascular disease, coronary heart disease,* and *coronary artery disease.*

Coronary Artery Disease

The heart muscle must have an adequate blood supply to contract properly. As mentioned, the coronary arteries carry oxygen and blood to the myocardium. When a coronary artery becomes narrowed or blocked, the area of the heart muscle supplied by that artery becomes ischemic and injured, and infarction may result.

Pathogenesis. Scientists have discovered a gene on chromosome 19, near the gene to the LDL (low-density lipoprotein) receptor used to remove LDL cholesterol from the blood (Tas, 1991). This gene is called the atherosclerosis susceptibility (ATHS) gene, and it may account for nearly half of all cases of atherosclerosis (Nishina et al., 1992). This gene causes a set of characteristics that triple a person's risk of myocardial infarction; the combination of factors includes upper body obesity, low concentrations of high-density lipoprotein in the blood, high blood concentrations of fatty compounds, and a preponderance of the small, dense form of low-density lipopro-

Table 3–1
CARDIAC DISEASES

Heart Muscle	Heart Valves	Cardiac Nervous System
Coronary artery disease	Rheumatic fever	Arrhythmias
Myocardial infarct	Endocarditis	Tachycardia
Pericarditis	Mitral valve prolapse	Bradycardia
Congestive heart failure	Congenital deformities	
Aneurysms		

teins in the blood. Together, these make up an atherogenic lipoprotein profile. About 30 per cent of Americans are estimated to have this profile.

The actual pathogenesis of coronary artery disease follows this process (Cohen and Michel, 1988):

- Injury to endothelial cell wall
- Fibroblastic proliferation in the intima
- Accumulation of lipids at the junction of the arterial intima and media, further obstructing blood flow
- Degeneration and hyalinization (conversion into a substance like glass) of atheromatous areas
- Calcium deposition at edges of hyaline areas

The major disorders due to insufficient blood supply to the myocardium are angina pectoris, congestive heart failure (CHF), and myocardial infarction (MI). These disorders are collectively known as coronary artery disease, also called coronary heart disease or ischemic heart disease.

Coronary artery disease (CAD) includes atherosclerosis (fatty build-up), thrombus (blood clot), and spasm (intermittent constriction).

Atherosclerosis. Atherosclerosis is the disease process often called *arteriosclerosis,* or *hardening of the arteries*. It is a progressive process that begins in childhood. It can occur in any artery in the body, but it is most common in medium-sized arteries, such as are found in the heart, brain, kidneys, and legs. From childhood on, the arteries begin to fill with a fatty substance, or lipids such as triglycerides and cholesterol, which then calcify or harden.

This filler, called *plaque,* is made up of fats, calcium, and fibrous scar tissue and lines the usually supple arterial walls (Fig. 3–3), progressively narrowing the arteries. These arteries carry blood rich in oxygen to the myocardium (middle layer of the heart consisting of the heart muscle), but the atherosclerotic process leads to ische-

mia and to necrosis of the heart muscle. Necrotic tissue gradually forms a scar, but before scar formation, the weakened area is susceptible to aneurysm development. Scarred tissue does not contribute to the contractile force of wall motion during systole (Sokolow et al., 1990).

When fully developed, plaque can cause bleeding, clot formation, and distortion or rupture of a blood vessel. Heart attacks and strokes are the most sudden and often fatal signs of the disease.

Thrombus. When plaque builds up on the artery walls, the blood flow is slowed and a clot (thrombus) may form on the plaque. When a vessel becomes blocked with a clot, it is called *thrombosis. Coronary thrombosis* refers to the formation of a clot in one of the coronary arteries, usually causing a heart attack.

The mechanism of blood clotting consists of a highly complex series of chemical reactions involving three phases of coagulation followed by a clot resolution phase (Table 3–2). Clot resolution follows the clot formation process by interaction of the fibrinolysin enzyme with fibrinogen to form fragments that have antithrombin action.

Spasm. Sudden constriction of a coronary artery is called a spasm; blood flow to that part of the heart is cut off or decreased. A brief spasm may cause mild symptoms that never return. A prolonged spasm may cause heart damage, such as an infarct. This process can occur in healthy persons who have no cardiac history, as well as in people who have known atherosclerosis. Although the causes are not well known, current studies indicate that chemicals like nicotine and cocaine may lead to coronary artery spasm (Christan et al., 1990; Majid et al., 1992). Other possible factors include anxiety and cold air.

Risk/Contributing Factors. In 1948, the United States government decided to investigate the etiology, incidence, and pathology of CAD by studying residents of a typical small town in the United States called Framingham, Massachusetts. Over the next 10, 20, and 30 years, the participants in the

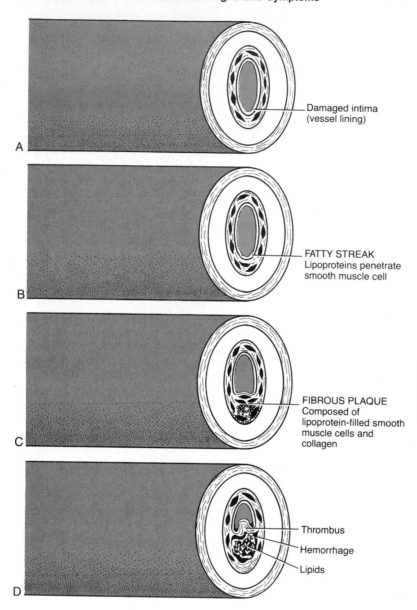

A

Damaged intima
(vessel lining)

B

FATTY STREAK
Lipoproteins penetrate
smooth muscle cell

C

FIBROUS PLAQUE
Composed of
lipoprotein-filled smooth
muscle cells and
collagen

D

Thrombus

Hemorrhage

Lipids

Figure 3–3

Hardening of the arteries. *A,* Atherosclerosis begins with an injury to the endothelial lining of the artery (intimal layer) that makes the vessel permeable to circulating lipoproteins. *B,* Penetration of lipoproteins into the smooth muscle cells of the intima produces "fatty streaks." *C,* A fibrous plaque large enough to decrease blood flow through the artery develops. *D,* Calcification with rupture or hemorrhage of the fibrous plaque is the final advanced stage. Thrombosis may occur, further occluding the lumen of the blood vessel.

study began to die, when possible postmortem examinations were conducted to ascertain the causes of death.*

* For an interesting social and medical critique of the Framingham Study, see Lynch, J.J.: The Broken Heart: The Medical Consequences of Loneliness. New York, Basic Books, 1977.

The research revealed important modifiable and nonmodifiable risk factors associated with death caused by CHD. Since that time, an additional category, *contributing factors,* has been added (Table 3–3). The three greatest risk factors for cardiovascular disease that can be controlled are cigarette smoking, high blood pressure,

Table 3–2
PHASES OF COAGULATION

Phase 1—Vascular Phase	Phase 2—Platelet Phase	Phase 3—Coagulation Phase
Trauma occurs	Intimal damage occurs	Plasma protein form prothrombin
Local vasoconstriction	Platelets become sticky	Prothrombin is converted to thrombin
Mechanical pressure from blood leaking out	Platelets adhere to collagen and vascular surfaces	Fibrin formation into fibrinogen in the presence of thrombin
	Blood flow slows down	Fibrinogen limits clot size

and high blood cholesterol. Most other risk factors can also be managed (obesity, lack of exercise, diabetes, stress), but a few are beyond control (family history of heart disease, age, sex, and race).

Family History. If one or more members of a family (parent, sister, or brother) have a history of cardiovascular disease, the chances of developing heart disease are increased.

Age and Sex. With aging, the risk of CVD increases, with increasing symptomatic CAD after age 40 years. Women generally develop CAD 10 years later than men and heart attacks another 10 years later, because of the hormonal protection estrogen offers women premenopausally. This "bio-logic protection factor" increases HDL, or "good cholesterol," and decreases LDL, "bad cholesterol" (see explanation under Laboratory Values later in this chapter).

Studies confirm that women with heart disease face bias and medical discrimination in their diagnosis and treatment. Their symptoms are more likely to be misinterpreted, overlooked, or dismissed as psychosomatic. Consequently, some women are never properly diagnosed and die unnecessarily (Diethrich and Cohen, 1992a).

By age 45 years, heart disease affects one woman in nine. By age 65, that ratio becomes one in three. Although heart disease is more prevalent among men, it is more deadly for women. Compared with a man, a

Table 3–3
RISK FACTORS AND CORONARY ARTERY DISEASE

Modifiable Risk Factors	Nonmodifiable Risk Factors	Contributing Factors
Physical inactivity	Age	Obesity
Cigarette smoking	Male gender	Response to stress
Elevated serum cholesterol	Family history	Personality
High blood pressure	Race	Diabetes
		Hormonal status

Adapted from Reigle, J., and Ringel, K.A.: Nursing care of clients with disorders of cardiac function. *In* Black, J.M., and Matassarin-Jacobs, E. (eds.): Luckmann and Sorenson's Medical-Surgical Nursing, 4th ed. Philadelphia, W.B. Saunders, 1993, p. 1140.

woman who has a heart attack is more likely to die. If she survives, she is more vulnerable to a second attack and chronic, disabling chest pain. If she has bypass surgery or balloon angioplasty, she is less likely to survive; if she does survive, she is less likely to recover fully (Diethrich and Cohen, 1992b).

Hormones circulating in the blood also alter the action of other body chemicals in both sexes. For example, the enzyme *cyclooxygenase* produces *thromboxane* in the presence of testosterone. Thromboxane constricts the blood vessels and encourages blood clotting. In the presence of estrogen, cyclooxygenase dilates the blood vessels and slows clotting (Diethrich and Cohen, 1992c).

Race. The risk of heart disease is higher among African-Americans than whites, but white men die more frequently from CAD than do nonwhites. Three times as many African-Americans have extremely high blood pressure, a major risk factor. Native Americans have an unusually high rate of diabetes and obesity, which would normally result in heart disease. However, in this population, lower total and LDL cholesterol levels offset the difference.

Hypertension. Hypertension, or high blood pressure, causes the heart to work harder and may injure the arterial walls, making them prone to atherosclerosis. Women who have undetected or uncontrolled hypertension have five times the risk of sudden death, heart attack, and angina than women with normal blood pressure. Hypertension is aggravated by obesity and is associated with diabetes and regular alcohol use. It can be initiated or aggravated by the use of oral contraceptives, especially for women who smoke. Preventive measures such as exercise, avoidance of salt and alcohol, and especially weight control deserve a high priority (Kannel et al., 1993).

Diabetes. More than 80 per cent of people who have diabetes die of some form of cardiovascular disease. Uncontrolled diabetes creates excess blood sugar that can be changed into triglycerides. Triglycerides, along with cholesterol, promote the development of atherosclerosis. Evidence shows that exercise can help control blood lipid abnormalities.

Sedentary Lifestyle. A sedentary lifestyle is nearly as dangerous as smoking and having high cholesterol and is far more prevalent. Lack of exercise causes poor circulation, loss of muscle tone and strength, and weight gain. Researchers still have not established the relationship between exercise and the risk of CAD, but it has been observed that people who seldom exercise do not recover from heart attacks as quickly or as easily as physically active people. Regular aerobic exercise lowers resting pulse rate and blood pressure, improves the ratio of "good" to "bad" cholesterol, and helps prevent and control diabetes and osteoporosis (Diethrich and Cohen, 1992c).

Serum Cholesterol. Cholesterol is a fatty substance (lipid) that is naturally present in the body's cells. Lipids measured are total cholesterol and triglycerides. Total cholesterol is broken into high-density lipoprotein (HDL), or "good" cholesterol, which carries cholesterol away from the cells, and low-density lipoprotein (LDL), or "bad" cholesterol, which carries cholesterol to the cells.

People who have abnormally high levels of cholesterol (between 200 and 240 mg/dl) circulating in their blood are at substantially greater risk for heart disease. This risk doubles when cholesterol levels exceed 240 mg/dl and the ratio of total cholesterol to HDL is more than 4.0. Cholesterol levels are influenced by heredity, diet, exercise, heavy alcohol consumption, weight, medications, menopausal status (Posner et al., 1993), and smoking.

A new analysis from the Framingham Heart Study, presented by Castelli (1992), shows that men and women who have high triglyceride levels (more than 1.7 mmol/L) and a low high-density lipoprotein (HDL) level (less than 1.03 mmol/L) have a significantly higher rate of CAD and can be identified.

As a risk factor, this risk group (high triglyceride–low HDL) is independently related to occurrence of CAD and produces twice as many cases of CAD as the next highest disease-producing lipid abnormality. This trait is associated with increased insulin resistance, higher blood sugar levels, higher uric acid levels, hypertension, and centrally mediated obesity.

Smoking. Cigarette smoking increases heart rate and blood pressure; decreases the oxygen-carrying capacity of blood; increases poisonous gases and elements of the blood such as carbon monoxide, cyanide, formaldehyde, and carbon dioxide; causes narrowing of blood vessels; and increases the work of the heart. Smoking enhances the process of atherosclerosis by a direct effect on the blood vessel wall, increasing the tendency for blood clot formation.

Male adult smokers have a 70 per cent higher mortality rate than do male nonsmokers, and all smokers have more than twice the risk of heart attack than do nonsmokers. People who quit smoking will lose their increased risk in 24 months (Waller, 1989).

Obesity. This alone can lead to CVD, because excess weight makes the heart work harder to pump blood throughout the body and is commonly associated with high blood pressure and high fat (triglyceride and cholesterol) levels. Obesity is defined medically as being 15 per cent above the normal weight for age and height (O'Toole, 1992) and can be caused by inactivity, overeating, or hypothyroidism.

Stress and Personality. Emotional stress raises the heart rate and blood pressure, increasing the workload on the heart. After emotional distress, the heart rate takes longer to slow down. Whether the controversial "Type A" personality characterized by hostility, anger, irritability, impatience, insecurity, and cynicism has a greater risk for CHD remains unclear. The anger component in the stress response is important; these factors may have more significance in women (Dimsdale, 1988; Stokes, 1990).

Clinical Signs and Symptoms. Atherosclerosis, by itself, does not necessarily produce symptoms. For manifestations to develop, there must be a critical deficit in blood supply to the heart in proportion to the demands of the myocardium for oxygen and nutrients (supply and demand imbalance). When atherosclerosis develops slowly, collateral circulation develops to meet the heart's demands. Often, symptoms of CAD do not appear until the lumen of the coronary artery narrows by 75 per cent.

Treatment and Prognosis. Coronary artery disease is a progressive disorder. If not prevented or treated in early stages, it will progress to more severe forms of cardiac disorders. Common sequelae of CAD include sudden cardiac death, angina pectoris, and myocardial infarction. In addition, clients may develop heart failure, chronic arrhythmias, conduction disturbances, and unstable angina.

As indicated, prevention, rather than treatment, is the goal for clients with CAD. Fatty streaks are capable of regressing and disappearing entirely if cholesterol and fat intake are reduced. Medications can be given to reduce cholesterol levels and reduce the risk of clotting. Cessation of cigarette smoking, controlling diet, and managing diabetes and hypertension can also decrease the risk of CAD.

Percutaneous transluminal coronary angioplasty (PTCA) is a surgical technique in which a balloon-tipped catheter is inserted into a blocked coronary artery. The balloon is inflated to compress the plaque and open the artery. At present, surgical methods only ease the symptoms and cannot halt the process of atherosclerosis.

Early experience with PTCA indicates that women have less short-term benefit and suffer more immediate complications than men (Eysmann and Douglas, 1992).

Higher procedural mortality is only partly explained by cardiovascular risk factors. Long-term results for women appear to be similar to, if not better than, those for men.

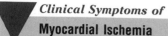

Clinical Symptoms of
Myocardial Ischemia

- Angina pectoris (chest pain)
- Eventual myocardial infarct (MI, i.e., necrosis or death of the heart muscle)

Angina Pectoris (Reigle and Ringel, 1993)

Acute pain in the chest, called *angina pectoris*, results from the imbalance between cardiac workload and oxygen supply to myocardial tissue. Although the primary cause of angina is CAD, angina can occur in people with normal coronary arteries and with other conditions affecting the supply/demand balance (see Causes of Myocardial Ischemia).

As vessels become lined with atherosclerotic plaque, symptoms of inadequate blood supply develop in the tissues supplied by these vessels. A growing mass of plaque in the vessel collects platelets, fibrin, and cellular debris. Platelet aggregations are known to release prostaglandin capable of causing vessel spasm. This in turn promotes platelet aggregation and a vicious spasm/pain cycle begins.

The present theory of heart pain suggests that pain occurs as a result of an accumulation of metabolites within an ischemic segment of the myocardium. The transient ischemia of angina or the prolonged, necrotic ischemia of a myocardial infarction sets off pain impulses secondary to rapid accumulation of these metabolites in the heart muscle.

The imbalance between cardiac workload and oxygen supply can develop as a result of disorders of the coronary vessels, disorders of circulation, increased demands on output of the heart, or damaged myocardium unable to utilize oxygen properly (see Causes of Myocardial Ischemia).

Clinical Signs and Symptoms. The client may indicate the location of the symptoms by placing a clenched fist against the ster-

---

CAUSES OF MYOCARDIAL ISCHEMIA

Decreased Blood Supply
Vessels
  Atherosclerotic narrowing
  Inadequate collateral circulation
  Spasm due to smoking, emotion, or cold
  Coronary arteritis
  Hypertension
  Hypertrophic cardiomyopathy
Circulatory Factors
  Arrhythmias (↓ BP)
  Aortic stenosis
  Hypotension
  Bleeding
Blood Factors (↑ Viscosity)
  Anemia
  Hypoxemia
  Polycythemia

Increased Blood Demand
Hyperthyroidism
Arteriovenous fistula
Thyrotoxicosis
Exercise/exertion
Emotion/excitement
Digestion of a large meal

num. Angina radiates most commonly to the left shoulder and down the inside of the arm to the fingers; but it can also refer pain to the neck, jaw, teeth, upper back, possibly down the right arm, and occasionally to the abdomen (see Fig. 3–8).

Recognizing heart pain in women is more difficult as the symptoms are less reliable and often do not follow the classic pattern described earlier. Many women describe the pain in ways consistent with unstable angina, suggesting that they first become aware of their chest discomfort or have it diagnosed only after it reaches more advanced stages. Some experience a sensation similar to inhaling cold air, rather than the more typical shortness of breath. Other women complain only of weakness and lethargy, and some have noted isolated pain in the midthoracic spine or throbbing and aching in the right biceps muscle (Diethrich and Cohen, 1992d).

Pain associated with the angina and myocardial infarction occurring along the inner aspect of the arm and corresponding to the ulnar nerve distribution results from common connections between the cardiac and brachial plexuses.

Cardiac pain referred to the jaw occurs through internuncial (neurons connecting other neurons) fibers from cervical spinal cord posterior horns to the spinal nucleus of the trigeminal nerve. Abdominal pain produced by referred cardiac pain is more difficult to explain and may be due to the overflow of segmental levels to which visceral afferent nerve pathways flow (see Fig. 6–3). This overflow increases the chances that final common pain pathways between the chest and the abdomen may occur.

The *sensation* of angina is described as squeezing, burning, pressing, choking, aching, or bursting. Angina is often confused with heartburn or indigestion, hiatal hernia, or gallbladder disease, but the pain of these other lesions is not described as sharp or knifelike. The client often says the pain feels like "gas" or "heartburn" or "indigestion." Referred pain from the external oblique abdominal muscle can cause heartburn in the anterior chest wall.

Clinical Signs and Symptoms of
Heartburn

- Frequent "heartburn" attacks
- Frequent use of antacids to relieve symptoms
- Heartburn wakes client up at night
- Acid or bitter taste in the mouth
- Burning sensation in the chest
- Discomfort after eating spicy foods
- Difficulty in swallowing

Clinical Signs and Symptoms of
Angina Pectoris

- Gripping, viselike feeling of pain or pressure behind the breast bone
- Pain that may radiate to the neck, jaw, back, shoulder, or arms (most often the left arm)
- Toothache
- Burning indigestion
- Dyspnea (shortness of breath)
- Nausea
- Belching

A physician must make the differentiation between angina and heartburn, hiatal hernia, and gallbladder disease.

Severity is usually mild or moderate. Rarely is the pain described as severe. As to *location,* 80 to 90 per cent of clients experience the pain as retrosternal or slightly to the left of the sternum. The *duration* of angina as a direct result of myocardial ischemia is typically 1 to 3 minutes and no longer than 3 to 5 minutes. However, attacks precipitated by a heavy meal or extreme anger may last 15 to 20 minutes. Angina is relieved by rest or nitroglycerin (a coronary artery vasodilator).

Severity of pain is not a good prognostic indicator; some people with severe discomfort live for many years, whereas others with mild symptoms may die suddenly. If the pain is not relieved by rest or up to 3 nitroglycerin tablets (taken one at a time at 5-minute intervals) in 10 to 15 minutes, the physician should be notified and the client taken to a cardiac care unit. (Nitroglycerin dilates the coronary arteries and improves collateral cardiac circulation, thus providing an increase in oxygen to the heart muscle and a decrease in symptoms of angina.)

The decreased blood supply to the heart makes it especially vulnerable to arrhythmias and myocardial infarction, which could be fatal. About one third of all those who suffer from angina pectoris die suddenly from myocardial infarction or arrhythmias (O'Toole, 1992).

Types of Anginal Pain. There are a number of types of anginal pain, including chronic stable angina (also referred to as "walk-through" angina), resting angina or angina decubitus, unstable angina, nocturnal angina, atypical angina, new-onset angina, and Prinzmetal's or "variant" angina.

Chronic stable angina occurs at a predictable level of physical or emotional stress and responds promptly to rest or to nitroglycerin. No pain occurs at rest, and the location, duration, intensity, and frequency of chest pain are consistent over time. *Resting angina* or *angina decubitus* is chest pain that occurs at rest in the supine position and frequently at the same time every day. The pain is neither brought on by exercise nor relieved by rest.

Unstable angina, also known as *crescendo angina, preinfarction angina,* or *progressive angina,* is an abrupt change in the intensity and frequency of symptoms or decreased threshold of stimulus, such as the onset of chest pain while at rest. The duration of these attacks is longer than the usual 1 to 5 minutes; they may last for up to 20 to 30 minutes. Such changes in the pattern of angina require immediate medical follow-up by the client's physician.

Nocturnal angina may awaken a person from sleep with the same sensation experienced during exertion. During sleep, this exertion is usually caused by dreams. This type of angina may be associated with underlying congestive heart failure. *Atypical angina* refers to unusual symptoms (e.g., toothache or earache) related to physical or emotional exertion. These symptoms subside with rest or nitroglycerin.

New-onset angina describes angina that has developed for the first time within the last 60 days. *Prinzmetal's* or *"variant" angina* produces symptoms similar to typical angina but is caused by coronary artery spasm. These spasms periodically squeeze arteries shut and keep the blood from reaching the heart. Coronary arteries are usually clear of plaque or physiologic changes causing obstruction of the blood vessels. This form of angina occurs at rest, especially in the early hours of the morning, and can be difficult to induce by exercise. It is cyclic and frequently occurs at the same time each day.

Variant angina is more common in women under age 50 years, whereas angina of effort is uncommon in women in this age group in the absence of severe hypercholesterolemia, hypertension, or diabetes mellitus. It is more commonly associated with various types of arrhythmias or conduction defects (Sokolow et al., 1990).

Treatment (O'Toole, 1992). Relief from pain and prevention of attacks by avoiding situations that precipitate them are the first steps in the care of someone with angina. Usually, changes in life style and breaking lifelong habits are required. Organic nitrates (e.g., Cardilate, Isordil, or nitroglycerin) may be administered orally or sublingually for relief from anginal pain. Beta-adrenergic receptor blockers, such as propranolol (Inderal) are used to treat clients who do not respond to weight control and treatment with vasodilators and whose angina significantly limits their activities. These agents decrease the heart rate, blood pressure, and myocardial oxygen consumption while increasing the client's exercise tolerance.

A group of drugs called calcium channel blockers (Procardia, Calan, Isoptin, Cardizem) are beneficial in relieving pain in those clients whose angina is the result of coronary artery spasm or constriction. Clients most likely to obtain dramatic relief from drugs of this kind are those who experience chest pain while resting or sleeping, upon exposure to cold, or during emotional stress. See Appendix at the end of this chapter for common medications used in treating diseases of the heart and circulatory system.

Myocardial Infarct

Myocardial infarct (MI), also known as a heart attack, coronary occlusion, or just "a coronary," is the development of ischemia and necrosis of myocardial tissue. It results from a sudden decrease in coronary perfusion or an increase in myocardial oxygen demand without adequate blood supply. If the requirements for blood are not eased (e.g., by decreased activity), the heart attempts to continue meeting the increased demands for oxygen with an inadequate blood supply, which leads to an MI. Myocardial tissue death is usually preceded by a sudden occlusion of one of the major coronary arteries (Canobbio, 1990).

The myocardium receives its blood supply from the two large coronary arteries and their branches. Occlusion of one or more of these blood vessels (coronary occlusion) is one of the major causes of myocardial infarction. The occlusion may result from the formation of a clot that develops suddenly when an atheromatous plaque ruptures through the sublayers of a blood vessel, or when the narrow, roughened inner lining of a sclerosed artery leads to complete thrombosis (O'Toole, 1992).

Although coronary thrombosis is the most common cause of infarction, many interrelated factors may be responsible, including coronary artery spasm, platelet aggregation and embolism, thrombus secondary to rheumatic heart disease, endocarditis, aortic stenosis, a thrombus on a prosthetic mitral or aortic valve, or a dislodged calcium plaque from a calcified aortic or mitral valve (Canobbio, 1990).

Coronary blood flow is affected by the tonus (tone) of the coronary arteries. Arteries "clogged" by plaque formation become rigid, and resultant spasm may be provoked by cold and by exercise, which explains the adverse effect of both factors on clients with angina (Bauwens and Paine, 1983).

Clinical Signs and Symptoms. The onset of an infarct may be characterized by severe fatigue for several days before the infarct. People who have MIs may not experience any pain and may be unaware that damage is occurring to the heart muscle as a result of prolonged ischemia.

They may have severe unrelenting chest pain described as "crushing pain" lasting 30 or more minutes, which is not alleviated by rest or by nitroglycerin. This chest pain may radiate to the arms, throat, and back, persisting for hours (see Fig. 3–9). Other symptoms include pallor, profuse perspiration, and possibly nausea and vomiting. The pain of an MI may be misinterpreted as indigestion because of the nausea and vomiting. A medical evaluation may be difficult because many clients have coexisting hiatal hernia, peptic ulcer, or gallbladder disease (Berkow and Fletcher, 1992).

Morris et al. (1990) noted that the shoulder-hand syndrome (more accurately termed reflex sympathetic dystrophy, or RSD) was a common complication of myocardial infarction when clients were treated with strict, prolonged bed rest and immobilization. The change from prolonged bed rest to early ambulation has almost eliminated this problem. Rarely, clients with preexisting disease of the shoulder and medical complications requiring prolonged

▼ *Clinical Signs and Symptoms of*

Myocardial Infarction

- Severe substernal chest pain or squeezing pressure
- Pain possibly radiating down both arms
- Feeling of indigestion
- Angina lasting for 30 minutes or more
- Angina unrelieved by rest or nitroglycerin
- Pain of infarct relieved by a change in position
- Nausea
- Sudden dimness or loss of vision or loss of speech
- Pallor
- Diaphoresis (heavy perspiration)
- Shortness of breath
- Weakness, numbness, and feelings of faintness
- Painful shoulder-hand syndrome (RSD)

bed rest develop the shoulder-hand syndrome. It begins 1 to 3 months after infarction with shoulder pain, stiffness, and marked limitation of motion of the shoulder joint, shoulder girdle, and arm. The hand may become swollen, shiny, stiff, and discolored (see Table 12–10).

Prognosis and Treatment (Reigle and Ringel, 1993). Because the infarction process may take up to 6 hours to complete, restoration of adequate myocardial perfusion is important if significant necrosis is to be limited (Canobbio, 1990). Since the advent of coronary care units and devices that aid in promptly recognizing and treating life-threatening arrhythmias, 70 to 80 per cent of those suffering from an acute MI survive the initial attack. Deaths generally result from severe dysrhythmias, cardiogenic shock, congestive heart failure, rupture of the heart, and recurrent MI.

Clients who survive an MI without developing complications require a period of 6 to 12 weeks for complete recovery. Unfortunately, 50 percent of those who completely recover from their first coronary will die within 5 years; 75 per cent will die within 10 years from massive infarctions (Stewart, 1992).

Treatment goals for clients with acute MI are successful resolution of the acute attack and prompt alleviation of manifestations, prevention of complications and further attacks, and rehabilitation and education. Medical management may include hospital admission, surgery, medications, thrombolytic therapy, and cardiac rehabilitation.

Pericarditis (Ott, 1993b)

Pericarditis is an inflammation of the parietal pericardium (fluid-like membrane between the [fibrous] pericardium and the epicardium) and the visceral (epicardium) pericardium (see Fig. 3–2). This inflammatory process may develop either as a primary condition or secondary to a number of diseases and circumstances (see Causes of Pericarditis).

Pericarditis may be acute or chronic (recurring); it is not known why pericarditis may be a single illness in some people and be recurrent in others. Chronic pericarditis is called *constrictive pericarditis*.

Clinical Signs and Symptoms. At first, pericarditis may have no external signs or symptoms. The symptoms of acute pericarditis vary with the cause but usually include chest pain and dyspnea, an increase in the pulse rate, and a rise in temperature. Malaise and myalgia may occur.

Over time, the inflammatory process may result in an accumulation of fluid in the pericardial sac, preventing the heart from expanding fully. The subsequent chest pain of pericarditis (see Fig. 3–10) closely mimics that of an MI as it is substernal, is associated with cough, and may radiate to the left shoulder or supraclavicular area. It can be differentiated from MI by the pat-

CAUSES OF PERICARDITIS

Infections

> Viral: Coxsackie, influenza
> Bacterial: tuberculosis, staph, strep, meningococcus, pneumonia
> Parasitic
> Fungal

Myocardial Injury

> Myocardial infarction
> Cardiac trauma: blunt or penetrating pericardium; rib fracture
> Postcardiac surgery

Hypersensitivity

> Collagen diseases: rheumatic fever, scleroderma, systemic lupus erythematosus, rheumatoid
>   arthritis
> Drug reaction
> Radiation/cobalt therapy

Metabolic Disorders

> Uremia
> Myxedema
> Chronic anemia

Neoplasm

> Lymphoma, lung or breast cancer

Aortic Dissection

Adapted from Ott, B.: Nursing care of clients with cardiac structure disorders. *In* Black, J.M., and Matassarin-Jacobs, E. (eds.): Luckmann and Sorensen's Medical-Surgical Nursing, 4th ed. Philadelphia, W.B. Saunders, 1993, p. 1221.

tern of relieving and aggravating factors (Table 3–4).

For example, the pain of an MI is unaffected by position, breathing, or movement, whereas the pain associated with pericarditis may be relieved by kneeling on all fours, leaning forward, or sitting upright. Pericardial chest pain is often worse with breathing, swallowing, or belching. The pain tends to be sharp or cutting and may recur in intermittent bursts that are usually precipitated by a change in body position. Pericarditis pain may diminish if the breath is held (Hurst, 1990).

Prognosis and Treatment. The prognosis in most cases of acute viral pericarditis is excellent, provided that myocardial involvement is minimal. However, in a person with cardiac involvement, without prompt treatment shock and death can result from decreased cardiac output.

In the constrictive form of chronic pericarditis, which may be tuberculous in origin, calcium and fibrous deposits may form

Table 3-4
CHARACTERISTICS OF CARDIAC CHEST PAIN

Angina	Myocardial infarct	Mitral Valve Prolapse	Pericarditis
1-5 minutes	30 minutes-hours	Hours	Hours to days
Moderate intensity	Severe (can be painless)	Rarely severe	Varies; mild to severe
Tightness; chest discomfort	Crushing pain; intolerable (can be painless)	May be asymptomatic; unlike angina in quality or quantity	Asymptomatic; varies; can mimic MI
Subsides with rest or nitroglycerin	Unrelieved by rest or nitroglycerin	Unrelieved by rest or nitroglycerin	Relieved by kneeling on all fours, leaning forward, or sitting upright
Pain related to tone of arteries (spasm)	Pain related to heart ischemia	Mechanism of pain unknown	Pain related to inflammatory process

around the heart and interfere with its movements. This form may be extremely serious and difficult to cure. Surgery may be the treatment of choice to remove constrictions and permit free heart action.

▼ *Clinical Signs and Symptoms of*
Pericarditis

- Substernal pain that may radiate to the neck, upper back, upper trapezius, left supraclavicular area, down the left arm to the costal margins
- Difficulty in swallowing
- Pain relieved by leaning forward or by sitting upright
- Pain aggravated by movement associated with deep breathing (laughing, coughing, deep inspiration)
- Pain aggravated by trunk movements (side bending or rotation)
- History of fever, chills, weakness, or heart disease. A recent MI accompanying the pattern of symptoms may alert the physical therapist to the need for medical referral to rule out cardiac involvement

When acute pericarditis is of known etiology, treatment of the underlying cause is indicated. Otherwise, symptomatic intervention is provided using pharmacologic agents, especially for fever and pain.

Congestive Heart Failure or Heart Failure (Reigle and Ringel, 1993)

Heart failure, also called *cardiac decompensation* and *cardiac insufficiency,* can be defined as a physiologic state in which the heart is unable to pump enough blood to meet the metabolic needs of the body (determined as oxygen consumption) at rest or during exercise, even though filling pressures are adequate.

The heart fails when, because of intrinsic disease or structural defects, it cannot handle a normal blood volume, or in the absence of disease cannot tolerate a sudden expansion in blood volume (e.g., exercise). Heart failure is not a disease itself; instead, the term denotes a group of manifestations related to inadequate pump performance from either the cardiac valves or myocardium.

Whatever the cause, when the heart fails to propel blood forward normally, congestion occurs in the pulmonary circulation as blood accumulates in the lungs. The right ventricle, which is not yet affected by congestive heart disease, continues to pump more blood into the lungs. The immediate result is shortness of breath and, if the process continues, actual flooding of the air spaces of the lungs with fluid seeping from the distended blood vessels. This last phenomenon is called pulmonary congestion or pulmonary edema (Urden et al., 1992).

Because a properly functioning heart depends on both ventricles, failure of one ventricle almost always leads to failure of the other ventricle. This is called ventricular interdependence. Right-sided ventricular failure (right-sided heart failure) causes congestion of the peripheral tissues and viscera. The liver may enlarge, the ankles may swell, and the client develops ascites (fluid accumulates in the abdomen).

Risk Factors. Some clients have preexisting mild-to-moderate heart disease with no evidence of congestive heart failure. However, when the heart undergoes undue stress from risk factors, compensatory mechanisms may be inadequate, and the heart fails. Conditions that precipitate or exacerbate heart failure include physical or emotional stress, dysrhythmia, fever, infection, anemia, thyroid disorders, pregnancy, Paget's disease, nutritional deficiency (e.g., thiamine deficiency secondary to alcoholism), pulmonary disease, and hypervolemia from poor renal function or medications such as steroids.

Clinical Signs and Symptoms

Left Ventricular Failure. Failure of the left ventricle causes either pulmonary congestion or a disturbance in the respiratory control mechanisms. These problems in turn precipitate respiratory distress. The degree of distress varies with the client's position, activity, and level of stress.

Dyspnea is subjective and does not always correlate with the extent of heart failure. To some extent, exertional dyspnea occurs in all clients. The increased fluid in the tissue spaces causes dyspnea, at first on effort and then at rest, by stimulation of stretch receptors in the lung and chest wall and by the increased work of breathing with stiff lungs (Sokolow et al., 1990). *Par-*

oxysmal nocturnal dyspnea (PND) resembles the frightening sensation of suffocation. The client suddenly awakens with the feeling of severe suffocation. Once the client is in the upright position, relief from the attack may not occur for 30 minutes or longer.

Orthopnea is a more advanced stage of dyspnea. The client often assumes a "three-point position," sitting up with both hands on the knees and leaning forward. Orthopnea develops because the supine position increases the amount of blood returning from the lower extremities to the heart and lungs. This gravitational redistribution of blood increases pulmonary congestion and dyspnea. The client learns to avoid respiratory distress at night by supporting the head and thorax on pillows. In severe heart failure, the client may resort to sleeping upright in a chair.

Cough is a common symptom of left ventricular failure and is often hacking, producing large amounts of frothy, blood-tinged sputum. The client coughs because a large amount of fluid is trapped in the pulmonary tree, irritating the lung mucosa.

Pulmonary edema may develop when rapidly rising pulmonary capillary pressure causes fluid to move into the alveoli, causing extreme breathlessness, anxiety, frothy sputum, nasal flaring, use of accessory breathing muscles, tachypnea, noisy and wet breathing, and diaphoresis.

Cerebral hypoxia may occur as a result of a decrease in cardiac output causing inadequate brain perfusion. Depressed cerebral function can cause anxiety, irritability, restlessness, confusion, impaired memory, bad dreams, and insomnia.

Fatigue and muscular weakness are often associated with left ventricular failure. Inadequate cardiac output leads to hypoxic tissue and slowed removal of metabolic wastes, which in turn causes the client to tire easily. Disturbances in sleep and rest patterns may aggravate fatigue.

Renal changes can occur in both right- and left-sided heart failure but are more evident with left-sided failure. During the day, the client is upright, blood flow is

▼ *Clinical Signs and Symptoms of*
Left-Sided Heart Failure

- Fatigue and dyspnea after mild physical exertion or exercise
- Persistent spasmodic cough, especially when lying down, while fluid moves from the extremities to the lungs
- Paroxysmal nocturnal dyspnea (occurring suddenly at night)
- Orthopnea (person must be in the upright position to breathe)
- Tachycardia
- Fatigue and muscle weakness
- Edema and weight gain
- Irritability/restlessness
- Decreased renal function or frequent urination at night

▼ *Clinical Signs and Symptoms of*
Right-Sided Heart Failure

- Increased fatigue
- Dependent edema (usually beginning in the ankles)
- Pitting edema (after 5 to 10 pounds of edema accumulate)
- Edema in the sacral area or the back of the thighs
- Right upper quadrant pain
- Cyanosis of nail beds

away from the kidneys, and the formation of urine is reduced. At night, urine formation increases as blood flow to the kidney improves. *Nocturia* may interfere with effective sleep patterns, which contributes to fatigue as mentioned. As cardiac output falls, decreased renal blood flow may result in oliguria (reduced urine output), a late sign of heart failure.

Right Ventricular Failure. Failure of the right ventricle results in peripheral edema and venous congestion of the organs. As the liver becomes congested with venous blood, it becomes enlarged and abdominal pain occurs. If this occurs rapidly, stretching of the capsule surrounding the liver causes severe discomfort. The client may notice either a constant aching or a sharp pain in the right upper quadrant.

Dependent edema is one of the early signs of right ventricular failure. Edema is usually symmetric and occurs in the dependent parts of the body where venous pressure is the highest. In ambulatory people, edema begins in the feet and ankles

and ascends up the lower legs. It is most noticeable at the end of a day and often decreases after a night's rest. In the recumbent person, pitting edema may develop in the presacral area and, as it worsens, progress to the genital area and medial thighs.

Cyanosis of the nail beds appears as venous congestion reduces peripheral blood flow. Clients with congestive heart failure often feel anxious, frightened, and depressed. Fears may be expressed as frightening nightmares, insomnia, acute anxiety states, depression, or withdrawal from reality.

Prognosis and Treatment (Sokolow et al., 1990). The overall prognosis of congestive, or cardiac, failure has improved considerably in recent years because of the therapeutic advances made, such as the availability of oral diuretics, ACE (angiotensin-converting enzyme) inhibitors, vasodilators, inotropic agents, and surgical and medical treatment of underlying causes.

However, prognosis remains poor because treatment is often delayed until cardiac failure is advanced when treatable conditions such as hypertensive heart failure and valvular heart disease with heart failure are not recognized and treated early.

In moderate, nonprogressive cardiac failure, the annual mortality rate is about 10 to 15 per cent, whereas in severe progressive cardiac failure, the annual mortality rate is 50 per cent or more. Treatment is directed toward the underlying cause and may include surgery, medications, or rest with activity as tolerated, unless the problem (e.g., ischemic or dilated cardiomyopathy) cannot be reversed, and then treatment is only palliative.

Case Example A 65-year-old man came to the clinic with a referral from his family doctor for "Hip pain—evaluate and treat." Past medical history included three total hip replacements of the right hip, open heart surgery 6 years ago, and persistent hypertension currently being treated with beta-blockers. During the interview, it was discovered that the client had experienced many bouts of hip pain, leg weakness, and loss of hip motion. He was not actually examined by his doctor but had contacted the physician's office by phone, requesting a new P.T. referral.

On examination, large, adhesed scars were noted along the anterior, lateral, and posterior aspects of the right hip, with significant bilateral hip flexion contractures. Pitting edema was noted in the right ankle, with mild swelling observed around the left ankle as well. The client was unaware of this swelling; further questions were negative for shortness of breath, difficulty in sleeping, cough, or other symptoms of cardiopulmonary involvement. The bilateral edema could have been from compromise of the lymphatic drainage system following the multiple surgeries and adhesive scarring.

However, with the positive history for cardiovascular involvement, *bilateral* edema, and telephone-derived referral, the physician was contacted by phone to notify him of the edema, and the client was directed by the physician to make an appointment. The client was diagnosed in the early stages of congestive heart failure. Physical therapy to address the appropriate hip musculoskeletal problems was continued.

Aneurysm (Dennison and Black, 1993)

An aneurysm is an abnormal dilatation (commonly a saclike formation) in the wall of an artery, a vein, or the heart. Aneurysms occur when the vessel wall becomes weakened from trauma, congenital vascular disease, infection, or atherosclerosis (Abraham et al., 1991).

Types of Aneurysms. Aneurysms are designated either venous or arterial and are also described according to the specific vessel in which they develop. *Thoracic aneurysms* usually involve the ascending, transverse, or descending portion of the aorta; *abdominal aneurysms* generally involve the aorta between the renal arteries and iliac branches; *peripheral arterial aneurysms* affect the femoral and popliteal arteries.

Thoracic and Peripheral Arterial Aneurysms. A dissecting aneurysm (most often a thoracic aneurysm) splits and penetrates the arterial wall, creating a false vessel. Thoracic aneurysms occur most frequently in hypertensive men between the ages of 40 and 70 years. Marked elevation of blood pressure may facilitate rapid disruption and final rupture of the aortic wall when a small tear in the intima has occurred (Bauwens and Paine, 1983).

The most common site for peripheral arterial aneurysms is the popliteal space in the lower extremities. Popliteal aneurysms cause ischemic symptoms in the lower limbs and an easily palpable pulse of larger amplitude. An enlarged area behind the knee may be present, seldom with discomfort.

Abdominal Aortic Aneurysms. Abdominal aortic aneurysms (AAAs) occur about four times more often than thoracic aneurysms. The natural course of an untreated AAA is expansion and rupture in one of several places, including the peritoneal cavity, the mesentery, behind the peritoneum, into the inferior vena cava, or into the duodenum or rectum. The most common site for an AAA is just below the kidney (just below the takeoff of the renal arteries), with referred pain to the thoraco-lumbar junction (see Fig. 3–11).

Clinical Signs and Symptoms. Most AAAs are asymptomatic; discovery occurs on physical or x-ray examination of the abdomen or lower spine for some other reason. The most common symptom is awareness of a pulsating mass in the abdomen, with or without pain, followed by abdominal pain and back pain. Groin pain and flank pain may be experienced because of increasing pressure on other structures.

The most frequent complication of AAA is rupture, which occurs most often in aneurysms 5 cm or larger. Rupture causes intense pain, typically in one or both flanks, with referred pain to the back at the level of the rupture and radiation to the lower abdomen, groin, or genitalia. Back pain may be the only presenting feature.

Extreme pain may be felt at the base of the neck along the back, particularly in the interscapular area, while dissection proceeds over the aortic arch and into the descending aorta (Bauwens and Paine, 1983).

Ruptured AAA presents with a triad of symptoms including abdominal pain combined with intense back and flank pain and possible scrotal pain for males, a pulsating abdominal mass, and shock, with systolic

▼ *Clinical Signs and Symptoms of*
Aneurysm

- Chest pain with any of the following:
  - Palpable, pulsating mass (abdomen, popliteal space)
  - Abdominal "heart beat" felt by the client when lying down
  - Dull ache in the midabdominal left flank or low back
  - Groin and/or leg pain
  - Weakness or transient paralysis of legs

▼ *Clinical Signs and Symptoms of*
Ruptured Aneurysm

- Sudden, severe chest pain with a tearing sensation (see Fig. 3–11)
- Pain may extend to the neck, shoulders, lower back, or abdomen but rarely to the joints and arms, which distinguishes it from myocardial infarction
- Pulsating abdominal mass
- Systolic blood pressure below 100 mm Hg
- Pulse rate more than 100 BPM
- Ecchymoses in the flank and perianal area
- Lightheadedness and nausea

blood pressure below 100 mm Hg and pulse rate over 100 beats per minute.

Other symptoms may include ecchymoses in the flank and perianal area; severe and sudden pain in the abdomen, paravertebral area, or flank; and lightheadedness and nausea with sudden hypotension.

Treatment and Prognosis. Treatment of aneurysms depends on the particular vessel involved, the size of the aneurysm, and the general health status of the client. Antihypertensive medications are recommended. Surgery is not usually performed on clients with an asymptomatic AAA smaller than 4 to 5 cm, but it is the only intervention for clients with a ruptured AAA.

When surgical clipping or repair is recommended, collateral circulation must be adequate. Aneurysms of the heart and great vessels should be repaired even if they are small. The risk of elective surgical repair ranges from 2 to 4 per cent, whereas operation after rupture is rarely successful in more than one third of clients.

The mortality following surgery performed before rupture is about 5 per cent. The 5-year survival rate after diagnosis is over 50 per cent, and myocardial infarction is the most common cause of death (Sokolow et al., 1990).

Diseases Affecting the Heart Valves

The second category of heart problems includes those that occur secondary to impairment of the valves caused by disease (e.g., rheumatic fever or coronary thrombosis), congenital deformity, or infection such as endocarditis. Three types of valve deformities may affect aortic, mitral, tricuspid, or pulmonic valves: *stenosis, insufficiency,* or *prolapse.*

Stenosis is a narrowing or constriction that prevents the valve from opening fully and may be caused by growths, scars, or abnormal deposits on the leaflets. *Insufficiency* (also referred to as regurgitation) occurs when the valve does not close properly and causes blood to flow back into the heart chamber. *Prolapse* affects only the mitral valve and occurs when enlarged valve leaflets bulge backward into the left atrium.

These valve conditions increase the workload of the heart and require the heart to pump harder to force blood through a stenosed valve or to maintain adequate flow if blood is seeping back. A further complication for people with a malfunctioning valve may occur secondary to a bacterial infection of the valves (endocarditis).

People affected by diseases of the heart valves may be asymptomatic, and extensive auscultation with a stethoscope and diagnostic study may be required to differentiate one condition from another. In early symptomatic stages, cardiac valvular disease causes the person to become fatigued easily. As stenosis or insufficiency progresses, the main symptom of heart failure (breathlessness or dyspnea) appears (Urden et al., 1992).

▼ *Clinical Signs and Symptoms of*
Cardiac Valvular Disease

- Easy fatigue
- Dyspnea
- Palpitation (subjective sensation of throbbing, skipping, rapid or forcible pulsation of the heart)
- Chest pain
- Pitting edema
- Orthopnea or paroxysmal dyspnea
- Dizziness and syncope (episodes of fainting or loss of consciousness)

Rheumatic Fever (Williams, 1991; Ott, 1993b)

Rheumatic fever is an infection caused by streptococcal bacteria that can be fatal or may lead to rheumatic heart disease, a chronic condition caused by scarring and deformity of the heart valves (Fig. 3–4). It is called rheumatic fever because two of the most common symptoms are fever and joint pain (O'Toole, 1992).

The infection generally starts with strep throat in children between the ages of 5 and 15 years and damages the heart in approximately 50 per cent of cases. Rheumatic fever produces a diffuse, proliferative, and exudative inflammatory process. The exact pathogenesis is unclear, but it is probably through an abnormal humoral and cell-mediated response to streptococcal cell membrane antigens. These antigens bind to receptors on the heart, tissue, and joints, which begins the autoimmune response, thus classifying rheumatic fever as an autoimmune disease.

The aggressive use of specific antibiotics in the United States had effectively removed

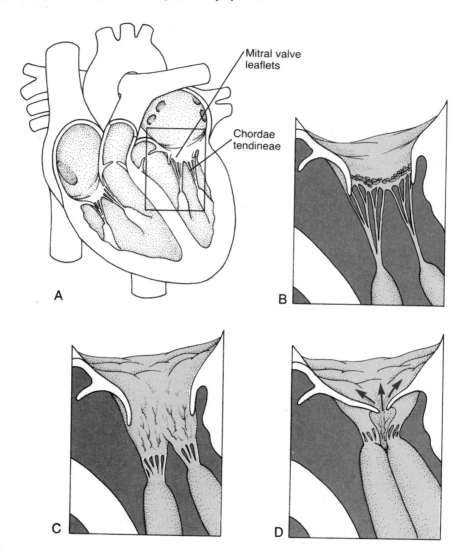

Figure 3–4

Cardiac valvular disease caused by rheumatic fever. *A,* Inflammation of the membrane over the mitral (and aortic) valves may cause edema and accumulation of fibrin and platelets on the chordae tendineae. *B,* This accumulation of inflammatory materials produces rheumatic vegetations that affect the support provided by the chordae tendineae to the AV valves. *C,* In this view, the mitral valve leaflets have become thickened with scar tissue so that the valves fail to close properly (mitral stenosis). *D,* Regurgitation or back flow of blood into the atrium develops when the scarred valve fails to close tightly. Prolonged, severe stenosis with mitral regurgitation leads to symptoms of congestive heart failure.

rheumatic fever as the primary cause of valvular damage. However, in 1985, a series of epidemics of rheumatic fever were reported in several widely diverse geographic regions of the continental United States (Odio, 1986; Veasy et al., 1987; Wald et al., 1987). Currently, the prevalence and incidence of cases have not approximated the 1985 record, but they have remained above baseline levels.

In most of the people affected by this epidemic (children as well as young adults aged 18 to 30 years and occasionally middle-aged individuals), the initial triggering streptococcal sore throat or pharyngitis did not cause extreme illness, if any discomfort at all. The onset of rheumatic fever 2 or 3 weeks later rapidly brought a carditis and in some instances acute congestive heart failure and even death.

The reasons for the recurrence of rheumatic fever that presented with mild migratory polyarthritis and rapidly increasing acute carditis, valvular damage, and severe pancarditis are unknown, although there are a number of possible explanations.

Perhaps there is a new, more insidious strain of the bacteria that cause strep throat, or there may have been a resurgence of particular strains of strep bacteria that cause rheumatic fever. Because of the previous decline in rheumatic fever, aggressive diagnosis and treatment of strep infections may be responsible. Some researchers speculate that strep bacteria strains may follow periodic cycles, as seen in other diseases such as measles.

Clinical Signs and Symptoms. The most typical clinical profile of a child or young adult with acute rheumatic fever is an initial cold or sore throat followed 2 or 3 weeks later by sudden or gradual onset of painful migratory joint symptoms in knees, shoulders, feet, ankles, elbows, fingers, and neck. Fever of 37.2°C to 39.4°C (99°F to 103°F) and palpitations and fatigue are also present. Malaise, weakness, weight loss, and anorexia may accompany the fever.

The migratory arthralgias may last only 24 hours, or they may persist for several weeks. Joints that are sore and hot and contain fluid completely resolve, followed by acute synovitis, heat, synovial space tenderness, swelling, and effusion present in a different area the next day. The persistence of swelling, heat, and synovitis in a single joint or joints for more than 2 to 3 weeks is extremely unusual in acute rheumatic fever.

In the acute, full-blown sequelae, short-ness of breath and increasing nocturnal cough will also occur. A rash on the skin of the limbs or trunk is present in fewer than 2 per cent of clients with acute rheumatic fever. Subcutaneous nodules over the extensor surfaces of the arms, heels, knees, or back of the head may occur.

All layers of the heart (epicardium, endocardium, myocardium, and pericardium) may be involved, and the heart valves are affected by this inflammatory reaction. The most characteristic and potentially dangerous anatomic lesion of rheumatic inflammation is the gross effect on cardiac valves, most commonly the mitral and aortic valves. As many as 25 per cent of clients will have mitral valvular disease 25 to 30 years later.

Rheumatic chorea (also called chorea or St. Vitus' dance) may occur 1 to 3 months after the strep infection and always occurs after polyarthritis. Chorea in a child, teenager, or young adult is almost always a manifestation of acute rheumatic fever. Other uncommon causes of chorea are systemic lupus erythematosus, thyrotoxicosis, and cerebrovascular accident, but these are unlikely in a child.

The client develops rapid, purposeless, nonrepetitive movements that may involve all muscles except the eyes. This chorea may last for 1 week or several months or

▼ *Clinical Signs and Symptoms of*
Rheumatic Fever

- Migratory arthralgias
- Subcutaneous nodules on extensor surfaces
- Fever and sore throat
- Flat, painless skin rash (short duration)
- Carditis
- Chorea
- Weakness, malaise, weight loss, and anorexia

may persist for several years without permanent impairment of the central nervous system (Williams, 1991; Berkow and Fletcher, 1992).

Prognosis and Treatment. Initial episodes of rheumatic fever last months in children and weeks in adults. Twenty per cent of children have recurrences within 5 years. Recurrences are uncommon after 5 years of good health and are rare after age 21 years. The immediate mortality rate is 1 to 2 per cent. Persistent rheumatic activity with a greatly enlarged heart, heart failure, and pericarditis indicates a poor prognosis. Otherwise, the prognosis for life is good (Sokolow et al., 1990).

Aspirin is generally the drug of choice in treating children or young adults with acute rheumatic fever. Aspirin is usually administered to treat the joint manifestations and fever and as a general antiinflammatory agent.

Children with acute chorea are generally treated with some form of central nervous system depressant such as phenobarbital. In most cases (barring known penicillin allergy), children and young adults are treated with penicillin. Corticosteroids are used when there is clear evidence of rheumatic carditis.

Throat cultures must be obtained on all close family members and others in close contact so that those who have positive cultures for group A beta-hemolytic streptococci can be treated with penicillin.

Endocarditis (Hunder, 1992)

Bacterial endocarditis, another common heart infection, causes inflammation of the cardiac endothelium (layer of cells lining the cavities of the heart) and damages the tricuspid, aortic, or mitral valve. This infection may be caused by bacteria, or it may occur as a result of abnormal growths on the closure lines of previously damaged valves. These growths consist of collagen fibers and may separate from the valve, embolize, and cause infarction in the myo-cardium, kidney, brain, spleen, abdomen, or extremities.

In addition to clients with previous valvular damage, injection drug users (IDUs) and postcardiac surgical clients are at high risk for developing endocarditis. Congenital heart disease and degenerative heart disease, such as calcific aortic stenosis, may also cause bacterial endocarditis. The prosthetic cardiac valve has become more important as a predisposing factor for endocarditis because cardiac surgery is performed on a much larger scale than in the past.

This infection is often the consequence of invasive diagnostic procedures, such as renal shunts and urinary catheters, long-term indwelling catheters, or dental treatment (due to the increased opportunities for normal oral microorganisms to gain entrance to the circulatory system by way of highly vascularized oral structures). People who are susceptible may take antibiotics as a precaution prior to undergoing any of these procedures.

This disease is more prevalent in men than in women, and half of all clients diagnosed as having bacterial endocarditis are older than 50 years; bacterial endocarditis rarely occurs in children.

Clinical Signs and Symptoms. Clinical manifestations can be divided into three groups: *systemic infection* (fever, chills, sweats, malaise, weakness, anorexia, weight loss), *intravascular involvement* (dyspnea, chest pain, cold and painful extremities, petechiae, and splinter hemorrhages), and *immunologic reaction to infection* (arthralgia, proteinuria, hematuria, acidosis) (Durack, 1990).

A significant number of clients (up to 45 per cent) with bacterial endocarditis initially have musculoskeletal symptoms, including arthralgia, arthritis, low back pain, and myalgias. Half these clients will have only musculoskeletal symptoms without other signs of endocarditis. The early onset of joint pain and myalgia is more likely if the client is older and has had a previously diagnosed heart murmur.

The most frequent musculoskeletal symptom in clients with bacterial endocarditis is *arthralgia,* generally in the proximal joints. The shoulder is the most commonly affected site, followed (in declining incidence) by the knee, hip, wrist, ankle, metatarsophalangeal and metacarpophalangeal joints, and acromioclavicular joints.

Most endocarditis clients with arthralgias have only one or two painful joints, although some may have pain in several joints. Painful symptoms begin suddenly in one or two joints, accompanied by warmth, tenderness, and redness. Symmetric arthralgia in the knees or ankles may lead to a diagnosis of rheumatoid arthritis. One helpful clue: as a rule, morning stiffness is not as prevalent in clients with endocarditis as in those with rheumatoid arthritis or polymyalgia rheumatica.

Almost one third of clients with bacterial endocarditis have *low back pain;* in many clients, it is the principal musculoskeletal symptom reported. Back pain is accompanied by decreased range of motion and spinal tenderness. Pain may affect only one side, and it may be limited to the paraspinal muscles. Endocarditis-induced low back pain may be very similar to that associated with a herniated lumbar disc: it radiates to the leg and may be accentuated by raising the leg or by sneezing. The key difference is that neurologic deficits are usually absent in clients with bacterial endocarditis.

Endocarditis may produce destructive changes in the *sacroiliac joint,* probably as a result of seeding the joint by septic emboli. The pain will be localized over the SI joint, and the physician will use roentgenograms and bone scans to verify this diagnosis

Widespread diffuse *myalgias* may occur during periods of fever, but these are not appreciably different from the general myalgia seen in clients with other febrile illnesses. More commonly, myalgia will be restricted to the calf or thigh. Bilateral or unilateral leg myalgias occur in approxi-

> ### Clinical Signs and Symptoms of
> ### Endocarditis
>
> - Constitutional symptoms
> - Dyspnea, chest pain
> - Cold and painful extremities
> - Petechiae/splinter hemorrhages
> - Musculoskeletal symptoms
> - Myalgias
> - Arthralgias
> - Low back/sacroiliac pain
> - Arthritis

mately 10 to 15 per cent of all clients with bacterial endocarditis.

The cause of back pain and leg myalgia associated with bacterial endocarditis has not been determined. Some suggest that concurrent aseptic meningitis may contribute to both leg and back pain. Others suggest that leg pain is related to emboli that break off from the infected cardiac valves. The latter theory is supported by biopsy evidence of muscle necrosis or vasculitis in clients with bacterial endocarditis.

The diagnosis of bacterial endocarditis is even more complex in the geriatric population. Elderly clients have a higher frequency of nonpathologic heart murmurs and are less likely to develop fever in response to infection.

Rarely, other musculoskeletal symptoms such as osteomyelitis, nail clubbing, tendinitis, hypertrophic osteoarthropathy, bone infarcts, and ischemic bone necrosis may occur.

Treatment and Prognosis. Once the diagnosis is established, treatment is with appropriate antibiotics given intravenously for 4 to 6 weeks. There are many complications, including congestive heart failure and arterial, systemic, or pulmonary emboli. Relapse can occur up to 2 or more weeks after therapy. During this time, the client is warned against excessive physical exertion, but normal activities of daily living can be resumed with the physician's approval.

Lupus Carditis (Stevens and Ziminski, 1992)

Except for pericarditis, clinically significant cardiac disease directly associated with systemic lupus erythematosus (SLE) is relatively infrequent, but because of the musculoskeletal involvement, it may be of major importance for the physical therapist. Primary lupus cardiac involvement may include pericarditis, myocarditis, endocarditis, or a combination of the three.

SLE is a multisystem clinical illness associated with the release of a broad spectrum of autoantibodies into the circulation (see Chapter 11). The inflammatory process mediated by the immune response can target the heart and vasculature of the client with SLE.

Pericarditis is the most frequent cardiac lesion associated with SLE, presenting with the characteristic substernal chest pain that varies with posture, becoming worse in recumbency and improving with sitting or bending forward.

Myocarditis may occur and is strongly associated with skeletal myositis in SLE (Borenstein et al., 1978). *Lupus endocarditis* has been reported in 32 to 44 per cent of clients in major clinicopathologic studies. Major lesions associated with SLE are mitral insufficiency, aortic insufficiency and mitral and aortic stenosis. These valves can be surgically replaced.

Secondary cardiac involvement for the client with SLE may include hypertension, which occurs in 25 per cent to 49 per cent of clients with SLE; renal failure; hypercholesterolemia (excess serum cholesterol); and infection (infective carditis, which is rare).

Congenital Valvular Defects

Congenital malformations of the heart occur in approximately 1 of every 100 babies born in the United States. The most common defects include ventricular or atrial septal defect (hole between the ventricles or atria), tetralogy of Fallot (combination of four defects), patent ductus arteriosus (shunt caused by an opening between the aorta and the pulmonary artery), and congenital stenosis of the pulmonary, aortic, and tricuspid valves (Fig. 3–5). These congenital defects require surgical correction and may be part of the client's *past medical history*. They are not conditions that are likely to mimic musculoskeletal lesions and are therefore not covered in detail in this text.

Only one condition, *mitral valve prolapse* (MVP), is included in this section because of its increasing prevalence in the physical therapy client population. Usually, the client with MVP presents with some other unrelated primary (musculoskeletal) diagnosis. During physical therapy treatment, the symptomatic MVP client may experience symptoms associated with MVP and require assurance or education regarding exercise and MVP.

Mitral Valve Prolapse (Frederickson, 1992; Ott, 1993b). In a little more than 10 per cent of the population, there is a slight variation in the shape or structure of the mitral valve of the heart that could cause mitral valve prolapse. There may be a genetic component, as it tends to be more common in young women (Lavie and Savage, 1987). This structural variation has many other names, including floppy valve syndrome, Barlow's syndrome, and click-murmur syndrome.

The incidence of MVP appears to be increasing dramatically in recent years, possibly attributed to nutritional changes and ever-increasing continual stress levels in our society, or possibly owing to better diagnostic testing documenting the true incidence for the first time.

Usually, this is a benign condition in isolation; however, it can be associated with a number of other conditions including endocarditis, myocarditis, atherosclerosis, systemic lupus erythematosus, muscular

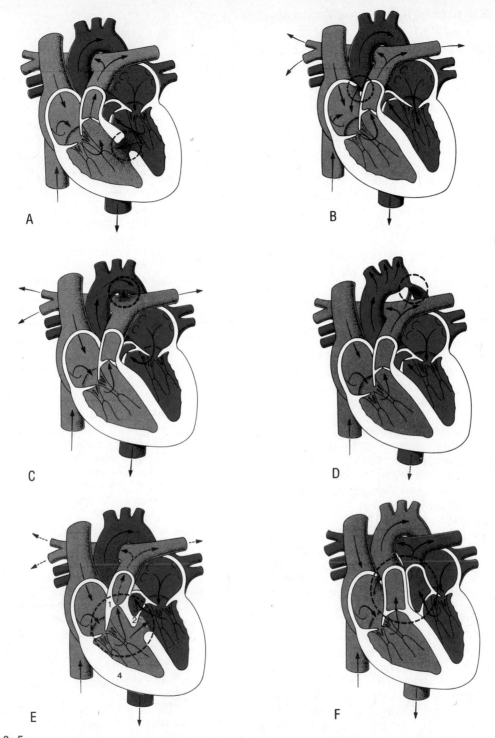

Figure 3–5

Congenital malformations of the heart. *A*, Ventricular septal defect. *B*, Atrial septal defect. *C*, Patent ductus arteriosus. *D*, Coarctation of the aorta. *E*, Tetralogy of Fallot: (1) Stenosis of the pulmonary valve; (2) ventricular septal defect; (3) aorta communicates with both ventricles; (4) enlargement of the right ventricle wall. *F*, Transposition of the great arteries.

dystrophy, acromegaly, and cardiac sarcoidosis.

MVP appears to be due to connective tissue abnormalities in the valve leaflets. Normally, when the lower part of the heart contracts, the mitral valve remains firm and allows no blood to leak back into the upper chambers. In MVP, the slight variation in shape of the mitral valve allows one part of the valve, the leaflet, to billow back into the upper chamber during contraction of the ventricle. One or both of the valve leaflets may bulge into the left atrium during ventricular systole.

Approximately 60 per cent of all clients with MVP experience no symptoms. Another 39 per cent experience occasional symptoms that are mildly to moderately uncomfortable enough to interfere with the person's ability to enjoy an unrestricted life; approximately 1 per cent suffer severe symptoms and life style restrictions.

Clinical Signs and Symptoms. Almost all the symptoms of MVP syndrome are due to an imbalance in the autonomic nervous system, called *dysautonomia*. This imbalance occurs because at the same time the mitral valve is formed in the unborn baby, the autonomic nervous system (ANS) is also being formed. Frequently, when there is a slight variation in structure of the heart valve, there is also a slight variation in the function or balance of the ANS. Symptoms include profound fatigue that cannot be correlated with exercise or stress, cold hands and feet, shortness of breath, chest pain, and heart palpitations. The most common triad of symptoms associated with MVP is fatigue, palpitations, and dyspnea (Fig. 3–6).

Although the fatigue that accompanies MVP is not related to exertion, deconditioning from prolonged inactivity may develop, further complicating the picture. Minor symptoms associated with MVP may include tremors, swelling of extremities, sleep disturbances, low back pain, irritable bowel syndrome, numbness in any part of the body, excessive perspiration or inability to perspire, skin rashes, muscular fas-

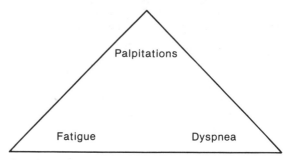

Figure 3–6
The triad of symptoms associated with mitral valve prolapse.

ciculations, visual changes or disturbances, difficulty in concentrating, memory lapses, and dizziness.

Although the chest pain associated with MVP can be severe, it differs from pain associated with myocardial infarct (see Table 3–4). One of the latest and probably best-known theories explaining the origin of MVP pain is that when there is an imbalance in the ANS, which controls contraction and relaxation of the chest wall muscles (the muscles of breathing), there may be inadequate relaxation between respirations. Over time, these chest wall muscles go into spasm, resulting in chest pain. Another possible origin of chest pain may be esophageal reflux (abnormal flow of stomach acid up the esophagus) and esophagitis, inflammation of the esophagus due to frequent flows of acid.

▼ Clinical Signs and Symptoms of
Mitral Valve Prolapse

- Profound fatigue
- Chest pain
- Palpitations or irregular heart beat
- Tachycardia
- Migraine headache
- Anxiety, depression, panic attacks
- Dyspnea

Frequently occurring musculoskeletal findings in clients with MVP include joint hypermobility, temporomandibular joint (TMJ) syndrome, and myalgias.

Prognosis and Treatment. MVP is not life threatening but may be life style threatening for the small number of people (rare) who have more severe structural problems that may progress to the point at which surgical replacement of the valve is required. For preventing infective endocarditis, the client may be given antibiotics prophylactically before any invasive procedures.

In addition to nutritional counseling and the use of medications, exercise is a key component in the treatment of MVP. MVP clients are often referred to an exercise physiologist for a treatment program, but more and more are showing up in physical therapy clinics for conditioning and exercise programs as well.*

Defects of the Cardiac Nervous System (Cohen and Michel, 1988; Erickson, 1991)

The third component of cardiac disease is caused by failure of the heart's nervous system to conduct normal electrical impulses. The heart has its own intrinsic conduction system that allows the orderly depolarization of cardiac muscle tissue. Dysrhythmias, also called *arrhythmias,* are disorders of the heart rate and rhythm caused by disturbances in the conduction system (Reigle and Ringel, 1993).

Dysrhythmias may cause the heart to beat too quickly (tachycardia), too slowly (bradycardia), or with extra beats and fibrillations. Dysrhythmias can lead to dramatic changes in circulatory dynamics, such as hypotension, heart failure, and shock.

Clients who are neurologically unstable owing to recent CVA, head trauma, or other central nervous system insult often exhibit new dysrhythmias during the period of instability. These may be due to elevation of intracranial pressure, and once this has been controlled and returned to normal range, dysrhythmias usually disappear.

However, in clients who have preexisting dysrhythmias, preexisting coronary artery disease, or congestive heart failure, these "transient dysrhythmias" may not disappear and may lead to serious complications. Dizziness and loss of consciousness may occur, owing to loss of brain perfusion (not caused by transient ischemic attacks [TIAs], as is often suspected) when the dysrhythmia results in a serious reduction in cardiac output.

The physical therapist working with a client who has had a stroke may be the first health care professional to identify a dysrhythmia that appears during exercise. In the early recovery period, the therapist should monitor for these dysrhythmias by taking the client's pulse. New dysrhythmias should be reported to the physician.

Fibrillation

The SA node (or cardiac pacemaker) initiates and paces the heart beat. During a myocardial infarct, damaged heart muscle cells, deprived of oxygen, release small electrical impulses that may disrupt the heart's normal conduction pathway between the ventricles. The heart attack may develop suddenly into ventricular fibrillation that can result in sudden death. Similarly, a heart damaged by coronary artery disease (with or without previous infarcts), can go into ventricular fibrillation.

Atrial fibrillation is characterized by a total disorganization of atrial activity without effective atrial contraction. This arrhythmia is seen commonly in clients who have thyrotoxicosis, cardiomyopathy, digitalis intoxication, rheumatic mitral stenosis, hypertensive heart disease, pericarditis, or congestive heart disease.

---

* Caution is advised in the use of weight training for the MVP client—gradual build-up using light weights and increased repetitions is recommended.

▼ *Clinical Signs and Symptoms of*
Fibrillation

- Subjective report of palpitations
- Sensations of fluttering, skipping, irregular beating or pounding, heaving action
- Dyspnea
- Chest pain
- Anxiety
- Pallor
- Nervousness
- Cyanosis

▼ *Clinical Symptoms of*
Sinus Tachycardia

- Palpitation (most common symptom)
- Restlessness
- Chest discomfort or pain
- Agitation
- Anxiety and apprehension

Clinical Signs and Symptoms. Symptoms of fibrillation vary depending on the functional state of the heart, and fibrillation may exist without symptoms. The patient is usually aware of the irregular heart action and reports feeling "palpitations." Careful questioning may be required to pinpoint the exact description of sensations reported by the patient.

Palpitation often results from emotional or psychic disturbance and does not necessarily imply an organic cardiac condition (Massie and Kleiger, 1983). Separate from disturbances of cardiac rhythm, palpitations may result from effort, excitement, tobacco, caffeine, alcohol, or infection.

Treatment. The physician will search for the precipitating cause the first time fibrillation occurs. Initial therapy is determined by the client's clinical status and is aimed at slowing the ventricular rate and restoring atrial systole. Medications such as quinidine, digitalis, and propranolol may be used.

Sinus Tachycardia (Kinney et al., 1991)

Sinus tachycardia, defined as abnormally rapid heart rate, usually taken to be over 100 beats per minute, is the normal physiologic response to such stressors as fever, hypotension, thyrotoxicosis, anemia, anxiety, exertion, hypovolemia, pulmonary emboli, myocardial ischemia, congestive heart failure, and shock.

Sinus tachycardia is usually of no physiologic significance; however, in clients with organic myocardial disease, the result may be reduced cardiac output, congestive heart failure, or dysrhythmias. Because heart rate is a major determinant of oxygen requirements, angina or perhaps an increase in the size of an infarction may accompany persistent tachycardia in clients with coronary artery disease.

Clinical Signs and Symptoms. The symptoms of tachycardia vary from one person to another and may range from an increased pulse to a group of symptoms that would restrict normal activity of the client. Anxiety and apprehension may occur depending on the pain threshold and emotional reaction of the client (Massie and Kleiger, 1983).

Treatment. Medical treatment should be directed toward correcting the underlying disease state that caused the sinus tachycardia. Elimination of tobacco, alcohol, coffee, tea, or other stimulants may be helpful.

Sinus Bradycardia (Kinney et al., 1991)

In sinus bradycardia, impulses travel down the same pathway as in sinus rhythm, but the sinus node discharges at a

▼ *Clinical Signs and Symptoms of*

Sinus Bradycardia

■ Reduced pulse rate
■ Syncope

rate less than 60 beats per minute. Bradycardia may be normal in athletes or young adults and is therefore asymptomatic.

In most cases, sinus bradycardia is a benign dysrhythmia and may actually be beneficial by producing a longer period of diastole and increased ventricular filling. In some clients who have acute myocardial infarction, it reduces oxygen demands and may help minimize the size of the infarction.

Eye surgery, meningitis, intracranial tumors, cervical and mediastinal tumors, and certain disease states such as MI, myxedema, obstructive jaundice, and cardiac fibrosis may produce sinus bradycardia.

Clinical Signs and Symptoms. Syncope may be preceded by sudden onset of weakness, sweating, nausea, pallor, vomiting, and distortion or dimming of vision. Signs and symptoms remit promptly when the client is placed in the horizontal position (Berkow and Fletcher, 1992).

Treatment. Treatment of sinus bradycardia is needed only when symptoms such as chest pain, dyspnea, lightheadedness, or hypotension occur. Medications or electric pacing may be utilized.

CARDIOVASCULAR DISORDERS

Peripheral Vascular Disorders

Impaired circulation may be caused by a number of acute or chronic medical conditions known as *peripheral vascular diseases* (PVDs). PVDs can affect the arterial, venous, or lymphatic circulatory system (Kisner and Colby, 1990).

Vascular disorders secondary to occlusive arterial disease usually have an underlying atherosclerotic process that causes disturbances of circulation to the extremities and can result in significant loss of function of either the upper or lower extremities.

Peripheral arterial occlusive diseases also can be caused by embolism, thrombosis, trauma, vasospasm, inflammation, or autoimmunity. The cause of some disorders is unknown.

Arterial Disease

Arterial diseases include acute arterial occlusion caused by (1) thrombus, embolism, or trauma to an artery, (2) arteriosclerosis obliterans, (3) thromboangitis obliterans or Buerger's disease, or (4) Raynaud's disease. Each of these disorders will be described more completely in the following sections.

Clinical manifestations of chronic arterial occlusion due to peripheral vascular disease may not appear for 20 to 40 years. The lower limbs are far more susceptible to arterial occlusive disorders and atherosclerosis than are the upper limbs (Dennison and Black, 1993).

Diabetes mellitus increases the susceptibility to CHD, but the specific mechanism by which this happens is poorly understood. People with diabetes have abnormalities that affect a number of steps in the development of atherosclerosis. Only the combination of factors, such as hypertension, abnormal platelet activation, and metabolic disturbances affecting fat and serum cholesterol, can account for all the increased risk (Wechsler, 1991).

Clinical Signs and Symptoms. The most important symptoms of chronic arterial occlusive disease are intermittent claudication (limping due to pain, ache, or cramp in the muscles of the lower extremities caused by ischemia or insufficient blood flow) and rest pain. The pain associated with arterial disease is generally felt as a dull, aching tightness deep in the muscle, but it may be described as a boring, stabbing, squeezing, pulling, or even burning sensation. Although the pain is sometimes referred to as a cramp, there is no actual spasm in the painful muscles.

The location of the pain is determined by the site of the major arterial occlusion. The most frequent lesion, which is present in about two thirds of clients, is occlusion of the superficial femoral artery between the groin and the knee, producing pain in the calf that sometimes radiates to the popliteal region and to the lower thigh.

Aortoiliac occlusive disease induces pain in the gluteal and quadriceps muscles, whereas occlusion of the popliteal or more distal arteries causes pain in the foot (Layzer, 1985).

In the typical case of superficial femoral artery occlusion, there is a good femoral pulse at the groin but arterial pulses are absent at the knee and foot, although resting circulation appears to be good in the foot. After exercise, the client may have numbness in the foot as well as pain in the calf. The foot may be cold and pale, which is an indication that the circulation has been diverted to the arteriolar bed of the leg muscles (Layzer, 1985).

Painful, cramping symptoms occur during walking and disappear quickly with rest. In most clients, the symptoms are constant and reproducible, i.e., the client who cannot walk the length of the house because of leg pain one day but is able to walk indefinitely the next does not have intermittent claudication (Dennison and Black, 1993).

Intermittent claudication is influenced by the speed, incline, and surface of the walk. Exercise tolerance decreases over time, so that episodes of claudication occur more frequently with less exertion.

Treatment. Treatment recommended for clients with intermittent claudication combines smoking cessation, daily walking exercise, dietary management, endovascular intervention (therapeutic catheter-based treatment), pain control, and pharmacologic management.

ARTERIOSCLEROSIS OBLITERANS

Arteriosclerosis obliterans, defined as arteriosclerosis in which proliferation of the intima has caused complete obliteration of the lumen of the artery, is also known as *atherosclerotic occlusive disease, chronic occlusive arterial disease, obliterative arteriosclerosis,* and *peripheral arterial disease.* It is the most common occlusive arterial disease that causes chronic ischemia of the lower extremities and accounts for about 95 per cent of cases. This disease is most often seen in elderly clients and is commonly associated with diabetes mellitus (Kisner and Colby, 1990).

Arterial Disease

- Intermittent claudication
- Burning, ischemic pain at rest
- Rest pain aggravated by elevating the extremity; relieved by hanging the foot over the side of the bed or chair
- Decreased skin temperature
- Dry, scaly, or shiny skin
- Poor nail and hair growth
- Possible ulcerations on weight-bearing surfaces (e.g., toes, heel)
- Vision changes (diabetic atherosclerosis)
- Fatigue on exertion (diabetic atherosclerosis)

Arteriosclerosis Obliterans

- Intermittent claudication
- Pain at rest
- Ulceration and gangrene

Other risk factors in arteriosclerosis obliterans are smoking, hypertension, obesity, and atherosclerosis in the coronary arteries. As with atherosclerosis elsewhere, arteriosclerosis obliterans develops slowly and insidiously over a period of years. Initially, the client is asymptomatic as collateral circulation develops. Over time, the collateral vessels may become occluded, causing more ischemia.

Treatment. Treatment is as described for arterial disease to arrest the progress of the disease, produce vasodilation, relieve pain, and provide supportive services. Treatment involves smoking cessation, daily walking exercise, dietary management, endovascular intervention, pain control, and pharmacologic management.

BUERGER'S DISEASE (Dennison and Black, 1993)

Buerger's disease, or *thromboangiitis obliterans,* is a vasculitis of small and medium-sized veins and arteries in the extremities of young adults. It is a disease seen predominantly in men aged 20 to 40 years who smoke cigarettes. The disease process is gradual; it starts distally, then progresses cephalad, involving both upper and lower extremities. The exact pathogenesis is unknown.

Clinical Signs and Symptoms. Pain is the outstanding symptom. Intermittent claudication is a common problem that occurs in almost all clients at some stage of the disease. It is often the first symptom noted by the client, usually in the arch of the foot.

Rest pain with persistent ischemia of one or more digits and coldness or cold sensitivity may be early symptoms. Various types of paresthesias may occur. Pulsations in the posterior tibial and dorsalis pedis arteries are weak or absent.

Ulceration and gangrene are frequent complications and may occur early in the course of the disease. Gangrene usually occurs in one extremity at a time. In advanced cases, the extremities may be abnormally red or cyanotic, particularly when

▼ *Clinical Signs and Symptoms of*

Buerger's Disease

- Pain
- Intermittent claudication
- Cold sensitivity
- Ulceration and gangrene (complications)
- Color, temperature, skin, nail bed changes
- Paresthesias

dependent. Edema of the legs is fairly common. Color or temperature changes involving only one extremity, only certain digits, or only portions of digits also may occur in advanced disease. Changes in nail beds and skin may also appear.

Prognosis and Treatment. Thromboangiitis is usually not life-threatening, but it does result in disability from pain and amputation. Intervention is generally the same as for atheroclerotic peripheral arterial disease. The need for smoking cessation is imperative. Pain control for clients with rest pain and ischemic lesions is essential. Regional sympathetic ganglionectomy and amputation may be necessary.

RAYNAUD'S PHENOMENON AND DISEASE

The term *Raynaud's phenomenon* refers to intermittent episodes during which small arteries or arterioles in extremities constrict, causing temporary pallor and cyanosis of the digits and changes in skin temperature. These episodes occur in response to cold temperature or strong emotion (anxiety, excitement). As the episode passes, the changes in color are replaced by redness. If the disorder is secondary to another disease or underlying cause, the term *Raynaud's phenomenon* is used.

Secondary Raynaud's phenomenon is often associated with connective tissue or collagen vascular disease such as scleroderma, polymyositis/dermatomyositis, systemic lupus erythematosus, or rheumatoid arthritis. Raynaud's phenomenon may occur after trauma or use of vibrating equipment such as jackhammers, or it may be related to various neurogenic lesions (e.g., thoracic outlet syndrome) and occlusive arterial diseases.

Raynaud's disease is a primary vasospastic disorder. It appears to be caused by (1) hypersensitivity of digital arteries to cold, (2) release of serotonin, and (3) congenital predisposition to vasospasm. Eighty per cent of clients with Raynaud's disease are women between the ages of 20 and 49 years. Primary Raynaud's disease rarely leads to tissue necrosis.

Idiopathic Raynaud's disease is differentiated from secondary Raynaud's phenomenon by a history of symptoms for at least 2 years with no progression of the symptoms and no evidence of underlying case (Berkow and Fletcher, 1992).

Clinical Signs and Symptoms. The typical progression of Raynaud's phenomenon is pallor in the digits, followed by cyanosis accompanied by feelings of cold, numbness, and occasionally pain, and finally, intense redness accompanied by tingling or throbbing.

The pallor is caused by vasoconstriction of the arterioles in the extremity, which leads to decreased capillary blood flow. Blood flow becomes sluggish and cyanosis appears; the digits turn blue. The intense redness or rubor results from the end of vasospasm and a period of hyperemia as

oxygenated blood rushes through the capillaries.

Treatment. Conservative protective measures, cessation from tobacco use, limiting caffeine intake, and stress management and biofeedback are the initial treatment choices. Drug therapy to induce smooth muscle relaxation, to relieve spasm, and to increase arterial flow may be recommended. Sympathectomy is sometimes performed, but the long-term results are disappointing as peripheral nerves regenerate and symptoms return.

Venous Disorders (Dennison and Black, 1993)

Venous disorders can be separated into acute and chronic conditions. Acute venous disorders include thromboembolism. Chronic venous disorders can be separated further into varicose vein formation and chronic venous insufficiency.

Acute venous disorders are due to formation of thrombi (clots), which obstruct venous flow. Blockage may occur in both superficial and deep veins. Superficial thrombophlebitis is often iatrogenic, resulting from careless insertion of intravenous catheters or inattentive care of intravenous sites.

Deep venous thrombosis is a common disorder affecting women more than men and adults more than children. Approximately one third of clients over 40 years of age who have had either major surgery or an acute myocardial infarction develop deep venous thrombosis (Wyngaarden et al., 1992).

Chronic venous insufficiency, also known as postphlebitic syndrome, is identified by chronic swollen limbs; thick, coarse, brownish skin around the ankles; and venous stasis ulceration. Chronic venous insufficiency is the result of dysfunctional valves that reduce venous return, which thus increases venous pressure and causes venous stasis and skin ulcerations.

Chronic venous insufficiency follows

▼ *Clinical Signs and Symptoms of*

Raynaud's Phenomenon and Disease

- Pallor in the digits
- Cyanotic, blue digits
- Cold, numbness, pain of digits
- Intense redness of digits

most severe cases of deep venous thrombosis but may take as long as 5 to 10 years to develop. Education and prevention are essential, and clients with a history of deep venous thrombosis must be monitored periodically for life.

Etiology. Thrombus formation is usually attributed to venous stasis, hypercoagulability, or injury to the venous wall. *Venous stasis* is caused by immobilization or absence of the calf muscle pump, surgery,* obesity, pregnancy, paralysis, and congestive heart failure.

Hypercoagulability often accompanies malignant neoplasms, especially visceral and ovarian tumors. Oral contraceptives and hematologic disorders also may increase the coagulability of the blood.

Vein wall trauma may occur as a result of intravenous injections, Buerger's disease, fractures and dislocations, certain antibiotics (e.g., chlortetracycline), sclerosing agents, and opaque mediator radiography.

Clinical Signs and Symptoms. Superficial thrombophlebitis presents as a local, raised, red, slightly indurated (hard), warm, tender cord along the course of the involved vein.

In contrast, symptoms of deep venous thrombosis are less distinctive; about one half of clients are asymptomatic. The most common symptoms are pain in the region of the thrombus and unilateral swelling distal to the site. Other symptoms include redness or warmth of the leg, dilated veins, or low-grade fever possibly accompanied by chills and malaise. Unfortunately, the first clinical manifestation may be pulmonary embolism. Frequently, clients have thrombi in both legs even though the symptoms are unilateral.

Homans' sign (discomfort in the upper calf during gentle, forced dorsiflexion of the foot) is commonly assessed during physical examination. Unfortunately, it is insensitive and nonspecific. It is present in less than

* Especially orthopedic surgery, gynecologic cancer surgery, major abdominal surgery, coronary artery bypass grafting, renal transplantation, and splenectomy.

Clinical Signs and Symptoms of
Superficial Venous Thrombosis

- Subcutaneous venous distention
- Palpable cord
- Warmth, redness
- Indurated (hard)

Clinical Signs and Symptoms of
Deep Venous Thrombosis

- Unilateral tenderness or leg pain
- Unilateral swelling (difference in leg circumference)
- Warmth
- Positive Homans' sign
- Discoloration
- Pain with placement of blood pressure cuff around calf inflated to 160 to 180 mm Hg

one third of clients with documented deep venous thrombosis. In addition, more than 50 per cent of clients with a positive finding of Homans' sign do not have evidence of venous thrombosis.

Prognosis and Treatment. Pulmonary emboli (see Chapter 4), most of which start as thrombi in the large deep veins of the legs, are an acute and potentially lethal complication of deep venous thrombosis. Symptoms of superficial thrombophlebitis are relieved by bed rest with elevation of the legs and the application of heat for 7 to 15 days. When local signs of inflammation subside, the client is usually allowed to ambulate wearing elastic stockings. Sometimes, antiinflammatory medications are required. Anticoagulants such as heparin and warfarin are used to prevent clot extension.

▼ *Clinical Signs and Symptoms of*
Lymphedema

- Edema of the dorsum of the foot or hand
- Usually unilateral
- Worse after prolonged dependency
- No discomfort or a dull, heavy sensation

Lymphedema

The third type of peripheral vascular disorder, lymphedema, is defined as an excessive accumulation of fluid in tissue spaces. Lymphedema typically occurs secondary to an obstruction of the lymphatic system from trauma, infection, radiation, or surgery (Kisner and Colby, 1990).

Postsurgical lymphedema is usually seen after surgical excision of axillary, inguinal, or iliac nodes, usually performed as a prophylactic or therapeutic measure for metastatic tumor. Lymphedema secondary to primary or metastatic neoplasms in the lymph nodes is common.

Treatment. There is no known cure for lymphedema once the swelling appears. Clients at high risk of lymphedema have the extremity elevated to improve lymphatic drainage, and range of motion exercises to decrease edema by activating the muscle pump are initiated.

The goal of treatment is to remove as much fluid as possible from the affected extremity. Physical therapy, diuretics, and elastic stockings are used in combination to accomplish this goal.

Hypertension (Dennison and Black, 1993)

Hypertension, or high blood pressure, is defined as a persistent elevation of systolic blood pressure above 140 mm Hg and of diastolic pressure above 90 mm Hg measured on at least two separate occasions at least 2 weeks apart; in other words, sustained elevation of blood pressure. Clients over 65 years of age often have systolic and diastolic measurements over these amounts, so for these clients, hypertension is redefined as systolic pressure over 160 mm Hg and/or diastolic pressure over 95 mm Hg.

Hypertension is often considered in conjunction with peripheral vascular disorders for several reasons. Both are disorders of the circulatory system; the courses of both diseases are affected by similar factors; and hypertension is a major risk factor in atherosclerosis, the largest single cause of peripheral vascular disease.

Hypertension can be classified according to type (systolic or diastolic), cause, and degree of severity. *Primary* (or *essential*) *hypertension* is also known as *idiopathic hypertension* and accounts for 90 to 95 per cent of all hypertensive clients.

Secondary hypertension results from an identifiable cause, including a variety of specific diseases or problems such as renal disease, use of oral contraceptives, Cushing's syndrome, or hyperthyroidism. Intermittent elevation of blood pressure interspersed with normal readings is called *labile hypertension* or *borderline hypertension*.

The severity of hypertension is classified by degrees as follows:

Class I **(mild)**	90–104 mm Hg
Class II **(moderate)**	105–114 mm Hg
Class III **(severe)**	115 mm Hg or greater

Risk Factors. Modifiable risk factors include stress, obesity, and insufficient intake of nutrients. Stress has been shown to cause increased peripheral vascular resistance and cardiac output and to stimulate sympathetic nervous system activity. Sodium is an important factor in essential hypertension. A high-salt diet may induce excessive release of natriuretic hormone, which may indirectly increase blood pressure. Potassium deficiency also can cause hypertension.

▼ *Clinical Signs and Symptoms of*
Hypertension

- Occipital headache
- Vertigo (dizziness)
- Flushed face
- Spontaneous epistaxis
- Vision changes
- Nocturnal urinary frequency

Nonmodifiable factors include family history, age, gender, and race. The incidence of hypertension increases with age, with a poorer prognosis for clients whose hypertension began at a young age. Men experience hypertension at higher rates and at an earlier age than do women until after age 60 years. After age 50 years, more women than men begin to develop hypertension. Hypertension is the most serious health problem for African-Americans in the United States. The reasons are unclear but may include higher salt intake, heredity, and greater environmental stress (Kaplan, 1991).

Clinical Signs and Symptoms. Hypertensive clients are usually asymptomatic in early stages, but when symptoms do occur, they include occipital headache (usually present in the early morning), vertigo, flushed face, nocturnal urinary frequency, spontaneous nosebleeds, and blurred vision.

Prognosis and Treatment. The advent of antihypertensive agents has dramatically reduced the mortality rate associated with hypertension. If untreated, nearly one half of hypertensive clients die of heart disease, one third die of stroke, and the remaining 10 to 15 per cent die of renal failure.

Normalizing high blood pressure is the goal of treatment, which may be accomplished by treating the underlying cause for secondary hypertension or nonpharmaco-

logic intervention as initial therapy for primary hypertension. Weight reduction; modification of dietary fat; restriction of sodium, caffeine, alcohol, and smoking; and nutritional supplements are all recommended before initiating pharmacologic intervention with antihypertensive medication.

Transient Ischemic Attack

Hypertension is a major cause of heart failure, stroke, and kidney failure. Aneurysm formation and congestive heart failure are also associated with hypertension (Walsh, 1991). Persistent, elevated diastolic pressure damages the intimal layer of the small vessels, which causes an accumulation of fibrin, local edema, and possibly, intravascular clotting.

Eventually, these damaging changes diminish blood flow to vital organs, such as the heart, kidneys, and brain, resulting in complications such as heart failure, renal failure, and cerebrovascular accidents or stroke. Many people have brief episodes of transient ischemic attacks (TIAs) before they have an actual stroke. The attacks occur when the blood supply to part of the brain has been temporarily disrupted. These ischemic episodes last from 5 to 20 minutes, although they may last for as long as 24 hours. TIAs are important warning signals that an obstruction exists in an artery leading to the brain.

▼ *Clinical Signs and Symptoms af*
Transient Ischemic Attack

- Slurred speech or sudden difficulty with speech
- Temporary blindness or other dramatic visual changes
- Paralysis or extreme weakness, usually affecting one side of the body

Orthostatic Hypotension

Orthostatic hypotension, an excessive fall in blood pressure of 20 mm Hg or more on assuming the erect position, is not a disease but a manifestation of abnormalities in normal blood pressure regulation. This condition may occur as a normal part of aging or secondary to the effects of drugs such as hypertensives, diuretics, and antidepressants; venous pooling (e.g., pregnancy, prolonged bed rest, or standing); or neurogenic origins. The latter includes diseases affecting the autonomic nervous system, such as Guillain-Barré syndrome, diabetes mellitus, or multiple sclerosis.

Orthostatic intolerance is the most common cause of lightheadedness in clients, especially those who have been on prolonged bed rest or those who have had prolonged anesthesia for surgery. When getting a person up out of bed for the first time, blood pressure and heart rate should be monitored in the supine position and repeated after the person is upright. With dangling the legs off the bed, a significant drop in blood pressure may occur with or without compensatory tachycardia. This drop may provoke lightheadedness, and standing may even produce loss of consciousness (Cohen and Michel, 1988).

These postural symptoms are often accentuated in the morning and are aggravated by heat, humidity, heavy meals, and exercise.

▼ *Clinical Signs and Symptoms of*
Orthostatic Hypotension

- Lightheadedness
- Syncope
- Mental or visual blurring
- Sense of weakness or "rubbery" legs

CHEST PAIN

The four types of pain discussed in Chapter 1, including cutaneous, deep somatic (or parietal), visceral, and referred pain, also apply to chest pain. The pathways and referral of pain in the thorax are not well understood. It is clear that within the chest cavity, parietal pleura (the cavity lining) has sensory nerve fibers that respond to chemical and mechanical forces exerted on this pleura. However, there are few nerve endings (if any) in the visceral pleurae (linings of the various organs), such as the heart or lungs. The exception to this statement is in the area of the pericardium (sac enclosed around the entire heart), which is adjacent to the diaphragm (see Fig. 3–2).

Experiments by Capps and Coleman (1932) showed that pain fibers do exist in the lower parietal pericardium, adjacent to the diaphragm. Stimulation of this portion of the parietal membrane results in sharp pain along the superior border of the trapezius muscle. This referral pattern is identical to the pattern that occurs as a result of stimulation of the central diaphragm and is postulated to be carried by the phrenic nerves that innervate the diaphragm (Fig. 3–7).

Extensive disease may occur within the body cavities without the occurrence of pain until the process extends to the parietal pleura lining of the chest or abdominal cavity wall). Neuritis (constant irritation of nerve endings) in the parietal pleura then produces pain (Bauwens and Paine, 1983).

Pain fibers, originating in the chest parietal pleura, are conveyed through the chest wall as fine twigs of the intercostal nerves. Irritation of these nerve fibers results in pain in the chest wall that is usually described by the client as knifelike and is sharply localized, occurring cutaneously (in the skin).

This pain may be aggravated by any respiratory movement involving the diaphragm, such as sighing, deep breathing, coughing, sneezing, laughing, or the hic-

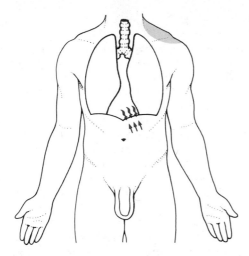

Figure 3–7
Irritation of the peritoneal (outside) or pleural (inside) surface of the central area of the diaphragm refers sharp pain to the upper trapezius muscle, neck, and supraclavicular fossa. The pain pattern is ipsilateral to the area of irritation. Irritation to the peripheral portion of the diaphragm refers sharp pain to the costal margins and lumbar region (not shown).

cups, and may be referred along the costal margins or into the upper abdominal quadrants.

Cardiac Causes

There are many causes of chest pain, both cardiac and noncardiac in origin (see Table 12–3). As discussed, cardiac-related pain may arise secondary to angina, myocardial infarction, pericarditis, endocarditis, or dissecting aortic aneurysm. Cardiac-related chest pain can also occur when there is normal coronary circulation, as in the case of clients with pernicious anemia (chronic, progressive reduction of red blood cells, and subsequent loss of oxygen). These clients may have angina on physical exertion because of the lack of nutrition to the myocardium.

Coronary disease may go unnoticed because the client has had no anginal or infarct pain associated with ischemia. This

situation occurs when a collateral circulation is established to counteract an obstruction of the blood flow to the heart muscle. Gradual occlusion of principal coronary vessels may be accompanied by anastomoses (connecting channels) between the branches of the right and left coronary arteries eliminating the person's perception of pain.

Noncardiac Causes

Pleuropulmonary disorders
   Pulmonary embolism
   Cor pulmonale
   Pulmonary hypertension
   Pleurisy with pneumonia
   Spontaneous pneumothorax
Musculoskeletal disorders
   Myalgia
   Postoperative pain
   Fractured ribs
   Myofascial trigger points
   Costochondritis
   Cervical spine disorders
Neurologic disorders
   Intercostal neuritis
   Dorsal nerve root radiculitis
   Thoracic outlet syndrome
Gastrointestinal disorders
Breast pain
Anxiety states

Pleuropulmonary Disorders

Pulmonary chest pain results usually from obstruction, restriction, dilation, or distention of the large airways or large pulmonary artery walls. Specific diagnoses include pulmonary hypertensive pain, pulmonary embolism, mediastinal emphysema, and spontaneous pneumothorax (Hurst, 1990). Pleuropulmonary disorders are discussed in detail in Chapter 4.

Musculoskeletal Disorders

Musculoskeletal disorders such as myalgia associated with muscle exertion, myofascial trigger points, costochondritis, or xiphoiditis can produce pain in the chest and arms. Compared with angina pectoris, the pain associated with these conditions may last for seconds or hours, and prompt relief does not occur with the ingestion of nitroglycerin.

Muscle exertion secondary to prolonged or repeated movement may create a condition of *myalgia,* or muscular pain. Myalgia of chest muscles caused by repeated coughing may be associated with a recent upper respiratory infection. This information is brought to the examiner's attention when reviewing the Family/Personal History form. Clients who have chest pain should be asked during the physical therapy interview about recent activities of a repetitive nature that could cause sore muscles (e.g., painting or washing walls; calisthenics, including pushups; or recent repetitive lifting of heavy boxes or weights).

Postoperative chest pain following cardiac transplantation is usually due to the sternal incision and musculoskeletal manipulation during surgery. Coronary insufficiency does not present as chest pain owing to cardiac denervation (Cohen and Michel, 1988).

Fractured ribs can cause sharp, localized pain at the level of the fracture with an increase in symptoms associated with respiratory movements, such as deep inspiration, laughing, sneezing, or coughing.

Myofascial trigger points (Travell and Simons, 1983), which are defined as hypersensitive spots in the skeletal musculature involving the serratus anterior, pectoralis, sternalis, or upper rectus abdominis muscles, may produce precordial (the region over the heart and lower part of the thorax) pain (see Fig. 3–12*A* to *D*). Abdominal muscles have multiple referred pain patterns that may reach up into the chest or midback and produce heartburn or deep epigastric (upper middle region of the abdomen, lower sternum) pain (see Table 12–1). The client may present with a history of prolonged, vigorous activity that requires forceful abdominal breathing, such as bending and lifting.

Chest pain from serratus anterior trigger points may present at rest in severe cases. Clients with this myofascial syndrome may report that they are "short of breath" or that they are in pain when they take a deep breath. Serratus anterior trigger points on the left side of the chest can contribute to the pain associated with myocardial infarction. This pain is rarely aggravated by the usual tests for range of motion at the shoulder but may result from a strong effort to protract the scapula. Palpation reveals tender points that increase symptoms, and there is usually a palpable taut band present within the involved muscles.

There may be a history of muscle strain from lifting weights overhead, pushups, prolonged running, or severe coughing. When active trigger points occur in the left pectoralis major muscle, the referred pain (anterior chest, to the precordium and down the inner aspect of the left arm) is easily confused with that due to coronary insufficiency. Chest pain that persists long after an acute myocardial infarction is often due to myofascial trigger points. As with all myofascial syndromes, inactivation of the trigger points eliminates the client's symptoms of chest pain.

Costochondritis or *xiphoiditis* involves local swelling and pain of the associated costochondral, chondrosternal, or xiphisternal joints. The second costocartilage on either side is the most common area of involvement, but any costochondral articulations can be involved. Pain and tenderness may be reproduced by palpation of the local areas. The condition may persist for months without fever or systemic symptoms (Smith, 1990). Clinical signs and symptoms of this disorder are reviewed in detail in Chapter 12.

Chest pain can occur as a result of *cervical spine disorders,* because nerves originating as high as C34 can extend as far as the nipple line. For example, pectoral, suprascapular, dorsal scapular, and long thoracic nerves originating in lower cervical levels can cause pain in the chest, midscapular regions, and post-scapular regions when irritated (Bauwens and Paine, 1983) (see Clues to Differentiating Chest Pain).

CLUES TO DIFFERENTIATING CHEST PAIN

- History of repetitive motion
- Presence of trigger points(s)
- Elimination of trigger point(s) eliminates symptoms
- Lack of musculoskeletal objective findings
- Presence of chronic cough
- Red flag–associated signs and symptoms
- Effect of food on symptoms or presence of GI symptoms
- History (e.g., flu, trauma, upper respiratory infection, herpes, shingles)
- Effect of exertion (total body versus upper body alone)

Neurologic Disorders

Neurologic disorders such as intercostal neuritis and dorsal nerve root radiculitis or a neurovascular disorder such as thoracic outlet syndrome can cause chest pain. The most commonly recognized neuritis is *herpes zoster (shingles)*.

Herpes Zoster (Nicol, 1993)

Herpes zoster is an infection caused by the same virus that causes chickenpox. There is an increased incidence of herpes zoster in clients with lymphoma, tuberculosis, leukemia, and acquired immunodeficiency syndrome (AIDS), probably because of their decreased immunologic response. It can be triggered by trauma, by injection of drugs, or for no known cause (O'Toole, 1992).

Clinical Signs and Symptoms. Clusters of grouped vesicles appear unilaterally along cranial or spinal nerve dermatomes after 1 to 2 days of pain, itching, and hyperesthesia. Neuritic chest wall conditions are usually dermatomal in distribution; pain and skin rash are confined to the somatic distribution of the involved spinal nerve. Because they follow nerve pathways, the lesions do not cross the body midline; however, the nerves of both sides may be involved.

Herpes zoster lesions evolve into crusts on the skin and ulcers on the superficial mucous membranes. The eruption clears in about 2 weeks, unless the period between the pain and the eruption is longer than 2 days.

The pain may be constant or intermittent and vary from light burning to a deep visceral sensation. The duration of pain may be weeks, months, or years. The pattern of the pain differs from coronary pain because the neuritis is unrelated to effort and lasts for prolonged periods. Unfortunately, in the elderly, the pain generally lasts months to years; because symptoms are poorly controlled, this condition is very exhausting for older people.

Treatment. Treatment is symptomatic, aimed at relieving pain and itching by use

▼ *Clinical Signs and Symptoms of*
Herpes Zoster (Shingles)

- Fever, chills
- Headache and malaise
- 1 to 2 days of pain, itching, and hyperesthesia
- Skin eruptions (vesicles) appear along dermatomes 4 or 5 days after the other symptoms

of analgesics and sedatives. Systemic corticosteroids are used to decrease the incidence of postherpetic neuralgia in clients over the age of 50 years. The antiviral agent acyclovir (Zovirax) can be used to treat localized herpes zoster infections (Deglin and Vallerand, 1993).

Herpes zoster is a communicable disease and requires some type of isolation. Specific precautions depend on whether the disease is localized or disseminated and on the condition of the client. Persons susceptible to chickenpox should avoid contact and stay out of the client's room (O'Toole, 1992).

Dorsal Nerve Root Irritation

Other conditions of neuritis involve the dorsal nerve roots of the thoracic spine and can refer pain to the lateral and anterior chest wall. This somatic pain can be localized to the point of irritation or is referred to any point along the peripheral nerve. Pain may be described as sharp or dull and aching, with referral possibly to one or both arms through branches of the brachial plexus.

Pain associated with dorsal nerve root irritation is accompanied commonly by a history of back pain, pain more superficial than cardiac pain, which is usually aggravated by exertion of just the upper body and is accompanied by other neurologic signs (e.g., numbness, tingling, and muscle atrophy). Lesions producing dorsal nerve root pain may be infectious (e.g., *radiculitis,* which is an inflammation within or beneath the dura mater [intradural] of the spinal nerve root). However, the pain is more likely to be the result of mechanical irritation of the root due to spinal disease or deformity (e.g., bony spurs secondary to osteoarthritis, or to the presence of cervical ribs placing pressure on the brachial plexus) (Bauwens and Paine, 1983).

Thoracic Outlet Syndrome (Smith, 1990)

Thoracic outlet syndrome refers to compression of the neural and vascular structures that leave, or pass over, the superior rim of the thoracic cage. Various names have been given to the condition, including first thoracic rib, cervical rib, scalenus anticus, costoclavicular, and hyperabduction syndromes according to the presumed site of major neurovascular compression.

Symptoms may be related to occupational activities, to poor posture, to sleeping with arms elevated over the head, or to acute injuries such as cervical whiplash. Most people become symptomatic in the third or fourth decade, and women are affected three times more often than men.

Most people with thoracic outlet syndrome experience pain in the upper extremity resulting from somatic nerve compression, usually in the distribution of the ulnar nerve. Paresthesias (burning, pricking sensation) and hypoesthesia (abnormal decrease in sensitivity to stimulation) are common; anesthesia and motor weakness are reported in only about 10 per cent of the cases.

Although the pain almost always involves the hand and arm, it may also radiate into the head and neck, the shoulder region, the scapula, or the axilla. In a few individuals, the pain associated with thoracic outlet syndrome may occur mainly in the anterior

▼ *Clinical Signs and Symptoms of*
Dorsal Nerve Root Irritation

- Lateral or anterior chest wall pain
- History of back pain
- Pain is aggravated by exertion of only the upper body
- May be accompanied by neurologic signs
  - Numbness
  - Tingling
  - Muscle atrophy

▼ *Clinical Signs and Symptoms of*

Thoracic Outlet Syndrome

- Mimics carpal tunnel syndrome (CTS)
- Paresthesia of fingers
- Weakness and atrophy of small muscles of the hand
- Positive Adson's sign
- Positive result from a hyperabduction test
- Positive result from a costoclavicular test
- Pain in the anterior chest wall
- Shoulder pain

chest wall and may occur in episodes suggestive of coronary heart disease.

Vascular compression is manifest as more diffuse pain in the limb, with associated fatigue and weakness. With more severe arterial compromise, the client may describe coolness, pallor, cyanosis, or symptoms of Raynaud's phenomenon.

Palpation of the supraclavicular space may elicit tenderness or may define a prominence indicative of a cervical rib. The effect on pulse of Adson's maneuver (deep inspiration with the neck fully extended and the head rotated toward the side of symptoms), the hyperabduction test (arm extended overhead), and the costoclavicular test (exaggerated military attention posture) should be compared in both arms. Other tests are described in orthopedic assessment texts.

Gastrointestinal Disorders

Gastrointestinal disorders may cause chest pain with radiation of pain to the shoulders and back (see Fig. 3–13). *Cholecystitis* (inflammation of the gallbladder) can be mistaken for angina pectoris and myocardial infarction.

Cholecystitis presents as discrete attacks of epigastric or right upper quadrant pain, associated with nausea, vomiting, and fever and chills. The pain has an abrupt onset, is either steady or intermittent, and is associated with tenderness to palpation in the right upper quadrant. The pain may be referred to the back and right scapular area. Rarely, left upper quadrant and anterior chest pain occur. Dark urine and jaundice indicate that the stone has obstructed the common duct. Symptoms of dyspepsia, flatulence, indigestion, and intolerance to fatty and spicy foods often lead to the discovery of gallstones, yet the gallbladder is often not responsible for these symptoms (Hurst, 1990).

Acute pancreatitis is more likely to be confused with acute myocardial infarction, and the hypotension that may occur with pancreatitis can produce a reduction of coronary blood flow with the production of angina pectoris. Acute pancreatitis causes pain in the upper part of the abdomen that radiates to the back (at the level of the tenth thoracic vertebra to the second lumbar vertebra) and may spread out over the lower chest. A fever may develop in 24 to 48 hours with abdominal tenderness, which is minimal compared with the degree of pain (Hurst, 1990).

Gastric duodenal peptic ulcer may occasionally cause pain in the lower chest rather than in the upper abdomen. Pain caused by an ulcer is often immediately relieved by antacids and food, such as milk and bland foodstuffs. Ulcer pain is not produced by effort and lasts longer than angina pectoris (Smith, 1990).

Pain in the lower substernal area may arise as a result of *reflux esophagitis* (regurgitation of gastroduodenal secretions). It may be gripping, squeezing, or burning, described as "heartburn" or "indigestion." Like that of angina pectoris, the discomfort of reflux esophagitis may be precipitated by recumbency or by meals; however, unlike angina, it is not precipitated by exercise and is relieved by antacids.

For a more thorough description of these conditions, refer to Chapter 6 in this text.

Symptoms Associated with

Gastrointestinal Disorders

- Chest pain (may radiate to back)
- Nausea
- Vomiting
- Blood in stools
- Pain on swallowing or associated with meals
- Jaundice
- Heartburn or indigestion
- Dark urine

Breast Pain

Breast pain (see Figs. 3–12 and 3–14) is caused most commonly by benign and malignant tumors, inflammatory breast disease such as mastitis (inflammation of the breast), trigger points, or mastodynia (mammary neuralgia).

Mastodynia is a unilateral breast pain caused by irritation of the upper dorsal intercostal nerves and is associated almost always with ovulatory cycles. This association between symptoms and menses may be discovered during the physical therapy interview when the client responds to Special Questions for Women. The pain occurs initially at the premenstrual period, and later it may become persistent.

Breast cancer and cysts develop more frequently in individuals who have a family history of the disease (Berkow and Fletcher, 1992). Any indication of such a family history on the Family/Personal History form in association with breast pain requires medical follow-up. The client's subjective report of family history of breast disease or report of palpable breast nodules or lumps and previous history of chronic mastitis is very important.

The skin surface over a tumor may be red, warm, edematous, firm, and painful.

There may be skin dimpling over the lesion, with attachment of the mass to surrounding tissues preventing normal mobilization of skin, fascia, and muscle. Jarring or movement of the breasts and movement of the arms may aggravate the pain with radiation of pain to the inner aspects of the arm(s).

The client who presents with a painful or tender breast may have *trigger points* in the lateral margin of the pectoralis major or pectoralis minor muscle. These hypersensitive spots in the skeletal musculature can refer pain to the chest in a manner that confusingly simulates the pain of coronary insufficiency in persons with no history or evidence of cardiac disease. Although these patterns strongly mimic cardiac pain, myofascial trigger point pain shows a much wider variation in its response to daily activity than does angina pectoris (Travell and Simons, 1983).

This breast pain pattern may be differentiated from the aching pain arising from the

Clinical Signs and Symptoms of

Breast Pathology

- Family history of breast disease
- Palpable breast nodules or lumps and previous history of chronic mastitis
- Breast pain with possible radiation to inner aspect of arm(s)
- Skin surface over a tumor may be red, warm, edematous, firm, and painful
- Firm, painful site under the skin surface
- Skin dimpling over the lesion with attachment of the mass to surrounding tissues, preventing normal mobilization of skin, fascia, and muscle
- Pain aggravated by jarring or by movement of the breasts
- Pain that is not aggravated by resistance to isometric movement of the upper extremities

pectoral muscles by a history of upper extremity overuse usually associated with pectoral myalgia. Resistance to isometric movement of the upper extremities reproduces the symptoms of a pectoral myalgia but does not usually aggravate pain associated with breast tissue.

Travell notes that in acute myocardial infarction, pain is commonly referred from the heart to the midregion of the pectoralis major and minor muscles. The injury to the heart muscle initiates a viscerosomatic process that activates trigger points in the pectoral muscles. After recovery from the acute infarction, these self-perpetuating trigger points tend to persist in the chest wall, unless they are inactivated.

Anxiety State/Panic Disorder
(Hurst, 1990)

An anxiety state producing chest pain, called *neurocirculatory asthenia,* is the most common noncardiovascular cause of chest pain. Psychogenic chest pain may be manifested in the form of cardiac or respiratory symptoms mimicking myocardial infarction.

There are several types of chest discomfort due to anxiety. The pain may be sharp, intermittent, lancinating, or stabbing and located in the region of the left breast. The area of pain is often no larger than the tip of the finger, and it is often associated with a local area of hyperesthesia of the chest wall.

Discomfort in the upper portion of the chest, neck, and left arm, again unrelated to effort, may occur. There may be a sense of persistent weakness and unpleasant awareness of the heart beat. Previously, radiation of chest discomfort to the neck or left arm was considered to be diagnostic of atherosclerotic coronary heart disease. Now, stress testing and coronary arteriography have shown that chest discomfort of

this type can occur in clients with normal coronary arteriograms.

The pain may last no longer than it takes to snap the fingers, or precordial aching pain may last for hours or days and is unrelated to effort. The area of discomfort is often the size of the hand. Retrosternal tightness of variable duration also may occur, unrelated to exercise, and distinguishing this sensation from myocardial ischemia may be impossible without extensive testing.

Some clients with anxiety may have a choking sensation in the throat caused by hysteria. There may be associated hyperventilation. Palpitation, claustrophobia, and occurrence of symptoms in crowded places is common. Acute hyperventilation occurs in people with and without heart disease and may be misleading. Such clients have numbness and tingling of the hands and lips and feel as if they are going to "pass out."

For a more detailed explanation of this condition, see Chapter 1.

▼ *Clinical Signs and Symptoms of*
Chest Pain Due to Anxiety

- Dull, aching discomfort in the substernal region and in the anterior chest
- Sinus tachycardia
- Fatigue
- Fear of closed-in places
- Diaphoresis
- Dyspnea
- Dizziness
- Choking sensation
- Hyperventilation: numbness and tingling of hands and lips

Overview CARDIAC CHEST PAIN PATTERNS

ANGINA (Fig. 3–8)

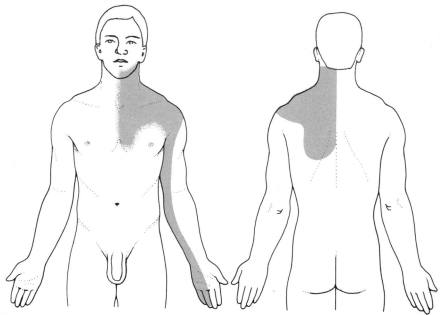

Figure 3–8

Pain patterns associated with angina. *Left,* Area of substernal discomfort projected to the left shoulder and arm over the distribution of the ulnar nerve. Referred pain may be present only in the left shoulder or in the shoulder and along the arm only to the elbow. *Right,* Occasionally, anginal pain may be referred to the back in the area of the left scapula or the interscapular region.

Location:	Substernal/retrosternal (beneath the sternum)
Referral:	Neck, jaw, back, shoulder, or arms (most commonly the left arm)
	May have only a toothache
	Occasionally to the abdomen
Description:	Viselike pressure, squeezing, heaviness, burning indigestion
Intensity:*	Mild to moderate
	Builds up gradually or may be sudden
Duration:	Usually less than 10 minutes
	Never more than 30 minutes
	Average: 3–5 minutes

* For each pattern reviewed throughout this text, intensity is related directly to the degree of noxious stimuli.

Associated Signs
and Symptoms: Shortness of breath (dyspnea)

                     Nausea

                     Diaphoresis (heavy perspiration)

                     Anxiety or apprehension

                     Belching (eructation)

Relieving
Factors: Rest or nitroglycerin

Aggravating
Factors: Exercise or physical exertion

                     Cold weather or wind

                     Heavy meals

                     Emotional stress

■ ■ ■ ■ ■ ■ ■ ■ ■ ■ ■

MYOCARDIAL INFARCTION (Fig. 3–9)

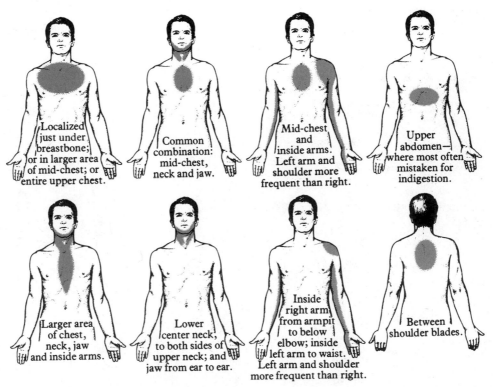

Figure 3–9
Early warning signs of a heart attack.

Location:	Substernal, anterior chest
Referral:	May radiate like angina, frequently down both arms
Description:	Burning, stabbing, viselike pressure, squeezing, heaviness
Intensity:	Severe
Duration:	Usually at least 30 minutes; may last 1 to 2 hours
	Residual soreness 1 to 3 days
Associated Signs and Symptoms:	Dizziness, feeling faint
	Nausea, vomiting
	Pallor
	Diaphoresis (heavy perspiration)
	Apprehension, severe anxiety
	Fatigue, sudden weakness
	Dyspnea
	May be followed by painful shoulder-hand syndrome (see text)
Relieving Factors:	None, unrelieved by rest or nitroglycerin taken every 5 minutes for 20 minutes
Aggravating Factors:	Not necessarily anything; may occur at rest or follow emotional stress or physical exertion

■ ■ ■ ■ ■ ■ ■ ■ ■ ■ ■ ■

PERICARDITIS (Fig. 3–10)

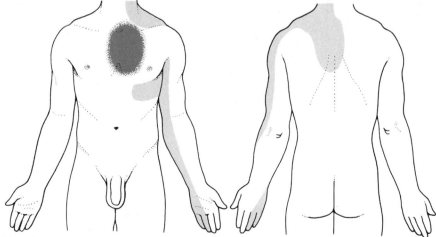

Figure 3–10

Substernal pain associated with pericarditis *(dark red)* may radiate anteriorly *(light red)* to the costal margins, neck, upper back, upper trapezius, and left supraclavicular area or down the left arm.

Location:	Substernal or over the sternum, sometimes to the left of midline toward the cardiac apex
Referral:	Neck, upper back, upper trapezius, left supraclavicular area, down the left arm, costal margins
Description:	More localized than pain of myocardial infarction
	Sharp, stabbing, knifelike
Intensity:	Moderate to severe
Duration:	Continuous, may last hours or days with residual soreness following
Associated Signs and Symptoms:	Usually medically determined associated symptoms (e.g., by chest auscultation using a stethoscope)
Relieving Factors:	Sitting upright or leaning forward
Aggravating Factors:	Muscle movement associated with deep breathing (e.g., laughter, inspiration, coughing)
	Left lateral (side) bending of the upper trunk
	Trunk rotation (either to the right or to the left)
	Supine position

■ ■ ■ ■ ■ ■ ■ ■ ■ ■ ■

DISSECTING AORTIC ANEURYSM (Fig. 3–11)

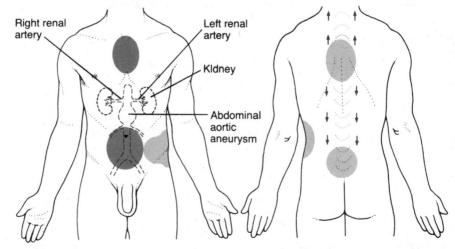

Figure 3–11

Most aortic aneurysms (more than 95 per cent) are located just below the renal arteries and extend to the umbilicus, causing low back pain. Chest pain *(dark red)* associated with thoracic aneurysms may radiate *(light red)* to the neck, interscapular area, shoulders, lower back, or abdomen. Early warning signs of an impending rupture may include an abdominal heart beat when lying down (not shown) or a dull ache in the midabdominal left flank or lower back *(light red)*.

Location:	Anterior chest (thoracic aneurysm)
	Abdomen (abdominal aneurysm)
Referral:	Thoracic area of back
	Pain may move in the chest as dissection progresses
	Pain may extend to the neck, shoulders, interscapular area, or lower back
Description:	Knifelike, tearing (thoracic aneurysm)
	Dull ache in the lower back or midabdominal left flank (abdominal aneurysm)
Intensity:	Severe, excruciating
Duration:	Hours
Associated Signs and Symptoms:	Pulses absent
	Person senses "heart beat" when lying down
	Palpable, pulsating abdominal mass
	Lower blood pressure in one arm
	Other medically determined symptoms
Relieving Factors:	None
Aggravating Factors:	Supine position accentuates symptoms

Overview   NONCARDIAC CHEST PAIN PATTERNS

MUSCULOSKELETAL DISORDERS (Fig. 3–12)

Location:	Variable
	Costochondritis (inflammation of the costal cartilage) may occur at the sternum or rib margins
	Upper rectus abdominis trigger points on the left side; pectoralis, serratus anterior, or sternalis muscles may produce precordial pain
Referral:	Variable, depending on the structure involved
	Abdominal oblique trigger points have multiple referred pain patterns that may reach up into the chest (Travell and Simons, 1983)
	Pectoralis trigger points refer pain down the inner aspect of the arms along the ulnar distribution to the fourth and fifth digits
Description:	Aching or soreness
Intensity:	Mild to severe; may depend on person's anxiety level—if fearful of a "serious" condition, the pain level may be accentuated and often decreases with medical reassurance that the condition is not an early sign of heart disease

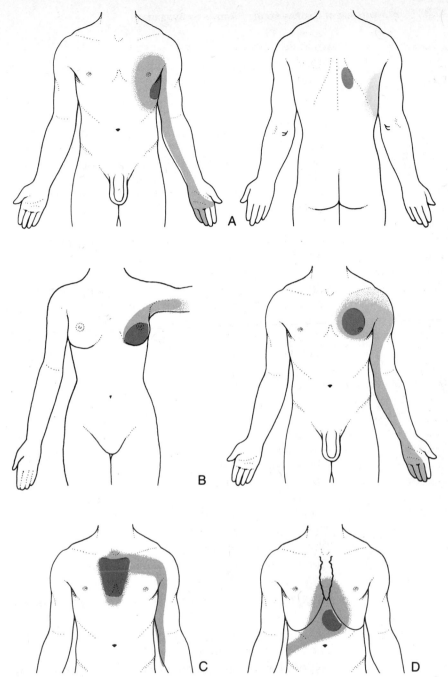

Figure 3–12

A, Referred pain pattern from the left serratus anterior muscle. *B*, Left pectoralis major muscle: referred pain pattern in a woman and a man. *C*, Referred pain pattern from the left sternalis muscle. *D*, Referred pain from the external oblique abdominal muscle can cause "heartburn" in the anterior chest wall. (*A, C,* and *D* from Travell, J.G., and Simons, D.G.: Myofascial Pain and Dysfunction: The Trigger Point Manual. Vol. 1. Baltimore, Williams and Wilkins, 1983. *B*, Adapted from Travell, J.G., and Simons, D.G.: Myofascial Pain and Dysfunction: The Trigger Point Manual. Vol. 1. Baltimore, Williams & Wilkins, 1983.)

Duration:

Minutes or hours

Days to weeks, may become chronic over months if continually aggravated

Associated Signs and Symptoms:

Usually none

History of muscle exertion often associated with prolonged or repeated coughing secondary to upper respiratory infection

Myofascial syndrome causing restricted chest expansion may be associated with shortness of breath, difficulty in taking a deep breath, or in finishing a single sentence without stopping to breathe (Travell and Simons, 1983)

Relieving Factors:

Heat, immobilization during acute phase; medication relief does *not* occur with ingestion of nitroglycerin

Aggravating Factors:

Chest wall movement such as coughing, deep inspiration

Tender to palpatory pressure; muscles involved ache when palpated or squeezed firmly

Myofascial syndrome may be aggravated by a strong effort to protract the scapula (Travell and Simons, 1983)

■ ■ ■ ■ ■ ■ ■ ■ ■ ■ ■ ■

NEUROLOGIC DISORDERS

Location:

May be localized around the precordium (upper central region of the abdomen, the diaphragm)

Referral:

May be localized along the course of the inflamed nerve at the sternum, in the axillary lines, or on either side of the vertebrae

May be referred to the lateral and anterior chest wall

Referral occasionally to one or both arms through branches of the brachial plexus; described as aching

Description: Burning, stabbing, knifelike, exquisite tenderness to pressure

Intensity: Usually intense

Duration: Days to weeks, condition usually persists if untreated

Associated Signs and Symptoms:

Vesicular (blister) rash accompanies herpes zoster or "shingles," a distinctive form of dorsal nerve root irritation

Hyperesthesia (increased sensitivity to touch or other sensory stimuli) may occur with herpes zoster

Chills, fever, headache, malaise with neuritis of the chest wall

Positive result on Adson's test, hyperabduction, or costoclavicular tests with thoracic outlet syndrome

Neurologic signs associated with dorsal nerve root irritation (e.g., numbness, tingling, muscle atrophy)

Relieving
Factors: Heat, medication

Aggravating
Factors: Cold, palpatory pressure, exertion of the upper body

■ ■ ■ ■ ■ ■ ■ ■ ■ ■

GASTROINTESTINAL DISORDERS (Fig. 3–13) (patterns described in greater detail in Chapter 6)

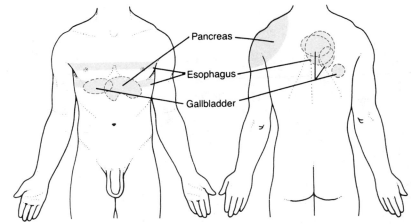

Figure 3–13
Chest pain caused by gastrointestinal disease with referred pain to the shoulder and back.

Location: Substernal, epigastric area of upper abdominal quadrants
Referral: May radiate around chest to shoulders, upper back
Description: Burning, knotlike pain, "heartburn"
Intensity: Mild to severe
Duration: Minutes to hours
Associated Signs
and Symptoms: Nausea, jaundice, vomiting, blood in stool (melena), pain on swallowing associated with esophageal disorders

Relieving
Factors: Belching, antacids, upright position

Aggravating
Factors: Supine position, meals

■ ■ ■ ■ ■ ■ ■ ■ ■ ■ ■

BREAST PAIN (Figs. 3–12, 3–14)

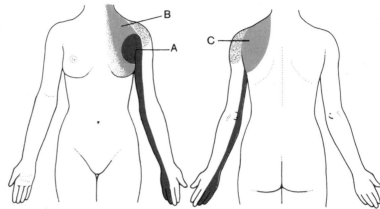

Figure 3–14

Pain arising from the breast. *A,* Mammary pain referred into the axilla along the medial aspect of the arm. *B,* Referral pattern to the supraclavicular level and into the neck. *C,* Breast pain may be diffuse around the thorax through the intercostal nerves. Pain may be referred to the back and to the posterior shoulder.

Location:	Specifically within the breast tissue
	May be localized in pectoral and supraclavicular areas
Referral:	Around the chest into the axilla, to the back at the level of the breast, occasionally into the neck and posterior aspect of the shoulder girdle
	Along the medial aspects of the arm(s) to fourth and fifth digits
Description:	Sharp, cutting, sharp aching
Intensity:	Mild to severe
Duration:	Intermittent to constant (may coincide with menstrual cycle)
Associated Signs and Symptoms:	May have no other symptoms
	May report change in breasts (e.g., discharge or bleeding from breasts, lumps, retracted nipple, distorted nipple or breast contour)
	Enlarged or tender lymph nodes
	Edematous and red, warm skin over the area of involvement
	Hypersensitivity of the nipple with intolerance to clothing
	Trigger points in the chest wall musculature associated with muscle exertion and resultant myalgia
	Previous history of myocardial infarct with resultant pectoral trigger points
Relieving Factors:	Temporary relief may be obtained from rest, heat, or ice

Aggravating
Factors:

Jarring or bouncing movement of the breasts

Movement of the upper extremities

Resistance to isometric movement of the upper extremities (pectoral myalgia)

■ ■ ■ ■ ■ ■ ■ ■ ■ ■ ■

ANXIETY STATES

Location:

Variable but commonly in the substernal region and anterior chest

Usually localized to a point

Referral: Does not radiate

Description: Sharp, stabbing, vague discomfort, pressure, burning, crushing

Intensity: Mild to severe

Duration: Usually brief, may last from minutes to hours

Associated Signs
and Symptoms:

Dyspnea

Fatigue

Sighing respirations (hyperventilation)

Chest wall tenderness

Tachycardia

Relieving
Factors:

Relaxation techniques, medications, rest

Aggravating
Factors:

Intense emotion (e.g., anger, fear, worry)

Crowded places

Not aggravated by deep inspiration

LABORATORY VALUES

The results of diagnostic tests can provide the therapist with information to assist in client education. The client often reports test results to the therapist and asks for information regarding the significance of those results. The information presented in this text discusses potential reasons for abnormal laboratory values relevant to clients with cardiovascular problems.

A basic understanding of laboratory tests

used specifically in the diagnosis and monitoring of cardiovascular problems can provide the therapist with additional information regarding the client's status. Some of the tests commonly used in the management and diagnosis of cardiovascular problems include lipid screening (cholesterol levels, low density lipoprotein/LDL levels, high density lipoprotein/HDL levels, and triglyceride levels), serum electrolytes, and arterial blood gases (see Chapter 4).

Other laboratory measurements of importance in the overall evaluation of the client with cardiovascular disease include red blood cell values (e.g., red blood cell count, hemoglobin, and hematocrit). Those values (see Chapter 5) provide valuable information regarding the oxygen-carrying capability of the blood and the subsequent oxygenation of body tissues, such as the heart muscle.

Cholesterol

Cholesterol is a waxy substance that is a normal constituent of bile. High levels of serum cholesterol have been associated with the development of atherosclerosis, the formation of fatty plaques within the surface of blood vessel walls. A build-up of such deposits can occlude blood circulation to the heart muscle and can result in death of the heart muscle (myocardial infarction).

Excessive dietary intake of cholesterol and saturated fats increases the total blood cholesterol level. There also seems to be an inherited tendency toward increased cholesterol levels. Cholesterol levels vary according to age and may be elevated at the time of testing because of external circumstances (e.g., pregnancy, medications, position, and ingestion of vitamins).

In the last few years, there has been disagreement among physicians with regard to the "normal" value of cholesterol. The literature has demonstrated *much* discussion and variation in the recommended normal values (Chernecky et al., 1993). Some researchers have suggested that normal cholesterol parameters should be lower than the currently recorded normals and that these lower values are more appropriate in the prevention and treatment of coronary artery disease. At this time, however, the lower values suggested are still under investigation. The cholesterol values presented in this text can serve as a reference guide for the physical therapist. The values listed in Table 3–5 are the *highest* norms found in the literature and account for variance according to age (Chernecky et al., 1993).

Table 3–5
BLOOD CHOLESTEROL LEVELS

Age (Years)	Values (mg/dl)
< 25	125–200
25–40	140–225
40–50	160–245
50–65	170–265
> 65	< 265

A client with a serum cholesterol level greater than 259 mg/dl is three times more likely to develop coronary artery disease than is a client with a level of 200 mg/dl or less (Reigle and Ringel, 1993). The mean level for clients with heart attacks appears to be 240 mg/dl, with the most heart attacks occurring in clients with levels in the 200 to 240 range (Diethrich and Cohen, 1992).

Triglycerides

Triglycerides are fats circulating in the bloodstream that are used in the body to provide energy for various metabolic activities. Excessive amounts of triglyceride are stored in adipose tissue. Triglyceride levels increase rapidly in response to foods high in calories, sugar, and fat. Triglyceride levels decrease with exercise. High levels of triglycerides are associated with increased risk of cardiovascular disease. Triglyceride levels tend to increase with age and are slightly different for men and women. The values listed in Table 3–6 are guidelines for reference and may vary according to the same variables described for serum cholesterol. Levels greater than 250 mg/dl are believed to carry a greater risk of heart disease (Cella and Watson, 1989).

Low-Density Lipoprotein/ High-Density Lipoprotein

LDL and HDL are the two major types of cholesterol circulating in the blood serum.

Table 3–6
TRIGLYCERIDE LEVELS

Age (Years)	Value (mg/dl)
Female Adult	
20–29	10–100
30–39	10–110
40–49	10–122
50–59	10–134
> 59	10–147
Female Child	
1–19	10–121
Male Adult	
20–29	10–157
30–39	10–182
40–49	10–193
50–59	10–197
> 59	10–199
Male Child	
1–19	10–103

From Chernecky, C., et al.: Laboratory Tests and Diagnostic Procedures. Philadelphia, W.B. Saunders, 1993, p. 932.

Table 3–7
SERUM ELECTROLYTE LEVELS

Test	Normal Values
Serum potassium	3.5–5.3 mEq/L
Serum sodium	136–145 mEq/L
Serum calcium	8.2–10.2 mg/dl (4.5–5.5 mEq/L)
Serum magnesium	1.8–3 mg/dl (1.5–2.5 mEq/L)

From Chernecky, C., et al.: Laboratory Tests and Diagnostic Procedures. Philadelphia, W.B. Saunders, 1993.

HDLs are thought to be formed in the liver and are the source of "good" or readily transportable cholesterol. Research has suggested that high levels of HDL and low levels of LDL are associated with a decreased risk of cardiovascular disease. HDL levels have been found to increase with exercise. Low levels of HDL and high levels of LDL are considered to be risk factors for the development of atherosclerotic heart disease (Cella and Watson, 1989).

Serum Electrolytes

Measurement of serum electrolyte values is particularly important in diagnosis, management, and monitoring of the client with cardiovascular disease, since electrolyte levels have a direct influence on the function of cardiac muscle (in a manner similar to that of skeletal muscle). Abnormalities in serum electrolytes, even in noncardiac clients, can result in significant cardiac dysrhythmias and even cardiac arrest. In addition, certain medications prescribed for cardiac clients can alter serum electrolytes in such a way that rhythm problems can occur as a result of the medication. The electrolyte levels most important to monitor include potassium, sodium, calcium, and magnesium (Table 3–7).

Potassium. Serum potassium levels can be lowered significantly as a result of diuretic therapy (particularly with loop diuretics such as Lasix [furosemide]), vomiting, diarrhea, sweating, and alkalosis. Low potassium levels cause increased electrical instability of the myocardium, life-threatening ventricular dysrhythmias, and increased risk of digitalis toxicity (Jacobsen, 1993). Serum potassium levels must be measured frequently by the physician in any client taking a digitalis preparation (such as Digoxin), since most of these clients are also on diuretic therapy. Low potassium levels in clients on digitalis can cause digitalis toxicity and precipitate life-threatening dysrhythmias.

Increased potassium levels most commonly occur owing to renal and endocrine problems or as a result of potassium replacement overdose. Cardiac effects of increased potassium levels include ventricular dysrhythmias and asystole/flat line (complete cessation of electrical activity of the heart).

Sodium. Serum sodium levels indicate the client's state of water/fluid balance, which is particularly important in congestive heart failure and other pathologic states related to fluid imbalances. A low serum sodium level can indicate water overload or extensive loss of sodium through diuretic use, vomiting, diarrhea, or diaphoresis. A high serum sodium level can indicate a water deficit state such as dehydration or water loss (e.g., lack of antidiuretic hormone [ADH]).

Calcium. Serum calcium levels can be decreased as a result of multiple transfusions of citrated blood, renal failure, alkalosis, laxative or antacid abuse, and parathyroid damage or removal. A decreased calcium level provokes serious and often life-threatening ventricular dysrhythmias and cardiac arrest.

Increased calcium levels are less common but can be caused by a variety of situations, including thiazide diuretic use (e.g., Diuril [chlorothiazide]), acidosis, adrenal insufficiency, immobility, and vitamin D excess. Calcium excess causes atrioventricular conduction blocks or tachycardia and ultimately can result in cardiac arrest (Jacobsen, 1993).

Magnesium. Serum magnesium levels are rarely changed in healthy individuals because magnesium is abundant in foods and water. However, magnesium deficits are often seen in alcoholic clients or in clients with critical illnesses that involve shifting of a variety of electrolytes. Magnesium deficits often accompany potassium and calcium deficits. A decrease in serum magnesium results in myocardial irritability and cardiac dysrhythmias, such as atrial or ventricular fibrillation or premature ventricular beats (PVCs) (Kee, 1993).

PHYSICIAN REFERRAL

The description and location of chest pain associated with pericarditis, myocardial infarction, angina, breast pain, gastrointestinal disorders, and anxiety are often similar. The physician is able to distinguish among these conditions through a careful history, medical examination, and medical testing.

For example, the severe substernal pain of pericarditis closely mimics the pain of acute myocardial infarction, but the two disorders differ in aggravating and relieving factors. Pain associated with gastrointestinal disorders involving the esophagus may create pain like that of angina pectoris, with discomfort precipitated by recumbency or by meals. However, the esophageal pain is not aggravated by exercise, whereas true angina is caused by exercise or by physical exertion and is relieved by rest. In both these examples, chest auscultation and an electrocardiogram (ECG) provide the physician with valuable diagnostic information.

It is not the physical therapist's responsibility to differentiate diagnostically among the various causes of chest pain, but rather to recognize the systemic origin of signs and symptoms that may mimic musculoskeletal disorders.

For example, compared with angina, the pain of true musculoskeletal disorders may last for seconds or for hours, is not relieved by nitroglycerin, and may be aggravated by exertion of just the upper body.

The physical therapy interview presented in Chapter 2 is the primary mechanism used to begin exploring a client's reported symptoms and is accomplished by carefully questioning the client to determine the location, duration, intensity, frequency, associated symptoms, and relieving or aggravating factors related to pain or symptoms.

When to Refer a Client to the Physician

When a client mentions signs and symptoms, these may be clues to systemic disease processes that mimic musculoskeletal pain and dysfunction. Clients often confide in physical therapists and describe symptoms of a more serious nature. Cardiac symptoms unknown to the physician may be mentioned to the therapist during the opening interview or in subsequent visits.

The materials presented in this chapter help prepare the therapist for making re-

---

GUIDELINES FOR PHYSICIAN REFERRAL

- When a client presents with any combination of systemic signs or symptoms
- Women with chest or breast pain who have a positive family history of breast cancer should always be referred to a physician for a follow-up examination
- Cardiac clients should be sent back to their physician under the following conditions:
  - Nitroglycerin tablets do not relieve anginal pain
  - Pattern of angina changes
  - Patient has abnormally severe chest pain
  - Anginal pain radiates to the jaw or to the left arm
  - Anginal pain is not relieved by rest
  - Upper back feels abnormally cool, sweaty, or moist to touch
  - Client has any doubt about his or her present condition

---

ferral decisions. An understanding of the nature of thoracic pain provides a knowledge base for recognizing cardiac and noncardiac chest pain patterns and the systemic signs and symptoms associated with these patterns.

Immediate Medical Attention

In the clinic setting, the onset of an anginal attack requires immediate cessation of exercise. If the client is currently taking nitroglycerin, self-administration of medication is recommended. Relief from pain should occur within 1 to 2 minutes. The dose may be repeated according to the prescribed direction. If anginal pain is not relieved in 20 minutes or if the client has nausea, vomiting, or profuse sweating, immediate medical intervention may be indicated.

Changes in the pattern of angina, such as increased intensity, decreased threshold of stimulus, or longer duration of pain, require immediate intervention by the physician. Clients in treatment under these circumstances should either be returned to the care of the nursing staff or, in the case of an outpatient, should be encouraged to contact their physicians by telephone for further instructions before leaving the physical therapy department. The client should be advised not to leave unaccompanied.

Systemic Signs and Symptoms Requiring Physician Referral

Referral by the therapist to the physician is recommended when the client presents with any combination of systemic signs or symptoms discussed throughout this chapter. These signs and symptoms should always be correlated with the client's history to rule out systemic involvement or to

---

GUIDELINES FOR IMMEDIATE MEDICAL ATTENTION

- If anginal pain is not relieved in 20 minutes
- If the client has nausea, vomiting, or profuse sweating

identify musculoskeletal or neurologic disorders that would be appropriate for physical therapy treatment.

Absent pulses	Difficulty in swallowing	Heart fibrillation	Persistent cough
Anxiety or apprehension	Distortion of vision or speech	Heart palpitations	Restlessness
Bradycardia		Hemoptysis	Skin rashes or petechiae
Breast lumps or nodules	Dyspnea	Homan's sign positive	Skipped heart beats
Chest pain caused by exertion	Edema and weight gain	Irritability	Sudden incoordination
Chest pressure	Eructation	Migratory joint pain	Sudden weakness
Claudication	Fatigue, severe	Nausea/vomiting	Syncope
Cold sweat	Fever	Night sweats	Tachycardia
Diaphoresis	"Heart beat" in the back or abdomen	Nocturnal dyspnea	Transient paralysis
		Orthopnea	
		Painful shoulder-hand syndrome	
		Pallor	

 Key Points to Remember

- Fatigue beyond expectations during or after exercise is a red flag symptom.

- Be on the alert for cardiac risk factors in older adults, especially women, and begin a conditioning program before an exercise program.

- The client with stable angina typically has a normal blood pressure; it may be low, depending on medications. BP may be elevated when anxiety accompanies chest pain or during acute coronary insufficiency; systolic BP may be low if there is heart failure.

- Cervical disc disease and arthritic changes can mimic atypical chest pain of angina pectoris, requiring screening through questions and musculoskeletal evaluation.

- If a client uses nitroglycerin, make sure she or he has a fresh supply, and check that the physical therapy department has a fresh supply in a readily accessible location.

- Make sure a client with cardiac compromise has not smoked a cigarette or eaten a large meal just before exercise.

- A person taking medications, such as beta-blockers or calcium channel blockers, may not be able to achieve a target heart rate (THR) above 90 beats per minute. To determine a safe rate of exercise, heart rate should return to the resting level 2 minutes after stopping exercise.

- A 3-pound or greater weight gain or gradual, continuous gain over several days, resulting in swelling of the ankles, abdomen, and hands, combined with shortness of breath, fatigue, and dizziness that persist despite rest, may be red flag symptoms of congestive heart failure.

- The pericardium (sac around the entire heart) is adjacent to the diaphragm. Pain of cardiac and diaphragmatic origin is often experienced in the shoulder, because the heart and the diaphragm are supplied by the C5–6 spinal segment. The visceral pain is referred to the corresponding somatic area.

SUBJECTIVE EXAMINATION	*Special Questions to Ask*

Past Medical History

- Has a doctor ever said that you have heart trouble?
- Have you ever had a heart attack?
  - If yes, when? Please describe.
- Do you associate your current symptoms with your heart problems?
- Have you ever had rheumatic fever, growing pains, twitching of the limbs called St. Vitus' dance, or rheumatic heart disease?
- Have you ever had an abnormal electrocardiogram (ECG)?
- Have you ever had an ECG taken while you were exercising (e.g., climbing up and down steps or walking on a treadmill) that was not normal?
- Do you have a pacemaker, artificial heart, or any other device to assist your heart?
- For the therapist: Remember to review smoking, diet, life style, exercise, and stress history (see Family/Personal History, Chapter 2).

Angina/Myocardial Infarct

- Do you have angina (pectoris) or chest pain or tightness?
  - If yes, please describe the symptoms and tell me when it occurs.
  - If yes, what makes it better?
  - If no, pursue further with the following questions.
- Do you ever have discomfort or tightness in your chest?
- Have you ever had a crushing sensation in your chest with or without pain down your left arm?
- Do you have pain in your jaw either alone or in combination with chest pain?
- If you climb a few flights of stairs fairly rapidly, do you have tightness or pressing pain in your chest?
- Do you get pressure or pain or tightness in the chest if you walk in the cold wind or face a cold blast of air?
- Have you ever had pain or pressure or a squeezing feeling in the chest that occurred during exercise, walking, or any other physical or sexual activity?

Associated Symptoms

- Do you ever have bouts of rapid heart action, irregular heart beats, or palpitations of your heart?
- Have you ever felt a heart beat in your abdomen when you lie down?
  - If yes, is this associated with low back pain or left flank pain?
  (Abdominal aneurysm)

- Do you ever notice sweating, nausea, or chest pain when your current symptoms (e.g., back pain, shoulder pain) occur?

- Do you have frequent attacks of heartburn or do you take antacids to relieve heartburn or acid indigestion? **(Noncardiac cause of chest pain, abdominal muscle trigger point, gastrointestinal disorder)**

- Do you get very short of breath during activities that do not make other people short of breath? **(Dyspnea)**

- Do you ever wake up at night gasping for air or have short breaths? **(Paroxysmal nocturnal dyspnea)**

- Do you ever need to sleep on more than one pillow to breathe comfortably? **(Orthopnea)**

- Do you ever get cramps in your legs if you walk for several blocks? **(Intermittent claudication)**

- Do you ever have swollen feet or ankles?

  - If yes, are they swollen when you get up in the morning? **(Edema/CHF)**

- Have you gained unexpected weight during a fairly short period of time (i.e., less than 1 week)? **(Edema, CHF)**

- Do you ever feel dizzy or have fainting spells? **(Valvular insufficiency, bradycardia, pulmonary hypertension, orthostatic hypotension)**

- Have you had any significant changes in your urine (e.g., increased amount, concentrated urine, frequency at night, or decreased amount)? **(CHF, diabetes, hypertension)**

- Do you ever have sudden difficulty with speech, temporary blindness, or other changes in your vision? **(Transient ischemic attacks)**

- Have you ever had sudden weakness or paralysis down one side of your body or just in an arm or a leg? **(Transient ischemic attacks)**

Medications

- Have you ever taken digitalis, nitroglycerin, or any other drug for your heart?

- Have you been on a diet or taken medications to lower your blood cholesterol?

- For the therapist: Any clients taking anticlotting drugs should be examined for hematoma, nosebleed, or other sites of bleeding. Protect client from trauma.

For clients taking nitroglycerin:

- Do you ever have headaches, dizziness, or a flushed sensation after taking nitroglycerin? (Most common side effects)

- How quickly does your nitroglycerin reduce or eliminate your chest pain? (Use as a guideline in the clinic when the client has angina during exercise; refer to a physician if angina is consistently unrelieved with nitroglycerin or rest after the usual period of time)

For Clients with Breast Pain

- Do you have any discharge from your breasts or nipples?
- Have you self-examined your breasts for any lumps or nodules?
- Have you noticed any unusual prominence of veins on your breasts?
- Have you been involved in any activities of a repetitive nature that could cause sore muscles (e.g., painting, washing walls, pushups or other calisthenics, heavy lifting or pushing, overhead movements, prolonged running, or fast walking)?
- Have you recently been coughing excessively?
- Have you ever had a heart attack? **(Residual trigger points)**

For Clients with Joint Pain

- Have you had any skin rashes or dotlike hemorrhages under the skin? **(Rheumatic fever, endocarditis)**
  - If yes, did this occur after a visit to the dentist? **(Endocarditis)**
- Do you notice any change in your chest/shoulder/upper back pain or symptoms when you take your medication? **(Allergic response)**

CASE STUDY*

REFERRAL

A 30-year-old woman with five children comes to you for an evaluation on the recommendation of her friend, who received physical therapy from you last year. She has not been to a physician since her last child was delivered by her obstetrician 4 years ago. Her chief complaint is pain in the left shoulder and left upper trapezius with pain radiating into the chest and referred pain down the medial aspect of the arm to the thumb and first two fingers. When the medical history is being taken, she mentions that she was told 5 years ago that she had a mitral valve prolapse secondary to rheumatic fever, which she had when she was 12 years old.

There is no reported injury or trauma to the neck or shoulder, and the symptoms subside with rest. Physical exertion, such as carrying groceries up the stairs or laundry outside, aggravates the symptoms, but she is uncertain whether just using her upper body has the same effect. She is not taking any medication, denies any palpitations, but complains of fatigue and has dyspnea after playing ball with her son for 10 or 15 minutes.

Despite the client's denial of injury or trauma, the neck and shoulder should be screened for any possible musculoskeletal or neurologic origin of symptoms. Your observation of the woman indicates that she is 30 to 40 pounds overweight. She confides that she is under physical and emotional stress by the daily demands made by seven people in her house. She is not involved in any kind of exercise program outside of her play activities with the children. These two factors (obesity and stress) could account for her chronic fatigue and dyspnea, but that determination must be made by a physician. Even if you can identify a musculoskeletal basis for this woman's symptoms, the past medical history of rheumatic heart disease and absence of medical follow-up would support your recommendation that the client should go to the physician for a medical checkup.

How do you rule the possibility that this pain is not associated with a mitral valve prolapse and is caused instead by true cervical spine or shoulder pain?

It should be pointed out here that the physical therapist is not equipped with the skills, knowledge, or expertise to determine that the mitral valve prolapse is the cause of the client's symptoms. However, a thorough subjective and objective evaluation can assist the therapist both in making a determination regarding the client's musculoskeletal condition and in providing clear and thorough feedback for the physician upon referral.

SCREENING FOR MITRAL VALVE PROLAPSE

- Pain of a mitral valve must be diagnosed by a physician
- Mitral valve may be asymptomatic
- Positive history for rheumatic fever
- Carefully ask the client about a history of possible neck or shoulder pain, which the person may not mention otherwise
- Musculoskeletal pain associated with the neck or shoulder is more superficial than cardiac pain
- Total body exertion causing shoulder pain may be secondary to angina or myocardial ischemia and subsequent infarction, whereas movements of just the upper extremity causing shoulder pain are more indicative of a primary musculoskeletal lesion
     Does your shoulder pain occur during exercise, such as walking, climbing stairs, mowing the lawn, or during any other physical or sexual activity that doesn't require the use of your arm or shoulder?
- Presence of associated signs and symptoms, such as dyspnea, fatigue, or heart palpitations
- X-ray findings, if available, may confirm osteophyte formation with decreased intraforaminal spaces, which may contribute to cervical spine pain
- History of neck injury or overuse
- History of shoulder injury or overuse
- Results of objective tests to clear or rule out the cervical spine and shoulder as the cause of symptoms
- Presence of other neurologic signs to implicate the cervical spine or thoracic outlet type of symptoms (e.g., abnormal deep tendon reflexes, subjective report of numbness and tingling, objective sensory changes, muscle wasting or atrophy)
- Pattern of symptoms: A change in position may relieve symptoms associated with a cervical disorder

References

Abraham, T., Bakamauskas, A., and Kavanaugh, J.: Management of persons with cardiovascular problems. *In* Phipps, W., Long, B., Woods, N., and Cassmeyer, V. (eds.): Medical-Surgical Nursing, Concepts and Clinical Practice, 4th ed. St. Louis, Mosby–Year Book, 1991, pp. 669–736.

Abraham, T., and Kavanaugh, J.: Assessment of the cardiovascular system. *In* Phipps, W., Long, B., Woods, N., and Cassmeyer, V. (eds.): Medical-Surgical Nursing, Concepts and Clinical Practice, 4th ed. St. Louis, Mosby-Year Book, 1991, pp. 599–630.

Ahrens, T., and Taylor, L.: Hemodynamic Waveform Analysis. Philadelphia, W.B. Saunders, 1992.

Arizona Heart Institute and Foundation: Heart Disease. Phoenix, Arizona, 1991.

Bauwens, D.B., and Paine, R.: Thoracic pain. *In* Blacklow, R.S. (ed.): MacBryde's Signs and Symptoms, 6th ed. Philadelphia, J.B. Lippincott, 1983, pp. 139–164.

Berkow, R., and Fletcher, A.J. (eds.): The Merck Manual of Diagnosis and Therapy, 16th ed. Rahway, New Jersey, Merck Sharp & Dohme Research Laboratory, 1992.

Borenstein, D.G., Fye, B., Arnett, F.C., et al.: The myocarditis of systemic lupus erythematosis: Association with myositis. Annals of Internal Medicine *89*:619–625, 1978.

Canobbio, M.M.: Cardiovascular Disorders. St. Louis, C.V. Mosby, 1990.

Capps, J.A., and Coleman, G.H.: An Experimental and Clinical Study of Pain in the Pleura, Pericardium and Peritoneum. New York, Macmillan, 1932.

Castelli, W.P.: Epidemiology of triglycerides: A view from Framingham. American Journal of Cardiology *70*(19):3H–9H, 1992.

Cella, J., and Watson, J.: Nurses' Manual of Laboratory Tests. Philadelphia, F.A. Davis, 1989.

Chernecky, C., Krech, R., and Berger, B.: Laboratory Tests and Diagnostic Procedures. Philadelphia, W.B. Saunders, 1993.

Christan, T., Turnbull, T., and Cline, D.: Cardiopulmonary abnormalities after smoking cocaine. Southern Medical Journal *83*(3):335–338, 1990.

Cohen, M., and Michel, T.H.: Cardiopulmonary symptoms in physical therapy practice. New York, Churchill Livingstone, 1988.

Deglin, J., and Vallerand, A.: Davis's Drug Guide for Nurses, 3rd ed. Philadelphia, F.A. Davis, 1993.

Dennison, P.D., and Black, J.M.: Nursing care of clients with peripheral vascular disorders. *In* Black, J.M., and Matassarin-Jacobs, E. (eds.): Luckmann and Sorensen's Medical-Surgical Nursing, 4th ed. Philadelphia, W.B. Saunders, 1993, pp. 1253–1314.

Diethrich, E.B., and Cohen, C.: Women and Heart Disease. New York, Times Book, Random House, 1992a, pp. xiv, 8.

Diethrich, E.B., and Cohen, C.: Women and Heart Disease. New York, Times Book, Random House, 1992b, p. 4.

Diethrich, E.B., and Cohen, C.: Women and Heart Disease. New York, Times Book, Random House, 1992c, pp. 66–67.

Diethrich, E.B., and Cohen, C.: Women and Heart Disease. New York, Times Book, Random House, 1992d, pp. 33–35.

Dimsdale, J.E.: A perspective on type A behavior and coronary disease. New England Journal of Medicine *318*(2):110–112, 1988.

Durack, D.T.: Infective and noninfective endocarditis. *In* Hurst, J.W. (ed.): The Heart. New York, McGraw-Hill, 1990.

Erickson, B.A.: Dysrhythmias. *In* Kinney, M.R., Packa, D.R., Andreoli, K.G., and Zipes, D.P. (eds.): Comprehensive Cardiac Care, 7th ed. St. Louis, Mosby–Year Book, 1991, pp. 105–252.

Eysmann, S. B., and Douglas, P.S.: Reperfusion and revascularization strategies for coronary artery disease in women. Journal of the American Medical Association *268*(14):1903–1907, 1992.

Frederickson, L.: Confronting Mitral Valve Prolapse Syndrome. New York, Warner Books, 1992.

Hunder, G.G.: When musculoskeletal symptoms point to endocarditis. Journal of Musculoskeletal Medicine *9*(3):33–40, 1992.

Hurst, J.W. (ed.): Atherosclerotic coronary heart diseae. *In* The Heart, 7th ed. New York, McGraw-Hill, 1990, pp. 961–1001.

Jacobsen, L.: Assessment of clients with cardiovascular disorders. *In* Black, J.M., and Matassarin-Jacobs, E. (eds.): Luckmann and Sorensen's Medical-Surgical Nursing, 4th ed. Philadelphia, W.B. Saunders, 1993, pp. 1105–1138.

Kannel, W.B., Garrison, R.J., and Dannenberg, A.L.: Secular blood pressure trends in normotensive persons: The Framingham study. American Heart Journal *125*(4): 1154–1158, 1993.

Kaplan, N.M.: Clinical Hypertension, 5th ed. Baltimore, Williams and Wilkins, 1991.

Kee, J.: Fluid and electrolyte balance. *In* Black, J.M., and Matassarin-Jacobs, E. (eds.): Luckmann and Sorensen's Medical-Surgical Nursing, 4th ed. Philadelphia, W.B. Saunders, 1993, pp. 259–296.

Kinney, M.R., Packa, D.R., Andreoli, K.G., and Zipes, D.P.: Comprehensive Cardiac Care, 7th ed. St. Louis, Mosby-Year Book, 1991.

Kisner, C., and Colby, L.A.: Therapeutic Exercise: Foundations and Techniques, 2nd ed. Philadelphia, F.A. Davis, 1990.

Lavie, D., and Savage, D.: Prevalence and clinical features of mitral valve prolapse. American Heart Journal *113*(5):1281, 1987.

Layzer, R.B.: Neuromuscular Manifestations of Systemic Disease. Philadelphia, F.A. Davis, 1985.

Majid, P.A., Cheirif, J.B., Rokey, R., Sanders, W.E., Patel, B., Zimmerman, J.L., and Dellinger, R.P.: Does cocaine cause coronary vasospasm in chronic cocaine abusers? A study of coronary and systemic hemodynamics. Clinical Cardiology *15*(4):253–258, 1992.

Massie, E., and Kleiger, R.E.: Palpitation and tachycardia. *In* Blacklow, R.S. (ed.): MacBryde's Signs and

Symptoms, 6th ed. Philadelphia, J.B. Lippincott, 1983, pp. 295–315.

Morris, D.C., Hurst, J.W., and Walter, P.F.: The recognition and treatment of myocardial infarction and its complications. *In* Hurst, J.W. (ed.): The Heart, 7th ed. New York: McGraw-Hill, 1990.

Nicol, N.H.: Nursing care of clients with integumentary disorders. *In* Black, J.M., and Matassarin-Jacobs, E. (eds.): Luckmann and Sorensen's Medical-Surgical Nursing, 4th ed. Philadelphia, W.B. Saunders, 1993, pp. 1955–1984.

Nishina, P.M., Johnson, J.P., Naggert, J.K., and Krauss, R.M.: Linkage of atherogenic lipoprotein phenotype to the low density lipoprotein receptor locus on the short arm of chromosome 19. Proceedings of the National Academy of Science USA *89*(2):708–712, 1992.

Odio, A.: The incidence of acute rheumatic fever in a suburban area of Los Angeles: A ten-year study. Western Journal of Medicine *144*:179–184, 1986.

O'Toole, M. (ed.): Miller-Keane Encyclopedia and Dictionary of Medicine, Nursing and Allied Health, 5th ed. Philadelphia, W.B. Saunders, 1992.

Ott, B.: Structure and function of the cardiovascular system. *In* Black, J.M., and Matassarin-Jacobs, E. (eds.): Luckmann and Sorensen's Medical-Surgical Nursing, 4th ed. Philadelphia, W.B. Saunders, 1993a, pp. 1091–1104.

Ott, B.: Nursing care of clients with cardiac structure disorders. *In* Black, J.M., and Matassarin-Jacobs, E. (eds.): Luckmann and Sorensen's Medical-Surgical Nursing, 4th ed. Philadelphia, W.B. Saunders, 1993b, pp. 1211–1252.

Posner, B.M., Cupples, L.A., Miller, D.R., Cobb, J.L., Lutz, K.J., and D'Agostino, R.B.: Diet, menopause, and serum cholesterol levels in women: The Framingham study. American Heart Journal *125*(2 Pt 1):483–489, 1993.

Reigle, J., and Ringel, K.A.: Nursing care of clients with disorders of cardiac function. *In* Black, J.M., and Matassarin-Jacobs, E. (eds.): Luckmann and Sorensen's Medical-Surgical Nursing, 4th ed. Philadelphia, W.B. Saunders, 1993, pp. 1139–1194.

Smith, R.B.: Neuromuscular-skeletal causes of chest discomfort: Thoracic outlet syndrome. *In* Hurst, J.W. (ed.): The Heart. New York, McGraw-Hill, 1990, pp. 992–993.

Sokolow, M., McIlroy, M.B., and Cheitlin, M.D.: Clinical Cardiology, 5th ed. Norwalk, Connecticut, Appleton and Lange, 1990.

Stevens, M.B., and Ziminski, C.M.: Heart disease in systemic lupus erythematosus. Journal of Musculoskeletal Medicine *9*(6):41–46, 1992.

Stewart, S.L.: Acute MI: A review of pathophysiology, treatment and complications. Journal of Cardiovascular Nursing *6*(4):1–25, 1992.

Stokes, J.: Cardiovascular risk factors. Cardiovascular Clinics *20*(3):3–20, 1990.

Tas, J.: Genetic predisposition to coronary heart disease and gene for apolipoprotein CIII. Lancet *337*(8733):113–114, 1991.

Travell, J.G., and Simons, D.G.: Myofascial Pain and Dysfunction: The Trigger Point Manual. Vol. 1. Baltimore, Williams & Wilkins, 1983.

Urden, L., Davie, J., and Thelan, L.: Essentials of Critical Care Nursing. St. Louis, Mosby-Year Book, 1992.

Veasy, L.G., Wiedmeier, S.E., Orsmond, G.S., et al.: Resurgence of acute rheumatic fever in the intermountain area of the United States. New England Journal of Medicine *316*:421–427, 1987.

Wald, E.R., Dashefsky, B., Feidt, C., et al.: Acute rheumatic fever in Western Pennsylvania and the Tristate Area. Pediatrics *80*:371–374, 1987.

Waller, B.F.: Atherosclerotic and nonatherosclerotic coronary artery factors in acute myocardial infarction. Cardiovascular Clinics *20*(1):29–104, 1989.

Walsh, M.E.: Management of persons with peripheral vascular problems. *In* Phipps, W., Long, B., Woods, N., and Cassmeyer, V. (eds.): Medical-Surgical Nursing, Concepts and Clinical Practice, 4th ed. St. Louis, Mosby-Year Book, 1991, pp. 737–774.

Wechsler, R.: Diabetes and Heart Disease. The Juvenile Diabetes Foundation International Countdown New York, Winter 1991, pp. 15–22.

Williams, R.C.: Recognizing and managing rheumatic fever in the 90s. Journal of Musculoskeletal Medicine *8*(4):18–27, 1991.

Wyngaarden, J.B., et al.: Cecil Textbook of Medicine, 19th ed. Philadelphia, W.B. Saunders, 1992.

Bibliography

Braunwald, E. (ed.): Heart Disease: A Textbook of Cardiovascular Medicine, 4th ed. Philadelphia, W.B. Saunders, 1992.

Irwin, S., and Tecklin, J.S.: Cardiopulmonary Physical Therapy, 2nd ed. St. Louis, C.V. Mosby, 1990.

Kaplan, N.M.: Clinical Hypertension, 5th ed. Baltimore, Williams & Wilkins, 1991.

Silver, M.D. (ed.): Cardiovascular Pathology, 2nd ed. Vols. 1 and 2. New York, Churchill Livingstone, 1991.

Strandness, D.E. (ed.): Peripheral Vascular Diseases: Current Research and Clinical Applications. Philadelphia, W.B. Saunders, 1987.

Appendix
Common Cardiovascular Medications

Medications	Indications/Side Effects
Trade/Generic Names	* = *Call doctor when possible* ** = *Call doctor immediately*
ACE Inhibitors	To treat high blood pressure and heart failure; prevent constriction of blood vessels and the retention of sodium and fluid. *Side Effects:* Cough, skin rash, loss of taste, weakness, headaches *palpitations, swelling of feet or abdomen **dizziness, fainting

Alpha-Blockers
  Capoten/captopril
  Lotensin/benazepril
  Vasotec/enalapril maleate
	To lower blood pressure by dilating blood vessels.
	
	Side Effects: Headache, palpitations, fatigue, nausea, weakness and drowsiness
	*palpitations
	**dizziness, fainting

Antiarrhythmics
  Cardioquin/quinidine
  Procan/procainamide
    hydrochloride
  Rhythmol/propafenone
    hydrochloride
	To alter conduction patterns in the heart.
	
	Side Effects: Nausea, palpitations, vomiting
	*rash
	*insomnia
	**dizziness
	**symptoms of congestive heart failure (shortness of breath, swollen ankles, coughing up blood)

Anticoagulants
  Coumadin/warfarin sodium
  Platelet inhibitors
  Asplrln
  Persantine/dipyridamole
	To prevent blood clot formation.
	
	Side Effects: Easy bruising
	*stomach irritation (aspirin and persantine)
	**joint or abdominal pain
	**difficulty in breathing or swallowing
	**paralysis
	**unexplained swelling, unusual or uncontrolled bleeding

Antihypertensives
  Aldomet/methyldopa
  Catapres/clonidine
  Wytensin/guanabenz acetate
	To lower high blood pressure by dilating the blood vessels.
	
	Side Effects: Drowsiness, depression, sexual dysfunction, fatigue, dry mouth, stuffy nose, fever, upset stomach, change in bowel habits, weight gain and fluid retention
	**dizziness

Beta-Blockers
  Inderal/propranolol hydrochloride
  Lopressor/metoprolol tartrate
  Tenormin/atenolol
	To block sympathetic conduction at beta-receptors and decrease blood pressure, dysrhythmias, and angina.
	
	Side Effects: Insomnia, nausea, fatigue, slow pulse, weakness, increased cholesterol and blood sugar levels
	*nightmares
	*sexual dysfunction
	**asthmatic attacks
	**dizziness

Medications	Indications/Side Effects
Calcium Channel Blockers Procardia/nifedipine Cardizem/diltiazem hydrochloride	To dilate coronary arteries to lower blood pressure and suppress some dysrhythmias. *Side Effects:* Fluid retention, palpitations, headache, flushes *rash **dizziness
Digitalis Compounds Lanoxin/digoxin Crystodigin/digitoxin	To strengthen the heart's pumping force and decrease electrical conduction. *Side Effects:* Fatigue, weakness, headache, irregular heart rhythms, nausea, vomiting **bradycardia
Diuretics *THIAZIDE DIURETICS* (e.g., Diuril/chlorothiazide) *POTASSIUM-SPARING DIURETICS* (e.g., Aldactone/spironolactone) *LOOP DIURETICS* (e.g., Lasix/furosemide)	To increase the excretion of sodium and water and control high blood pressure and fluid retention. *Side Effects:* Drowsiness, dehydration, electrolyte imbalances, gout, nausea, pain, hearing loss, blood sugar abnormalities, elevated cholesterol and lipoprotein levels *muscle cramps **dizziness, light-headness
Lipid-Lowering Drugs Lopid/gemfibrozil Mevacor/lovastatin Questran/cholestyramine Zocor/simvastatin Nia-Bid, Niacor, Nicobid/niacin	To interfere with the metabolism of blood fats in various ways by lowering cholesterol, low-density lipoproteins, and/or triglyceride levels in the blood. *Side Effects:* Nausea, vomiting, diarrhea, constipation, flatulence, and abdominal discomfort
Nitrates Nitrostat, Nitro-bid/nitroglycerin Iso-Bid, Isodril/isosorbide dinitrate	For dilation of coronary arteries. *Side Effects:* Headache, dizziness *orthostatic hypotension *tachycardia
Vasodilators Apresoline/hydralazine hydrochloride Loniten/minoxidil	To dilate the peripheral blood vessels (used in combination with diuretics). *Side Effects:* Headache, drowsiness, nausea, vomiting, diarrhea, hair growth (minoxidil only) *increased heart rate *swollen ankles **dizziness **difficulty in breathing

4

Overview of Pulmonary Signs and Symptoms

■ ■ ■ ■ ■ ■ ■ ■ ■ ■ ■

Clinical Signs and Symptoms of:

Respiratory Acidosis
Respiratory Alkalosis
Acute Bronchitis
Chronic Bronchitis
Emphysema
Asthma
Pneumonia
Bronchiectasis
Tuberculosis
Systemic Sclerosis Lung Disease
Lung Cancer
Paraneoplastic Syndrome

Brain Metastasis
Metastasis to the Spinal Cord
Cystic Fibrosis
Pulmonary Involvement in Cystic Fibrosis
Occupational Lung Diseases
Deep Venous Thrombosis
Pulmonary Embolism
Cor Pulmonale
Pleurisy
Spontaneous Pneumothorax

Pulmonary pain patterns are usually localized in the substernal or chest region over involved lung fields that may include the anterior chest, side, or back. However, pulmonary pain can radiate to the neck, upper trapezius, costal margins, thoracic back, scapulae, or shoulder. Shoulder pain may radiate along the medial aspect of the arm, mimicking other neuromuscular causes of neck or shoulder pain. Pulmonary pain usually increases with inspiratory movements, such as laughing, coughing, sneezing, or deep breathing, and the client notes the presence of associated symptoms, such as dyspnea (exertional or at rest), persistent cough, fever, and chills.

For the client presenting with neck, shoulder, or back pain, it may be necessary to consider the possibility of a pulmonary cause requiring medical referral. The material in this chapter will assist the physical therapist in treating both the client with a known pulmonary problem and the client presenting with musculoskeletal signs and symptoms that may have an underlying systemic basis (see Case Example).

147

Case Example. A 67-year-old woman with a known diagnosis of rheumatoid arthritis has been treated as needed in a physical therapy clinic for the last 8 years. She has reported occasional chest pain described as "coming on suddenly, like a knife pushing from the inside out—it takes my breath away." She missed 2 days of treatment because of illness, and when she returned to the clinic, the physical therapist noticed that she had a newly developed cough and that her rheumatoid arthritis was much worse. She says that she missed her appointments because she had the "flu."

Further questioning to elicit the potential development of chest pain on inspiration, the presence of ongoing fever and chills, and the changes in breathing pattern is recommended. Positive findings beyond the reasonable duration of influenza (7 to 10 days) or an increase in pulmonary symptoms (shortness of breath, hacking cough, hemoptysis, wheezing or other change in breathing pattern) raises a red flag indicating the need for medical referral. This clinical case points out that clients currently undergoing physical therapy for a known musculoskeletal problem may be describing signs and symptoms of systemic disease.

In the case of pleuropulmonary disorders, the client's recent personal medical history may include a previous or recurrent upper respiratory infection, or pneumonia. Central nervous system (CNS) symptoms, such as muscle weakness, muscle atrophy, headache, loss of lower extremity sensation, and localized or radicular back pain may be associated with lung cancer and must be investigated by a physician for diagnosis.

PULMONARY PHYSIOLOGY

The primary function of the respiratory system is to provide oxygen to and to remove carbon dioxide from cells in the body. The act of breathing, in which the oxygen and carbon dioxide exchange occurs, involves the two interrelated processes of ventilation and respiration. Ventilation is the movement of air from outside the body to the alveoli of the lungs. Respiration is the process of oxygen uptake and carbon dioxide elimination between the body and the outside environment (Guyton, 1992).

The structures involved in breathing are divided into two main categories—upper airway and lower airway. The upper airway consists of the nose, sinuses, pharynx, tonsils, and larynx, and the lower airway consists of the conducting airways (trachea, right and left main stem bronchi) and respiratory units (respiratory bronchioles, alveolar ducts, and alveoli). The structures of the upper airway function to warm, moisten, and filter the air that enters the lungs.

The larynx forms the upper portion of the trachea and consists of several cartilaginous structures held together by muscles and ligaments. The chief functions of the larynx are to serve as an airway between the trachea and pharynx and to protect the vocal cords. The epiglottis, a leaf-shaped lid of fibrocartilage, closes the entrance to the larynx during swallowing so that food and fluid are not aspirated (inhaled) into the trachea. The closing of the entrance into the trachea (glottis) also allows for an increase in intrathoracic pressure needed for lifting and coughing (Guyton, 1992).

The conducting airway structures have three primary functions: filtering, warming, and humidifying air. Air inspired through a normal respiratory tree is filtered of all particles before reaching the alveoli. This filtration occurs because goblet cells in the epithelial layer of the airways secrete copious amounts of mucus that coat the airways and trap foreign particles. In addition, cilia, which are found as far into the respiratory tree as the bronchi, then propel the mucus up the airway so that the foreign material can be removed by coughing, sneezing, or swallowing.

Respiration occurs within the alveoli (minute sacs that arise from the walls of the respiratory bronchioles) and within the alveolar ducts. The alveoli consist of a single layer of squamous epithelium and an elastic basement membrane. These two layers in conjunction with the layers of capillary endothelium form the alveolar-capillary membrane across which diffusion of oxygen and carbon dioxide occurs. The alveoli, in addition to functioning in respiration, produce surfactant, which is a substance that prevents lung collapse.

The right lung is divided into three lobes: upper, middle, and lower; the left lung has only two lobes: upper and lower. The right bronchus (airway leading to the lung) is wide and short and extends from the trachea at a straighter angle than does the left bronchus. The left bronchus is narrower and lies at more of an angle from the trachea (Guyton, 1992).

The lungs lie in and are protected by the thoracic cavity, which consists of the sternum and ribs anteriorly, and the ribs, scapulae, and vertebral column posteriorly. The thoracic cavity is lined with pleura, or serous membrane. One surface of the pleura lines the inside of the rib cage (parietal pleura), and the other surface, the visceral pleura, covers the lungs (Guyton, 1992).

Pulmonary Ventilation

Air moves in and out of the lungs as a result of changes in pressure. At the beginning of inspiration, the atmospheric air pressure is greater than alveolar pressure, so air moves into the alveoli. When the alveolar pressure is greater than atmospheric pressure, expiration occurs and air moves out of the lungs. The pressure gradient between the atmosphere and the alveoli is created by changes in the size of the thoracic cavity. As the thorax increases in size, pressure in the thorax decreases and air flows in from the atmosphere. The size of the thorax increases by contraction of the diaphragm and the external intercostal muscles. As the thorax expands, it pulls the lungs with it because the moist surfaces of the lungs and chest wall are bound together. Expiration is a passive process that is caused by the elastic recoil of the lungs and thoracic muscles (Guyton, 1992).

Gas Movement

Oxygen diffuses across the alveolar-capillary membrane from the alveoli into the blood because the pressure of oxygen of the alveolar air is greater than that of venous blood. Carbon dioxide diffuses in the opposite direction because the pressure of carbon dioxide in the venous blood is greater than the pressure of carbon dioxide in the alveolar air. Diffusion of oxygen can be decreased by the following factors (Guyton, 1992):

- Decreased atmospheric oxygen
- Decreased alveolar ventilation
- Decreased alveolar-capillary surface area
- Increased alveolar-capillary membrane thickness

Breathing is an automatic process by which sensors detecting changes in the levels of carbon dioxide continuously direct data to the medulla. The medulla then directs respiratory muscles that adjust ventilation. Breathing patterns can be altered voluntarily when this automatic response is overridden by conscious thought. The major sensors mentioned here are the central chemoreceptors (located near the medulla) and the peripheral sensors (located in the carotid body and aortic arch). The central chemoreceptors respond to increases in carbon dioxide and decreases in pH in cerebrospinal fluid. As carbon dioxide increases, the medulla signals a response to increase respiration. The peripheral chemoreceptor system responds to low arterial blood oxygen and is believed to function only in pathologic situations, such as when there are chronically elevated carbon dioxide levels (e.g., chronic obstructive pulmonary disease [COPD]).

ACID-BASE REGULATION

The proper balance of acids and bases in the body is essential to life. This balance is very complex and must be kept within the

Table 4–1

LABORATORY VALUES: UNCOMPENSATED AND COMPENSATED RESPIRATORY ACIDOSIS AND ALKALOSIS

	Normal pH Level	Normal pCO_2 Level	Normal HCO_3 Level
Arterial Blood	pH (7.35–7.45)	pCO_2 (35–45 mm Hg)	HCO_3 (22–26 mEq/L)
Respiratory Acidosis—Uncompensated	<7.35	>45	Normal
Compensated	Normal	>45	>26
Respiratory Alkalosis—Uncompensated	>7.45	<35	Normal
Compensated	Normal	<35	<22

narrow parameters of a pH of 7.35 to 7.45 in the extracellular fluid (Table 4–1). This number (or pH value) represents the *hydrogen ion* concentration in body fluid. A reading of less than 7.35 is considered "acidosis," and a reading greater than 7.45 is called "alkalosis." Life cannot be sustained if the pH values are less than 7.0 or greater than 7.8 (Lehman, 1991).

There are two ways in which hydrogen ions (or acids) circulate throughout the body:

■ Volatile hydrogen of carbonic acid

■ Nonvolatile hydrogen in organic acids, such as lactic, sulfuric, pyruvic, and phosphoric acids

Normal body metabolism results in the production of many of these acids. The lungs excrete a large amount of the *volatile* hydrogen in the carbonic acid as carbon dioxide (CO_2) and water (H_2O), and the lungs excrete a smaller amount of the *nonvolatile* acids (Lehman, 1991).

Living human cells are extremely sensitive to alterations in body fluid pH (hydrogen ion concentration); thus various mechanisms are in operation to keep the pH at a relatively constant level. Acid-base regulatory mechanisms include chemical buffer systems, the respiratory system, and the renal system. These systems interact very closely to maintain a normal acid-base ratio of 20 parts of bicarbonate to 1 part of carbonic acid and thus to maintain normal body fluid pH.

The carbonic acid/bicarbonate system is the primary extracellular fluid (ECF) chemical buffer system. This system responds immediately to changes in extracellular fluid pH. Carbonic acid is formed by the combination of CO_2 and H_2O. When a strong base is added to body fluids, it is buffered by carbonic acid. When a strong acid is added to the system, a bicarbonate buffer changes it to a salt and carbonic acid. The carbonic acid then further dissociates into CO_2 and H_2O and is excreted by the lungs.

The respiratory control center in the brain responds to increases in CO_2 and hydrogen ions in the body fluids by increasing or decreasing the rate and depth of respiration. When the body pH decreases or becomes more acid, respiratory rate and depth increase so that the lungs can increase the breakdown of carbonic acid to CO_2 and H_2O and can then exhale both the CO_2 and hydrogen. With increased respiratory rate, less CO_2 is available for the formation of carbonic acid. Conversely, when the pH rises or becomes more alkaline, the rate and depth of respiration decrease so that CO_2 is retained and more carbonic acid is formed.

However, long-term correction of acid-base disturbances is controlled by the renal excretion of hydrogen and by the renal production of bicarbonate. Even though this mechanism occurs more slowly (in hours to days) than buffer (immediately) or respiratory changes (in minutes to hours), renal action is more thorough and selective than is that of the other acid-base regulators. The primary mechanism of renal control in acid-base balance is the

Table 4–2
ARTERIAL BLOOD GAS VALUES

pH	7.35–7.45
pCO_2 (partial pressure of carbon dioxide)	35–45 mm Hg
HCO_3 (bicarbonate ion)	22–26 mEq/L
pO_2 (partial pressure of oxygen)	80–100 mm Hg
O_2 saturation (oxygen saturation)	95%–100%
Critical Values	
pH	<7.25 or >7.55
pCO_2	<20 or >60 mm Hg
HCO_3	<15 or >40 mEq/L
pO_2	<40 mm Hg
O_2 saturation	<75%

Adapted from Pagana, D., and Pagana, T.: Mosby's Diagnostic and Laboratory Test Reference. St. Louis, Mosby–Year Book, 1992, p. 104.

increase or decrease in the production of bicarbonate.

The blood test used most often to measure the effectiveness of ventilation and oxygen transport is the arterial blood gas (ABG) test (Table 4–2). The measurement of arterial blood gases is important in the diagnosis and treatment of ventilation, oxygen transport, and acid-base problems. The arterial blood gas test measures the amount of dissolved oxygen and carbon dioxide in arterial blood and indicates acid-base status by measurement of the arterial blood pH.

The pH is inversely proportional to the hydrogen ion concentration in the blood. Therefore, as the hydrogen ion concentration increases (acidosis), the pH decreases, and as the hydrogen ion concentration decreases (alkalosis), the pH increases.

The pCO_2 is a measure of the partial pressure of carbon dioxide in the blood. pCO_2 is termed the respiratory component in acid-base measurement, since the carbon dioxide level is primarily controlled by the lungs. As the carbon dioxide level increases, the pH decreases (respiratory acidosis), and as the carbon dioxide level

decreases, the pH increases (respiratory alkalosis) (Pagana and Pagana, 1992).

The bicarbonate ion (HCO_3) is a measure of the metabolic portion of acid-base function that involves the renal excretion of acid or the renal production of base (which is HCO_3). As the bicarbonate value increases, the pH increases (metabolic acidosis), and as the bicarbonate value decreases, the pH decreases (metabolic acidosis).

The pO_2 is a measure of the partial pressure of oxygen in the blood and represents the status of alveolar gas exchange. Oxygen saturation (O_2 sat.) is an indication of the percentage of hemoglobin saturated with oxygen. When 95 per cent to 100 per cent of the hemoglobin binds and carries oxygen, the tissues are adequately perfused with oxygen. As the pO_2 level decreases, the percentage of hemoglobin saturation also decreases. When the pO_2 level drops significantly (less than 60 mm Hg), small decreases in the pO_2 level will cause large decreases in the percentage of hemoglobin saturated with oxygen. At oxygen saturation levels of less than 70 per cent, the tissues are unable to carry out vital functions (Pagana and Pagana, 1992).

Respiratory Acidosis

Any condition that decreases pulmonary ventilation increases the retention and concentration of CO_2, hydrogen, and carbonic acid; this results in an increase in the amount of circulating hydrogen and is called respiratory acidosis. If ventilation is severely compromised, CO_2 levels become extremely high and respiration is depressed even further, causing hypoxia as well. During respiratory acidosis, potassium moves out of cells into the extracellular fluid to exchange with circulating hydrogen. This results in hyperkalemia (abnormally high potassium concentration in the blood) and cardiac changes that can cause cardiac arrest.

Respiratory acidosis can result from

▼ *Clinical Signs and Symptoms of*
Respiratory Acidosis

- Decreased ventilation
- Confusion
- Sleepiness and unconsciousness
- Diaphoresis
- Shallow rapid breathing
- Restlessness
- Cyanosis

▼ *Clinical Signs and Symptoms of*
Respiratory Alkalosis

- Lightheadedness
- Dizziness
- Numbness and tingling of the face, fingers, and toes
- Syncope (fainting)

pathologies that decrease the efficiency of the respiratory system. These pathologies can include damage to the medulla, which controls respiration, obstruction of airways (e.g., neoplasm, foreign bodies, pulmonary disease such as COPD, pneumonia), loss of lung surface ventilation (e.g., pneumothorax, pulmonary fibrosis), weakness of respiratory muscles (e.g., poliomyelitis, spinal cord injury, Guillain-Barré syndrome), or overdose of respiratory depressant drugs (Lehman, 1991).

As hypoxia becomes more severe, diaphoresis, shallow rapid breathing, restlessness, and cyanosis may appear. Cardiac arrhythmias may also be present as the potassium level in the blood serum rises.

Treatment is directed at restoration of efficient ventilation. If the respiratory depression and acidosis are severe, injection of intravenous sodium bicarbonate and use of a mechanical ventilator may be necessary. Any client with symptoms of inadequate ventilation or CO_2 retention needs immediate medical referral.

Respiratory Alkalosis

Increasesd respiratory rate and depth decrease the amount of available CO_2 and hydrogen and create a condition of increased pH, or alkalosis. By increasing pulmonary ventilation, CO_2 and hydrogen are eliminated from the body too quickly and are not available to buffer the increasingly alkaline environment.

Respiratory alkalosis is usually due to *hyperventilation*. Rapid, deep respirations are often caused by neurogenic or psychogenic problems, including anxiety, pain, and cerebral trauma or lesions. Other causes can be related to conditions that greatly increase metabolism (e.g., hyperthyroidism) or overventilation of patients with a mechanical ventilator (Lehman, 1991).

If the alkalosis becomes more severe, muscular tetany and convulsions can occur. Cardiac arrhythmias due to serum potassium loss through the kidneys may also occur. The kidneys keep hydrogen in exchange for potassium.

Treatment of respiratory alkalosis includes reassurance, assistance in slowing breathing and facilitating relaxation, sedation, pain control, CO_2 administration, and use of a rebreathing device such as a rebreathing mask or paper bag. A rebreathing device allows the patient to inhale and "rebreathe" the exhaled CO_2 (Lehman, 1991).

Respiratory alkalosis related to hyperventilation is a relatively common condition and might be present more often in the physical therapy setting than is respiratory acidosis. Pain and anxiety are common causes of hyperventilation, and treatment needs to be focused toward reduction

Table 4–3
RESPIRATORY DISEASES: SUMMARY OF DIFFERENCES

Disease	Primary Area Affected	Result
Bronchitis	Membrane lining bronchial tubes	Inflammation of lining
Bronchiectasis	Bronchial tubes (bronchi or air passages)	Bronchial dilation with inflammation
Pneumonia	Alveoli (air sacs)	Causative agent invades alveoli with resultant outpouring from lung capillaries into air spaces and continued healing process
Emphysema	Air spaces beyond terminal bronchioles (alveoli)	Breakdown of alveolar walls Air spaces enlarged
Asthma	Bronchioles (small airways)	Bronchioles obstructed by muscle spasm, swelling of mucosa, thick secretions
Cystic fibrosis	Bronchioles	Bronchioles become obstructed and obliterated. Later, larger airways become involved. Plugs of mucus cling to airway walls, leading to bronchitis, bronchiectasis, atelectasis, pneumonia, or pulmonary abscess

of both these interrelated elements. If hyperventilation continues in the absence of pain or anxiety, serious systemic problems may be the cause, and immediate physician referral is necessary.

If either respiratory acidosis or alkalosis persists for hours to days in a chronic, not life-threatening manner, the kidneys then begin to assist in the restoration of normal body fluid pH by selective excretion or retention of hydrogen ions or bicarbonate. This process is called "renal compensation." When the kidneys compensate effectively, blood pH values are within normal limits (7.35 to 7.45) even though the underlying problem may still cause the respiratory imbalance.

PULMONARY PATHOPHYSIOLOGY

Chronic Obstructive Pulmonary Disease

COPD, also called chronic obstructive lung disease (COLD), refers to a number of disorders that affect movement of air in and out of the lungs. The most important of these disorders are obstructive bronchitis, emphysema, and asthma. Although bronchitis, emphysema, and asthma may occur in a "pure form," they most commonly coexist. Although the term COPD is commonly used, specialists in pulmonary medicine believe it is not completely accurate, and the term *chronic airflow limitation (CAL)* may be used in its place (Cronin, 1993).

Factors predisposing to COPD include cigarette smoking, air pollution, occupational exposure to irritating dusts or gases, hereditary factors, infection, allergies, aging, and potentially harmful drugs and chemicals. COPD rarely occurs in nonsmokers. Air pollution, combined with the effects of cigarette smoking, exacerbates COPD by inducing bronchospasm and mucosal edema, which in turn increase airway resistance (Cronin, 1993).

In all forms of COPD, narrowing of the airways obstructs airflow to and from the lungs (Table 4–3). This narrowing impairs ventilation by trapping air in the bronchioles and alveoli. The obstruction increases the resistance to airflow. Trapped air hinders normal gas exchange and causes distention of the alveoli. Other mechanisms of COPD vary with each form of the disease.

Bronchitis

Acute. Acute bronchitis is an inflammation of the trachea and bronchi (tracheobronchial tree) that is self-limiting and of short duration with few pulmonary signs. Acute bronchitis may result from chemical irritation (e.g., smoke, fumes, gas) or may occur with viral infections such as influenza, measles, chickenpox, or whooping cough. These predisposing conditions may become apparent during the subjective examination (i.e., Personal/Family History form or the Physical Therapy Interview). Although bronchitis is usually mild, it can become complicated in elderly clients and in clients with chronic lung or heart disease. Pneumonia is a critical complication (Berkow and Fletcher, 1992).

Treatment. Treatment is symptomatic, involving cough suppressants, rest, and hydration (Liles and Ramsey, 1993).

Chronic. Chronic bronchitis is a condition associated with prolonged exposure to nonspecific bronchial irritants and is accompanied by mucus hypersecretion and by structural changes in the bronchi (large air passages leading into the lungs) (Berkow and Fletcher, 1992). This irritation of the tissue usually results from exposure to cigarette smoke, long-term inhalation of dust, or air pollution and causes hypertrophy of mucus-producing cells in the

▼ *Clinical Signs and Symptoms of*
Acute Bronchitis

- Mild fever from 1 to 3 days
- Malaise
- Back and muscle pain
- Sore throat
- Cough with sputum production, followed by wheezing
- Possibly laryngitis

▼ *Clinical Signs and Symptoms of*
Chronic Bronchitis

- Persistent cough with production of sputum (worse in the morning and evening than at midday)
- Reduced chest expansion
- Wheezing
- Fever
- Dyspnea (shortness of breath)
- Cyanosis (blue discoloration of skin and mucous membranes)
- Decreased exercise tolerance

bronchi. The swollen mucous membrane and thick sputum obstruct the airways, causing wheezing, and the client develops a cough to clear the airways. The clinical definition of a person with chronic bronchitis is anyone who coughs for at least 3 months per year for 2 consecutive years without having had a precipitating disease.

In bronchitis, partial or complete blockage of the airways from mucous secretions causes insufficient oxygenation in the alveoli. This combination of cyanosis from insufficient arterial oxygenation and edema from ventricular failure may result in the person known as a "blue bloater" (Fig. 4–1).

Diagnosis, Treatment, and Prognosis. To confirm that the condition is chronic bronchitis, tests are performed to determine whether the airways are obstructed and to exclude other diseases that may cause similar symptoms, such as silicosis, tuberculosis, or a tumor in the upper airway. Sputum samples will be analyzed, and lung function tests may be performed.

Treatment is aimed at keeping the airways as clear as possible. Smokers are encouraged and helped to stop smoking. A

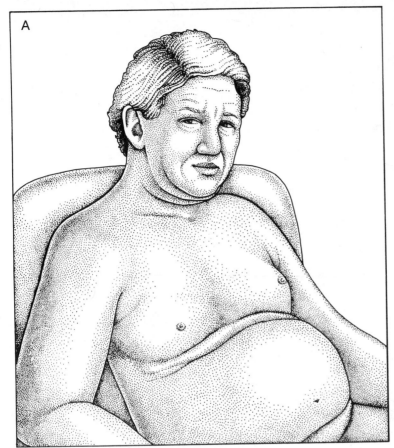

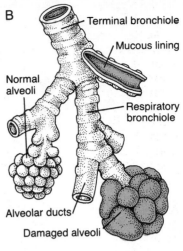

Figure 4–1

A, The client with chronic bronchitis may develop cyanosis and pulmonary edema, which cause a characteristic look, the "blue bloater." *B*, Chronic bronchitis may lead to the formation of misshapen or large alveolar sacs with reduced space for oxygen and carbon dioxide exchange.

combination of drugs may be prescribed to relieve the symptoms, including bronchodilators to open the obstructed airways and to thin the obstructive mucus so that it can be coughed up more easily.

Chronic bronchitis may develop slowly over a period of years, but it will not go away untreated. Eventually, the bronchial walls thicken, and the number of mucus glands increases. The client is increasingly susceptible to respiratory infections, during which the bronchial tissue becomes inflamed and the mucus becomes even thicker and more profuse. Antibiotics may be prescribed when the person with chronic bronchitis develops a secondary bacterial respiratory infection. Chronic bronchitis can be incapacitating and lead

to more serious and potentially fatal lung disease. Influenza and pneumococcal vaccines are recommended for these clients (Liles and Ramsey, 1993).

Emphysema (Cronin, 1993)

Emphysema may develop in a person after a long history of chronic bronchitis in which the alveolar walls are destroyed, which leads to permanent overdistention of the air spaces. Air passages are obstructed as a result of these changes (rather than as a result of mucus production, as in chronic bronchitis). Difficult expiration in emphysema is due to the destruction of the walls

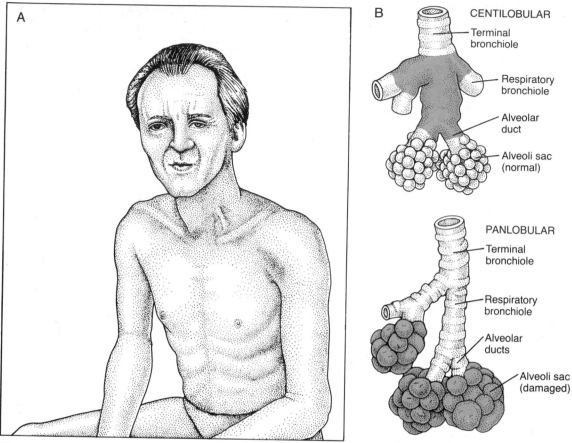

Figure 4–2

A, Emphysema traps air in the lungs, so that expelling air becomes increasingly difficult. The resultant physical features cause the client to be referred to as a "pink puffer." *B,* Centrilobular emphysema affects the upper airways and produces destructive changes in the bronchioles. Panlobular emphysema affects the lower airways and is more diffusely scattered throughout the alveoli.

(septa) between the alveoli, partial airway collapse, and loss of elastic recoil.

As the alveoli and septa collapse, pockets of air form between the alveolar spaces (called blebs) and within the lung parenchyma (called bullae). This process leads to increased ventilatory "dead space," or areas that do not participate in gas or blood exchange. The work of breathing is increased because there is less functional lung tissue to exchange oxygen and carbon dioxide. Emphysema also causes destruction of the pulmonary capillaries, further decreasing oxygen perfusion and ventilation.

There are three types of emphysema. *Centrilobular* emphysema (Fig. 4–2), the most common type, destroys the bronchioles, usually in the upper lung regions. Inflammation develops in the bronchioles, but usually the alveolar sac remains intact. *Panlobular* emphysema destroys the more distal alveolar walls, most commonly involving the lower lung. This destruction of alveolar walls may occur secondary to infection or to irritants (most commonly, cigarette smoke). These two forms of emphysema, collectively called centriacinar emphysema, occur most often in smokers. *Paraseptal* (or panacinar) emphysema destroys the alveoli in the lower lobes of the lungs, resulting in isolated blebs along the lung periphery. Paraseptal emphysema is believed to be the likely cause of spontaneous pneumothorax.

Clinical Signs and Symptoms. The irreversible destruction reduces elasticity of the lungs and increases the effort to exhale trapped air, causing marked dyspnea on exertion that later progresses to dyspnea at rest. Cough is uncommon. The client is often thin, has tachypnea with prolonged expiration, and uses the accessory muscles for respiration. The client often leans forward with the arms braced on the knees to support the shoulders and chest for breathing. The combined effects of trapped air and alveolar distention change the size and shape of the client's chest, causing a barrel chest and increased expiratory effort. The client is known as a "pink puffer" (see Fig. 4–2).

Prognosis and Treatment. As the disease progresses, there is a loss of surface area available for gas exchange. In the final stages of emphysema, cardiac complications, especially enlargement and dilatation of the right ventricle, may develop (O'Toole, 1992). The overloaded heart reaches its limit of muscular compensation and begins to fail (cor pulmonale).

The most important factor in the treatment of emphysema is cessation of smoking. The main goals for the client with emphysema are to improve oxygenation and decrease carbon dioxide retention. Pursed-lip breathing causes resistance to outflow at the lips, which in turn maintains intrabronchial pressure and improves the mixing of gases in the lungs. This type of breathing should be encouraged to help the client get rid of the stale air trapped in the lungs. Exercise will not improve pulmonary function but is used to enhance cardiovascular fitness and train skeletal muscles to function more effectively. Routine,

▼ **Clinical Signs and Symptoms of**

Emphysema

- Shortness of breath
- Dyspnea on exertion
- Orthopnea (only able to breathe in the upright position) immediately after assuming the supine position
- Chronic cough
- Barrel chest
- Weight loss
- Malaise
- Use of accessory muscles of respiration
- Prolonged expiratory period (with grunting)
- Wheezing
- Pursed-lip breathing
- Increased respiratory rate
- Peripheral cyanosis

progressive walking is the most common form of exercise.

Inflammatory/Infectious Disease

Asthma (Cronin, 1993)

Asthma is a medical term that comes from the Greek word for "panting" and means shortness of breath (Gershwin and Klingelhofer, 1992). It is a disorder of the bronchial airways, characterized by periods of bronchospasms (spasms of prolonged contraction of the airway) that are accompanied by edema (Fig. 4–3). Asthma is a complex disorder involving biochemical, immunologic, endocrine, infectious, autonomic, and psychologic factors. Respiratory symptoms can be caused by infections, hypersensitivity to irritants such as pollutants or allergens, psychologic stress, cold air, exercise, or drug use.

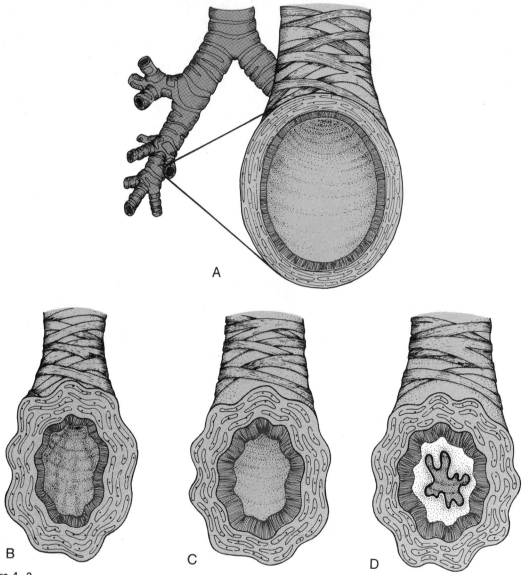

Figure 4–3

A, Cross-section of a normal bronchus, with mucous membrane in color. *B*, Bronchospasm: The smooth muscle surrounding the bronchus contracts and causes narrowing of the airway. *C*, Edema of the mucous membrane further narrows airways. *D*, Increased mucous secretion by the submucosal glands. (From Foster, R.L., Hunsberger, M.M., and Anderson, J.J.: Family-Centered Nursing Care of Children. Philadelphia, W.B. Saunders, 1989.)

Incidence. Asthma affects 2 to 3 per cent of the United States population (4 per cent of all children), and the prevalence, morbidity, and mortality of asthma are increasing in the United States (MMWR, 1990). The reason for the increase nationwide is unknown. Asthma is the most common chronic disease in children and adults. Ten to fifteen million Americans experience various degrees of asthma, from occasional bouts of shallow breathing to episodes severe enough to cause hypoxia (reduction of oxygen in body tissues) and cyanosis. According to the National Center for Health Statistics (NCHS), asthma is the leading cause of morbidity (illness resulting in loss of time at work or school) in the United States. It is found most often in urban, industrialized settings; in colder climates; and among the urban disadvantaged, especially African-Americans.

Asthma can occur at any age, although it is more likely to occur for the first time before the age of 5 years. In childhood, it is three times more common and more severe in boys; however, after puberty, the incidence in the sexes is equal. Asthma occurs in families, which indicates that it is an inherited disorder. Apparently environmental factors (e.g., viral infection) interact with inherited factors to produce disease.

Pathophysiology. Asthma may be categorized according to the precipitating cause(s): *extrinsic* bronchial asthma (or allergic asthma) refers to attacks that follow exposure to allergens, such as airborne pollens, molds, lint, dust, animal dander (skin and hair shedding), smoke, medications, foods, insect bites, and mold spores. This form of asthma usually begins in childhood. It is associated with high serum levels of the special antibody called IgE, which is a hereditary allergic mechanism, and represents a true allergic reaction.

Intrinsic bronchial asthma (nonallergic) does not have easily identifiable allergens and is triggered by many internal disorders, such as the common cold or upper respiratory infection, or even exercise. This form of asthma usually begins in adults over the age of 35 years. Clients with intrinsic asthma also may have nasal polyps and aspirin allergy (called triad disease).

Most asthmatic people have manifestations of both intrinsic and extrinsic disease. Asthma should be considered a syndrome with intrinsic, extrinsic, and occupational aspects (Mengert and Albert, 1993). Both forms of asthma can be triggered by changes in environmental temperature, strong odors (perfumed soaps and cosmetics), stress, emotion, and exercise. Physical exertion is a well-known trigger for asthma and causes exercise-induced bronchospasm (EIB). The attack typically comes a few minutes after the workout, when the body's output of adrenaline (which dilates the airways) subsides or when breathing through the mouth circulates cold, dry air through the airways. Mouth breathing causes degranulated mast cells to release bronchoconstrictive mediators inducing EIB.

In both forms of asthma, the airway is hyperreactive. Once the airway is in spasm, mucus plugs the airway, trapping distal air. Hyperventilation eventually occurs as the lung attempts to respond to the increased volume and pressure.

Clinical Signs and Symptoms. Asthma symptoms are commonly worse at night. During asthma attacks, clients are dyspneic and have marked respiratory effort. The

---

Clinical Signs and Symptoms of Asthma

Clinical signs and symptoms of asthma differ in degree (Table 4–4) and frequency among people, but the primary symptoms are

- Episodes of dyspnea
- Prolonged expiration
- Cough with or without sputum production, especially 5 to 10 minutes after exercise begins
- Skin retraction (clavicles, ribs, sternum)
- Abnormal fatigue
- Tickle in the back of the throat accompanied by a cough
- Tickle occasionally at the back of the neck
- Wheezing (advanced asthma)
- Nostril flaring (advanced)

Table 4–4

STAGES OF ASTHMA

Mild	Moderate	Severe
Symptoms reverse with cessation of activity	Audible wheezing Use of accessory muscles of respiration Leaning forward to catch breath	Blue lips/fingernails Tachypnea (30–40 breaths per minute) despite cessation of activity Cyanosis-induced seizures Skin and rib retraction

client prefers to sit upright or lean forward, using accessory muscles of respiration. Sternocleidomastoid retraction and intercostal retractions are evident during inspiration, along with nasal flaring. As the airway obstruction becomes more severe, the client may become anxious, which in turn increases the body's metabolic demands, inducing fatigue and further respiratory distress.

At the beginning of an attack, there is a sensation of chest constriction, inspiratory and expiratory wheezing, nonproductive coughing, prolonged expiration, tachycardia, and tachypnea. The severity of asthma can be classified as mild, moderate, or severe, depending on the symptoms.

Treatment and Prognosis. The effects of asthma are reversible with treatment, which has three components: environmental control, pharmacologic therapy for airflow obstruction (using beta-adrenergic agents such as bronchodilators) and inflammation, and immunotherapy. The goal in treatment is to manage acute exacerbations aggressively, minimize the number of exacerbations, and minimize the number of medications the client must take (Mays et al., 1990; Mitchell, 1992).

Physical therapists working with asthmatic clients should encourage them to maintain hydration by drinking fluids to prevent mucus plugs from hardening and to take prescribed medications (e.g., antihistamines, bronchodilators) before exercising to minimize exercise-induced asthma attacks. Exercise or hyperventilation-induced asthma can potentially be prevented by exercising in a moist, humid environment and by grading exercise per client tolerance using diaphragmatic breathing.

Complications. Status asthmaticus is a severe, life-threatening complication of asthma. With severe bronchospasm, the workload of breathing increases five to ten times, which can lead to acute cor pulmonale. When air is trapped, a severe paradoxic pulse develops as venous return is obstructed. This condition is seen as a blood pressure drop of over 10 mm Hg during inspiration.

Pneumothorax commonly develops. If status asthmaticus continues, hypoxemia worsens and acidosis begins. If the condition is untreated or not reversed, respiratory or cardiac arrest will occur. An acute asthma episode may constitute a medical emergency requiring emergency management with inhaled beta-adrenergics and intravenous theophylline and corticosteroids.

Pneumonia (Cronin, 1993)

Pneumonia is an inflammation of the lungs and can be caused by (1) aspiration of food, fluids, or vomitus; (2) inhalation of toxic or caustic chemicals, smoke, dust, or gases; or (3) a bacterial, viral, or mycoplasmal infection. It may be primary or secondary (a complication of another disease); it often follows influenza.

The common feature of all types of pneumonia is an inflammatory pulmonary response to the offending organism or agent. This response may involve one or both

Risk factors predisposing a client to pneumonia are

■ Smoking

■ Air pollution

■ Upper respiratory infection (URI)

■ Altered consciousness: alcoholism, head injury, seizure disorder, drug overdose, general anesthesia

■ Tracheal intubation

■ Prolonged immobility

■ Immunosuppressive therapy: corticosteroids, cancer chemotherapy

■ Nonfunctional immune system: AIDS

■ Severe periodontal disease

■ Prolonged exposure to virulent organisms

■ Malnutrition

■ Dehydration

■ Chronic diseases: diabetes mellitus, heart disease, chronic lung disease, renal disease, cancer

■ Prolonged debilitating disease

■ Inhalation of noxious substances

■ Aspiration of oral/gastric material

■ Aspiration of foreign materials (e.g., petroleum products)

■ Chronically ill, elderly clients who have poor immune systems, often residing in group-living situations

lungs at the level of the lobe (lobar pneumonia) or more distally beginning in the terminal bronchioles and alveoli (bronchopneumonia). Bronchopneumonia is seen more frequently than lobar pneumonia and is common in clients postoperatively and in clients with chronic bronchitis, particularly when these two situations coexist (Gaskell and Webber, 1980).

Infectious agents responsible for pneumonia are typically present in the upper respiratory tract and cause no harm unless resistance is lowered severely by some other factor, such as a severe cold, disease, alcoholism, or generally poor health (e.g., poorly controlled diabetes, chronic renal problems). Elderly or bedridden clients are particularly at risk due to physical inactivity and immobility. Limited mobility causes normal secretions to pool in the airways and facilitates bacterial growth (O'Toole, 1992).

Pneumocystis carinii is a protozoan organism rarely causing pneumonia in healthy individuals. *Pneumocystis carinii* pneumonia (PCP) has been the most common life-threatening opportunistic infection in persons with AIDS. PCP also has been shown to be the first indicator of conversion from HIV infection to the designation of AIDS in 60 per cent of individuals with HIV disease (Flaskerud and Ungvarski, 1992).

Clinical Signs and Symptoms. The onset of all pneumonias is generally marked by any of the following: fever, chills, sweats, pleuritic chest pain, cough, sputum production, hemoptysis, dyspnea, headache,

▼ *Clinical Signs and Symptoms of*

Pneumonia

■ Sudden and sharp pleuritic chest pain that is aggravated by chest movement

■ Hacking, productive cough (rust-colored or green, purulent sputum)

■ Dyspnea

■ Tachypnea (rapid respirations associated with fever or pneumonia) accompanied by decreased chest excursion on the affected side

■ Cyanosis

■ Headache

■ Fever and chills

■ Generalized aches and myalgia that may extend to the thighs and calves

■ Fatigue

or fatigue. The elderly client can have full-blown pneumonia and may present with altered mental status rather than fever or respiratory symptoms because of the changes in temperature regulation as we age.

The clinical manifestations of PCP are slow to develop; they include fever, tachypnea, tachycardia, dyspnea, nonproductive cough, and hypoxemia. A diffuse, bilateral pattern of alveolar infiltration is apparent on chest radiograph.

Treatment. The primary treatment for most forms of pneumonia is antibiotic therapy. Treatment for PCP consists of a 14-day course of trimethoprim-sulfamethoxazole (Bactrim) as the primary agent and pentamidine isethionate, recently FDA-approved for treatment of PCP. The mortality rate for PCP is about 50 per cent; if untreated, it is 100 per cent. Since such a high mortality is associated with this disease, clients at risk (e.g., clients with AIDS or hematologic malignancies) are treated prophylactically with trimethoprim-sulfamethoxazole. Aerosols of pentamidine isethionate also have shown encouraging results as a treatment option and prophylactic measure for PCP (Mitchell, 1992). Hospitalization may be required for the immunocompromised client. Otherwise, if the client has an intact defense system and good general health, recuperation can take place at home with rest and supportive treatment. In the hospital, rigorous handwashing by medical personnel is essential for reducing the transmission of infectious agents.

Bronchiectasis

Bronchiectasis is a chronic pulmonary condition that occurs after infections, such as childhood pneumonia or cystic fibrosis. Once a common disease because of measles, pertussis, tuberculosis, and poorly treated bacterial pneumonias, the prevalence of bronchiectasis has diminished greatly since the introduction of antibiot-

▼ *Clinical Signs and Symptoms of*
Bronchiectasis

Clinical signs and symptoms of bronchiectasis vary widely, depending on the extent of the disease and on the presence of complicating infection, but may include

- Chronic, "wet" cough with copious foul-smelling secretions; generally worse in the morning after the individual has been recumbent for a length of time
- Hemoptysis (bloody sputum)
- Occasional wheezing sounds
- Dyspnea
- Sinusitis (inflammation of one or more paranasal sinuses)
- Weight loss
- Anemia
- Malaise
- Recurrent fever and chills
- Fatigue

ics. It is characterized by abnormal dilatation of the large air passages leading into the lungs (bronchi) and by destruction of bronchial walls. Bronchiectasis is caused by repeated damage to bronchial walls. The resultant destruction and bronchial dilatation reduce bronchial wall movement so that secretions cannot be removed effectively from the lungs, and the person is predisposed to frequent respiratory infections. Ventilation is eventually obstructed, and advanced bronchiectasis may cause pneumonia, cor pulmonale, or right-sided ventricular failure.

Treatment. All pulmonary irritants, especially cigarette smoke, should be avoided. Postural drainage, adequate hydration, good nutrition, and bronchodilator therapy in bronchospasm are important components in treatment. Antibiotics are used during disease exacerbations (e.g., increased cough, purulent sputum, hemoptysis, malaise, and weight loss) (Mengert and Albert, 1993).

Tuberculosis (Cronin, 1993)

Tuberculosis (TB) is a bacterial infectious disease transmitted by the gram-positive, acid-fast bacillus *Mycobacterium tuberculosis*. Despite improved methods of detection and treatment, TB remains a worldwide health problem with an estimated 3 million new cases diagnosed each year (Perez-Stable and Hopewell, 1989).

Before the development of anti-TB drugs in the late 1940s, TB was the leading cause of death in the United States. Drug therapy, along with improvements in public health and general living standards, resulted in a marked decline in incidence. However, recent influxes of immigrants from developing Third World nations, rising homeless populations, and the emergence of HIV led to an increase in reported cases in the mid-1980s, reversing a 40-year period of decline.

Risk Factors. Although TB can affect anyone, certain segments of the population have an increased risk of contracting the disease:

- elderly people, who constitute nearly half of the newly diagnosed cases of TB in the United States
- certain racial and ethnic groups, such as Native Americans, Eskimos, and African-Americans, especially the economically disadvantaged or homeless
- people who are incarcerated
- immigrants from Southeast Asia, Ethiopia, Mexico, and Latin America
- clients dependent on alcohol or other chemicals with resultant malnutrition, debilitation, and poor health
- infants and children under the age of 5 years

- clients with reduced immunity (e.g., those with HIV infection, with malnutrition, or on cancer chemotherapy or steroid therapy)
- people with diabetes mellitus and/or end-stage renal disease

The following precautions must be followed by all health care personnel when in contact with a client diagnosed with TB:

Guidelines for Physical Therapists for
Preventing Transmission of Tuberculosis

- Doors to isolation rooms must be kept closed
- Client must wear a mask when leaving the room
- Anyone entering the room must wear a mask properly
- Staff and employees attending clients must be tested for TB
- Handwashing is required before and after contact with client

Pathophysiology. The mycobacterium is usually spread by airborne droplet nuclei, which are produced when infected persons sneeze, speak, sing, or cough. Once released into the atmosphere, the organisms are dispersed and can be inhaled by a susceptible host. Brief exposure to a few bacilli rarely causes an infection. More commonly, it is spread with repeated close contact with an infected person.

After the bacilli are inhaled, they pass into the respiratory system and implant themselves on the bronchioles or alveoli. After implantation, the organisms multiply with no initial resistance from the host. While a cellular immune response is being activated, the bacilli can spread via lymph channels to circulating blood and thus throughout the body, so that significant spread can occur before the body can mount a defense. Eventually, acquired cell-mediated immunity limits further multiplication, and a characteristic tissue reaction called an epithelioid cell tubercle results. The central portion of this lesion undergoes necrosis and can produce a cavity in the bronchi. Tubercular material may then enter the bronchial system and can be transmitted via airborne droplets.

This lesion heals, and calcification and scarring take place. These changes can be seen by x-ray. When the lesion heals, the infection enters a latent period, in which it may persist without producing a clinical illness. The infection may remain dormant or may develop into a clinical disease if persistent organisms begin to multiply rapidly (Smeltzer and Bare, 1992).

Tuberculosis most often involves the lungs, but extrapulmonary TB (XPTB) can also occur in the kidneys, bone growth plates, lymph nodes, and meninges and can be disseminated throughout the body (Smeltzer and Bare, 1992). Widespread dissemination throughout the body is termed *miliary tuberculosis* and is more common in people 50 years or older and very young children with unstable or underdeveloped immune systems. On rare occasions, TB will affect the hip joints and vertebrae, resulting in severe, arthritis-like damage, possibly even avascular necrosis of the hip. Tuberculosis of the spine, referred to as Pott's disease, can result in compression fracture of the vertebrae.

Tuberculous Spondylitis (Pott's disease). Tuberculosis of a peripheral joint is usually a chronic, monarticular, purulent arthritis involving the hip, knee, elbow, or wrist. Symptoms are variable. Nagging local back pain may be present and may be referred to the anterior abdominal wall (mistaken for appendicitis). A tender, prominent spinal process may develop because of anterior wedging of two vertebral bodies. A paraspinal abscess may extend and present as a mass in the groin or supraclavicular space. A paraspinal abscess that compresses the spinal cord or granulation tissue that intrudes on the anterior

> ### Clinical Signs and Symptoms of Tuberculosis
>
> - Fatigue
> - Malaise
> - Anorexia
> - Weight loss
> - Low-grade fevers (especially in late afternoon)
> - Night sweats
> - Frequent, productive cough
> - Dull chest pain, tightness, or discomfort
> - Dyspnea

aspects of the cord may cause symptoms ranging from minor loss of bowel and urinary sphincter control to abrupt and irreversible paraplegia (Berkow and Fletcher, 1992).

Clinical Signs and Symptoms. Clinical signs and symptoms are absent in the early stages of TB. Many cases are found incidentally when routine chest radiographs are made for other reasons. When systemic manifestations of active disease initially present, the clinical signs and symptoms listed here may appear.

Tuberculin skin testing is done to determine whether the body's immune response has been activated by the presence of the bacillus. A positive reaction develops 3 to 10 weeks after the initial infection. A positive skin test reaction indicates the presence of a tuberculous infection but does not show whether the infection is dormant or is causing a clinical illness. Chest x-ray films and sputum cultures are done as a follow-up to positive skin tests. All cases of active disease are treated, and certain cases of inactive disease are treated prophylactically.

Treatment and Prognosis. Pharmacologic management through medication is the primary treatment of choice. Treatment has been complicated by multidrug resistant TB, present in at least 13 states (Snider and Roper, 1992). The disease is 50 per cent to 80 per cent fatal, even with intensive treatment. Noncompletion of treatment among inner city residents and the homeless presents an additional factor in the failure to eradicate TB (Brudney and Dobkin, 1991).

Preventing the transmission of tuberculosis by using such simple measures as covering the mouth and nose with a tissue when coughing and sneezing reduces the number of organisms excreted into the air. Adequate room ventilation and preventing overcrowding such as in homeless shelters and prisons are also well-known preventive measures. Drug therapy to prevent reactivation of latent TB infection is under investigation (Centers for Disease Control, 1989; Claremont et al., 1991;).

Vaccination is at least 60 per cent effective in preventing tuberculosis in certain populations and also prevents disseminated disease in children if they become infected with TB. There is no evidence at present regarding the efficacy of vaccination in HIV-infected children (Mann et al., 1992).

Treatment of Pott's disease follows the same chemotherapy regimen, with prompt response. Immobilization and avoidance of weight bearing may be required to relieve pain, with attention to maintaining strength and range of motion.

Systemic Sclerosis Lung Disease
(Silver, 1990)

Systemic sclerosis (SS) (scleroderma) is a disease of unknown etiology characterized by excessive connective tissue deposition (see also Chapter 11). Fibrosis affecting the skin and the visceral organs is the hallmark of SS. The lungs, highly vascularized and composed of abundant connective tissue, are a frequent target organ, ranking second only to the esophagus in visceral involvement.

Even though pulmonary complaints are rarely the presenting symptoms of SS, lung involvement develops in more than 70 per cent of clients with SS (Silver and LeRoy, 1988). As better treatments are developed for the other potentially fatal visceral manifestations, lung involvement is becoming the most frequent cause of death in SS clients.

The most common pulmonary manifestation of SS is interstitial fibrosis, which is clinically apparent in more than 50 per cent of cases. Autopsy results suggest a prevalence of 75 per cent, indicating the insensitivity of traditional tests such as pulmonary function tests and chest radiographs.

Clinical Signs and Symptoms. As discussed in Chapter 11, skin changes associated with SS generally precede visceral alterations. Dyspnea on exertion and nonproductive cough are the most common clinical findings associated with SS. Rarely, these symptoms precede the occurrence of cutaneous changes of scleroderma. Clubbing of the nails rarely occurs in SS because of the nearly universal presence of sclerodactyly (hardening and shrinking of connective tissues of fingers and toes). Peripheral edema may develop secondary to cor pulmonale, which occurs as the pulmonary fibrosis becomes advanced. Pulmonary manifestations in systemic sclerosis include

Common: Interstitial pneumonitis and fibrosis and pulmonary vascular disease

Less Common: Pleural disease, aspiration pneumonia, pneumothorax, neoplasm, pneumoconiosis, pulmonary hemorrhage, and drug-induced pneumonitis

Pleural effusions may appear with orthopnea, edema, and paroxysmal nocturnal dyspnea if congestive heart failure occurs. Cystic changes in the parenchyma may progress to form pneumatoceles (thin-walled air-containing cysts) that may rupture spontaneously and produce a pneumothorax. Clients with SS have an increased

▼ *Clinical Signs and Symptoms of*

Systemic Sclerosis Lung Disease

- Dyspnea on exertion
- Nonproductive cough
- Peripheral edema (secondary to cor pulmonale)
- Orthopnea
- Paroxysmal nocturnal dyspnea (congestive heart failure)
- Hemoptysis

incidence of lung cancer. Hemoptysis is usually the first signal of pulmonary malignancy.

Treatment and Prognosis. Successful medical treatment of SS lung disease is a major challenge, because lung disease is becoming the most frequent cause of death from SS. With the advent of converting enzyme inhibitors, renovascular hypertension usually can be treated successfully and its complications avoided. The course of SS is unpredictable, from a mild, protracted course to rapid respiratory failure and death.

There are no predictive tests to aid in the successful management of this disorder. There is no standard drug therapy currently effective with all SS, and each case is treated individually. Immunosuppressive drugs, plasmapheresis, oxygen therapy, and vasodilator therapy are used in addition to selected procedures such as antiinflammatory therapy for pleural disease, chest tube for recurrent pneumothorax, and antibiotics for aspiration pneumonia. Neither unilateral lung nor heart-lung transplantation is feasible in clients with end-stage lung disease secondary to systemic sclerosis.

NEOPLASTIC DISEASE

Lung Cancer (Bronchogenic Carcinoma) (Cronin, 1993)

Lung cancer is malignancy in the epithelium of the respiratory tract. At least a dozen different cell types of tumors are included under the classification of lung cancer. The four major types of lung cancer include small cell carcinoma (oat cell carcinoma), squamous cell carcinoma, adenocarcinoma, and large cell carcinoma. Clinically, lung cancers are grouped into two divisions: small cell lung cancer and non–small cell lung cancer. The term *lung cancer* excludes other disorders such as sarcomas, lymphomas, blastomas, and mesotheliomas.

The frequency of the various histologic types of lung cancer is changing. Adenocarcinoma has become the most frequent histologic type and is responsible for about 50 per cent of all lung cancers. Squamous cell carcinoma accounts for one third of all lung cancers; small cell carcinoma, 15 per cent; and large cell carcinoma, less than 5 per cent (Martini et al., 1987).

Incidence (Martini, 1993). Since the mid-1950s, lung cancer has been the most common cause of death from cancer in men, and in 1987, it overtook breast cancer to become the most common cause of death from cancer in women in the United States. Today, the American Cancer Society estimates that 56,000 women will die of lung cancer and 46,000 of breast cancer in 1993. Eighty per cent or more of the deaths attributed to lung cancer were attributable to smoking and were therefore preventable (Gritz, 1993). Cigarette smoking remains the risk factor with the largest influence on the incidence of lung cancer, with 85 per cent to 90 per cent of all lung cancers occurring in smokers.

Risk Factors. Compared with nonsmokers, heavy smokers (i.e., those who smoke more than 25 cigarettes a day) have a 20-fold greater risk of developing lung cancer.

Quitting smoking lowers the risk, but the decrease is gradual, and the risk does not approach that of a nonsmoker until 15 to 20 years later. Recent studies also have suggested that passive smoke (i.e., smoke inhaled from the environment surrounding an active smoker) may be responsible for up to 5 per cent of all lung cancers (Lesmes and Donofrio, 1992; Sexton, 1990; White et al., 1991).

The risk of lung cancer is increased in the smoker who is also exposed to other carcinogenic agents, such as radioactive isotopes, polycyclic hydrocarbons, vinyl chloride, metallurgic ores, and mustard gas. Whether these occupational factors increase the risk of cancer development in the nonsmoker is still unclear. The inhalation of asbestos fibers is associated with higher cancer risks for both smokers and nonsmokers. The rate of lung cancer in clients who live in urban areas is 2.3 times greater than that of those living in rural areas, thus implicating air pollution in increasing the risk of lung cancer; however, the exact role of air pollution is unknown.

Staging. Cancers of the lung are staged at the time of their initial presentation. The American Joint Committee for Cancer's tumor, nodes, metastasis (TNM) staging system is used (see explanation in Chapter 10). Tumors 3 cm or smaller in diameter are defined as T_1, and those larger than 3 cm are T_2 tumors. Tumors confined to the lung without any metastases, regional or distant, are classified as Stage I, and tumors associated with only hilar or peribronchial lymph node involvement (N_1) are classified as Stage II. Locally advanced tumors with mediastinal or cervical lymph node metastases and those with extension to the chest wall, mediastinum, diaphragm, or carina are classified as Stage III tumors. Finally, tumors presenting with distant metastases (M_1) are classified as Stage IV tumors (Martini, 1993).

Metastases. Metastatic spread of pulmonary tumors is usually to the long bones, vertebral column (especially the thoracic vertebrae), liver, and adrenal glands. Brain metastasis is also common, occurring in as much as 50 per cent of cases.

Local metastases by direct extension may involve the chest wall, pleura, pulmonary parenchyma, or bronchi. Further local tumor growth may erode the first and second ribs and associated vertebrae, causing bone pain and paravertebral pain associated with involvement of sympathetic nerve ganglia.

The lungs are the most frequent site of metastases from other types of cancer, because any tumor cells dislodged from a primary neoplasm into the circulation or lymphatics are usually filtered by the lungs. Carcinomas of the kidney, breast, pancreas, colon, and uterus are especially likely to metastasize to the lungs (Mitchell, 1992).

Paraneoplastic syndromes (remote effects of a malignancy—see explanation in Chapter 10) occur in 10 to 20 per cent of lung cancer clients. These usually result from the secretion of hormones by the tumor acting on target organs, producing a variety of symptoms. Occasionally, symptoms of paraneoplastic syndrome occur before detection of the primary lung tumor.

Clinical Signs and Symptoms. Clinical signs and symptoms of lung cancer often remain silent until the disease process is at an advanced stage. In many instances, lung cancer may mimic other pulmonary conditions or may present as chest, shoulder, or arm pain. Chest pain is a vague aching, and depending on the type of cancer, the client may have pleuritic pain on inspiration that limits lung expansion.

Hemoptysis (coughing or spitting up blood) may occur secondary to ulceration of blood vessels. Wheezing occurs when the tumor obstructs the bronchus. Dyspnea, either unexplained or out of proportion, is a red flag indicating the need for medical screening.

Centrally located tumors cause increased cough, dyspnea, and diffuse chest pain that can be referred to the shoulder, scapulae, and upper back. This pain is the result of peribronchial or perivascular nerve involvement. Other symptoms may include postobstructive pneumonia with fever, chills, malaise, anorexia, hemoptysis, and fecal breath odor (secondary to infection within a necrotic tumor mass). If these tumors extend to the pericardium, the client may develop a sudden onset of arrhythmia (tachycardia or atrial fibrillation), weakness, anxiety, and dyspnea.

Peripheral tumors are most often asymptomatic until the tumor extends through visceral and parietal pleura to the chest wall. Irritation of the nerves causes localized sharp, pleuritic pain that is aggravated by inspiration. Metastases to the mediastinum (tissues and organs between the sternum and the vertebrae, including the heart and its large vessels; trachea; esophagus; thymus; lymph nodes) may cause hoarseness or dysphagia secondary to vocal cord paralysis as a result of entrapment or local compression of the laryngeal nerve.

▼ *Clinical Signs and Symptoms of*
Lung Cancer

- Any change in respiratory patterns
- Recurrent pneumonia or bronchitis
- Hemoptysis
- Persistent cough
- Change in cough or development of hemoptysis in a chronic smoker
- Hoarseness or dysphagia
- Sputum streaked with blood
- Dyspnea (shortness of breath)
- Wheezing
- Sharp, pleuritic pain aggravated by inspiration
- Sudden, unexplained weight loss
- Chest, shoulder, or arm pain
- Atrophy and weakness of the arm and hand muscles

▼ *Clinical Signs and Symptoms of*
Paraneoplastic Syndrome

- Hypercalcemia
- Mental changes
- Gynecomastia
- Cushing's syndrome
- Hyponatremia (syndrome of inappropriate antidiuretic hormone)
- Trousseau's syndrome (migratory thrombophlebitis)

Apical (Pancoast's) tumors of the lung apex do not usually cause symptoms while confined to the pulmonary parenchyma. They can extend into surrounding structures and frequently involve the eighth cervical and first thoracic nerves within the brachial plexus. This nerve involvement produces sharp pleuritic pain in the axilla, shoulder, and subscapular area on the affected side, with atrophy of the upper extremity muscles.

Trigger points of the serratus anterior muscle (see Fig. 3–11) also mimic the distribution of pain caused by the eighth cervical nerve root compression. Trigger points can be ruled out by palpation and lack of neurologic deficits and may be confirmed by elimination with appropriate physical therapy treatment (Reynolds, 1981).

Prognosis and Treatment. The curability of lung cancer remains low. Currently, the overall 5-year survival rate ranges from 10 to 13 per cent (Boring et al., 1993). Survival without treatment is rarely possible, and most untreated clients die within 1 year of diagnosis, with a mean survival of less than 6 months. The key to increasing the survival rate of clients with lung cancer is early detection, but a tumor must be 1 cm in diameter before it is detectable on chest film. Unfortunately, invasion and metastasis usually have already occurred.

Clinical Symptoms of
Brain Metastasis

About 10 per cent of all people with lung cancer have central nervous system involvement at the time of diagnosis. Major clinical symptoms of brain metastasis result from increased intracranial pressure and include

- Headache
- Nausea and vomiting
- Malaise
- Anorexia
- Weakness
- Alterations in mental processes

Other prognostic factors include male sex, age greater than 70 years, prior chemotherapy, elevated serum lactic dehydrogenase levels, low serum sodium levels, and elevated alkaline phosphatase levels (Hansen et al., in press; Hinson and Perry, 1993).

Radiation therapy may be used as a potentially curative treatment in clients with locally advanced disease who are poor surgical risks, who have technically inoperable

Clinical Signs and Symptoms of
Metastasis to the Spinal Cord

Metastasis to the spinal cord produces signs and symptoms of cord compression, including

- Back pain (localized or radicular)
- Muscle weakness
- Loss of lower extremity sensation
- Bowel and bladder incontinence
- Diminished or absent lower extremity reflexes (unilateral or bilateral)

tumors, or who refuse thoracotomy. Radiation therapy may be used in combination with surgery or chemotherapy to improve treatment outcomes. Chemotherapy is commonly used in clients treated with surgery or radiation who experience recurrent disease or distant metastasis. However, large-scale studies have failed to demonstrate a significantly improved overall survival rate for these clients (Engelking, 1987). The decision to use chemotherapy is made on an individual basis, depending on the client's previous history, current condition, and acceptance of the risks and side effects involved.

Surgical resection is the treatment of choice in early stages of non–small cell lung cancer (NSCLC). Cure is possible if the disease is still localized to the thoracic cavity and no metastases are present. However, only 20 to 25 per cent of clients with NSCLC meet these criteria at the time of diagnosis.

GENETIC DISEASE OF THE LUNG

Cystic Fibrosis

Cystic fibrosis (CF) is an inherited disease of the exocrine ("outward-secreting") glands primarily affecting the digestive and respiratory systems. CF is the most common inherited genetic disease in the Caucasian population, affecting approximately 1 in 2000 white newborn infants in the United States.

The disease is inherited as a recessive trait: both parents must be carriers. In America, 5 per cent of the population, or 12 million people, carry a single copy of the CF gene. Because cysts and scar tissue on the pancreas were observed during autopsy when the disease was first being differentiated from other conditions, it was given the name cystic fibrosis of the pancreas. Although this term describes a secondary rather than primary characteristic, it has been retained (O'Toole, 1992).

Pathophysiology. In 1989, scientists isolated the cystic fibrosis gene located on chromosome 7. In healthy people, a protein called cystic fibrosis transmembrane conductance regulator (CFTR) provides a channel by which chloride (a component of salt) can pass in and out of cells. Clients with CF have a defective copy of the gene that normally enables cells to construct that channel. As a result, salt accumulates in the cells lining the lungs and digestive tissues, making the surrounding mucus abnormally thick and sticky. These secretions, which obstruct ducts in the pancreas, liver, and lungs, and abnormal secretion of sweat and saliva are the two main features of CF. Obstruction of the bronchioles by mucus plugs and trapped air predisposes the client to infection, which starts a destructive cycle of increased mucus production with increased bronchial obstruction and damage and eventually destroys lung tissue.

Clinical Signs and Symptoms. Pulmonary involvement is the most common and severe manifestation of CF. Obstruction of the airways leads to a state of hyperinflation. In time, fibrosis develops, and restrictive lung disease is superimposed on the obstructive disease. Over time, pulmonary obstruction leads to chronic hypoxia, hypercapnia, and acidosis. Pneumothorax,

▼ *Clinical Signs and Symptoms of*
Cystic Fibrosis

Clinical signs and symptoms of cystic fibrosis in the early or undiagnosed stages:
- Persistent coughing and wheezing
- Recurrent pneumonia
- Excessive appetite but poor weight gain
- Salty skin/sweat
- Bulky, foul-smelling stools (undigested fats due to a lack of amylase and tryptase enzymes)

▼ *Clinical Signs and Symptoms of*
Pulmonary Involvement in Cystic Fibrosis

- Tachypnea (very rapid breathing)
- Sustained chronic cough with mucus production and vomiting
- Barrel chest (caused by trapped air)
- Use of accessory muscles of respiration and intercostal retraction
- Cyanosis and digital clubbing
- Exertional dyspnea with decreased exercise tolerance

Further complications include
- Pneumothorax
- Hemoptysis
- Right-sided heart failure secondary to pulmonary hypertension

pulmonary hypertension, and eventually cor pulmonale may develop (Berkow and Fletcher, 1992).

Prognosis and Treatment. Advances in treatment, including antibiotics, chest physical therapy, enzyme supplements, and nutrition programs, have extended the average life expectancy for CF sufferers into their early 20s, with maximal survival estimated at 30 to 40 years. Because the genetic abnormality has been identified, gene therapy eventually may correct the disease (Wang and Viggiano, 1993).

Finding a way to deliver the normal copy of the gene into the lung cells remains a challenge. It is possible that delivery through an aerolized technique will incorporate sufficient quantities of the CFTR gene into the cells to offset the presence of the abnormal protein. The expectation is that the normal CFTR will reverse the physiologic defect in cystic fibrosis cells.

The course of CF varies from one client to another depending on the degree of pulmonary involvement. Deterioration is inevitable, leading to debilitation and eventually death.

OCCUPATIONAL LUNG DISEASES
(Cronin, 1993)

Lung diseases are among the most common occupational health problems. They are caused by the inhalation of various chemicals, dusts, and other particulate matter that are present in certain work settings. Not all clients exposed to occupational inhalants will develop lung disease. Harmful effects depend on the (1) nature of the exposure; (2) duration and intensity of the exposure; (3) presence of underlying pulmonary disease; (4) smoking history; and (5) particle size and water-solubility of the inhalant. The larger the particle, the lower the probability of its reaching the lower respiratory tract; highly water-soluble inhalants tend to dissolve and react in the upper respiratory tract, whereas poorly soluble substances may travel as far as the alveoli.

The most commonly encountered occupational lung diseases are occupational asthma, hypersensitivity pneumonitis, pneumoconioses, and acute respiratory irritation. The greatest number of occupational agents causing *asthma* are those with known or suspected allergic properties such as plant and animal proteins (e.g., wheat, flour, cotton, flax, and grain mites). In most cases, the asthma will resolve after exposure is terminated.

Hypersensitivity pneumonitis, or allergic alveolitis, is most commonly due to the inhalation of organic antigens of fungal, bacterial, or animal origin. *Pneumoconioses,* or "the dust diseases," result from inhalation of minerals, notably silica, coal dust, or asbestos. These diseases are most commonly seen in miners, construction workers, sandblasters, potters, and foundry and quarry workers. Pneumoconioses usually develop gradually over a period of years, eventually leading to diffuse pulmonary fibrosis that diminishes lung capacity and produces restrictive lung disease. Early symptoms may include cough and dyspnea on exertion. Chest pain, productive cough, and dyspnea at rest develop as the condition progresses.

Acute respiratory irritation results from the inhalation of chemicals such as ammonia, chlorine, and nitrogen oxides in the form of gases, aerosols, or particulate matter. If such irritants reach the lower airways, alveolar damage and pulmonary edema can result. Although the effects of these acute irritants are usually short-lived, some may cause chronic alveolar damage or airway obstruction.

Treatment and Prognosis. In most cases, treatment consists of prevention of exposure, with respiratory support as needed. Medications for asthma and steroids for hypersensitivity pneumonitis are helpful treatment tools. Cessation of smoking is important. When the irritants are removed, symptoms resolve in several days, and pulmonary functions normalize in a few weeks. Permanent damage or persistent hypersensitivity depends on the cause of the lung disease.

PLEUROPULMONARY DISORDERS

Pulmonary Embolism and Deep Venous Thrombosis

Pulmonary embolism (PE) involves pulmonary vascular obstruction by a displaced thrombus (blood clot), an air bubble, a fat globule, a clump of bacteria, amniotic fluid, vegetations on heart valves that develop with endocarditis, or other particulate matter (Mengert and Albert, 1993). Once dislodged, the obstruction travels to the lungs, causing shortness of breath, tachypnea (very rapid breathing), tachycardia, and chest pain.

The most common cause of PE is deep venous thrombosis (DVT) originating in the proximal deep venous system of the lower legs. The embolism causes an area of blockage, which then results in a localized area of ischemia known as a *pulmonary infarct*. The infarct may be caused by small emboli that extend to the lung surface (pleura) and result in acute pleuritic chest pain.

Risk Factors. The three major risk factors linked with DVT are blood stasis (e.g., immobilization due to bed rest, such as with burn patients, obstetric and gynecologic clients, and elderly or obese populations), endothelial injury (secondary to surgical procedures, trauma, or fractures of the legs or pelvis), and hypercoagulable states.

Other people at increased risk for DVT and PE include those with congestive heart failure, trauma, operation (especially hip, knee, and prostate surgery), age over 50 years, previous history of thromboembolism, malignant disease, infection, diabetes mellitus, inactivity or obesity, pregnancy, clotting abnormalities, and oral contraceptive use.

A careful review of the Personal/Family History form (outpatient) or hospital medical chart (inpatient) may alert the therapist to the presence of factors that predispose a client to have a PE.

Deep Venous Thrombosis (see also Chapter 3). Signs and symptoms include tenderness, leg pain, swelling (a difference in leg circumference of 1.4 cm in men and 1.2 cm in women is significant), and warmth. One may also see a positive Homans' sign,* subcutaneous venous distention, discoloration, a palpable cord, and/or pain upon placement of a blood pressure cuff around the calf (considerable pain with the cuff inflated to 160 to 180 mm

Hg). Unfortunately, at least half the cases of deep venous thrombosis are asymptomatic, and in up to 30 per cent of clients with clinical evidence of DVT, no DVT is demonstrable (Mengert and Albert, 1993).

Pulmonary Embolism. Signs and symptoms are nonspecific and vary greatly, depending on the extent to which the lung is involved, the size of the clot, and the general condition of the client. Dyspnea, pleuritic chest pain, and cough are the most common. Pleuritic pain is caused by an inflammatory reaction of the lung parenchyma or by pulmonary infarction or ischemia caused by obstruction of small pulmonary arterial branches. Typical pleuritic chest pain is sudden in onset and aggravated by breathing. The client may also report hemoptysis, apprehension, tachypnea, and fever (temperature as high as 39.5° C, or 103.5° F). The presence of hemoptysis indicates that the infarction or areas of atelectasis have produced alveolar damage (Cronin, 1993).

Prognosis and Treatment (Mengert and Albert, 1993). PE is responsible for about 10 per cent to 20 per cent of all hospital deaths, including up to 15 per cent of postoperative deaths, and is the leading cause of pregnancy-related mortality in the United States. Gangrene can result from embolization of a thrombus from the heart, aorta, or femoral arteries.

Heparin remains the treatment of choice in acute DVT or PE. It prevents further propagation of the thrombus but does not reduce the immediate embolic risk or enhance clot lysis.

Given the mortality of PE and the difficulties involved in its clinical diagnosis, prevention of DVT and PE is crucial. Heparin is also the most common agent for prophylaxis in clients undergoing general surgery who are at risk for DVT or PE and clients with myocardial infarction or congestive heart failure. For clients undergoing total hip replacement, major knee surgery, prostate surgery, and neurosurgery, and for women undergoing cesarean section, pneumatic calf compression, often in conjunc-

---

* Physical evidence of phlebitis is *Homans' sign,* which is deep calf pain on slow dorsiflexion of the foot or gentle squeezing of the affected calf. The inflamed nerves in the veins within the muscle are stretched. Only half of all people with deep venous thrombosis experience pain (Purtilo and Purtilo, 1989). Homans' sign is not specific for this condition because it also occurs with Achilles tendinitis and gastrocnemius and plantar muscle injury (Jarvis, 1992).

▼ *Clinical Signs and Symptoms of*
Deep Venous Thrombosis (DVT)

- Unilateral tenderness or leg pain
- Unilateral swelling (difference in leg circumference)
- Warmth
- Positive Homans' sign
- Subcutaneous venous distention (superficial thrombus)
- Discoloration
- Palpable cord (superficial thrombus)
- Pain with placement around calf of blood pressure cuff inflated to 160 to 180 mm Hg

▼ *Clinical Signs and Symptoms of*
Pulmonary Embolism (PE)

- Dyspnea
- Pleuritic (sharp, localized) chest pain
- Diffuse chest discomfort
- Persistent cough
- Hemoptysis (bloody sputum)
- Apprehension, anxiety, restlessness
- Tachypnea (increased respiratory rate)
- Fever

tion with gradient elastic stockings (not simple compressive stockings), is a preventive measure.

Although frequent changing of position, exercise, and early ambulation are necessary to prevent thrombosis and embolism, sudden and extreme movements should be avoided. Under no circumstances should the legs be massaged to relieve "muscle cramps," especially when the pain is located in the calf and the client has not been up and about (O'Toole, 1992). Restrictive clothing and prolonged sitting or standing should be avoided. Elevating the legs should be accomplished with caution to avoid severe flexion of the hips, which will slow blood flow and increase the risk of new thrombi.

Cor Pulmonale

When a pulmonary embolus has been sufficiently massive to obstruct 60 per cent to 75 per cent of the pulmonary circulation, the client may have central chest pain, and acute cor pulmonale occurs. Cor pulmonale is a serious cardiac condition and an emergency situation arising from a sudden dilatation of the right ventricle as a result of pulmonary embolism.

As cor pulmonale progresses, edema and other signs of right-sided heart failure develop. Symptoms are similar to those of congestive heart failure from other causes: dyspnea, edema of the lower extremities, distention of the veins of the neck, and liver distention. The hematocrit is increased as the body attempts to compensate for impaired circulation by producing more erythrocytes (Newman and Ross, 1990).

Treatment. Treatment is aimed at relief of the lung disorder causing the condition and relieving the pulmonary insufficiency.

▼ *Clinical Signs and Symptoms of*
Cor Pulmonale

- Peripheral edema (bilateral legs)
- Chronic cough
- Central chest pain
- Exertional dyspnea or dyspnea at rest
- Distention of neck veins
- Fatigue
- Wheezing
- Weakness

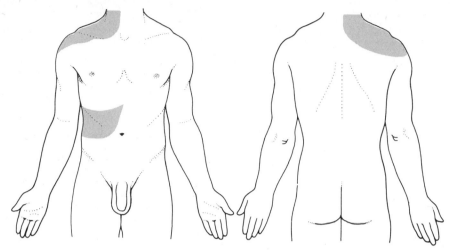

Figure 4–4
Chest pain over the site of pleuritis is usually perceived by the client (not shown). Referred pain *(light red)* associated with pleuritis may occur on the same side as the pleuritic lesion affecting the shoulder, upper trapezius muscle, neck, lower chest wall, or abdomen.

Pleurisy

Pleurisy is an inflammation of the pleura (serous membrane enveloping the lungs) and is caused by infection, injury, or tumor. The membranous pleura that encases each lung consists of two close-fitting layers: the visceral layer encasing the lungs and the parietal layer lining the inner chest wall. A lubricating fluid lies between these two layers.

If the fluid content remains unchanged by the disease, the pleurisy is said to be dry. If the fluid increases abnormally, it is a wet pleurisy or pleurisy with effusion (pleural effusion). If the wet pleurisy becomes infected with formation of pus, the condition is known as purulent pleurisy or empyema (O'Toole, 1992).

Pleurisy may occur as a result of many factors, including pneumonia, tuberculosis, lung abscess, influenza, systemic lupus erythematosus (SLE), rheumatoid arthritis, and pulmonary infarction. Pleurisy, with or without effusion associated with SLE, may be accompanied by acute pleuritic pain and dysfunction of the diaphragm (Gaskell and Webber, 1980).

Clinical Signs and Symptoms. The chest pain is sudden and may vary from vague discomfort to an intense stabbing or knife-like sensation in the chest. The pain is aggravated by breathing, coughing, laughing, or other similar movements associated with deep inspiration. The visceral pleura is insensitive; pain results from inflammation of the parietal pleura. Because the latter is innervated by the intercostal nerves, chest pain is usually felt over the site of the pleuritis, but pain may be referred to the lower chest wall, abdomen, neck, upper trapezius muscle, and shoulder because of irritation of the central diaphragmatic pleura (Fig. 4–4) (Berkow and Fletcher, 1992).

▼

Clinical Signs and Symptoms of **Pleurisy**

- Chest pain
- Cough
- Dyspnea
- Fever, chills
- Tachypnea (rapid, shallow breathing)

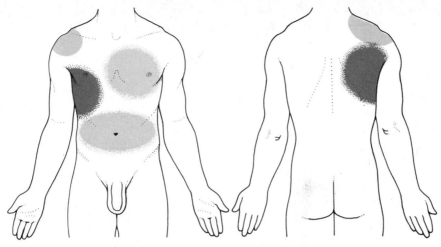

Figure 4–5
Possible pain patterns associated with spontaneous pneumothorax: upper and lateral thoracic wall with referral to the ipsilateral shoulder, across the chest, or over the abdomen.

Treatment. The most effective measures against pleurisy are those directed at the cause of the inflammation, such as the administration of antibiotics (O'Toole, 1992).

Spontaneous Pneumothorax

Spontaneous pneumothorax, or free air in the pleural cavity between the visceral and parietal pleurae, may occur secondary to pulmonary disease (e.g., when an emphysematous bulla or other weakened area on the lung ruptures) or as a result of trauma and subsequent perforation of the chest wall.

Air may enter the pleural space directly through a hole in the chest wall (open pneumothorax) or diaphragm. Air may escape into the pleural space from a puncture or tear in an internal respiratory structure (e.g., bronchus, bronchioles, or alveoli). This form of pneumothorax is called closed or spontaneous pneumothorax (Strohmyer, 1993).

Clinical Signs and Symptoms. Symptoms of spontaneous pneumothorax vary depending on the size of the pneumothorax

and on the extent of lung disease. When air enters the pleural cavity, the lung collapses, producing dyspnea and a shift of tissues and organs to the unaffected side. The client may have severe pain in the upper and lateral thoracic wall, which is aggravated by any movement and by the cough and dyspnea that accompany it.

The pain may be referred to the ipsilateral shoulder (corresponding shoulder on the same side as the pneumothorax), across the chest, or over the abdomen (Fig. 4–5). The client may be most comfortable when sitting in an upright position.

Clinical Signs and Symptoms of Spontaneous Pneumothorax

- Dyspnea
- Sudden, sharp chest pain
- Shoulder pain
- Weak and rapid pulse
- Fall in blood pressure
- Dry, hacking cough

Other symptoms may include a fall in blood pressure, a weak and rapid pulse, and cessation of normal respiratory movements on the affected side of the chest.

Treatment. When the pneumothorax is small, the lung often expands again in several days. Treatment may involve only bed rest and the administration of oxygen to relieve dyspnea.

If the lung fails to expand again or collapses further, air must be withdrawn from the pleural cavity through the use of a chest tube. The chest catheter permits the continuous escape of air and blood from the pleural space. This helps the lung expand by reestablishing subatmospheric pressure (i.e., negative pressure) in the pleural space, which is necessary for normal ventilation. Sometimes thoracotomy (surgical opening into the chest cavity) is done to explore the chest surgically and repair the site of origin of the pneumo- or hemothorax (Strohmyer, 1993).

PULMONARY PAIN PATTERNS
(Bauwens and Paine, 1983)

As discussed earlier in the section on chest pain in Chapter 3, the parietal pleura is sensitive to painful stimulation, but the visceral pleura is insensitive. Within the pulmonary system, the trachea and large bronchi are innervated by the vagus trunks, whereas the finer bronchi and lung parenchyma appear to be free of pain innervation.

Tracheobronchial pain is referred to sites in the neck or anterior chest at the same levels as the points of irritation in the air passages (Fig. 4–6). This irritation may be caused by inflammatory lesions, irritating foreign materials, or cancerous tumors.

Extensive disease may occur in the periphery of the lung without occurrence of pain until the process extends to the parietal pleura. Pleural irritation then results in sharp, localized pain that is aggravated by any respiratory movement. Clients usually note that the pain is alleviated by lying on the affected side, which diminishes the movement of that side of the chest ("autosplinting") (Scharf, 1989).

Debate continues concerning the mechanism by which pain occurs in the parietal membrane. It has been long thought that friction between the two pleural surfaces (when the membranes are irritated and covered with fibrinous exudate) causes sharp pain. Other theories suggest that intercostal muscle spasm due to pleurisy or stretching of the parietal pleura causes this pain.

Pleural pain is present in pulmonary disease processes including pleurisy, pneumonia, pulmonary infarct (when it extends to the pleural surface thus causing pleurisy), tumor (when it invades the parietal pleura), and spontaneous pneumothorax. Tumor, especially bronchogenic carcinoma, may be accompanied by severe, continuous pain when the tumor tissue, extending to the parietal pleura through the lung, constantly irritates the pain nerve endings in the pleura.

The *diaphragmatic pleura* receives dual pain innervation through the phrenic and intercostal nerves. Damage to the phrenic nerve produces paralysis of the corresponding half of the diaphragm. The phrenic nerves are sensory and motor from both surfaces of the diaphragm.

Stimulation of the peripheral portions of the diaphragmatic pleura results in sharp pain felt along the costal margins, which can be referred to the lumbar region by the lower thoracic somatic nerves. Stimulation of the central portion of the diaphragmatic pleura results in sharp pain referred to the upper trapezius muscle and shoulder on the ipsilateral side of the stimulation (see Fig. 3–7).

Pain of cardiac and diaphragmatic origin is often experienced in the shoulder because the heart and diaphragm are supplied by the C5–C6 spinal segment, and the visceral pain is referred to the corresponding somatic area (Scharf, 1989).

Diaphragmatic pleurisy secondary to pneumonia is common and refers sharp

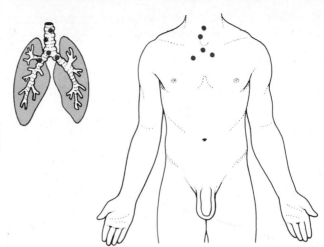

Figure 4–6
Tracheobronchial pain is referred to sites in the neck or anterior chest at the same levels as the points of irritation in the air passages. The points of pain are on the same side as the areas of irritation.

pain along the costal margins or upper trapezius, which is aggravated by any diaphragmatic motion, such as coughing, laughing, or deep breathing.

There may be tenderness to palpation along the costal margins, and sharp pain occurs when the client is asked to take a deep breath. A change in position (side bending or rotation of the trunk) does not reproduce the symptoms, which would be the case with a true intercostal lesion or tear. Forceful, repeated coughing can result in an intercostal lesion in the presence of referred intercostal pain from diaphragmatic pleurisy, which can make differentiation between these two entities impossible without a medical referral and further diagnostic testing.

Overview PULMONARY PAIN PATTERNS

PLEUROPULMONARY DISORDERS (Fig. 4–7)

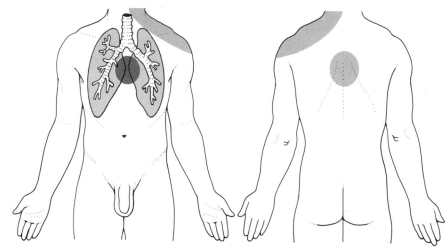

Figure 4–7

Primary pain patterns *(dark red)* associated with pleuropulmonary disorders, such as pulmonary embolus, cor pulmonale, pleurisy, or spontaneous pneumothorax, may vary but usually include substernal or chest pain. Pain over the involved lung fields (anterior, lateral, or posterior) may occur (not shown). Pain may radiate *(light red)* to the neck, upper trapezius muscle, ipsilateral shoulder, thoracic back, costal margins, or upper abdomen (the latter two areas are not shown).

Location:	Substernal or chest over involved lung fields—anterior, side, and back
Referral:	Often well localized (client can point right to the exact site of pain) without referral
	May radiate to neck, upper trapezius muscle, shoulder, costal margins, or upper abdomen
	Thoracic back pain occurs with irritation of the posterior parietal pleura
Description:	Sharp ache, stabbing, angina-like pressure, or crushing pain with pulmonary embolism
	Angina-like chest pain with severe pulmonary hypertension
Intensity:	Moderate
Duration:	Hours to days
Associated Signs and Symptoms:	Preceded by pneumonia or upper respiratory infection
	Wheezing
	Dyspnea (exertional or at rest)
	Hyperventilation

Tachypnea (increased respirations)

Fatigue, weakness

Tachycardia (increased heart rate)

Fever, chills

Edema

Apprehension or anxiety, restlessness

Persistent cough or cough with blood (hemoptysis)

Dry hacking cough (occurs with the onset of spontaneous pneumothorax)

Medically determined signs and symptoms (e.g., by chest auscultation and chest radiograph)

Relieving Factors:

Sitting

Some relief when at rest, but most comfortable position varies (pneumonia)

Pleuritic pain may be relieved by lying on the affected side

Aggravating Factors:

Breathing at rest

Increased inspiratory movement (e.g., laughter, coughing, sneezing)

Symptoms accentuated with each breath

■ ■ ■ ■ ■ ■ ■ ■ ■ ■ ■

LUNG CANCER

Location: Anterior chest

Referral: Scapulae, upper back, ipsilateral shoulder radiating along the medial aspect of the arm

First and second ribs and associated vertebrae and paravertebral muscles (apical or Pancoast's tumors)

Description: Localized, sharp pleuritic pain (peripheral tumors)

Dull, vague aching in the chest

Neuritic pain of shoulders/arm (apical or Pancoast's tumors)

Bone pain due to metastases to adjacent bone or to the vertebrae

Intensity: Moderate to severe

Duration: Constant

Associated Signs and Symptoms:

Hemoptysis (coughing up or spitting up blood)

Dyspnea or wheezing

Fever, chills, malaise, anorexia, and weight loss

Fecal breath odor

Tachycardia or atrial fibrillation (palpitations)

Muscle weakness or atrophy (e.g., Pancoast's tumor may involve the shoulder and the arm on the affected side)

Associated CNS symptoms:
Headache
Nausea
Vomiting
Malaise

Signs of cord compression:
Localized or radicular back pain
Weakness
Loss of lower extremity sensation
Bowel/bladder incontinence
Hoarseness, dysphagia (peripheral tumors)

Relieving
Factors: None without medical intervention

Aggravating
Factors: Inspiration: deep breathing, laughing, coughing

PHYSICIAN REFERRAL

It is more common for a physical therapist to be treating a client with a previously diagnosed musculoskeletal problem who now has chronic, recurrent pulmonary symptoms than to be the primary evaluator and health care provider of a client with pulmonary symptoms. In either case, the physical therapist needs to know what further questions to ask and which of the client's responses represent serious symptoms that require medical follow-up.

Shoulder or back pain can be referred from diseases of the diaphragmatic or parietal pleura, or secondary to metastatic lung cancer. When clients have chest pain, they usually fall into two categories: those who demonstrate chest pain associated with pulmonary symptoms and those who have true musculoskeletal problems, such as intercostal strains and tears, myofascial trigger points, fractured ribs, or myalgias secondary to overuse.

Clients with chronic, persistent cough, whether that cough is productive or dry and hacking, may develop sharp, localized intercostal pain similar to pleuritic pain.

Both intercostal and pleuritic pain are aggravated by respiratory movements, such as laughing, coughing, deep breathing, or sneezing. Clients who have intercostal pain secondary to insidious trauma or repetitive movements, such as coughing, can benefit from physical therapy.

For the client with asthma, it is important to maintain contact with the physician if the client develops signs of asthma or any bronchial activity during exercise. The doctor must be informed to help alter the dosage or the medications to maintain optimal physical performance.

The physical therapist will want to screen for medical disease through a series of questions to elicit the presence of associated systemic (pulmonary) signs and symptoms. Aggravating and relieving factors may provide further clues that can assist in making treatment or referral decisions.

In all these situations, the referral of a client to a physician is based on the family history of pulmonary disease, the presence of pulmonary symptoms of a systemic nature, or the absence of substantiating objective findings indicating a musculoskeletal lesion.

Systemic Signs and Symptoms Requiring Physician Referral

Anorexia

Apprehension

Anxiety

Arthralgias, myalgias

Barrel chest

Bowel/bladder incontinence

Bulky, foul-smelling stools

Chest pain

Chronic laryngitis

Cough with sputum

Cyanosis

Digital clubbing

Dysphagia

Dyspnea

Fecal breath odor

Fever, chills

Hacking cough

Headache

Hemoptysis

Hoarseness

Malaise, fatigue

Muscle weakness

Nausea, vomiting

Orthopnea

Pursed-lip breathing

Restlessness

Salty skin and sweat

Skin rash, pigmentation

Sore throat

Syncope

Tachypnea

Unexplained weight loss

Wheezing

 Key Points to Remember

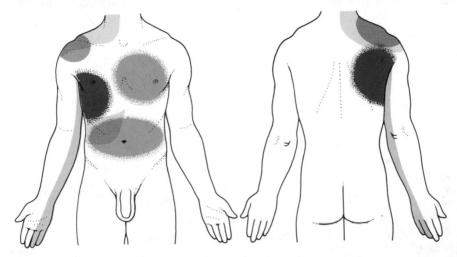

- Pulmonary pain patterns are usually localized in the substernal or chest region over involved lung fields that may include the anterior chest, side, or back.

- Pulmonary pain can radiate to the neck, upper trapezius, costal margins, thoracic back, scapulae, or shoulder.

- Shoulder pain caused by pulmonary involvement may radiate along the medial aspect of the arm mimicking other neuromuscular causes of neck or shoulder pain.

- Pulmonary pain usually increases with inspiratory movements, such as laughing, coughing, sneezing, or deep breathing.

- Shoulder pain that is relieved by lying on the involved side may be "autosplinting," a sign of a pulmonary cause of symptoms.

- Shoulder pain that is aggravated when lying supine (arm/elbow supported) may be an indication of a pulmonary cause of symptoms.

- For anyone presenting with pain patterns described above, especially in the absence of trauma or injury, check the client's personal medical history for previous or recurrent upper respiratory infection or pneumonia.

- Central nervous system (CNS) symptoms, such as muscle weakness, muscle atrophy, headache, loss of lower extremity sensation, and localized or radicular back pain, may be associated with lung cancer.

- Any CNS symptom may be the silent presentation of a lung tumor.

- Posterior leg or calf pain postoperatively may be caused by a thrombus and must be reported to the physician before physical therapy begins or continues.

- Always follow guidelines for preventing transmission of tuberculosis.

- Hemoptysis or exertional/at rest dyspnea, either unexplained or out of proportion to the situation or person, is a red flag symptom requiring medical referral.

- Any client with chest pain should be evaluated for trigger points and intercostal tears.

SUBJECTIVE EXAMINATION   *Special Questions to Ask*

- Have you ever had trouble with breathing or lung disease such as bronchitis, emphysema, asthma, or pneumonia?

- Are you having difficulty breathing now?

- Do you ever have shortness of breath or breathlessness or can't quite catch your breath?

    - If yes, when does this happen? When you rest? When you lie flat, walk on level ground, or walk up stairs?

    - Are the shortness of breath episodes associated with night sweats, cough, chest pain, or bluish color around your lips or fingernails?

    - Does your breathlessness seem to be related to food, pollen, dust, animals, season, or emotion? **(Asthma)**

    - Does your breathlessness occur when you are under stress or tension, and how long does it last?

    - What do you do to get your breathing back to normal?

- How far can you walk before you feel breathless?

- What symptoms stop your walking (e.g., shortness of breath, heart pounding, or weak legs)?

- Do you have any breathing aids (e.g., oxygen, nebulizer, humidifier, or intermittent positive pressure breathing)?

- Do you have a cough? (Note whether the client smokes, for how long and how much: Do you have a smoker's hack?)

    - If yes, to cough separate from smoker's cough, when did it start?

    - Do you cough anything up? If yes, please describe the color, amount, and frequency?

    - Are you taking anything to prevent this cough? If yes, does it seem to help?

■ Are there occasions when you can't seem to stop coughing?

■ Do you ever cough up blood?

  ■ If yes, what color is it? (Bright red = fresh blood; brown or black = older blood)

  ■ If yes, has this condition been treated?

■ Have you strained a muscle from coughing?

■ Have you ever injured your chest?

■ Does it hurt to touch your chest or take a deep breath (e.g., coughing, sneezing, sighing, or laughing)?

■ Have you ever been treated for a lung problem?

  ■ If yes, please describe what this problem was, when it occurred, and how it was treated.

■ Have you ever had a blood clot in your lungs?

  ■ If yes, when did it occur and how was it treated?

■ Have you had a chest x-ray film taken in the last 5 years?

  ■ If yes, when and where was it done? Give the results.

■ Do you work around asbestos, coal, dust, chemicals, or fumes?

  ■ If yes, please describe.

  ■ Do you wear a mask at work? If yes, approximately how much of the time do you wear a mask?

■ If the client is a farmer, ask what kind of farming: Some agricultural products may cause respiratory irritation.

■ Have you ever had tuberculosis?

  ■ If yes, when did it occur and how was it treated? What is your current status?

■ When was your last test for tuberculosis? Was the result normal?

■ (If the person indicated *asthma* on the Personal/Family History form): How can you tell when you are having an asthma attack?

  ■ What triggers an asthma attack for you? (Correlate this question with the core interview questions in the physical therapy interview concerning stressors and stress levels.)

  ■ Do you use medications during an attack?

  ■ If yes, which ones?

  ■ Do you exercise?

  ■ If yes, determine the amount and the intensity of exercise.

  ■ Do you have trouble with asthma during exercise?

  ■ Do you time your medications with your exercise to prevent an asthma attack during exercise?

■ Have you gained or lost a lot of weight recently?

- Gained **(Pulmonary edema, congestive heart failure, fat deposits under the diaphragm in the obese patient reduce ventilation)**
- Lost **(Emphysema, cancer)**
- Do your ankles swell? **(Congestive heart failure)**
- Have you been unusually tired lately? **(Congestive heart failure, emphysema)**
- Have you noticed a change in your voice? **(Pathology of left hilum or trachea)**
- Have you ever broken your nose or been told that you have a deviated septum (nasal passageway)?
  - If yes, does this seem to affect your breathing? **(Hypoxia)**
- Do you have nasal polyps?
  - If yes, does this seem to affect your breathing?
- Have you ever had lung or heart surgery?
  - If yes, what and when? **(Decreased vital capacity)**

CASE STUDY

REFERRAL

A 65-year-old man has come to you for an evaluation of low back pain, which he attributes to lifting a heavy box 2 weeks ago. During the course of the medical history, you notice that the client has a persistent cough and that he sounds hoarse. After reviewing the Personal/Family History form, you note that the client smokes two packs of cigarettes each day and that he has smoked at least this amount for at least 50 years. (One pack per day for one year is considered "one pack year.") This person has smoked an estimated 100 pack years; anyone who has smoked for 20 pack years or more is considered to be at risk for the development of serious lung disease. What questions will you ask to decide for yourself whether this back pain is systemic?

PHYSICAL THERAPY INTERVIEW

Introduction to Client

It is important for me to make certain that your back pain is not caused by other health problems, such as prostate problems or respiratory infection, so I will ask a series of questions that may not seem to be related to your back pain, but I want to be very thorough and cover every possibility in order to obtain the best and most effective treatment for you.

Pain

From your history form I see that you associate your back pain with lifting a heavy box 2 weeks ago. When did you first notice your back pain (sudden or gradual onset)?

Have you ever hurt your back before or have you ever had pain similar to this episode in the past? (Systemic disease: recurrent and gradually increases over time)

Please describe your pain (supply descriptive terms if necessary)

How often do you have this pain?
   FUPs   How long does it last when you have it?

What aggravates your pain/symptoms?

What relieves your pain/symptoms?

How does rest affect your pain?

Have you noticed any changes in your pain/symptoms since they first started up to the present time?

Do you have any numbness in the groin or inside your legs? (Saddle anesthesia: cauda equina)

Pulmonary

I notice you have quite a cough and you sound hoarse to me. How long have you had this cough and hoarseness (when did it first begin)?

Do you have any back pain associated with this cough? Any other pain associated with your cough? If yes, have the person describe where, when, intensity, aggravating and relieving factors.

How does it feel when you take a deep breath? Does your low back hurt when you laugh or take a deep breath?

When you cough, do you produce phlegm or mucus? If yes, have your ever noticed any red streaks or blood in it?

Does your coughing or back pain keep you awake at night?

Have you been examined by a physician for either your cough or your back pain?

Have you had any recent chest or spine x-rays taken? If yes, when and where. What were the results?

General Systemic

Have you had any night sweats, daytime fevers, or chills?

Do you have difficulty in swallowing or experience recurrent laryngitis? **(Oral cancer)**

Urologic

Have you ever been told that you have a prostate problem or prostatitis? If yes, determine when this occurred, how it was treated, and whether the person had the same symptoms at that time that he is now describing to you.

Have you noticed any change in your bladder habits?

FUPS: Have you had any difficulty in starting to urinate?

If you start urinating, does the flow start and stop without your being able to control it?

Is there any burning or discomfort on urination?

Have you noticed any blood in your urine?

Have you recently had any difficulty with kidney stones or bladder or kidney infections?

Gastrointestinal

Have you noticed any change in your bowel pattern?

Have you had difficulty having a bowel movement or find that you have soiled yourself without even realizing it? (**Cauda equina lesion**—this would require immediate referral to a physician)

Does your back pain begin or increase when you are having a bowel movement?

Is your back pain relieved after having a bowel movement?

Have you noticed any association between when you eat and when your pain/symptoms increase or decrease?

Final Question

Is there anything about your current back pain or your general health that we have not discussed that you think is important for me to know?

Refer to Special Questions to Ask for other questions that may be pertinent to this client, depending on the answers to these questions.

PHYSICIAN REFERRAL

As always, correlation of findings is important in making a decision regarding medical referral. If the client has a positive family history for respiratory problems (especially lung cancer) and if clinical findings indicate pulmonary involvement, the client should be strongly encouraged to see a physician for a medical check-up. If there are positive systemic findings, such as difficulty in swallowing, persistent hoarseness, shortness of breath at rest, night sweats, fevers, bloody sputum, recurrent laryngitis, or upper respiratory infections *either in addition to or in association with* the low back pain, the client should be advised to see a physician, and the physician should receive a copy of your findings. This guideline covers the client who has a true musculoskeletal problem but also has other health problems, as well as the client who may have back pain of systemic origin that is unrelated to the lifting injury 2 weeks ago.

References

Bauwens, D.B., and Paine, R.: Thoracic pain. *In* Backlow, R.S. (ed.). MacBryde's Signs and Symptoms, 6th ed. Philadelphia, J.B. Lippincott, 1983, pp. 139–164.

Berkow, R., and Fletcher, A.J. (eds.): The Merck Manual of Diagnosis and Therapy, 16th ed. Rahway, New Jersey, Merck Sharp & Dohme Research Laboratory, 1992.

Boring, C.C., Squires, T.S., and Tong, T.: Cancer statistics, CA: A Cancer Journal for Clinicians *43*:7–26, 1993.

Brudney, K., and Dobkin, J.: Resurgent tuberculosis in New York City: HIV, homeless and the decline of tuberculosis control programs. American Review of Respiratory Disease *144*:745–749, 1991.

Centers for Disease Control: Tuberculosis and human immunodeficiency virus infections: Recommendations of the Advisory Committee for the Elimination of Tuberculosis (ACET). Morbidity and Mortality Weekly Report *38*:236–250, 1989.

Claremont, H., Johnson, M., Coberly, J., et al.: Tolerance of short course tuberculosis chemoprophylaxis in HIV-infected individuals. Presented at the VII International Conference on AIDS, Florence, Italy, June 1991.

Cronin, S.N.: Nursing care of clients with lower airway disorders. *In* Black, J.M., and Matassarin-Jacobs, E. (eds.): Luckmann and Sorensen's Medical-Surgical Nursing, 4th ed. Philadelphia, W.B. Saunders, 1993, pp. 1021–1088.

Engelking, C.: Lung cancer: Chemotherapy. American Journal of Nursing *87*(11):1434, 1987.

Flaskerud, J., and Ungvarski, P.: HIV/AIDS, A Guide to Nursing Care, 2nd ed. Philadelphia, W.B. Saunders, 1992.

Gaskell, D.V., and Webber, B.A.: The Brompton Hospital Guide to Chest Physiotherapy, 4th ed. Oxford, Blackwell Scientific Publications, 1980.

Gershwin, M.E., and Klingelhofer, E.L.: Asthma: Stop Suffering, Start Living, 2nd ed. Reading, Massachusetts, Addison-Wesley Publishing Company, 1992.

Gritz, E.R.: Lung cancer: Now, more than ever, a feminist issue. CA: A Cancer Journal for Clinicians *43*(4):197–199, 1993.

Guyton, A.: Human Physiology and Mechanisms of Disease. Philadelphia, W.B. Saunders, 1992.

Hansen, H., Perry, M.C., Arriagada, A., et al.: Treatment evaluation: II IASLC workshop on combined radiotherapy and chemotherapy modalities in lung cancer. Lung Cancer, in press.

Hinson, J.A., and Perry, M.C.: Small cell lung cancer. CA: A Cancer Journal for Clinicians *43*(4):216–225, 1993.

Jarvis, C: Physical Examination and Health Assessment. Philadelphia, W.B. Saunders, 1992.

Lehman, M.K.: Acid-base imbalance. *In* Phipps, W., Long, B., Woods, N., and Cassmeyer, V. (eds.): Medical-Surgical Nursing Concepts and Clinical Practice. St. Louis, Mosby–Year Book, 1991, pp. 569–576.

Lesmes, G.R., and Donofrio, K.H.: Passive smoking: The medical and economic issues. American Journal of Medicine *93*(1A):38S–42S, 1992.

Liles, W.C., and Ramsey, P.G.: Infectious diseases. *In* Ramsey, P.G., and Larson, E.B. (eds): Medical Therapeutics, 2nd ed. Philadelphia, W.B. Saunders, 1993, pp. 62–127.

Mann, J., Tarantola, D.J.M., and Netter, T.W. (eds.): AIDS in the World: A Global Report. Cambridge, Massachusetts, Harvard University Press, 1992, p. 162.

Martini, N.: Operable lung cancer. CA: A Cancer Journal for Clinicians *43*(4):201–214, 1993.

Martini, N., Bains, M.S., McCormack, P.M., et al.: Surgical treatment in non-small cell carcinoma of the lung: The Memorial Sloan–Kettering experience. *In* Hoogstraten, B., Addis, B.J., Hansen, H.H., et al. (eds.): Treatment of Lung Tumors. Heidelberg, Germany, Springer-Verlag, 1987, pp. 111–132.

Mays, P. H., Richman, J., and Harris, H. W.: Results of a program to reduce admissions for adult asthma. Annals of Internal Medicine *112*:864–871, 1990.

Mengert, T.J., and Albert, R.K.: Pulmonary conditions. *In* Ramsey, P.G., and Larson, E.B. (eds.): Medical Therapeutics, 2nd ed. Philadelphia, W.B. Saunders, 1993, pp. 238–293.

Mitchell, J.: Nursing in management: Lower respiratory problems. *In* Lewis, S., and Collier, I. (eds.): Medical-Surgical Nursing, Assessment and Management of Clinical Problems, 3rd ed. St. Louis, Mosby–Year Book, 1992, pp. 500–556.

Morbidity and Mortality Weekly Report: Incidence of asthma: Rising rates of prevalence, morbidity, and mortality in the United States. MMWR *39*:493–497, 1990.

Newman, J.H., and Ross, J.C.: Chronic cor pulmonale. *In* Hurst, J.W. (ed.): The Heart, 7th ed. New York, McGraw-Hill, 1990, pp. 1220–1229.

O'Toole, M. (ed.): Miller-Keane Encyclopedia and Dictionary of Medicine, Nursing and Allied Health, 5th ed. Philadelphia, W.B. Saunders, 1992.

Pagana, D., and Pagana, T.: Mosby's Diagnostic and Laboratory Test Reference. St. Louis, Mosby–Year Book, 1992.

Perez-Stable, E.J., and Hopewell, P.C.: Current tuberculosis treatment regimens: Choosing the right one for your patient. Clinics in Chest Medicine, *10*(3):323, 1989.

Purtilo, D.T., and Purtilo, R.B.: A Survey of Human Diseases, 2nd ed. Boston, Little, Brown, 1989.

Reynolds, M.D.: Myofascial trigger point syndromes in the practice of rheumatology. Archives of Physical Medicine and Rehabilitation *62*:111, 1981.

Scharf, S.M.: History and physical examination. *In* Baum, G.L., and Wolinsky, E. (eds.): Textbook of Pulmonary Diseases, 4th ed. Boston, Little, Brown, 1989, pp. 213–226.

Sexton, D.L.: Nursing Care of the Respiratory Patient. Norwalk, Connecticut, Appleton and Lange, 1990.

Silver, R.M.: Pulmonary manifestations of systemic sclerosis: Evaluation and management. Journal of Musculoskeletal Medicine *7*(4):33–46, 1990.

Silver, R.M., and LeRoy, E.C.: Systemic sclerosis (scleoderma). *In* Samter, M., Talmage, D.W., Frank, M.M., et al. (eds.): Immunological Diseases. Boston, Little, Brown, 1988, pp. 1459–1499.

Smeltzer, S., and Bare, B.: Brunner and Suddarth's Textbook of Medical-Surgical Nursing, 7th ed. Philadelphia, J.B. Lippincott, 1992.

Snider, D.E., and Roper, W.L.: The new tuberculosis. New England Journal of Medicine *332*:703–705, 1992.

Strohmyer, L.L.: Nursing care of clients during medical-surgical emergencies. *In* Black, J.M., and Matassarin-Jacobs, E. (eds.): Luckmann and Sorensen's Medical-Surgical Nursing, 4th ed. Philadelphia, W.B. Saunders, 1993, pp. 2217–2253.

Wang, K.K., and Viggiano, T.: Gastrointestinal diseases. *In* Ramsey, P.G., and Larson, E.B. (eds.): Medical Therapeutics, 2nd ed. Philadelphia, W.B. Saunders, 1993, pp. 294–329.

White, J.R., Froeb, H.F., and Kulik, J.A.: Respiratory illness in nonsmokers chronically exposed to tobacco smoke in the work place. Chest *100*(1):39–43, 1991.

Bibliography

Asthma: Reading and Resource List. National Asthma Education Program. Washington, D.C., National Heart, Lung and Blood Institute, 1990.

Bauchner, H., and Rappaport, L.: Asthma self-management programs: A guide to proper selection. American Journal of Asthma and Allergy for Pediatricians *4*(1):8–13, 1990.

Bierman, C.W.: Management of exercise-induced asthma. Annals of Allergy *68*:119–122, 1992.

Clark, C.J.: The role of physical training in asthma. Chest *10*(5)(Suppl.):293S–298S, 1992.

Kerem, E., Canny, G., Tibshirani, R., et al.: Clinical-physiologic correlations in acute asthma of childhood. Pediatrics *87*(4):481–486, 1991.

Rampulla, C., Baiocchi, S., Dacosto, E., and Ambrosino, N.: Dyspnea on exercise; Pathophysiologic mechanisms. Chest *10*(5)(Suppl.):248S–252S, 1992.

Overview of Hematologic Signs and Symptoms

Hematology is defined as the study of blood. The blood consists of two major components: plasma, a pale yellow or gray-yellow fluid; and formed elements, erythrocytes (red blood cells, or RBCs), leukocytes (white blood cells, or WBCs), and platelets (thrombocytes). Blood is the circulating tissue of the body; the fluid and its formed elements circulate through heart, arteries, capillaries, and veins.

The erythrocytes carry oxygen to tissues and remove carbon dioxide from them. Leukocytes act in inflammatory and immune responses. The plasma carries antibodies and nutrients to tissues and removes wastes from tissues. Coagulation factors in plasma, together with platelets, control the clotting of blood.

Primary hematologic diseases are uncommon, but hematologic manifestations secondary to other diseases are common (Purtilo and Purtilo, 1989).

BLOOD COMPOSITION AND PHYSIOLOGY

The total blood volume in an adult is about 6 liters (5.5 quarts) or about 7.5 per cent of the body weight. Approximately 45 per cent of blood consists of formed elements: erythrocytes, leukocytes, and platelets (thrombocytes). The remaining 55 per cent of the

189

blood is the fluid portion, which is called plasma. Approximately 90 per cent of plasma consists of water. The remaining 10 per cent consists of proteins (albumin, immunoglobulin and other globulins, and fibrinogen), carbohydrates, vitamins, hormones, enzymes, lipids, and salts.

The proteins exert a powerful osmotic pull so that water can move from tissues into the blood. The globulins (alpha, beta, and gamma) transport other proteins; gamma globulin (consisting primarily of immunoglobulins) functions as antibodies and specifically gives the body immunity to disease. Fibrinogen is a protein in the plasma that is converted into fibrin (also known as clotting factor I) and used in the formation of a blood clot.

The term *hematopoiesis* means the production of blood cells. The hematopoietic system consists of the circulating blood, the bone marrow, the spleen, the thymus, and the lymph nodes, supplemented by the reticuloendothelial (capable of engulfing or phagocytosing particles) cells lining blood sinuses and found in most organs of the body.

Blood Formation

Stem cells are precursor or mother cells for blood cells with the capacity for both blood cell replication and differentiation. Stem cells are the precursor cells for various morphologically different blood cells through a process called differentiation. The stem cell is stimulated to change into clearly recognizable forms of the various cell types (Table 5–1).

Blood cells must go through stages of development in the same way that a human matures during development. In a healthy person, only mature adult cells are seen in the blood, whereas in many diseases, the immature and abnormal forms of the cells may be present. In the human embryo, hematopoiesis begins within 2 weeks after conception. Initially, the primitive stem cells arise in blood islands within the yolk

Table 5–1

FORMATION OF BLOOD CELLS

Stem Cells (Precursors)	Mature Cells
Monoblasts or promonocytes	Monocytes
Monocytes	Macrophages
Erythroblasts	Erythrocytes
Myeloblasts	Granulocytes
Lymphoblasts	Lymphocytes
Megakaryocytes	Platelets

sac of the embryo. Later (still during the gestational period), hematopoiesis takes place at different times in the liver, spleen, thymus, lymph nodes, and bone marrow. At birth, and continuing during life, hematopoiesis is confined to the bone marrow.

In the child, hematopoietic (red) bone marrow is located in the flat bones of the skull, clavicle, sternum, ribs, and pelvis and also in the long bones of the extremities and in the vertebrae. By 18 years of age (and for the remainder of adult life), the red bone marrow is normally confined to the flat bones only.

Control of Hematopoiesis

Erythrocyte, leukocyte, and platelet production is thought to be controlled by hormones and feedback mechanisms that maintain an ideal number of cells. The number of individual blood cells is controlled by specific hormones. Erythropoietin governs erythrocyte production; thrombopoietin governs platelet production; and leukopoietin theoretically controls granulocyte production (Purtilo and Purtilo, 1989).

Erythropoeisis, for example, is regulated by cellular oxygen requirements and general metabolic oxygen needs. The main function of the erythrocyte is to carry hemoglobin, which transports oxygen to the tissues. When the hemoglobin level is below normal (less than 12 g/dl in women; less than 14 g/dl in men) (Table 5–2A), the tissues do not receive an adequate supply

Table 5–2

A. TOTAL RED BLOOD CELL (RBC) COUNT; HEMOGLOBIN AND HEMATOCRIT VALUES FOR ADULTS

	Total RBC Count	Hematocrit	Hemoglobin
Women	4 to 5.5 million/mm^3	35–47%	12–15 g/dl
Men	4.5 to 6.2 million/mm^3	42–52%	14–16.5 g/dl

B. TOTAL WHITE BLOOD CELL (LEUKOCYTE) COUNT AND DIFFERENTIAL COUNT IN ADULTS AND CHILDREN OVER 2 YEARS OF AGE

Total WBC Count	4500–11,000/mm^3

Differential Count

Granulocytes	
Segs (segmented neutrophils; mature)	54–62%
Bands or stabs (immature neutrophils)	3–5%
EOs (eosinophils)	1–3%
BASOs (basophils)	0–.75%
Monos (monocytes)	3–7%
Lymphs (lymphocytes)	25–33%

C. PLATELET (THROMBOCYTE) COUNT

Adult and Child (over one year of age)	150,000–400,000/mm^3
Critical low	Less than 30,000/mm^3
Critical high	Greater than 1,000,000/mm^3

of oxygen, and a state of hypoxia exists. The lowered oxygen concentration in the blood stimulates the kidneys to produce the hormone erythropoietin. Erythropoietin is released from the kidneys and stimulates bone marrow stem cells to produce new erythrocytes. A decrease in or a lack of erythropoietin, such as occurs in both acute and chronic renal failure, results in severe anemia.

Normally, the rate of production of erythrocytes determines the hemoglobin level or erythrocyte count in the peripheral blood and shows little variation among normal individuals.

Production of erythrocytes can be limited by the availability of essential nutrients (e.g., iron, protein, folate, vitamins B$_{12}$ and B$_6$). Deficiency of these essential nutrients prevents normal maturation of the primitive red blood cells (erythroblasts) into erythrocytes, resulting in a nutritional deficiency anemia.

Erythrocytes

Erythrocytes outnumber leukocytes by 600 to 1. The average number of erythrocytes per cubic millimeter (mm^3) of circulating blood is about 5 million. Women are a few per cent below this value, and men are a few per cent above it (Guyton, 1992). This difference in erythrocyte values between men and women may be due to the erythropoietic stimulation that androgenic hormones have on the bone marrow. In addition, the altitude at which the person lives and the person's level of exercise affect the number of erythrocytes produced.

At high altitudes, where the quantity of oxygen in the air is decreased, insufficient amounts of oxygen are carried to the tissues, and erythrocytes are produced rapidly, so that the number of erythrocytes available for oxygen transport increases. The degree of a person's physical activity also helps determine the rate at which erythrocytes are produced. The athlete may have an erythrocyte count as high as 6.5 million/mm^3, whereas a sedentary person may have a count as low as 3 million/ mm^3 (Guyton, 1992).

Five days are required for the production of mature erythrocytes from stem cells. These erythrocytes live approximately 120 days in the bloodstream before being filtered through the spleen into the liver, where damaged erythrocytes are engulfed by reticuloendothelial cells. The mature erythrocyte consists primarily of hemoglobin and functions to supply oxygen to the tissues, removing carbon dioxide. Because of its biconcave disclike shape and flexibility, the erythrocyte is capable of squeezing through the narrow capillaries without rupturing. Abnormalities in either the shape or flexibility of erythrocytes are important components of some blood disorders, such as sickle cell anemia. Disorders of erythrocytes are classified as follows:

- Anemia (too few erythrocytes)
- Polycythemia (too many erythrocytes)
- Poikilocytosis (abnormally shaped erythrocytes)
- Anisocytosis (abnormal variations in size of erythrocytes)
- Hypochromia (deficient in hemoglobin)

Hemoglobin

Hemoglobin consists of an iron-containing molecule, heme, and a protein, globin.

Synthesis of hemoglobin begins in the mitochondria and continues in the cytoplasm of the cell. No hemoglobin synthesis takes place in the mature erythrocyte. The hemoglobin molecule within the erythrocyte is responsible for supplying the tissues with oxygen. The normal hemoglobin molecule has an attraction for oxygen as the oxygen binds to the iron in the hemoglobin. However, the iron of heme bonds more readily with carbon monoxide than with oxygen—a bond so tight that none of the body's chemistry can break it up (Pavel et al., 1993). Carbon monoxide poisoning and iron deficiency (e.g., in diet) are the two primary factors that can adversely affect hemoglobin's ability to bind with oxygen.

Leukocytes

Blood contains three major groups of leukocytes:

- Lymphoid cells (lymphocytes, plasma cells)
- Monocytes
- Granulocytes (neutrophils, eosinophils, and basophils)

Lymphocytes produce antibodies and react with antigens, thus initiating the immune response to fight infection. *Monocytes* are the largest circulating blood cells and represent an immature cell until they leave the blood and travel to the tissues. Once migrated, monocytes form macrophages when activated by foreign substances such as bacteria. The monocytes are active phagocytes. *Granulocytes* (granular leukocytes) contain within their granules lysing agents capable of digesting various foreign materials. Granulocytes assist in initiating the inflammatory response and defend the body against infectious agents by phagocytosing bacteria and other infectious substances.

Generally, the *neutrophils* (the most plentiful of the granulocytes) are the first phagocytic cells to reach an infected area, followed by monocytes; neutrophils and monocytes work together to phagocytose all foreign material present. The capacity of corticosteroids or alcohol to diminish the accumulation of neutrophils in inflamed areas may be due to their ability to reduce cell adherence.

Eosinophils, usually active in the later stages of inflammation, have some phagocytic properties, but they are generally weaker than neutrophils. One of the primary functions of eosinophils is to surround and engulf antigen-antibody complexes formed during an allergic response. In addition, they are also able to defend against parasitic infections (Jennings, 1992). Eosinophilia (abnormally large number of eosinophils in the blood) can occur as a result of allergic reactions such as asthma; pernicious anemia; and neoplastic conditions such as leukemia.

Basophils have a high content of heparin and histamine and have an important role in acute systemic allergic reactions. In the presence of bacteria or other infectious agents, the basophils erupt and distribute chemicals that trigger inflammation. At this point, neutrophils, eosinophils, or monocytes arrive to engulf or phagocytose the alien particle. Little else is known of the function of basophil cells.

The leukocyte count denotes the number of leukocytes in 1 cubic millimeter (mm^3) of whole blood. The leukocyte in a normal, healthy individual is usually between 5 to 10,000 leukocytes/mm^3. The leukocyte count may be elevated *(leukocytosis)* in bacterial infections, appendicitis, leukemia, pregnancy, hemolytic disease of the newborn, uremia, ulcers, and normally at birth. The leukocyte count may drop below normal values *(leukopenia)* in viral diseases (e.g., measles), brucellosis, typhoid fever, infectious hepatitis, rheumatoid arthritis, cirrhosis of the liver, and lupus erythematosus. Radiation and chemotherapy also may severely lower the leukocyte count.

Laboratory Procedures for Detecting Leukocyte Abnormalities. Only a few laboratory procedures are useful for diagnosing abnormalities of leukocytes—tests for total leukocyte count, leukocyte differential (Table 5–2B), peripheral blood morphology, and bone marrow morphology.

A differential leukocyte count is often done to determine whether a person has an infection or disease of the blood such as leukemia, and it is a routine component of the complete blood cell count (CBC). The differential white blood cell count examines the leukocyte distribution of 100 white blood cells. These are then classified (differentiated) according to their type, and a relative percentage of each cell type is reported (Chernecky et al., 1993). If the percentage of any one type of cell is significantly increased, the percentage of other types will be decreased, because the differential records a total of 100 cells.

In addition, an increase in band or stab cells (immature neutrophils) is called a "shift to the left," because young cells are illustrated on the left side of a cell-counting area while mature cells are on the right. It is common to see a shift to the left when infectious states are occurring in the body and when the total white cell count is elevated. However, a shift to the left in the presence of a low total white blood cell count indicates bone marrow depression or failure (Chernecky et al., 1993).

Platelets (Thrombocytes)

Platelets are the smallest formed element in blood, formed from megakaryocytes in the bone marrow. Platelets function primarily in hemostasis (stopping bleeding) and in maintaining capillary integrity (Guyton, 1992) (Table 5–2C). They are important in the coagulation (blood clotting) mechanism by forming hemostatic plugs in small ruptured blood vessels or by adhering to any injured lining of larger blood vessels. A number of substances derived from the platelet that function in blood coagulation have been labeled "platelet factors." Platelets survive approximately 8 to 10 days in circulation and are then removed by the reticuloendothelial cells. *Thrombocytosis* refers to a condition in which the number of platelets is abnormally high, whereas *thrombocytopenia* refers to a condition in which the number of platelets is abnormally low.

Platelets are affected by anticoagulant drugs, including aspirin and heparin, by diet (presence of lecithin preventing coagulation or vitamin K from promoting coagulation), by exercise that boosts the production of chemical activators that destroy unwanted clots, and by liver disease that affects the supply of vitamin K. Platelets are also easily suppressed by radiation and chemotherapy.

Normal Hemostasis and Coagulation (Bithell, 1987; Reich, 1989)

Hemostasis may be defined as the process that arrests the flow of blood from vessels containing blood under pressure and leads to the control of bleeding through the formation of platelet and fibrin clots at the site of injury (Baldy, 1992). Hemostasis is initiated by vascular injury and results in the formation of a firm platelet-fibrin barrier that prevents the escape of blood from the damaged vessel. In humans, hemostasis is the result of three interrelated phenomena:

- Various reactions intrinsic to blood vessels
- The formation of platelet plugs
- The formation of fibrin, the result of the processes of blood coagulation

The processes of platelet aggregation and blood coagulation are intrinsically "self-propagating." They constitute a threat to the organism if they extend beyond the wound site into the general circulation. This process normally does not happen because of homeostatic regulatory phenomena.

Vascular Phase

The vascular phenomenon associated with normal hemostasis and coagulation in humans is not clearly understood. The endothelium may release or secrete several substances that are active in the vascular phase of the hemostatic process. These substances include

- Tissue factor (activates the extrinsic pathway of coagulation)
- Adenosine diphosphate (ADP; mediates platelet aggregation)
- Bradykinin (vasodilator; important in inflammation)

The first step in the vascular phase is the constriction of arterioles at the edges of the wound while platelets clump together (platelet phase) to form a clot or thrombus, which in turn applies mechanical pressure by plugging the site of bleeding and by preventing further bleeding (Guyton, 1992).

Platelet Phase

After vascular injury, ADP is released from injured tissues or erythrocytes as the major factor in the initiation of the platelet phase. Platelets are first seen to adhere to exposed subendothelial structures, particularly collagen fibers. This phenomenon, called *platelet adhesion,* produces biochemical activation of the platelets. Various prostaglandins (fatty acids) and thromboxanes, which induce platelet aggregation and constrict arterial smooth muscle, are then synthesized. Other substances from storage sites within the platelet are released into the external environment to aid in vasoconstriction. Activated platelets become "sticky" and attach to each other to form clumps or plugs that increase progressively in size *(platelet aggregation).*

Plugs consisting entirely of platelets may stop bleeding in small injuries, but permanent hemostasis requires the presence of fibrin, which is the protein end-product of blood coagulation.

Coagulation Phase

The coagulation of blood involves the interaction of several plasma coagulation factors that leads to the conversion of a plasma protein, fibrinogen, into fibrin. The fibrin forms a mesh that then traps platelets and erythrocytes to plug blood vessels (Purtilo and Purtilo, 1989).

By international agreement and common usage, the coagulation proteins are designated as the following Roman numeral ordering system (Pavel et al., 1993):*

Factor I	fibrinogen
Factor II	prothrombin
Factor III	tissue thromboplastin
Factor IV	calcium
Factor V	labile factor, proaccelerin
Factor VII	proconvertin, stable factor
Factor VIII	antihemophilic factor
Factor IX	plasma thromboplastin, Christmas factor
Factor X	Stuart-Prower factor
Factor XI	plasma thromboplastin antecedent, antihemophilic factor C
Factor XII	Hageman factor
Factor XIII	fibrin-stabilizing factor

Plasma-clotting factors are inactive until substances released by injured tissues trigger activation of these factors. For example, fibrin is a strong polymer (protein) that is the physical basis of permanent hemostatic plugs formed in all blood clots. Thrombin (an enzyme) converts circulating fibrinogen into fibrin polymers. Thrombin generation occurs through two different re-

---

* Numeral VI is not used, and the numeric order of the factors does not reflect reaction sequence.

action sequences, the intrinsic and extrinsic coagulation pathways, which are not discussed in further detail in this text. The reader is referred to a more comprehensive hematologic textbook for a greater understanding of these pathways (see Bibliography).

CLASSIFICATION OF BLOOD DISORDERS

Erythrocyte Disorders

Anemia

Anemia is a reduction in the oxygen-carrying capacity of the blood owing to an abnormality in the quantity or quality of erythrocytes. The World Health Organization (WHO) has defined anemia in terms of the level of hemoglobin: less than 14 g/dl for men and less than 12 g/dl for women. "Low" levels may be appropriate if tissue oxygen requirements are decreased (e.g., in hypothyroidism) or if tissue delivery is enhanced by a decrease in hemoglobin oxygen affinity. "Normal" levels may be inadequate if tissue oxygen delivery is impaired by pulmonary insufficiency, cardiac disorders, or an increase in hemoglobin oxygen affinity (Price and Solomon, 1993).

Deficiency in the oxygen-carrying capacity of blood may result in disturbances in the function of many organs and tissues. These disturbances may lead to various symptoms that can also differ from one person to another. Slowly developing anemia in young, otherwise healthy individuals is well tolerated, and there may be no symptoms until hemoglobin concentration and hematocrit fall below one half of normal (see Table 5–2A). This person might make an appointment with a physician because many people have commented on the person's pale appearance. However, anemia of rapid onset may result in additional symptoms of dyspnea and palpitations even before severely low levels of he-

CLASSIFICATIONS OF ANEMIA

1. Acute or Chronic Loss of Blood

- Hemorrhage
- Excessive menstruation
- Bleeding hemorrhoids
- Bleeding peptic ulcers
- Renal failure (hemodialysis)

2. Destruction of Erythrocytes

- Mechanical or autoimmune hemolysis
- Hemoglobin abnormalities (e.g., sickle cell anemia)
- Enzyme defects (e.g., G6PD deficiency)
- Parasites (e.g., malaria)
- Hypersplenism
- Hereditary spherocytosis*
- Chronic inflammatory diseases

3. Decreased Production of Erythrocytes Due to Nutritional Deficiency

- Iron, B_{12}, folic acid deficiency

4. Decreased Production of Erythrocytes Due to Cellular Maturational Defects

- Thalassemias†
- Cytotoxic drugs (e.g., antineoplastic drugs)

5. Decreased Production of Erythrocytes Due to Decrease or Loss of Bone Marrow Function

- Decreased marrow stimulation (e.g., hypothyroidism, decreased erythropoietin production)
- Marrow failure (e.g., leukemia, aplasia)

---

* Erythrocytes have small spheres instead of the normal flexible biconcave disc shapes. These spheres rupture easily.

† Hemolytic anemia marked by a decreased rate of synthesis of one or more hemoglobin polypeptide chains.

Table 5–3
CHANGES ASSOCIATED WITH HEMATOLOGIC DISORDERS

Changes	Causes
Skin	
Light, lemon-yellow tint	Untreated pernicious anemia
White, waxy appearance	Severe anemia secondary to acute hemorrhage
Gray-green yellow	Chronic blood loss
Gray tint	Leukemia
Pale hands or palmar creases	Anemia
Nail Bed	
Brittle	Long-standing iron deficiency anemia
Concave (rather than convex)	Long-standing iron deficiency anemia
Oral Mucosa/Conjunctiva	
Pale or yellow color	Anemia

matocrit and hemoglobin have been reached.

A blood test is required to diagnose anemia medically, but it is sometimes difficult to define the borderline between normal blood and a state of anemia. All measures that determine numbers of red blood cells, hematocrit, and hemoglobin must take into account the variation and ranges in values among normal, healthy subjects.

Causes. Anemia is not a disease but is instead a symptom of any number of different blood disorders. It can be caused by factors such as poor diet (nutritional anemia); blood loss; exposure to industrial poisons such as chlorine gas; or diseases of the bone marrow (O'Toole, 1992). Anemias are usually classified on the basis of erythrocyte appearance (morphology) or etiology of the disease. Most anemias are caused by (1) loss of erythrocytes, (2) hemolysis (increased destruction of erythrocytes), or (3) decreased production of erythrocytes (see Classification of Anemia).

Clinical Signs and Symptoms. Although anemia is not the most common cause of weakness and fatigue, rapid onset of listlessness characterized by weakness and fatigue is an early sign of anemia and reflects the lack of oxygen transport to the lungs and muscles. Many people can have moderate-to-severe anemia without these symptoms. Because of the wide normal variations in skin color, changes in skin color, oral mucosae, and conjunctivae are more important than just pale skin. Changes in the hands and fingernail beds (Table 5–3; Fig. 5–1) are more reliable signs in observing anemia than facial skin. Although there is no difference in normal blood volume associated with severe anemia, there is a redistribution of blood so that organs most sensitive to oxygen deprivation (e.g., the brain, heart, and muscles) receive more blood than, for example, the hands and kidneys (Guyton, 1992).

During the inspection/observation portion of the objective examination, the physical therapist should look for pale palms

▼
Clinical Signs and Symptoms of
Anemia

- Skin pallor (palms, nail beds)
- Fatigue and listlessness
- Dyspnea on exertion accompanied by heart palpitations and rapid pulse (more severe anemia)

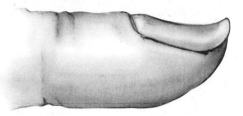

Figure 5–1

Abnormal condition of the nails associated with anemia. Thin, depressed nails with lateral edges tilted up, forming a concave profile called koilonychia (spoon nails), may also be due to a congenital or hereditary trait. (From Jarvis, C.: Physical Examination and Health Assessment. Philadelphia, W.B. Saunders, 1992, p. 271.)

with normal-colored creases (severe anemia causes pale creases as well). Observation of the hands should be done at the level of the client's heart. In addition, the anemic client's hands should be warm; if they are cold, the paleness is due to vasoconstriction. Pallor in dark-skinned people may be observed by the absence of the underlying red tones that normally give brown or black skin its luster. The brown-skinned individual demonstrates pallor with a more yellowish-brown color, and the black-skinned person will appear ashen or gray (Jarvis, 1992). The physician will also look at the conjunctivae of the eyes, mouth, pharynx, and lips for paleness or yellow color as additional confirming signs of anemia. Specific skin and nail changes are listed in Table 5–3.

Systolic blood pressure may not be affected, but diastolic pressure may be lower than normal, with an associated increase in the resting pulse rate. Resting cardiac output is usually normal in people with anemia, but cardiac output increases with exercise more than in nonanemic persons. As the anemia becomes more severe, resting cardiac output increases and exercise tolerance progressively decreases until dyspnea, tachycardia, and palpitations occur at rest.

Diminished exercise tolerance is expected in the client with anemia. Research has shown that people with chronic renal failure who have severe anemia are able to exercise but must exercise at a lower intensity than that of the normal population. The $\dot{V}O_{2max}$ for this type of anemic client is at least 20 per cent less than that for the normal population (Painter, 1993). Exercise testing and prescribed exercise(s) in anemic clients must be instituted with extreme caution and should proceed very gradually to tolerance and/or perceived exertion levels (Painter, 1993). In addition, exercise for any anemic client should be first approved by his or her physician.

Treatment. Treatment for anemia is determined according to the cause of the anemia and can include the following:

- Red blood cell transfusion (replacement of blood loss)
- Bone marrow transplantation (replacement of damaged marrow)
- Vitamin B_{12}; folic acid; iron (replacement of nutritional needs)
- Corticosteroids and androgens (stimulation of marrow to produce RBCs)
- Splenectomy (decrease destruction of RBCs)
- Erythropoietin replacement

Treatment of the severe anemia associated with renal failure has benefited from the recent availability of recombinant human erythropoietin (EPO; Epogen). The client with chronic renal failure who has a hematocrit of less than 30 per cent usually experiences significant symptoms of anemia and is a candidate for this new therapy. Human erythropoietin stimulates erythropoiesis and may elevate red blood cell counts enough to decrease the need for blood transfusions in this population. Currently this drug is recommended only for the treatment of anemia associated with chronic renal failure and the anemia secondary to zidovudine (AZT) therapy in HIV-infected persons (Deglin and Vallerand, 1993).

Table 5–4

LABORATORY VALUES ASSOCIATED WITH POLYCYTHEMIA

	Men	Women
Hemoglogin	> 17.5 g/dl	> 15.5 g/dl
Erythrocytes	> 6.0 × 10^{12}/L	> 5.5 × 10^{12}/L
Hematocrit	42–52%	37–47%

Polycythemia (O'Toole, 1992)

Polycythemia (also known as erythrocytosis) is defined as an increase in the total erythrocyte mass of the blood, characterized by an excessive number of erythrocytes and an increased concentration of hemoglobin. These increases in both the number of red blood cells and the concentration of hemoglobin result in an increased hematocrit (measure of the volume of packed red blood cells) and an increased hemoglobin level (Table 5–4). People with polycythemia have increased whole blood viscosity and increased blood volume.

The increased erythrocyte production results in this thickening of the blood and an increased tendency toward clotting. The viscosity of the blood limits its ability to flow easily, diminishing the supply of blood to the brain and to other vital tissues. Increased platelets in combination with the increased blood viscosity may contribute to the formation of intravascular thrombi. In the normal, healthy person, the number of erythrocytes is maintained at a stable level corresponding to the oxygen demand of the tissues. Any factors that reduce the supply of oxygen stimulate the production of the hormone erythropoietin, which is responsible for the control of erythrocyte production. The resultant increase in erythrocytes enables the blood to carry more oxygen to the tissues.

Types. There are two distinct forms of polycythemia:

■ Primary polycythemia (also known as polycythemia vera)

■ Secondary polycythemia

Polycythemia Vera. This disorder is one of a group of disorders collectively called myeloproliferative diseases. In this condition, production of erythrocytes is no longer under the control of erythropoietin. The effects of this form of polycythemia are well known: hyperplasia of the cell-forming tissues of the bone marrow with resultant elevation of the erythrocyte count and hemoglobin level and increase in the number of leukocytes and platelets. The etiology is unknown.

Polycythemia vera is a blood disorder that occurs in older people between 50 and 60 years of age; it is rarely diagnosed before 40 years of age. Men and women are affected equally. The increase in blood volume may be two to three times that of normal. Because of the increased concentration of erythrocytes and the resultant increased blood viscosity, the client shows increased skin coloration and elevated blood pressure. Gout is sometimes a complication of this form of polycythemia, and a typical attack of acute gout may be the first symptom.

Secondary Polycythemia. This disorder is a physiologic condition resulting from a decreased oxygen supply to the tissues, caused by situations such as normal acclimatization to high altitudes or heavy tobacco smoking. It also may be seen in association with severe, chronic lung and heart disorders, especially congenital heart defects. The body attempts to compensate for the reduced oxygen by manufacturing more hemoglobin and more erythrocytes. In some conditions, the production of erythropoietin is inappropriately increased, resulting in polycythemia.

Clinical Signs and Symptoms. The symptoms of this disease are often insidious in onset with vague complaints, and the client may be diagnosed only secondary to a sudden complication (e.g., a stroke or throm-

Clinical Signs and Symptoms of

Polycythemia

Clinical signs and symptoms of polycythemia (whether primary or secondary) are directly related to the increase in blood viscosity described earlier and may include

- Headache
- Dizziness
- Irritability
- Blurred vision
- Fainting
- Decreased mental acuity
- Feeling of fullness in the head
- Disturbances of sensation in the hands and feet
- General malaise and fatigue
- Weight loss
- Easy bruising
- Intolerable pruritus (skin itching) **(polycythemia vera)***
- Cyanosis (blue hue to the skin)
- Clubbing of the fingers
- Splenomegaly (enlargement of spleen)
- Gout
- Hypertension

---

* This condition of skin itching is particularly related to warm conditions, such as in bed at night or in a bath and is called the "hot bath sign" (Callender, 1986).

bosis). Blockage of the capillaries supplying the digits of either the hands or the feet may cause a peripheral vascular neuropathy with decreased sensation, burning, numbness, or tingling. This small blood vessel occlusion can also contribute to the development of cyanosis and clubbing. If the underlying disorder is not rec-ognized and treated, the person may develop gangrene and have subsequent loss of tissue.

Prognosis and Treatment. Because of the threat of complications from a thrombosis or hemorrhage, treatment is essential and directed toward reducing erythrocytes and platelets to normal values and suppressing the overactive bone marrow. In secondary polycythemia, successful treatment of the causative condition relieves the polycythemia. Mild cases can be treated with periodic phlebotomy (removal of excess blood), although this does not stop the rapid regeneration of erythrocytes and may cause iron deficiency. More serious cases require myelosuppressive therapy with radioactive agents. Injected into a vein, these agents localize in the bone marrow and irradiate the overactive marrow cells. The prognosis is good for 15 to 20 years after diagnosis, but enlargement of the spleen and replacement of the bone marrow by fibrous tissue results eventually in a condition called myelofibrosis, which may develop into an atypical leukemia-like disorder.

Sickle Cell Anemia

Sickle cell disease is a serious, hereditary, chronic disease. The sickle cell defect occurs in hemoglobin, the oxygen-carrying constituent of erythrocytes. Hemoglobin contains four chains of amino acids, the compounds that make up proteins. Two of the amino acid chains are known as alpha chains, and two are called beta chains. In normal hemoglobin, the amino acid in the sixth position on the beta chains isglutamic acid. But in people with sickle cell anemia, that sixth position is instead occupied by another amino acid, valine.This single amino acid substitution hasdevastating consequences (Gaston, 1990).

After releasing oxygen, hemoglobin molecules that contain the beta chain defect stick to one another instead of staying separate, forming long, rigid rods or tubules inside red blood cells. The rods cause the normally smooth, doughnut-shaped red cells to take on a sickle or curved shape and to lose their vital ability to deform and squeeze through tiny blood vessels. The sickled cells, which become stiff and sticky, clog small blood vessels, depriving tissue of an adequate blood supply. Most of the problems associated with sickle cell anemia, including pain from ulcers, strokes, and blindness, stem from this blockage (Gaston, 1990).

Risk Factors. Sickle cell anemia is most common among tropical Africans (as much as 30 per cent) and their descendants. Approximately 1 in 12 African-Americans carry the abnormal gene, and about 1 in 625 persons develop actual sickle cell anemia. Sickle cell anemia can also occur in persons of Mediterranean ancestry (Adams and Zanderer, 1993).

Individuals with the mutant gene from only one parent are said to have sickle cell trait. About 40 per cent of the hemoglobin in these individuals is hemoglobin S (HbS), the abnormal sickle cell hemoglobin. Under normal circumstances, there appear to be no clinical signs and symptoms associated with this amount of HbS. Sickle cell disease occurs when the individual inherits the mutant gene from each parent; thus almost all the hemoglobin is HbS. Approximately 50,000 individuals have sickle cell disease in the United States, and there is a correspondingly higher number in Africa.

Pathogenesis. Researchers postulate that in the arterial system, the erythrocytes contain an oxygenated solution of HbS (Mozzarelli et al., 1987). When the cell squeezes through a narrow capillary to reach the venous system, it releases its oxygen to the tissues. The sickle hemoglobin transports oxygen normally, but when it loses its oxygen, the hemoglobin molecules align themselves in such a way that the erythrocytes become stiff and sickle cell–shaped. For a time, this sickling is reversible because the cells are reoxygenated in arterial blood; however, eventually the change becomes irreversible.

In the process of sickling and unsickling, the erythrocyte membrane becomes damaged. In addition, the abnormally stiff cells do not pass easily through capillaries and veins and tend to cause obstruction to the blood flow (Callender, 1986). Under stress, oxygen is released too soon and the cell sickles while it is in the capillary, thus blocking this small vessel. Oxygen deprivation takes place, and damage to tissue occurs. The sooner the oxygen is released, the more severe (clinically) is the sickle cell disease. This release time can be shortened even more by the presence of acidosis, dehydration, trauma, strenuous physical exertion, emotional stress, pregnancy, extremes of heat and cold, and increased body temperatures (fever) (Adams and Zanderer, 1993).

Sickle cell anemia is characterized by a series of "crises" that result from early destruction of the abnormal cells and obstruction of blood flow to the tissues. Stress from viral or bacterial infection, hypoxia, dehydration, emotional disturbance, extreme temperatures, or fatigue may precipitate a crisis. Clinical crises in sickle cell disease can be either acute or chronic and usually fit into one of three categories based on mechanism (Thomas and Holbrook, 1987):

- Vasoocclusion

- Infection

- Erythrocyte destruction or sequestration

Clinical Signs and Symptoms. Clinical symptoms may be observed in the first year of life (Ahulu-Konotey, 1974).

Pain is caused by blockage of red blood cells forming sickle cell clots. This vasoocclusive crisis (painful episodes of ischemic tissue damage) typically lasts for 5 or 6 days. Older clients more often report extremity and back pain during vascular crises. Compared with hand-foot syndrome, the pain is usually asymmetric and is not associated with swelling. Sickle cell disease

▼ *Clinical Signs and Symptoms of*
Sickle Cell Anemia

- Pain
  - Abdominal
  - Chest
  - Headaches
- Bone and joint crises from the ischemic tissue, lasting for hours to days and subsiding gradually
  - Low-grade fever
  - Extremity pain
  - Back pain
  - Periosteal pain
  - Joint pain, especially in the shoulder and hip
- Vascular complications
  - Cerebrovascular accidents (affects children and young adults most often)
  - Chronic leg ulcers
  - Avascular necrosis of the femoral head
  - Bone infarcts
- Pulmonary crises
  - Bacterial pneumonia
  - Pulmonary infarction (less common)
- Neurologic manifestations
  - Convulsions

- Drowsiness
- Coma
- Stiff neck
- Paresthesias
- Cranial nerve palsies
- Blindness
- Nystagmus
- Hand-foot syndrome
  - Fever
  - Pain
  - Dactylitis (painful swelling of the dorsum of hands and feet)
- Splenic sequestration crisis (occurs before adolescence)
  - Liver and spleen enlargement due to trapped erythrocytes
  - Subsequent spleen atrophy due to repeated blood vessel obstruction
- Renal complications
  - Enuresis (bed-wetting)
  - Nocturia (excessive urination at night)
  - Hematuria (blood in the urine)
  - Pyelonephritis
  - Renal papillary necrosis
  - End-stage renal failure (elderly population)

in a young child often presents as the hand-foot syndrome in a symmetric pattern. Occlusion of small vessels supplying the metacarpal and metatarsal bones causes painful swelling, which is often accompanied by a low-grade fever. Vasoocclusive crises other than hand-foot syndrome are less common in children under 5 years of age (Vichinsky et al., 1988).

Cerebrovascular accidents (CVAs) are a frequent and severe manifestation of sickle cell anemia, and they affect 6 per cent to 12 per cent of clients, most commonly children. Recovery may be complete in some cases, or serious neurologic damage may result. A second CVA occurs in up to 70 per cent of those who have the initial neurologic insult.

Prognosis and Treatment. The prognosis for persons with sickle cell disease is poor. Some people with the disease have only a few symptoms, whereas others are affected severely and have a short life span. Very few people who are affected severely live beyond the age of 20 years, and some people die in infancy or early childhood (O'Toole, 1992). Cerebral hemorrhage or shock causes death in many children with this disorder. Early diagnosis, especially newborn screening for the abnormal hemoglobins, is important in the long-term preventive care of these people.

Although there is no cure for sickle cell anemia, significant decreases in morbidity and mortality have been achieved by early diagnosis, intensive medical supervision, and advances in the treatment of complications. With advances in the treatment of sickle cell disease, some people may survive beyond age 60 years (Adams and Zanderer, 1993).

Investigators at the National Institutes of Health and Johns Hopkins University School of Medicine have investigated the use of fetal hemoglobin as a treatment possibility. Fetal hemoglobin is the hemoglobin present in the unborn fetus. After birth, the body stops making fetal hemoglobin and begins to produce adult hemoglobin. It has been observed that people with sickle cell anemia have a lower than normal amount of fetal hemoglobin. Significantly increased fetal hemoglobin levels can decrease the ability of cells to sickle. A new prescription drug (hydroxyurea) is being tested as a way to increase the level of fetal hemoglobin in red blood cells, thereby preventing the complications of sickle cell anemia. Serious side effects hamper general use of this treatment.

At the present time, treatment of sickle cell anemia is symptomatic, and preventive measures are used to reduce the incidence of crises and to avoid dehydration, cold, and infections. When the crisis is due to inflammatory changes, medications such as analgesics or corticosteroids are sometimes administered to relieve musculoskeletal pain (O'Toole, 1992). Exchange transfusions to reduce hemoglobin S levels below 40 per cent may be used therapeutically (for neurologic, cardiac, or retinal symptoms; hypoxemia; severe prolonged or infarctive crises; acute splenic sequestration [infants]; and chronic leg ulcers). These transfusions also can be used prophylactically (during pregnancy or before general anesthesia). Long-term exchange transfusion may be useful in selected clients with severe neurologic retinal or cardiac symptoms (Jarvis, 1992).

Specific physical therapy treatment of the person with sickle cell disease (whether a child or an adult) is outlined by McLaurin (1985).

Case Example. A 20-year-old African-American woman came to physical therapy with severe right knee joint pain. She could recall no traumatic injury but reported hiking 2 days previously in the Rocky Mountains with her brother, whom she was visiting (she was from New York City). A general screen for systemic illness revealed frequent urination over the past 2 days. She also complained of stomach pain, but she thought this was related to the stress of visiting her family. Past medical history included one other similar episode when she had acute pneumonia at the age of 11 years. She stated that she usually felt fatigued but thought it was due to her active social life and busy professional career.

On examination, the right knee was enlarged and inflamed, with joint range of motion limited by the local swelling. In fact, pain, swelling, and guarded motion in the joint prevented a complete evaluation. Given that restraint, there were no other physical findings, but not all special tests were completed. The neurologic screen was negative.

This woman was treated for local joint inflammation, but the combination of change in altitude, fatigue, increased urination, and stomach pains alerted the therapist to the possibility of a systemic process despite the client's explanation for the fatigue and stomach upset. Because the client was from out of town and did not have a local physician, the therapist telephoned the hospital emergency department for a telephone consultation. It was suggested that a blood sample be obtained for preliminary screening while the client continued to receive physical therapy. Laboratory results included the following:

Hct	30%	(normal = 35 to 47%)
Hb	10 g/dl	(normal = 12 to 15 g/dl)
WBC	20,000/mm^3	(normal = 4500 to 11,000/mm^3)

Based on these findings, the client was admitted to the hospital and diagnosed as having sickle cell anemia. It is likely that the change in altitude, the emotional stress of visiting family, and the physical exertion precipitated a "crisis." She received continued physical therapy treatment during her hospital stay and was discharged with further follow-up planned in her home city.

Adapted from Jennings, B.: Nursing role in management: Hematological problems. *In* Lewis, S., and Collier, I. (eds.): Medical-Surgical Nursing: Assessment and Management of Clinical Problems. St. Louis, Mosby—Year Book, 1992, pp. 664–714. Used with permission.

Leukocyte Disorders

Leukocytosis

Leukocytosis characterizes many infectious diseases and is recognized by a count of more than 10,000 leukocytes/mm³. It can be associated with an increase in circulating neutrophils (neutrophilia). Leukocytosis is a common finding and may be caused by the following (Griffin, 1986):

- Bacterial infections
- Inflammation or tissue necrosis (e.g., infarction, myositis, vasculitis)
- Metabolic intoxications (e.g., uremia, eclampsia, acidosis, gout)

▼ ***Clinical Signs and Symptoms of***
Leukocytosis

These clinical signs and symptoms are usually associated with symptoms of the conditions listed earlier and may include

- Fever
- Symptoms of localized or systemic infection
- Symptoms of inflammation or trauma to tissue

- Neoplasms (especially bronchogenic carcinoma, lymphoma, melanoma)
- Acute hemorrhage
- Splenectomy
- Acute appendicitis
- Pneumonia
- Intoxication by chemicals
- Acute rheumatic fever

Leukopenia

Leukopenia, or reduction of the number of leukocytes in the blood below 5000 per microliter, can be caused by a variety of factors. It can occur in many forms of bone marrow failure such as that following antineoplastic chemotherapy or radiation therapy, in overwhelming infections, in dietary deficiencies, and in autoimmune diseases (Pagana and Pagana, 1992). Mild reduction in the white blood cell count can be caused by viral infections. Infection in the immunosuppressed person is a major problem. It is important for the physical therapist to be aware of the client's most recent white blood cell count prior to and during the course of physical therapy if the client is immunosuppressed.

Nadir, or the lowest point the white blood count reaches, usually occurs 7 to 14 days after chemotherapy or radiation therapy. At this time, the client is extremely

▼ ***Clinical Signs and Symptoms of***
Leukopenia

- Sore throat, cough
- High fever, chills, sweating
- Ulcerations of mucous membranes (mouth, rectum, vagina)
- Frequent or painful urination
- Persistent infections

susceptible to opportunistic infections and severe complications. The importance of good handwashing and hygiene practices cannot be overemphasized when treating any of these people.

Treatment. Treatment is directed toward elimination of the cause of the reduced leukocytes and control of any infections. Pharmacologic therapy includes the use of antibiotics, antifungal agents, and colony-stimulating drugs such as filgrastim (Neupogen). This relatively new drug is a glycoprotein that binds to and stimulates immature neutrophils to divide and differentiate and also activates mature neutrophils. This drug markedly assists in decreasing the incidence of infection in people who have received bone marrow–depressing antineoplastic agents (Deglin and Vallerand, 1993).

Leukemia

Leukemia is a disease arising from the bone marrow and involves the uncontrolled growth of blood cells; a complete discussion of this cancer is found in Chapter 10.

Platelet Disorders

Thrombocytosis

Thrombocytosis is a platelet count of more than 1 million per microliter. It is usually temporary and may occur as a compensatory mechanism after severe hemorrhage, surgery, and splenectomy; in iron deficiency and polycythemia vera; and as a manifestation of an occult (hidden) neoplasm (e.g., lung cancer). It is associated with a tendency to clot as well as a tendency to bleed. These manifestations can occur simultaneously because the excessive concentration of platelets is thought to interfere with the production of thromboplastin, which is necessary for normal coagulation (Schumann, 1992). Blood viscosity is increased by the very high platelet count, resulting in intravas-

cular clumping (or thrombosis) of the sludged platelets (Reich, 1989).

Thrombocytopenia

Thrombocytopenia, a decrease in the number of platelets (less than 150,000/mm³) (see Table 5–2C) in circulating blood, can result from decreased or defective platelet production or from accelerated platelet destruction. A major concern with this disorder is the prevention of excessive bleeding from trauma to the mucous membranes, skin, and underlying tissues, including muscles (O'Toole, 1992). Severe bleeding may occur from any mucous membrane, including the nose, uterus, gastrointestinal tract, urinary tract, and respiratory tract (Pavel et al., 1993). Causes of thrombocytopenia (Griffin, 1986) include

- Bone marrow infiltration by malignant cells (e.g., leukemia, metastatic carcinoma)
- Viral infections
- Prosthetic heart valves
- Nutritional deficiency
- Drugs (e.g., cytotoxic agents, gold, sulfonamides, ethanol/alcohol)
- Hemorrhage
- Disseminated intravascular coagulation (DIC): widespread formation of thromboses primarily in the capillaries
- Hypersplenism (condition of exaggerated hemolytic processes within the spleen)
- Aplastic anemia (deficiency of erythrocytes because of arrested development of erythrocytes in the bone marrow)
- Autoantibody-mediated platelet injury (e.g., idiopathic thrombocytopenic purpura, or ITP)
- Drug-induced platelet reduction or damage (e.g., from aspirin, quinidine, quinine, and sulfonamides)

Clinical Signs and Symptoms. Severe thrombocytopenia results in the appear-

▼ *Clinical Signs and Symptoms of*
Thrombocytopenia

- Bleeding after minor trauma
- Spontaneous bleeding
  - Petechiae (small red dots)
  - Ecchymoses (bruises)
  - Purpura spots (bleeding under the skin)
- Menorrhagia (excessive menstruation)
- Bleeding of the gums and nose

ance of multiple petechiae (small, purple, pinpoint hemorrhages into the skin), most often observed on the lower legs. Gastrointestinal bleeding and bleeding into the central nervous system associated with severe thrombocytopenia may be life-threatening manifestations of thrombocytopenic bleeding. These severe consequences of thrombocytopenia are not usually encountered by the physical therapist, and this disorder does not cause massive bleeding into the tissues or the joints.

However, the physical therapist must be alert for obvious skin or mucous membrane symptoms of thrombocytopenia, which include severe bruising, external hematomas, and the presence of multiple petechiae. These symptoms usually indicate a platelet count well below 100,000/mm³. Strenuous exercise or any exercise that involves straining or bearing down could precipitate a hemorrhage, particularly of the eyes or brain. People with undiagnosed thrombocytopenia need immediate physician referral.

Treatment. Treatment for thrombocytopenia depends on the precipitating cause. If the thrombocytopenia is caused by chemical agents such as cancer chemotherapy or radiation, then the agent may need to be stopped until the platelet count elevates. Platelet transfusions also can be administered when the count becomes dangerously low (less than 20,000/mm³; see

Table 5–2C). Methods of treatment for immune related thrombocytopenia, such as ITP, include corticosteroids, attenuated androgens (danazol), and plasmapheresis (Jennings, 1992; Pavel et al., 1993). Plasmapheresis is a procedure that removes blood from the body, separates the portion containing the antiplatelet antibodies, then returns the "cleansed" blood to the body.

Coagulation Disorders

Hemophilia (Cotta et al., 1986)

Hemophilia is a hereditary blood-clotting disorder caused by an abnormality of functional plasma-clotting proteins known as factors VIII and IX. In most cases, the hemophiliac person has normal amounts of the deficient factor circulating, but it is in a functionally inadequate state. Persons with hemophilia bleed longer than those with normal levels of functioning factors VIII or IX, but the bleeding is not any faster than would occur in a normal person with the same injury.

Etiology. This disease is sex-linked recessive, with bleeding manifested only in men; women carry and transmit the abnormal genes. The disease affects approximately 1 in 10,000 men from all races and socioeconomic groups. The female hemophilia carriers will transmit the gene to half of their daughters and half of their sons. Males with hemophilia transmit the gene to all of their daughters but to none of their sons (Pavel et al., 1993). Although in most cases of hemophilia there is a known family history, this disorder can occur in families without a previous history of blood-clotting disorders.

Types. The most common forms of hemophilia are hemophilia A (classic hemophilia), which affects the factor VIII gene, and hemophilia B (Christmas disease), which affects the factor IX gene. Both forms produce similar clinical bleeding patterns, but hemophilia A is the more common type, affecting approximately 80 per

Table 5–5
CLASSIFICATION OF HEMOPHILIA

Hemophilia	Clotting Activity Level *(% of Normal)	Hemorrhages
Mild	5 to 50	Spontaneous hemorrhages: rare
Moderate	>1 but <5	Spontaneous bleeding: not usually; major episodes after minor trauma
Severe	<1	Spontaneous bleeding or with minor trauma

* Normal concentrations of coagulation factors are between 50% and 150%. Level of severity remains constant throughout a person's life. The level of clotting factor and clinical symptoms present are usually similar among family members.
    Data from Cotta, S., Jutra, M., and McQuarrie, A.: Physical Therapy in Hemophilia. New York, The National Hemophilia Foundation, 1986.

cent of all hemophiliacs. Another clotting disorder is von Willebrand's disease, which is a rare deficiency or defect of a glycoprotein (von Willebrand factor)* and is frequently confused with hemophilia A. Von Willebrand's disease can also affect women (Pavel et al., 1993).

Hemophilia can be described as being mild, moderate, or severe based on the amount of active clotting factor present in the blood. The level of severity remains constant throughout a person's life. The level of clotting factor and clinical symptoms present are usually similar among family members. Normal concentrations of coagulation factors are between 50 per cent and 150 per cent (Cotta et al., 1986).

Persons with *mild hemophilia* have a clotting activity level of 5 per cent to 50 per cent. Spontaneous hemorrhages are rare, and joint and deep muscle bleeding is uncommon. These people bleed with surgical or other major trauma and must then be treated like people with severe hemophilia. Persons with *moderate hemophilia* have clotting factor levels greater than 1 per cent but less than 5 per cent. Spontaneous bleeding is usually not a problem

with these people; however, they can still have major bleeding episodes after minor trauma. *Severe hemophilia* is defined as a factor level activity in the blood less than 1 per cent of normal. These persons are likely to bleed spontaneously or with only slight trauma (Cotta et al., 1986) (Table 5–5).

Primary treatment goals for the hemophiliac client during bleeding episodes are to stop any bleeding that is occurring as quickly as possible and to transfuse the missing factors VIII and IX until the bleeding stops. Prophylactic transfusion of factors VIII and IX to a level of 50 per cent above normal is recommended prior to minor surgery and dental extractions or in case of minor injury (Pavel et al., 1993). Over time, the hemophiliac client may develop an inhibitor for the administered factors VIII or IX, which is an acquired circulating antibody that destroys these factors when they are transfused as a method of treatment. An inhibitor is found in approximately 10 per cent to 20 per cent of people with factor VIII deficiency and in 2 to 3 per cent of those with factor IX deficiency. Inhibitors usually develop in severe hemophiliacs before the age of 20 years and often result in complications in treatment (Cotta et al., 1986).

Clinical Signs and Symptoms. Usually diagnosed in childhood, hemophilia is demonstrated in the following ways (Pavel et al., 1993):

---

* For further information, refer to Hilgartner, M., and Montgomery, R.: Understanding von Willebrand's Disease. New York, The National Hemophilia Foundation, 1985.

- Slow persistent bleeding from cuts, scratches, and other minor trauma
- Delayed hemorrhage that follows minor injuries (hours to days after injury)
- Severe hemorrhaging from the gums after dental extraction
- Bleeding after brushing teeth with a hard-bristled toothbrush
- Sometimes fatal nosebleeds after injury to the nose
- Gastric hemorrhage
- Bleeding into deep subcutaneous tissue, muscle tissue, and around peripheral nerves
- Recurrent hemarthrosis

Bleeding into the joint spaces (hemarthrosis) is one of the most common clinical manifestations of hemophilia, most often affecting the knee, elbow, ankle, hip, and shoulder (in order of most common appearance). Recurrent hemarthrosis results in hemophiliac arthopathy (joint disease). Bleeding may result from an identifiable trauma or stress or may be spontaneous (most common with the severe hemophiliac). Hemarthroses are not common in the first year of life but increase in frequency as the child begins to walk. The severity of the hemarthrosis may vary (depending on the degree of injury) from mild pain and swelling, which resolves without

treatment within 1 to 3 days, to severe pain with an excruciatingly painful, swollen joint that persists for several weeks and resolves slowly with treatment.

Pain usually occurs before any other evidence of bleeding, and medical referral should be made even before there are physical signs. There must be a high level of suspicion that any unexplained symptom is an episode of bleeding (Price and Solomon, 1993). Coughing up blood is not a finding associated with hemophilia and should be reported to the physician immediately.

Bleeding into the joints eventually results in chronic joint changes, with a progressive loss of motion, muscle atrophy, and flexion contractures. Bleeding episodes must be treated early with factor replacement and joint immobilization during the period of pain. This type of affected joint is particularly susceptible to being injured again, setting up a cycle of vulnerability to trauma and repeated hemorrhages.

Bleeding into the muscles is the second most common site of bleeding in persons with hemophilia. Muscle hemorrhages can be more insidious and massive than joint hemorrhages. They may occur anywhere but are common in the flexor muscle groups, predominantly the iliopsoas, gastrocnemius, and flexor surface of the forearm, and they result in deformities such as hip flexion contractures, equinus

▼ *Clinical Signs and Symptoms for*
Acute Hemarthrosis

- Aura, tingling, or prickling sensation
- Stiffening into the position of comfort
- Decreased range of motion
- Pain
- Swelling
- Tenderness
- Heat

▼ *Clinical Signs and Symptoms for*
Muscle Hemorrhage

- Gradually intensifying pain
- Protective spasm of the muscle
- Limitation of movement at the surrounding joints
- Muscle assumes the position of comfort (usually shortened)
- Loss of sensation

▼ *Clinical Signs and Symptoms of*
Gastrointestinal Involvement

■ Abdominal pain and distention
■ Melena (blood in stool)
■ Hematemesis (vomiting blood)
■ Fever
■ Low abdominal/groin pain due to bleeding into wall of large intestine or iliopsoas muscle
■ Flexion contracture of the hip due to spasm of the iliopsoas muscle secondary to retroperitoneal hemorrhage

position of the foot, or Volkmann's deformity of the forearm.

When bleeding into the psoas or iliacus muscle puts pressure on the branch of the femoral nerve supplying the skin over the anterior thigh, loss of sensation occurs. Distention of the muscles with blood causes pain that can be felt in the lower abdomen, possibly even mimicking appendicitis when bleeding occurs on the right side. In an attempt to relieve the distention and reduce the pain, a position with hip flexion is preferred.

Two tests are used to distinguish an iliopsoas bleed from a hip bleed:

1. When the client flexes the trunk, severe pain is produced in the presence of *iliopsoas bleeding,* whereas only mild pain is found with a hip hemorrhage.

2. When the hip is gently rotated in either direction, severe pain is experienced with a *hip hemorrhage,* which is absent or mild with iliopsoas bleeding.

Gastrointestinal bleeding involvement may occur gradually or suddenly and may last for several weeks.

Over time, the following complications may occur:

■ Vascular compression causing localized ischemia and necrosis

■ Replacement of muscle fibers by nonelastic fibrotic tissue causing shortened muscles and thus producing joint contractures

■ Peripheral nerve lesions from compression of a nerve that travels in the same compartment as the hematoma, most commonly affecting the femoral, ulnar, and median nerves

■ Pseudotumor formation with bone erosion

Treatment. Effective treatment is based on an accurate diagnosis of the deficient clotting factor and its level in the blood. This requires a battery of common blood tests for bleeding time, partial thromboplastin time, factor assays, and tests to monitor the liver, kidney, immune function, and hepatitis status.

Current treatment relies on infusion of human plasma-derived clotting factor that is produced using one of several processing methods. Although transmission of the human immunodeficiency (HIV) virus (precursor for the acquired immunodeficiency syndrome [AIDS]) has almost been eliminated, the transmission of the hepatitis virus is still a problem. Recently improved methods of viral inactivation (pasteurization; solvent-detergent treatment) have resulted in a reduced risk of hepatitis transmission.

With the advent of genetic engineering, the FDA has now approved two recombinant factor VIII products. Unlike human plasma–derived factors made from plasma pooled from thousands of donors, recombinant factor VIII is now derived from a nonhuman source. With recombinant factor, human viruses will not be transmitted through factor use, and the chance of any other contaminants' being transmitted appears unlikely (National Hemophilia Foundation, 1993).

Comprehensive medical management of hemophilia may involve the use of drugs to control pain in acute bleeding and chronic arthropathies. The common pain reliever aspirin and any of its derivatives cannot be used by persons with hemophilia because these agents inhibit platelet function. Antiinflammatory nonsteroidal drugs can contain derivatives of aspirin and must be used cautiously. Corticosteroids are used occasionally for the treatment of chronic synovitis.

Physical therapy treatment has been effective in preventing spontaneous bleeding through the protective strengthening of the musculature surrounding affected joints and through client education. Physical therapy is used during episodes of acute hemorrhage to control pain and additional bleeding and to maintain positioning and prevent further deformity (Cotta et al., 1986).

PHYSICIAN REFERRAL

Understanding the components of a client's past medical history that can affect hematopoiesis can provide the physical therapist with valuable insight into the client's present symptoms, which are usually already well known to the attending physician. For example, the effects of certain drugs, exposure to radiation, or recent cytotoxic cancer chemotherapy can affect bone marrow. Whenever uncertain, the physical therapist is encouraged to contact the physician by telephone for discussion and clarification of the client's medical symptoms.

A history of excessive menses, a folate-poor diet, alcohol abuse, drug ingestion, family history of anemia, and family roots in geographic areas where red blood cell enzyme or hemoglobin abnormalities are prevalent represent some important findings. The presence of any one or more of these factors should alert the physical therapist to the need for medical referral when the client is not already under the care of a physician or when new signs or symptoms develop.

In addition, exercise for *anemic* clients must be instituted with extreme caution and should first be approved by the client's physician. Clients with undiagnosed thrombocytopenia need immediate medical referral. The physical therapist must be alert for obvious skin or mucous membrane symptoms of *thrombocytopenia*. The presence of severe bruising, hematomas, and multiple petechiae usually indicates a platelet count well below normal. With clients who have been diagnosed with *hemophilia,* medical referral should be made when any painful episode develops in the muscle(s) or joint(s). Pain usually occurs before any other evidence of bleeding. Any unexplained symptom may be a signal of bleeding.

Systemic Signs and Symptoms Requiring Physician Referral

Any client who has any of the generalized symptoms in the following list, without obvious or already known cause, should be further evaluated by a physician. At the very least, these signs and symptoms should be documented and a copy sent to the physician.

Abdominal/chest/back pain	Evidence of hemarthrosis/muscle hemorrhage
Blurred vision	Fainting
Changes in hands and fingernails	Fatigue and listlessness
Changes in skin color	Fever
Cyanosis	Feeling of fullness in head
Dactylitis	Headache
Decreased mental acuity	Irritability
Digital clubbing	Palpitations
Disturbances of sensation in hands/feet	Petechiae
	Pruritus
Dizziness	Rapid pulse
Dyspnea on exertion	Weakness
Easy bruising	Weight loss

Key Points to Remember

- Anemia may have no symptoms until hemoglobin concentration and hematocrit fall below one half of normal.

- Weakness, fatigue, and dyspnea are early signs of anemia.

- Exercise for anemic clients must be instituted with physician approval and gradually per tolerance and/or perceived exertion levels.

- Platelet level below 20,000/mm³ (thrombocytopenia) can be lethal. Multiple bruises and petechiae may be the only sign.

- For clients with known thrombocytopenia, exercise programs must avoid the Valsalva or bearing down movement, and caution must be used to avoid further injury by bumping against objects.

- During the inspection/observation portion of the objective examination, screen both hands for skin or nail bed changes indicative of hematologic involvement.

- For the client with hemophilia, bleeding episodes must be treated early with factor replacement and joint immobilization during the period of pain. Never apply heat to a bleeding or suspected bleeding area.

- Pain may be the only symptom of a joint or muscle bleed for the client with hemophilia. Any painful symptom in this population must be screened medically.

- The National Hemophilia Foundation (NHF) publishes an excellent pamphlet for physical therapists treating hemophiliacs: *Physical Therapy in Hemophilia* (1986), written by S. Cotta et al. This can be ordered by calling the NHF at (212) 219-8180.

SUBJECTIVE EXAMINATION *Special Questions to Ask*

- Is there a known history of anemia in your family?

- Have you recently had a serious blood loss (possibly requiring transfusion)? (**Anemia**; also consider **jaundice/hepatitis posttransfusion**)

- Do you experience shortness of breath or heart palpitations with slight exertion (e.g., climbing stairs) or even just at rest? (**Anemia**)

- **For persons at elevations above 3500 feet:** Have you recently moved from one geographic location to another? (**Polycythemia**)

- Have you ever been told that you have a congenital heart defect (also chronic lung/heart disorders)? (**Polycythemia: also possible with history of heavy tobacco use**)

- Do you ever have episodes of dizziness, blurred vision, headaches, fainting, or feeling of fullness in your head? (**Polycythemia**)

- Do you have a history of bruising easily or excessive blood loss? (**Polycythemia, hemophilia, thrombocytopenia**)

- For example, do you ever notice tiny, round (nonraised) red spots on your skin that later change color to blue or yellow? **(Petechiae associated with thrombocytopenia)**

- For example, do you usually notice excessive bruising, bleeding, or bleeding into the joints spontaneously or after minor trauma, surgery, or dental procedures?

- Do you have recurrent infections and low-grade fever, such as colds, influenza-like symptoms, other upper respiratory infections? **(Abnormal leukocytes)**

- Do you tend to have frequent nosebleeds? **(Epistaxis)**

- If yes to either of the last two questions, ask more about the initial onset of these bleeding episodes.*

- Do you have black, tarry stools **(bleeding into the gastrointestinal tract)** or blood in urine **(genitourinary tract)?**

- Has any previous bleeding been severe enough to require blood transfusions?

- Have you been exposed to occupational or industrial gases, such as chlorine gas, mustard gas, Agent Orange, napalm? **(Chemical and biologic warfare)**

- **For women (anemia, thrombocytopenia):** Do you frequently have prolonged or excessive bleeding in association with your menstrual flow? (Excessive may be considered to be measured by the use of more than four tampons each day; prolonged menstruation usually refers to more than 5 days—both these measures are subjective and must be considered along with other factors, such as the presence of other symptoms, personal menstrual history, placement in the life cycle [i.e., in relation to menopause].)

---

* Symptoms beginning in infancy or childhood suggest a congenital hemostatic defect, whereas symptoms beginning later in life indicate an acquired disorder, such as secondary to drug-induced defect of platelet function, a common cause of easy bruising and excessive bleeding. This bruising or bleeding occurs usually in association with trauma, menstruation, dental work, or surgical procedures. Drug-induced bruising or bleeding may also occur with use of aspirin and aspirin-containing compounds; nonsteroidal antiinflammatory agents like ibuprofen (Motrin), fenoprofen (Nalfon), and naproxen (Naprosyn); and penicillins, because these drugs inhibit platelet function to some extent (Reich, 1989).

■ ■ ■ ■ ■   ■ ■ ■ ■ ■ ■

CASE STUDY*

REFERRAL

You are working in a hospital setting and you have received a physician's referral to "evaluate and treat" a patient who was involved in a serious automobile accident 10 days ago. The patient had internal injuries that required immediate abdominal surgery and 600 ml of blood transfused within 24 hours postoperatively. His condition is considered to be medically "stable."

CHART REVIEW

What specific medical information should you look for in the patient's chart before beginning your evaluation?

■ ■ ■ ■ ■ ■   ■ ■ ■ ■ ■

Patient's name, age, and occupation

Past medical history: Previous myocardial infarcts, history of heart disease, diabetes (type)

Surgical report: Type of surgery, locations of scar, any current contraindications

Were there any other injuries?   If yes, what were these and what is the current status of each injury?

Body weight

Pulmonary status: Is the patient a cigarette or pipe smoker?

Is the patient currently receiving oxygen or respiratory therapy?

What is the patient's current pulmonary status after the accident and postoperatively?

Laboratory report: Hematocrit/hemoglobin levels

Anemia?

Current status: Nursing reports of the patient's complaints of any kind (e.g., symptoms of dyspnea or heart palpitations from rapid loss of blood)

Vital signs: Blood pressure

Presence of fever

Resting pulse rate

Current medications: Be aware of the purpose for each medication and its potential side effects.

Has the patient been up at all yet?

If yes, when? How far did he walk? How much assistance was required? Did he have symptoms of orthostatic hypotension?

Does the patient have any gastrointestinal symptoms?

Patient's orientation to time, place, and person

Are there any dietary or fluid restrictions while the patient is in the physical therapy department? Is he on an intravenous line?

Are there any known discharge plans at this time?

References

Adams, P., and Zanderer, B.: Sickle cell anemia. Med-Surg Nursing Quarterly *1*(4):1–21, Spring 1993.

Ahulu-Konotey, F.I.D.: The sickle cell diseases. Archives of Internal Medicine *133*:611, 1974.

Baldy, C.: Coagulation. *In* Price, S., and Wilson, L. (eds.): Pathophysiology: Clinical Concepts of Disease Processes. St. Louis, Mosby-Year Book, 1992, pp. 209–220.

Bithell, T.C.: Normal hemostasis and coagulation. *In* Thorup, O.A. (ed.): Leavell and Thorup's Fundamentals of Clinical Hematology, 5th ed. Philadelphia, W.B. Saunders, 1987, pp. 126–162.

Callender, S.T.: Blood Disorders. Oxford, Oxford University Press, 1986.

Chernecky, C., Krech, R., and Berger, B.: Laboratory Tests and Diagnostic Procedures. Philadelphia, W.B. Saunders, 1993.

Cotta, S., Jutra, M., and McQuarrie, A.: Physical Therapy in Hemophilia. New York, The National Hemophilia Foundation, 1986.

Deglin, J., and Vallerand, A.: Davis's Drug Guide for Nurses, 3rd ed. Philadelphia, F.A. Davis, 1993.

Gaston, M.: Sickle Cell Anemia. Washington, D.C., U.S. Department of Health and Human Services, National Institutes of Health, June 1990.

Griffin, J.P.: Hematology and Immunology. Norwalk, Connecticut, Appleton-Century-Crofts, 1986.

Guyton, A.: Human Physiology and Mechanisms of Disease, 5th ed. Philadelphia, W.B. Saunders, 1992.

Jarvis, C.: Physical Examination and Health Assessment. Philadelphia, W.B. Saunders, 1992, p. 236.

Jennings, B.: Nursing role in management: Hematological problems. In Lewis, S., and Collier, I. (eds.): Medical-Surgical Nursing: Assessment and Management of Clinical Problems. St. Louis, Mosby-Year Book, 1992, pp. 664–714.

McLaurin, S.E.: Sickle cell disease: A need for physical therapy intervention. Clinical Management, 6:12, 1985.

Mozzarelli, A., Hofrichter, J., and Eaton, W.A.: Delay time of hemoglobin S polymerization prevents most cells from sickling in vivo. Science 237:500, 1987.

National Hemophilia Foundation: AIDS Update. Revised recommendations by medical and scientific advisory council concerning HIV infection, AIDS and hepatitis in the treatment of hemophilia following the FDA approval of recombinant factor VIII. New York, Medical Bulletin #176, 1993.

O'Toole, M. (ed.): Miller-Keane Encyclopedia and Dictionary of Medicine, Nursing and Allied Health, 5th ed. Philadelphia, W.B. Saunders, 1992.

Pagana, K., and Pagana, T.: Mosby's Diagnostic and Laboratory Test Reference. St. Louis, Mosby-Year Book, 1992.

Painter, P.: End stage renal disease. In Skinner, J. (ed.): Exercise Testing and Exercise Prescription for Special Cases: Theoretical Basis and Clinical Application, 2nd ed. Philadelphia, Lea and Febiger, 1993, pp. 351–362.

Pavel, J., Plunkett, A., and Sink, B.: Nursing care of clients with hematologic disorders. In Black, J., and Matassarin-Jacobs, E. (eds.): Luckman and Sorensen's Medical-Surgical Nursing: A Psychophysiologic

Approach, 4th ed. Philadelphia, W.B. Saunders, 1993, pp. 1335–1402.

Price, R.H., and Solomon, L.R.: Hematology and transfusion medicine. In Ramsey, P.G., and Larson, E.B. (eds.): Medical Therapeutics, 2nd ed. Philadelphia, W.B. Saunders, 1993, pp. 346–373.

Purtilo, D.T., and Purtilo, R.B.: A Survey of Human Diseases, 2nd ed. Boston, Little, Brown, 1989.

Ramsey, P.G., and Larson, E.B.: Medical Therapeutics, 2nd ed. Philadelphia, W.B. Saunders, 1993.

Reich, P.R.: Hematology: Physiopathologic Basis for Clinical Practice, 2nd ed. Boston, Little, Brown, 1989.

Schumann, M.: Hemorrhagic disorders: Abnormalities of platelet and vascular functions. In Wyngaarden, J.B., Smith, L.H., and Bennett, J.C.: Cecil Textbook of Medicine, 19th ed. Philadelphia, W.B. Saunders, 1992, pp. 987–998.

Thomas, R., and Holbrook, T.: Sickle cell disease. Postgraduate Medicine 81:265, 1987.

Vichinsky, E.P., Hurst, D., and Lubin, B.: Update on sickle cell disease: Basic concepts. Hospital Medicine, Sept: 128–158, 1983.

Vichinsky, E.P., Hurst, D., and Lubin, B.: Update on sickle cell disease. Hospital Medicine, Feb:131–149, 1988.

Bibliography

Delamore, I.W.: Hematological Effect of Systemic Diseases. Philadelphia, W.B. Saunders, 1990.

Hoffbrand, A.V., and Brenner, M.K. (eds.): Recent Advances in Hematology. New York, Churchill-Livingstone, 1992.

Hoffbrand, A.V., and Pettit, J.E.: Essential Hematology, 3rd ed. Cambridge, England, Blackwell Science, 1992.

Holdredge, S.A., and Cotta, S.: Physical therapy and rehabilitation in the care of the adult and child with hemophilia. In Hilgartner, M., and Pochedly, C. (eds.): Hemophilia in the Child and Adult. New York, Raven Press, 1989, pp. 235–262.

Hoots, W.K., Buchanan, G.R., Parmley, R.T., Alperin, J.B., Kletzel, M., and Sexauer, C.L.: Comprehensive care for patients with hemophilia: An expanded role in reducing risk for human immunodeficiency virus. Texas Medicine 87(6):73–75, June 1991.

Lee, G.R., et al.: Wintrobe's Clinical Hematology, 9th ed. Vols. 1 and 2. Philadelphia, Lea & Febiger, 1993.

Spivak, J.L., and Eichner, E.R. (eds.): The Fundamentals of Clinical Hematology, 3rd ed. Baltimore, Johns Hopkins Press, 1993.

6

Overview of Gastrointestinal Signs and Symptoms

Gastrointestinal (GI) disorders can refer pain to the sternal region, shoulder, scapular region, midback, lower back, and hip. This pain can mimic primary musculoskeletal lesions, causing confusion for the physical therapist or for the physician assessing the clients' chief complaints. Although these musculoskeletal symptoms can occur alone, the client usually has other systemic signs and symptoms associated with GI disorders. A careful interview to screen for systemic illness is essential when assessing the client who has musculoskeletal pain of unknown etiology. The physical therapy interview should include a few important questions concerning the client's history and the presence of any associated signs or symptoms that would immediately alert the physical therapist about the need for medical follow-up.

The most common intraabdominal diseases to refer pain to the musculoskeletal system from ulceration or infection of the mucosal lining. Although pain can be experienced far from the actual site of the disorder, the GI system offers patterns of pain and accompanying symptoms that should give the physical therapist who does a thorough investigation grounds for suspicion.

This chapter presents the most clinically meaningful GI symptoms and their most common underlying causes.

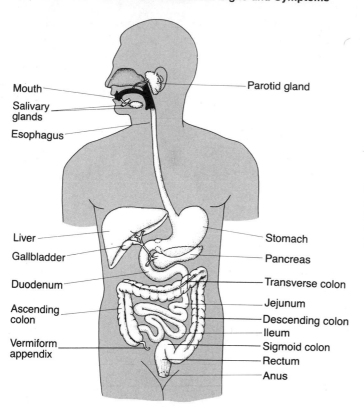

Mouth
Salivary glands
Esophagus
Liver
Gallbladder
Duodenum
Ascending colon
Vermiform appendix

Parotid gland
Stomach
Pancreas
Transverse colon
Jejunum
Descending colon
Ileum
Sigmoid colon
Rectum
Anus

Figure 6–1

Organs of the digestive system. (From Guyton, A.C.: Textbook of Medical Physiology, 8th ed. Philadelphia, W.B. Saunders Company, 1991.)

GASTROINTESTINAL PHYSIOLOGY
(Long, 1991)

The upper GI tract consists of structures that aid in the ingestion and digestion of food, namely the mouth, esophagus, stomach, and duodenum (Fig. 6–1). The lower GI tract consists of the small and large intestines. Digestion is completed in the small intestine, and most of the nutrients are absorbed in this organ. The large intestine serves primarily to absorb water and electrolytes and to eliminate the waste products of digestion.

Esophagus

The esophagus is a hollow tube; the upper one third consists of skeletal muscle and the remainder of smooth muscle. It is lined with a mucous membrane that secretes a mucoid substance for protection. Swallowing consists of three phases: a voluntary phase in which the tongue forces the bolus of food into the pharynx, an involuntary pharyngeal phase in which the food moves into the upper esophagus, and an esophageal phase during which food moves from the pharynx and down into the stomach. The cardiac sphincter prevents reflux (backward flow) of the contents of the stomach back into the lower esophagus. Food is prevented from passing into the trachea by the closing of the trachea and the opening of the esophagus.

Stomach

The stomach and the remainder of the GI tract are made up of five layers of smooth muscle that have two types of contractions: tonus contractions and rhythmic contractions. These contractions assist the peristaltic movement of food and are responsible for the mixing of the food. The food bolus enters the stomach and continues to move through the stomach and intestines by peristalsis (muscular contraction that causes a wave to push food along). As the food moves toward the pyloric sphincter, peristaltic waves increase in force and intensity. The fluid mass now becomes known as chyme (semifluid mass of partly digested food). Chyme is pumped through the pyloric sphincter into the duodenum.

Intestines

The small intestine is about 2.5 cm (1 inch) wide and 6 m (20 feet) long and fills most of the abdomen. It consists of three parts—the duodenum, which connects to the stomach; the jejunum or middle portion; and the ileum, which connects to the large intestine.

The large intestine is about 6 cm (2.5 inches) wide and 1.5 m (5 feet) long. It consists of three parts—the cecum, which connects to the small intestine; the colon; and the rectum. The ileocecal valve prevents backward flow of fecal contents from the large intestine to the small intestine. The vermiform appendix, which has no function, is an appendage close to the ileocecal valve. The colon consists of four parts—the ascending, transverse, descending, and sigmoid colons. The rectum is 17 to 20 cm (7 to 8 inches) long, ending in the 2- to 3-cm anal canal. The opening (anus) is controlled by a smooth muscle internal sphincter and by a striated muscle external sphincter.

Contents of the small intestine (chyme) are propelled toward the anus by peristaltic movement, which also mixes the intestinal contents. Chyme moves slowly and normally takes 3 to 10 hours to move from the stomach to the ileocecal valve. The major portion of digestion occurs in the small intestine by the action of pancreatic and intestinal secretions and of bile (liver secretion that breaks down fats). Ninety per cent of absorption of nutrients occurs within the small intestine. Reabsorption of water, electrolytes, and the bile salts occurs predominantly in the ascending colon. The colon has the capacity to absorb six to eight times more fluid than is delivered to it daily.

Pancreas (O'Toole, 1992)

The pancreas is a large, elongated gland that is located transversely behind the stomach between the spleen and the duodenum (Fig. 6–2). The pancreas is both an exocrine gland and an endocrine gland. Its function in digestion is primarily an exocrine activity. The pancreas secretes digestive enzymes and pancreatic juice, which are transported through the hepatic duct to the duodenum, where proteins, carbohydrates, and fats are broken down. Bicarbonate ions in the pancreatic secretion help neutralize the acidic chyme that is passed along from the stomach to the duodenum.

Because of the pancreas' dual function as both an exocrine and endocrine gland, the pancreas and the disorders of the pancreas, including diabetes mellitus, digestive disorders, pancreatic carcinoma, pancreatitis, and cystic fibrosis, are discussed in various chapters throughout the text. This chapter focuses primarily on the digestive disorders associated with the pancreas.

ABDOMINAL PAIN (Ridge and Way, 1993; Guyton, 1992)

Pain is a subjective sensation resulting from the central transmission of peripherally received noxious stimuli. It usually indicates damage to tissue unless the stimulus is removed.

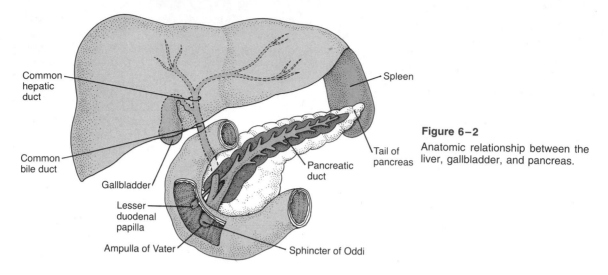

Common hepatic duct

Common bile duct

Gallbladder

Lesser duodenal papilla

Ampulla of Vater

Spleen

Tail of pancreas

Pancreatic duct

Sphincter of Oddi

Figure 6–2

Anatomic relationship between the liver, gallbladder, and pancreas.

Afferent nerve impulses transmit pain from the esophagus to the spinal cord by small, unnamed sympathetic nerves. Visceral afferent nerves from the liver, diaphragm, and pericardium are derived from dermatomes C3 to C5 and reach the central nervous system (CNS) via the phrenic nerve.

Afferent nerves from the gallbladder, stomach, pancreas, and small intestine travel through the celiac plexus (network of ganglia and nerves supplying the abdominal viscera) and the greater splanchnic nerves and enter the spinal cord from T6 to T9.

Afferent stimuli from the colon, appendix, and pelvic viscera enter the 10th and 11th thoracic segments through the mesenteric plexus and lesser splanchnic nerves. Finally, the sigmoid colon, rectum, ureters, and testes are innervated by fibers that reach T11 to L1 segments through the lower splanchnic nerve.

Stimuli for Abdominal Pain

The abdominal viscera are ordinarily insensitive to many stimuli, such as cutting, tearing, or crushing, that when applied to the skin evoke severe pain. Visceral pain fibers are sensitive only to stretching or tension in the wall of the gut from neoplasm, distention, or forceful muscular contractions secondary to bowel obstruction or spasm.

The rate that tension develops must be rapid enough to produce pain; gradual distention, such as with malignant obstruction, may be painless unless ulceration occurs.

Inflammation may produce visceral pain and ischemia (deficiency of blood) that subsequently produces pain by increasing the concentration of tissue metabolites in the region of the sensory nerve. Pain associated with ischemia is steady pain, whether this ischemia is secondary to vascular disease or due to obstruction causing strangulation of tissue. Other causes of abdominal pain are shown in Table 6–1.

Types of Abdominal Pain

Visceral

Visceral pain (internal organs) occurs in the midline because the abdominal organs receive sensory afferents from both sides

Table 6–1
CAUSES OF ABDOMINAL PAIN

Intraabdominal		Extraabdominal
Generalized Peritonitis	Biliary obstruction	*Thoracic*
Perforated viscus: peptic ulcer	Gallstone	Pneumonitis
Primary bacterial peritonitis	Stricture	Pulmonary embolism
Pneumococcal	Tumor	Pneumothorax
Streptococcal	Parasites	Empyema
Enteric bacillus	Ureteral obstruction: calculi (kidney stone)	Myocardial ischemia
Tuberculosis	Hepatic capsule distention	Myocarditis
Nonbacterial peritonitis	Acute hepatitis (toxic or viral)	Endocarditis
Ruptured ovarian cyst	Common duct obstruction	Esophagitis
Ruptured follicle cyst	Budd-Chiari syndrome	Esophageal spasm
	Renal capsule distention	Esophageal rupture
Localized Peritonitis*	Pyelonephritis	
	Ureteral obstruction	*Neurogenic*
Appendicitis	Uterine obstruction	Radiculitis
Cholecystitis	Neoplasm	Spinal cord tumors
Peptic ulcer	Pregnancy/childbirth	Peripheral nerve tumors
Regional enteritis (Crohn's disease)	Ruptured ectopic pregnancy	Spinal arthritis
Colitis: ulcerative, amebic, bacterial	Rupturing arterial aneurysm	Herpes zoster
Abdominal abscess	Aortic	Tabes dorsalis
Postoperative	Iliac	
Hepatic	Visceral	*Metabolic*
Pancreatic		Uremia
Splenic	*Ischemia*	Diabetes mellitus
Diverticular		Porphyria
Tuboovarian	Intestinal angina or infarction	Acute renal insufficiency
Pancreatitis	Arterial stenosis	
Hepatitis: viral, toxic	Embolism	*Hematologic*
Pelvic inflammatory disease	Polyarteritis	Sickle cell anemia
Endometriosis	Splenic infarction	Hemolytic anemia
Lymphadenitis	Torsion	
	Gallbladder	*Miscellaneous*
Pain from Increased Visceral Tension	Spleen	Muscular contusion
	Ovarian cyst	Hematoma
Intestinal obstruction	Testicle	Tumor
Adhesions	Appendix	Toxins
Hernia	Hepatic infarction: toxemia	Hypersensitivity reactions
Tumor	Tissue necrosis: uterine fibroid, hepatoma	Insect bites
Fecal impaction		Reptile venoms
Intestinal hypermotility	*Retroperitoneal Neoplasms*	Drugs
Irritable colon		Lead poisoning
Gastroenteritis		

* Many types of local peritonitis may become generalized by rupture into the free peritoneal cavity.
From Sleisenger, M.H., and Fordtran J.S. (eds.): Gastrointestinal Disease, 5th ed. Philadelphia, W.B. Saunders, 1993.

of the spinal cord. The site of pain corresponds to dermatomes from which the diseased organ receives its innervation (Fig. 6–3). Pain is not well localized because innervation of the viscera is multisegmental with few nerve endings.

Additionally, although the viscera experience pain, the visceral peritoneum (membrane enveloping organs) is insensitive to pain. Except in the presence of widespread inflammation or ischemia, it is possible to have extensive disease without pain until

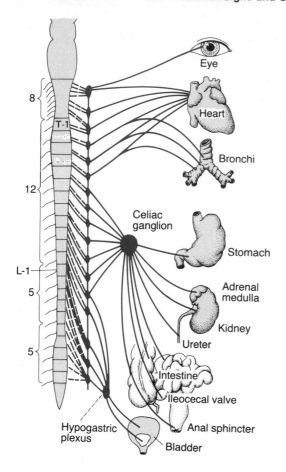

Figure 6–3

Diagram of the autonomic nervous system. The visceral afferent fibers mediating pain travel with the sympathetic nerves, except for those from the pelvic organs that follow the parasympathetics of the pelvic nerve. Sympathetics are represented here by *solid lines;* parasympathetics are represented by *dashed lines.* (From Guyton, A.C.: Textbook of Medical Physiology, 8th ed. Philadelphia, W.B. Saunders, 1991.)

the disease progresses enough to involve the parietal peritoneum.

Location: (Fig. 6–4):	Midline
	Dermatomal levels
Referral:	Poorly localized (the person cannot point to the specific site)
	No specific referral patterns
Description:	Cramping, burning, and gnawing
Intensity:	Dull
Duration:	Constant

Associated Signs and Symptoms:	Sweating
	Pallor
	Restlessness
	Nausea
	Emesis (vomiting)

Parietal

Parietal (somatic) relates to the wall of any cavity, such as the chest or pelvic cavities. Whereas the visceral peritoneum is insensitive to pain, the parietal peritoneum is well supplied with pain nerve end-

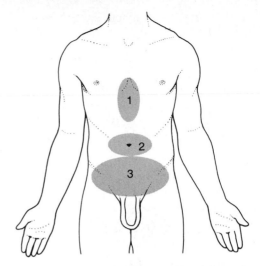

Figure 6-4

Visceral pain: (1) the epigastric region; (2) the periumbilical region; and (3) the lower midabdominal region.

ings. Parietal pain may be unilateral (rather than midline only), because at any given point the parietal peritoneum obtains innervation from only one side of the nervous system.

Location:	Midline or unilateral pelvic region
	Localized more precisely to the site of the lesion than is visceral pain
Referral:	Pelvic cavity: Wide variety of pain patterns depending on the organs involved—referred to abdomen, lower back, or legs
Description:	Knifelike, cutting, stabbing
Intensity:	More intense than visceral pain
Duration:	Constant
Associated Signs and Symptoms:	Aggravated by coughing or by respiratory movement

Referred

Location:	Pain occurs in *remote areas*

supplied by the same neurosegment as the diseased organ by way of shared central pathways for afferent neurons.

Pain may be felt in skin or deeper tissues.

Client can point precisely to the area that hurts (well-localized).

Referral:	Referred pain occurs *when noxious visceral stimulus becomes more intense.*
	Referred pain *can occur alone* (without accompanying visceral pain), but usually visceral pain precedes the development of referred pain.
	Hyperesthesia (excessive sensibility to sensory stimuli) of skin and *hyperalgesia* (excessive sensibility to painful stimuli) of muscle may develop in the referred pain-distribution.
Description:	Tenderness, burning, aching
Intensity:	Dull to exquisite
Duration:	Constant

Associated Signs and Symptoms:

Muscle spasm

Vasoconstriction

Radial pulse difficult to palpate*

Increased pulse rate*

Increased blood pressure (systolic and diastolic)

Pallor

Vasodilation

Profuse sweating

Subjective report of feeling excessively warm

Flushed appearance of skin

- Constipation
- Diarrhea
- Fecal incontinence
- Referred shoulder pain
- Tenderness over McBurney's point (see Appendicis)

GASTROINTESTINAL PATHOPHYSIOLOGY

Gastrointestinal Organ Symptoms
(Ridge and Way, 1993)

It is very important for the physical therapist to assess carefully the client's complaints, because GI tract symptoms can sometimes imitate musculoskeletal dysfunction. Symptoms, including pain, can be related to various GI organ disturbances and differ in character depending on the affected organ. The most clinically meaningful GI symptoms reported in a physical therapy practice include:

- Dysphagia
- Odynophagia
- Melena
- Epigastric pain with radiation to the back
- Symptoms affected by food
- Early satiety with weight loss

Dysphagia

Dysphagia is the sensation of food catching or sticking in the esophagus. This sensation may occur (initially) just with coarse, dry foods and may eventually progress to include anything swallowed, even thin liquids and saliva. Achalasia is a process by which the circular and longitudinal muscular fibers of the lower esophageal sphincter do not relax. This disorder contributes to esophageal stricture. Closure *(achalasia)* of the esophageal sphincter may also create an obstruction of the esophagus. Other possible causes of dysphagia include peptic esophagitis (inflammation of the esophagus) with stricture (narrowing) and neoplasm (Ruder, 1993a). The presence of dysphagia requires prompt attention by the physician. Treatment is based on a subsequent endoscopic examination.

Case Example An obese 88-year-old woman with a total knee replacement (TKR) was referred for rehabilitation because of loss of motion, joint swelling, and persistent knee pain. She was accompanied to the clinic for each session by one of her three daughters. Over a period of 2 or 3 weeks, each daughter commented on how much weight the mother had lost. When questioned, the client complained of a loss of appetite and difficulty in swallowing, but she had been evaluated and treated only for her knee pain by the orthopedist. She was encouraged to contact her family doctor for evaluation of these red flag symptoms and was subsequently diagnosed with esophageal cancer. Knowing the right questions to ask and making the referral resulted in early diagnosis of her condition.

---

* Changes in pulse associated with pain can occur with visceral pain, parietal pain, or referred pain because of the autonomic nervous system's response to pain in general. Whenever there is a sympathetic response of magnitude, pulse rate will increase; however, because of vasoconstriction, amplitude may decrease, making palpation and auscultation more difficult.

Odynophagia

Odynophagia, or pain during swallowing, can be caused by esophagitis or esophageal spasm. Esophagitis may occur secondary to the herpes simplex virus or fungus caused by the prolonged use of strong antibiotics. Pain after eating may occur with esophagitis or may be associated with coronary ischemia (Ruder, 1993a).

To differentiate esophagitis from coronary ischemia: *esophagitis pain* is relieved by upright positioning and is intensified by supine positioning, whereas *cardiac pain* is relieved by nitroglycerin or by supine positioning. Both conditions require medical attention.

Melena

Melena, or black, tarry stool, occurs as a result of large quantities of·blood in the stool. When asked about changes in bowel function, clients may describe black, tarry stools that have an unusual odor. The odor is caused by the presence of blood, and the black color arises as the digestive acids in the bowel oxidize red blood cells. Melena is very sticky and does not clean well. Clients may describe bowel smears on their undergarments.

Upper GI tract (e.g., esophageal, stomach, or duodenal) lesions produce melena. The lesion may be caused by a bleeding ulcer, esophageal varices, or vascular abnormalities of the stomach that break open and bleed easily.

Esophageal varices are dilated blood vessels, usually secondary to cirrhosis of the liver. Blood that would normally be pumped back to the heart must bypass the damaged liver. The blood then "backs up" through the esophagus (Matassarin-Jacobs and Strasburg, 1993). Vascular abnormalities of the stomach causing bleeding may include ulcers.

The client should be asked about the presence of any blood in the stool to determine whether it is melenotic (from the upper GI tract) or bright red (from the distal colon or rectum). Bleeding from internal or external *hemorrhoids* (enlarged veins inside or outside the rectum) is a common cause of bright red blood in the stools.

Epigastric Pain with Radiation

Epigastric pain with radiation to the back may occur secondary to long-standing ulcers. For example, the client may be aware of an ulcer but does not relate the back pain to the ulcer. Close questioning related to GI symptoms can provide the physical therapist with knowledge of underlying systemic disease processes.

Diagnostic interviewing is especially helpful when clients have neglected medical treatment for so long that back pain caused by an ulcer may in turn have created biomechanical changes in muscular contractions and spinal movement. These changes eventually create pain of a biomechanical nature (Rose and Rothstein, 1982). The client then presents with enough true musculoskeletal findings that a diagnosis of back dysfunction can be supported. However, the symptoms may be associated with a systemic problem. A good medical history can be a valuable tool in revealing the actual cause of the back pain.

Symptoms Affected by Food

Clients may or may not be able to relate pain to meals. Pain associated with gastric ulcers (located more proximally in the GI tract) may begin within 30 to 90 minutes after eating, whereas pain associated with duodenal or pyloric ulcers (located distally beyond the stomach) may occur 2 to 4 hours after meals (i.e., between meals). Alternatively stated, food is not likely to relieve the pain of a gastric ulcer, but it may relieve the symptoms of a duodenal ulcer (Ruder, 1993b).

The client with a duodenal ulcer may re-

Table 6–2
CAUSES OF CONSTIPATION

Neurogenic	Muscular	Mechanical	Rectal Lesions	Drugs/Diet

Cortical, voluntary, or involuntary evacuation
Central nervous system lesions
  Multiple sclerosis
  Cord tumors
  Tabes dorsalis
  Traumatic spinal cord lesions
	Atony (loss of tone)
	Severe malnutrition
	Metabolic defects
	Hypothyroidism
	Hypercalcemia
	Potassium depletion
	Hyperparathyroidism
	Inactivity
		Bowel obstruction
		  Neoplasm
		  Volvulus (intestinal twisting)
		  Diverticulitis
		Extraalimentary tumors (including pregnancy)
		Colostomy
			Thrombosed hemorrhoids
			Perirectal abscess
				Anesthetic agents (recent general surgery)
				Antacids (containing aluminum or calcium)
				Anticholinergics
				Anticonvulsants
				Antidepressants
				Antihistamines
				Antipsychotics
				Barium sulfate
				Diuretics
				Iron compounds
				Narcotics
				Lack of dietary bulk
				Renal failure (due to fluid restriction, phosphate binders)
				Myocardial infarction (narcotics for pain control)

Adapted from Blacklow, R.S. (ed.): MacBryde's Signs and Symptoms, 6th ed. Philadelphia, J.B. Lippincott, 1983.

port pain during the night between 12 midnight and 3:00 a.m. This pain should be differentiated from the nocturnal pain associated with cancer by its intensity and duration. More specifically, the *gnawing pain of an ulcer* may be relieved by eating, but the *intense, boring pain associated with cancer* is not relieved by any measures.

Early Satiety

Early satiety occurs when the client feels hungry, takes one or two bites of food, and feels full. The sensation of being full is out of proportion with the time of the previous meal and the initial degree of hunger experienced.

Constipation (DeVroede, 1993)

Constipation is defined clinically as being a condition of prolonged retention of fecal content in the GI tract resulting from decreased motility of the colon or difficulty in expelling stool.

Changes in bowel habit may be a response to many other factors, such as diet (decreased fluid and bulk intake), side effects of medication, acute or chronic diseases of the digestive system, extraabdominal diseases, personality, mood (depression), emotional stress, inactivity, prolonged bed rest, and lack of exercise (Table 6–2). Commonly implicated medications include narcotics, aluminum- or calcium-containing antacids, tricyclic antidepressants, phenothiazines, calcium channel blockers, and iron salts (Dugdale et al., 1993).

Constipation is almost a universal problem for clients with chronic renal failure. For these people, fluid restrictions, inability to eat most high-fiber foods, and activity intolerance reduce the effectiveness of customary measures for preventing constipation (Butera, 1993).

Diets that are high in refined sugars and low in fiber discourage bowel activity. Transit time of the alimentary bolus from the mouth to the anus is influenced mainly by dietary fiber and is decreased with increased fiber intake. Additionally, motility can be decreased by emotional stress that has been correlated with personality. Constipation associated with severe depression can be improved by exercise (Tucker et al., 1981).

People with low back pain may develop constipation as a result of muscle guarding and splinting that causes reduced bowel motility. Pressure on sacral nerves from stored fecal content may cause an *aching discomfort in the sacrum, buttocks, or thighs.*

Complications of constipation can include any or all of the following problems (Smeltzer and Bare, 1992):

- Decreased pulse, decreased cardiac output, and increased intrathoracic and intracranial pressure from increased use of the Valsalva maneuver (straining maneuver)
- Fecal impaction (accumulation of dry fecal material that cannot be expelled)
- Megacolon (dilated, atonic colon caused by a fecal mass that obstructs movement of colon contents, leading to perforation of the bowel)
- Cathartic colon (mucosal atrophy of the colon with muscle thickening and fibrosis, from chronic laxative use resulting in electrolyte imbalance and seepage of fecal liquid)

In addition, some researchers have proposed that metabolic and bacterial end-products of stool formation are carcinogenic, and that constipation causes a longer contact of these products with the bowel wall. The longer contact then increases the probability of cancer development (Ruder and Matassarin-Jacobs, 1993).

The group of associated problems that comprise constipation may be interpreted in a different manner by each individual. Common manifestations of this problem are hard stools, stools that are difficult to expel, infrequent stools or a feeling of incomplete evacuation after defecation, and general discomfort. Intractable constipation is called *obstipation* and can result in a fecal impaction that must be removed.

Because there are many specific organic causes of constipation, it is a symptom that may require further medical evaluation. It is considered a red flag symptom when clients with unexplained constipation have sudden and unaccountable changes in bowel habits or blood in the stools (Knauer, 1993a).

Diarrhea (Fine et al., 1993)

Diarrhea, by definition, is an abnormal increase in stool liquidity and daily stool weight associated with increased stool frequency (i.e., more than three times per day). This may be accompanied by urgency, perianal discomfort, and fecal incontinence. The causes of diarrhea vary widely from one person to another, but food, alcohol, use of laxatives and other drugs, medication side effects, and travel may contribute to the development of diarrhea (Table 6–3).

The intestine of the normal bowel contains 9 liters of fluid: 2 liters are from ingested foods and liquids, and the remainder is from digestive secretions (Guyton, 1992). It is well known that the first 3 to 5 pounds of weight loss for most people starting a diet occurs as a result of water loss from the intestines. The volume of chyme in the small bowel depends on the type of food eaten. Chyme increases with sugar intake and decreases with protein ingestion. Ingestion of alcohol (sugar) can produce diarrhea secondary to a decrease in enzymes and vitamins and hypermobility of the intestines.

Acute diarrhea, especially when associated with fever, cramps, and blood or pus in the stool, can accompany invasive enteric infection. Chronic diarrhea associated with weight loss is more likely to indicate

Table 6–3
CAUSES OF DIARRHEA

Malabsorption	Neuromuscular	Mechanical	Infectious	Nonspecific
Pancreatitis	Irritable bowel	Incomplete	Viral	Ulcerative
Pancreatic	syndrome	obstruction	Bacterial	colitis
carcinoma	Diabetic enteropathy	Neoplasm	Parasitic	Diverticulitis
Crohn's disease	Hyperthyroidism	Adhesions	Protozoal *(Giardia)*	Diet
	Caffeine	Stenosis		Laxative abuse
		Fecal impaction		Food allergy
		Muscular		Antibiotics
		incompetency		Lactose (milk)
		Postsurgical effect		intolerance
		(ileal bypass)		

Adapted from Blacklow, R.S. (ed): MacBryde's Signs and Symptoms, 6th ed. Philadelphia, J.B. Lippincott, 1983.

neoplastic or inflammatory bowel disease. Extraintestinal manifestations such as arthritis or skin or eye lesions are often present in idiopathic inflammatory bowel disease (Ockner, 1992). Any of these combinations of symptoms must be reported to the physician by the client.

Laxative abuse contributes to the production of diarrhea and begins a vicious cycle as chronic laxative users experience excessive secretion of aldosterone and resultant edema when they attempt to stop using laxatives. This edema and increased weight forces the person to continue to rely on laxatives.

The tremendous use of laxatives in the American population is substantiated by the more than 225 million dollars spent on laxatives annually (Darlington, 1966; Pharmacology, 1992; Product Management Drugs Cosmetics, 1975). The abuse of laxatives is common in the anorectic (loss of appetite due to emotional state) and bulimic (eating disorder) populations; affected persons may ingest up to 100 laxatives at a time.

For the client describing chronic diarrhea, it may be necessary to probe further about the use of laxatives as a possible contributor to this condition. These questions can be asked tactfully during the core interview when asking about medications, including over-the-counter drugs such as laxatives. Encourage the client to discuss bowel management without drugs at the next appointment with the physician.

Drug-induced diarrhea is associated most commonly with antibiotics. Gastrointestinal symptoms resolve when the drug is discontinued. Diarrhea may occur as a direct result of antibiotic use but may also develop 6 to 8 weeks after first ingestion of an antibiotic.

Bloody Diarrhea. Bloody diarrhea is usually associated with a sense of urgency (the person senses that he or she must find a bathroom immediately and cannot wait), frequency, and cramping pain.

Among the many potential causes of bloody diarrhea are ulcerative colitis, Crohn's disease, colitis (secondary to overgrowth of bacteria after a long course of antibiotics), benign or malignant colonic obstruction (stools must be liquid to pass by the obstruction), amebic colitis (the person has a recent history of travel outside the United States), and angiodysplasia, a vascular lesion in which clusters of vessels (capillaries) break open and bleed.

Medical diagnosis is made by fiberoptic endoscopy (visual examination of the interior structures of the intestines with an instrument) and by barium enema.

Fecal Incontinence

Fecal incontinence may be described as an inability to control evacuation of stool and is associated with a sense of urgency, diarrhea, and abdominal cramping. Causes include partial obstruction of the rectum (cancer), colitis, and radiation therapy, especially in the case of women treated for cervical or uterine cancer. The radiation may cause trauma to the rectum that results in incontinence and diarrhea. Anal distortion secondary to traumatic childbirth, hemorrhoids, and hemorrhoidal surgery may also cause fecal incontinence.

Pain in the Left Shoulder

Pain in the left shoulder (Kehr's sign) can occur as a result of free air or blood in the abdominal cavity, such as a ruptured spleen causing distention. The core interview may help the client recall any precipitating trauma or injury, such as a sharp blow during an athletic event, a fall, or perhaps an automobile accident. The client may not connect these seemingly unrelated events with the present shoulder pain.

Case Example. A 23-year-old soccer player sustained a blow from the side as he was moving down the soccer field. He fell on his left side with the full force of his own body weight and the weight of the other player on top of him. He reported having "the wind knocked out of me" and sat out on the sidelines for 20 minutes. He resumed playing and completed the game. The next morning, he woke up with severe left shoulder pain and stopped by the office of a physical therapist located in the same building as his office. The objective examination was unremarkable for shoulder movement dysfunction, which was inconsistent with the client's complaint of "constant pain." The client was treated symptomatically and instructed in pendulum exercises to maintain the joint motion.

He made a follow-up appointment with the therapist for the next day, but before noon, he collapsed at work and was taken to a hospital emergency department. A diagnosis of ruptured spleen was made during emergency surgery. A ruptured spleen would have sent the typical adult for medical care much sooner, but this client was in excellent physical condition with a high tolerance for pain. Physical therapy treatment was not appropriate in this situation; an immediate medical referral was indicated given the history of trauma, sudden onset of symptoms, left shoulder pain (Kehr's sign), and constancy of pain.

Peptic Ulcer (O'Toole, 1992)

Peptic ulcer is a loss of tissue lining the lower esophagus, stomach, and duodenum. Gastric and duodenal ulcers are considered together in this section. Acute lesions that do not extend through the mucosa are called erosions. Chronic ulcers involve the muscular coat, destroying musculature and replacing it with permanent scar tissue at the site of healing.

The etiology of peptic ulcers is not entirely understood. Originally, all ulcers in the upper gastrointestinal tract were believed to be caused by the aggressive action of hydrochloric acid and pepsin on the mucosa. They thus became known as "peptic ulcers," which is actually a misnomer (Richardson, 1992). Although acid and pepsin are secreted by most ulcers, it is not clear why mucosal resistance to them becomes impaired.

These secretions are not the only causes of ulcers. Heredity, socioeconomic status, psychologic profile, cigarette smoking, and use of nonsteroidal antiinflammatory drugs have a known correlation with peptic ulcers. Both gastric and duodenal ulcers tend to occur in families. Relatives (individually) of persons with gastric ulcers have three times the expected number of gastric ulcers.

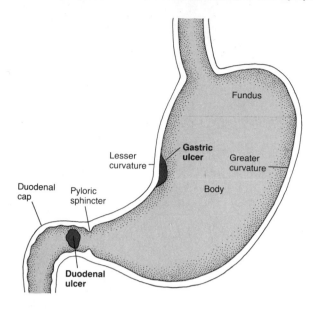

Figure 6–5

Most common sites for peptic ulcers. (Adapted from Ignatavicius, D.D., and Bayne, M.V.: Medical-Surgical Nursing. Philadelphia, W.B. Saunders, 1991.)

Although gastric ulcers are more likely to occur in the lower socioeconomic group, possibly due to poor nutrition, there is no direct evidence that either diets or particular foods cause ulcers. Psychologic stress can and does alter gastric function. Prolonged physiologic or psychologic stress produces *stress ulcers*. A stress ulcer differs from a chronic peptic ulcer by being more acute and more likely to hemorrhage. Perforation occurs occasionally, and pain is rare.

The most important exogenous factors associated with peptic ulcer disease are cigarette smoking and the use of nonsteroidal antiinflammatory drugs (NSAIDs). Alcohol and caffeine-containing beverages stimulate acid secretion, but there is no evidence that either causes gastric or duodenal ulcers (Richardson, 1992).

Whether cigarette smoking is related to the pathogenesis of ulcer disease is still unclear. Epidemiologic data support the following findings: Smoking is more common among clients with ulcers than among control subjects. There is a positive correlation between the quantity of cigarettes smoked and the prevalence of ulcer disease. Death due to peptic ulcer disease is more likely among clients who smoke than among those who do not. Duodenal ulcers are less likely to heal in cigarette smokers than in nonsmokers, and they recur more frequently in smokers than in nonsmokers. Whether these factors apply to people with gastric ulcers is not known (Richardson, 1992).

The average age at onset is 33 years, but duodenal ulcers may occur at any time from infancy to later years. Gastric ulcers are more likely to occur during the fifth and sixth decades of life; for men, duodenal ulcers more commonly occur during the fourth and fifth decades (Ruder, 1993b). In the past, men were more likely than women to develop gastric and duodenal ulcers. Now these ulcers are almost equally common in both sexes (Knauer, 1993a).

Duodenal ulcers are two to three times more common than gastric ulcers. About 95 per cent of duodenal ulcers occur in the duodenal bulb or cap (Fig. 6–5). About 60 per cent of benign gastric ulcers are located at or near the lesser curvature and most frequently on the posterior wall (Knauer, 1993a), which accounts for back pain as an associated symptom.

Clinical Signs and Symptoms. The cardinal symptom of peptic ulcer is epigastric

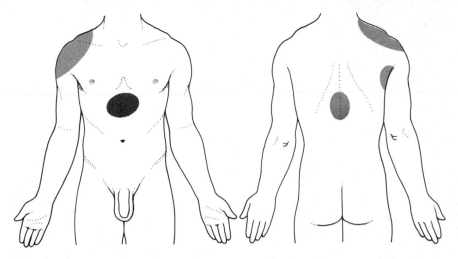

Figure 6–6

Stomach or duodenal pain *(dark red)* may occur anteriorly in the midline of the epigastrium or upper abdomen just below the xiphoid process. Referred pain *(light red)* to the back may occur at the level of the abdominal lesion (T6–T10). Other patterns of referred pain *(light red)* may include the right shoulder and upper trapezius or the lateral border of the right scapula.

pain that may be described as "heartburn" or as burning, gnawing, cramping, or aching located over a small area near the midline in the epigastrium near the xiphoid. Gastric ulcer pain often occurs in the upper epigastrium with localization to the left of the midline, whereas duodenal pain is in the right epigastrium.

The pain comes in waves that last several minutes (rather than hours) and may radiate below the costal margins, into the back, or rarely, to the right shoulder (Knauer, 1993a). The daily pattern of pain is related to the secretion of acid and the presence of food in the stomach to act as a buffer. The pain is diminished in the morning when secretion is low and after meals when food is present. The pain is most severe before meals and at bedtime. Symptoms often appear for 3 or 4 days or weeks and then subside, reappearing weeks or months later.

Other symptoms of uncomplicated peptic ulcer include nausea, loss of appetite, sometimes weight loss, and occasionally back pain. In duodenal ulcers, steady pain near the midline of the back (Fig. 6–6) between T6 and T10 with radiation to the right upper quadrant may indicate perforation of the posterior duodenal wall (Ruder, 1993b).

Complications of hemorrhage, perforation, and obstruction may lead to additional symptoms that the client does not relate to the back pain. Back pain may be the first and only symptom. Bleeding may occur when the ulcer erodes through a blood vessel. It may present as vomited bright red blood or coffee-ground vomitus and by tarry stools. The bleeding may vary from massive hemorrhage to occult (hidden) bleeding that occurs over a long period of time.

Prognosis and Treatment. Duodenal and gastric ulcers tend to have a chronic course with remissions and exacerbations. Many ulcers can be adequately controlled by medical management (Knauer, 1993a). The primary goals of medical treatment include relief of symptoms, promotion of healing, and prevention of complications and recurrences. Because each client re-

Table 6–4

NONSTEROIDAL ANTIINFLAMMATORY DRUGS (NSAIDs)

Generic	Brand Name
diclofenac sodium	Voltaren
diflunisal	Dolobid
etodolac	Lodine
fenoprofen calcium	Nalfon
flurbiprofen	Ansaid
ibuprofen	Motrin, Advil, Nuprin
indomethacin	Indocin
ketoprofen	Orudis
ketorolac tromethamine	Toradol
meclofenamate sodium	Meclomen
mefenamic acid	Ponstel
naproxen	Naprosyn
phenylbutazone	Butazolidin
piroxicam	Feldene
sulindac	Clinoril
tolmetin sodium	Tolectin

Adapted from Babb, R.R.: Gastrointestinal complications of nonsteroidal anti-inflammatory drugs. Western Journal of Medicine *157*:444–447, 1992. The listing of these drugs does not imply endorsement.

sponds differently to various treatment modes, the medical regimen is planned according to individual needs and responses. Treatment may include use of antacids, anticholinergic drugs, dietary modifications, stress management, and, in some cases, surgery.

Gastrointestinal Complications of NSAIDs

NSAIDs (Table 6–4) have become increasingly popular by virtue of their analgesic, antiinflammatory, antipyretic, and platelet-inhibitory actions. More than 90 million prescriptions are written annually (Babb, 1992). The association of aspirin and other NSAID use and ulcer disease is evident from numerous studies (Fries et al., 1991; Jaszewski, 1990; Silverstein, 1991). Drug-induced ulcers are most commonly caused by the ingestion of aspirin, with alcohol running a close second (O'Toole, 1992).

NSAIDs have deleterious effects on the entire gastrointestinal tract from the esophagus to the colon, although the most obvious clinical effect is on the gastroduodenal mucosa. Gastrointestinal complications of NSAID use include ulcerations, hemorrhage, perforation, stricture formation, and exacerbation of inflammatory bowel disease. A recent study (Allison et al., 1992) proposed that NSAIDs may be responsible for a large proportion of previously unexplained ulcers of the small intestine. Each NSAID has its own pharmacodynamic characteristics, and clients' responses to each drug may vary greatly (Babb, 1992).

NSAIDs may cause or may precipitate peptic ulcers, but little is known about the actual pathophysiologic mechanisms involved (Soll, 1992). Theoretically, these drugs break down the mucous membrane (which protects the GI tract) by inhibiting the intracellular cyclooxygenase enzyme system. This interference with normal mucosal protective mechanisms leads to local injury by allowing stomach acids to dissolve the intestine.

Many people diagnosed with painful musculoskeletal conditions rely on NSAIDs to relieve pain and improve function. Modi-

Clinical Signs and Symptoms of
Peptic Ulcer

- Epigastric pain 45 to 60 minutes after meals, relieved by food, milk, antacids, or vomiting
- Night pain (12 midnight to 3:00 A.M.)—same relief as for epigastric pain
- Radiating back pain
- Right shoulder pain (rare)
- Nausea
- Anorexia
- Weight loss
- Bloody stools
- Black, tarry stools

fication in diet combined with medications to neutralize stomach acids can help reduce one's chances of developing an ulcer.

Appendicitis (O'Toole, 1992)

Appendicitis is an inflammation of the vermiform appendix that occurs most commonly in adolescents and young adults. It is a serious disease usually requiring surgery. When the appendix becomes obstructed, inflamed, and infected, rupture may occur, leading to peritonitis.

Diseases that can be mistaken for appendicitis include Crohn's disease (regional enteritis), perforated duodenal ulcer, gallbladder attacks, and kidney infection on the right side, and for women, ruptured ectopic pregnancy, twisted ovarian cyst, or a hemorrhaging ovarian follicle at the middle of the menstrual cycle. Right lower lobe pneumonia sometimes is associated with prominent right lower quadrant pain (Knauer, 1993a).

Clinical Signs and Symptoms. The classic symptoms of appendicitis are pain preceding nausea and vomiting and low-grade fever in adults. Children tend to have higher fevers. Other symptoms may include coated tongue and bad breath.

The pain usually begins in the umbilical region and eventually localizes in the right lower quadrant of the abdomen over the site of the appendix. In retrocecal appendicitis, the pain may be referred to the thigh or right testicle (Sleisenger, 1992). The pain comes in waves, becomes steady, and is aggravated by motion, causing the client to bend over and tense the abdominal muscles or to lie down and draw the legs up to relieve abdominal muscle tension.

McBurney's Point

Parietal pain caused by inflammation of the peritoneum in acute appendicitis or peritonitis is localized at McBurney's point (Fig. 6–7). McBurney's point is located by palpation with the client in a supine position. Isolate the anterior superior iliac spine (ASIS) and the umbilicus: the physical therapist palpates for tenderness halfway between these two surface landmarks.

This method differs from palpation of the iliopsoas muscle, because the position used to locate the iliopsoas muscle is with the client in a supine position, with hips and knees flexed and fully supported in a 90-degree position. The physical therapist palpates one third of the distance between

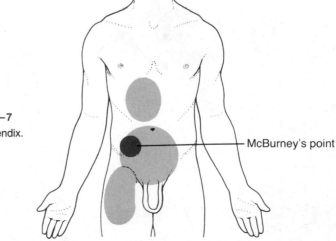

Figure 6–7
The appendix.

McBurney's point

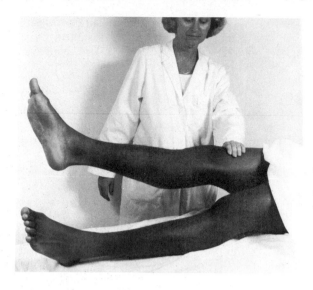

Figure 6-8

Iliopsoas muscle test. In the supine position, have the client actively perform a straight leg raise; apply resistance to the distal thigh as the client tries to hold the leg up. When the test is negative, the client feels no change. When the test is positive, painful symptoms are reproduced in the right lower quadrant. (From Jarvis, C.: Physical Examination and Health Assessment. Philadelphia, W.B. Saunders, 1992.)

the ASIS and the umbilicus. The client is asked to flex the hip gently to assist in isolating the iliopsoas muscle. Both McBurney's point and the iliopsoas muscle are palpated for reproduction of symptoms to rule out iliopsoas abscess associated with appendicitis or peritonitis.

Two other tests that can be performed to assess the possibility of a systemic origin of painful symptoms include the *iliopsoas muscle test* and the *obturator test*. The iliopsoas muscle test (Fig. 6–8) is performed when the acute abdominal pain of appendicitis is a possible cause of hip pain. When the iliopsoas muscle is inflamed by an inflamed or perforated appendix, the iliopsoas muscle test causes pain felt in the right lower quadrant.

The obturator test (Fig. 6–9) is also performed when the appendix could be the

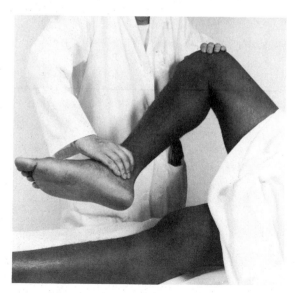

Figure 6-9

Obturator test. In the supine position, perform active assisted motion, flexing at the hip and 90 degrees at the knee. Hold the ankle and rotate the leg internally and externally. A negative or normal response is no pain. A positive test for appendicitis reproduces right lower quadrant pain. (From Jarvis, C.: Physical Examination and Health Assessment. Philadelphia, W.B. Saunders, 1992.)

Clinical Signs and Symptoms of
Appendicitis

- Periumbilical and/or epigastric pain
- Right lower quadrant pain
- Right thigh or testicle pain
- Positive McBurney's point
- Nausea and vomiting
- Dysuria (painful/difficult urination)
- Fever
- Coated tongue and bad breath

cause of referred pain to the hip. A perforated appendix irritates the obturator muscle, producing pain during the obturator test.

Prognosis and Treatment. Accurate diagnosis and early surgical removal of the appendix are essential. Delay of diagnosis produces significant mortality and morbidity rates if complications occur.

> **Case Example.** Remember the 32-year-old female university student featured in Figure 1–3? She had been referred to physical therapy with the provisional diagnosis: *Possible right oblique abdominis muscle tear/possible right iliopsoas muscle tear.* Her history included the sudden onset of "severe pain" in the right lower quadrant with accompanying nausea and abdominal distention. Aggravating factors included hip flexion, sit-ups, fast walking, and movements such as reaching, turning, and bending. Painful symptoms could be reproduced by resisted hip or trunk flexion, and tenderness/tightness was elicited on palpation of the right iliopsoas muscle as compared with the left. A neurologic screen was negative. Screening questions for general health revealed constitutional symptoms including fatigue, night sweats, nausea, and repeated episodes of severe, progressive pain in the right lower abdominal quadrant.
>
> Although she presented with a musculoskeletal pattern of symptoms at the time of her initial evaluation with the physician, by the time she entered the physical therapy clinic her symptoms had taken on a definite systemic pattern. She was returned for further medical follow-up, and a diagnosis of appendicitis complicated by peritonitis was established. This client recovered fully from all her symptoms following emergency appendectomy surgery.

Pancreatitis (O'Toole, 1992)

Pancreatitis is an inflammation of the pancreas that may result in autodigestion of the pancreas by its own enzymes. Pancreatitis can be acute or chronic, but the physical therapist is most likely to see acute pancreatitis.

Acute pancreatitis can arise from a variety of etiologic factors, but in most instances, the specific cause is unknown. Chronic alcoholism or toxicity from some other agent, such as glucocorticoids, thiazide diuretics, or acetaminophen, can bring on an acute attack of pancreatitis. A mechanical obstruction of the biliary tract may be present, usually because of gallstones in the bile ducts. Viral infections (e.g., mumps, herpesviruses, hepatitis) also may cause an acute inflammation of the pancreas.

Chronic pancreatitis is caused by long-standing alcohol abuse in more than 90 per cent of adult cases. Chronic pancreatitis is characterized by the progressive destruction of the pancreas with accompanying irregular fibrosis and chronic inflammation (Scarpelli, 1994).

Acute Pancreatitis

Clinical Signs and Symptoms (Kallsen, 1993). Symptoms in clients presenting with *acute pancreatitis* can vary from mild, nonspecific abdominal pain to profound shock with coma and, ultimately, death. Abdominal pain begins abruptly in the midepigastrium, increases in intensity for several hours, and can last from days to more than a week (Steinberg, 1992). The pain has a penetrating quality and radiates to the

▼ *Clinical Signs and Symptoms of*

Acute Pancreatitis

- Epigastric pain radiating to the back
- Nausea and vomiting
- Fever and sweating
- Tachycardia
- Malaise
- Weakness
- Jaundice

back. Pain is made worse by walking and lying supine and is relieved by sitting and leaning forward (Knauer, 1993b).

Chronic Pancreatitis

In clients with alcohol-associated pancreatitis, the pain often begins 12 to 48 hours after an episode of inebriation. Clients with gallstone-associated pancreatitis typically experience pain after a large meal. Nausea and vomiting accompany the pain. Other symptoms include fever, tachycardia, jaundice, and malaise.

Symptoms associated with *chronic pancreatitis* include persistent or recurrent episodes of epigastric and left upper quadrant pain with referral to the upper left lumbar region. Anorexia, nausea, vomiting, constipation, flatulence, and weight loss are common. Attacks may last only a few hours or

▼ *Clinical Signs and Symptoms of*

Chronic Pancreatitis

- Epigastric pain radiating to the back
- Upper left lumbar region pain
- Nausea and vomiting
- Constipation
- Flatulence
- Weight loss

as long as 2 weeks; pain may be constant (Knauer, 1993b).

Prognosis and Treatment. The clinical course of up to 90 per cent of clients with acute pancreatitis follows a self-limited pattern. However, a severe form of illness can develop in 10 to 15 per cent of clients, resulting in complications and requiring lengthy hospitalization (Kallsen, 1993). Chronic pancreatitis is a serious disease and often leads to chronic invalidism (Knauer, 1993b). Treatment for pancreatitis is largely symptomatic and designed to provide rest for the organ. Analgesics, fluid management, surgical removal of gallstones, and cessation of drinking alcohol are components of medical treatment.

Pancreatic Carcinoma

Pancreatic carcinoma is the fifth most common cause of death from cancer, exceeded only by lung, colorectal, breast, and prostate cancer. It appears to be linked to diabetes mellitus, use of alcohol, history of previous pancreatitis, and ingestion of a high-fat diet. Cancer of the pancreas is more common in African-Americans than whites, smokers than nonsmokers, and men than women (Kallsen, 1993).

Clinical Signs and Symptoms. The most common symptoms of pancreatic cancer are weight loss, epigastric/upper abdominal pain with radiation to the back, and jaundice secondary to obstruction of the bile duct. Epigastric pain is often vague and diffuse. Radiation of pain into the back is common and sometimes is the only symptom. Sitting up and leaning forward may provide some relief, and this usually indicates that the lesion has spread beyond the pancreas and is inoperable (Knauer, 1993b). Other signs and symptoms include light-colored stools, constipation, vomiting, and weakness (DiMagno, 1992).

Prognosis and Treatment. Ninety per cent of pancreatic cancer clients die within the first year after diagnosis. Only surgical resection offers any chance of cure (Di-

▼ *Clinical Signs and Symptoms of*

Pancreatic Carcinoma

- Epigastric/upper abdominal pain radiating to the back
- Back pain may be the only symptom
- Jaundice
- Weight loss
- Light-colored stools
- Constipation
- Vomiting
- Weakness

Magno, 1992). Carcinoma of the head of the pancreas has a very poor prognosis. Lesions of the ampulla, common duct, and duodenum have a better prognosis, with a reported 5-year survival rate of 20 per cent to 40 per cent after resection (Knauer, 1993b).

INFLAMMATORY/IRRITABLE BOWEL CONDITIONS

Any disruption of the digestive system can create symptoms such as pain, diarrhea, and constipation. The bowel is susceptible to altered patterns of normal motility caused by food, alcohol, tobacco, caffeine, drugs, physical and emotional stress, and life style (e.g., lack of regular exercise). Gastrointestinal effects of chemotherapy include nausea and vomiting, anorexia, taste alteration, weight loss, oral mucositis, diarrhea, and constipation.

During the course of evaluation and treatment with physical therapy, the conversation with the client may be directed toward the client's daily life. Physical therapists are often aware of daily stresses affecting a client—stresses that may aggravate the client's emotional perception of pain.

Use of the McGill Pain Questionnaire provided in Chapter 2, along with a knowledge of underlying types and causes of abdominal pain, can be very helpful in understanding the basis for a client's subjective report of pain. This knowledge can help the physical therapist recognize musculoskeletal complaints of a systemic origin that require referral to a physician.

Inflammatory Bowel Disease

Inflammatory bowel disease (IBD) refers to two inflammatory conditions:

- Ulcerative colitis (UC)
- Crohn's disease (CD) (also referred to as regional enteritis or ileitis)

Crohn's disease and ulcerative colitis are disorders of unknown etiology involving genetic and immunologic influences on the GI tract's ability to distinguish foreign from self-antigens and to "down-regulate" the mucosal immune response, allowing persistent increase of the tissue-damaging process. These two diseases share many epidemiologic, clinical, and therapeutic features. Both are chronic, medically incurable conditions (Hanauer, 1992).

Ulcerative colitis and Crohn's disease occur in all age groups but have a peak incidence in the second and third decades. The incidence of CD has risen over the past 20 years, and the combined prevalence of the two diseases is approximately 100 per 100,000 population (Hanauer, 1992).

Both UC and CD are discussed separately in the next section.

Stress-related bowel conditions are considered to be autoimmune diseases in which either the antibodies or other defense mechanisms are directed against the body. These chronic bowel conditions may occur suddenly or gradually and have no known etiology. A possible correlation of the onset of disease with life stresses and poor adaptation to those stresses is cited

Table 6–5

SYMPTOMS ASSOCIATED WITH NUTRITIONAL DEFICIENCIES

Symptoms	Nutritional Deficit
Generalized malnutrition, as shown by muscle wasting and growth retardation	Malabsorption of proteins, fats, carbohydrates; insufficient calories
Diarrhea, bloating, gas	Impaired absorption of salt and water caused by carbohydrate and fat malabsorption
Weakness	Anemia; electrolyte (sodium, potassium, bicarbonate, chloride, calcium, magnesium) imbalance
Anemia	Impaired absorption of iron, vitamin B_{12}, folic acid
Sore mouth and lips	Deficiency of iron and B vitamins
Numbness and tingling	Deficiency of vitamin B_{12} or other B vitamins; electrolyte imbalance
Swelling	Protein depletion
Absent menstrual periods	Protein and calorie depletion; rapid loss of weight
Bone pain	Protein depletion; vitamin D and calcium deficiency
Muscle spasms	Electrolyte imbalance (especially low calcium); pregnancy
Easy bleeding or bruising	Vitamin K deficiency

Adapted from Banks, P.A., Present, D.H., and Steiner, P.: The Crohn's Disease and Ulcerative Colitis Fact Book. National Foundation for Ileitis and Colitis. New York, Scribner & Sons, 1983.

in the majority of the literature referenced in this section, but this has not been proved conclusively.

Extraintestinal manifestations occur frequently in clients with inflammatory bowel disease and complicate its management. Manifestations involve the joints most commonly but also the skin, eyes, and mouth (Ruder and Matassarin-Jacobs, 1993). Skin lesions may occur as either erythema nodosum (red bumps/purple knots over the ankles and shins) or pyoderma (deep ulcers or canker sores) of the shins, ankles, and calves. Uveitis may cause red and painful eyes that are sensitive to light, but this condition does not affect the person's vision.

Nutritional Aspects of Inflammatory Bowel Disease (Ruder and Matassarin-Jacobs, 1993)

Nutritional deficiencies are the most common complications of IBD. Inflammation alone, along with the decrease in functioning surface area of the small intestine, increases food requirements, causing poor absorption.

The disease may progress to the point that the GI tract is no longer able to absorb enough nutrients to sustain life (Table 6–5). Intravenous nutritional support is then required. This method of intravenous feeding is known as hyperalimentation or total parenteral nutrition (TPN). Nutritional problems may occur associated with the medical treatment of IBD. The use of prednisone decreases vitamin D metabolism, impairs calcium absorption, decreases potassium supplies, and increases the nutritional requirement for protein and calories. Decreased vitamin D metabolism and impaired calcium absorption subsequently result in bone demineralization and osteoporosis.

Crohn's Disease (Ruder and Matassarin-Jacobs, 1993)

CD is an inflammatory disease that most commonly attacks the terminal end (or distal portion) of the small intestine (ileum) and the colon. However, it can occur anywhere along the alimentary canal from the mouth to the anus. It occurs more commonly in young adults and adolescents but can appear at any age (Smeltzer and Bare, 1992).

CD may have acute manifestations, but the condition is usually slow and nonaggressive. The client may present with mild intermittent symptoms months before the diagnosis is made. Fever may occur, with acute inflammation, abscesses, or rheumatoid manifestations.

Terminal ileum involvement produces pain in the periumbilical region with possible referred pain to the corresponding segment of the low back. Pain of the ileum is intermittent and felt in the lower right quadrant with possible associated iliopsoas abscess causing hip pain. A constant, aching soreness or tenderness usually indicates advanced disease. The client may experience relief of discomfort after passing stool or flatus. For this reason, it is important to ask whether low back pain is relieved after passing stool or gas.

Twenty-five per cent of people with CD may present with arthritis or migratory arthralgias (joint pain). The person may present with monoarthritis (i.e., asymmetric pattern affecting one joint at a time), usually involving an ankle or knee, although elbows and wrists can be included. Polyarthritis (involving more than one joint) or sacroiliitis (arthritis of the lower spine and pelvis) is common and may lead to ankylosing spondylitis in rare cases. Whether monoarthritic or polyarthritic, this condition comes and goes with the disease process and may precede repeat episodes of bowel symptoms by 1 to 2 weeks. With proper medical treatment, there is no permanent joint deformity.

Prognosis and Treatment. The mortality rate is not high, but recurrence and complications can result in disability. Because the inflammatory process in CD involves deeper layers of the bowel wall and is more chronic, healing may occur more slowly than in ulcerative colitis. Medical treatment is aimed at controlling the symptoms through antiinflammatory therapy (including steroids) and stress and dietary management. Surgical therapy is limited to management of complications.

Ulcerative Colitis (Ruder and Matassarin-Jacobs, 1993; Jewell, 1993)

By definition, UC is an inflammation and ulceration of the inner lining of the large intestine (colon) and rectum. When inflammation is confined to the rectum only, the condition is known as ulcerative proctitis. UC is not the same as irritable bowel syndrome (IBS) or spastic colitis (another term for IBS).

Clinical Signs and Symptoms. The predominant symptom of UC is rectal bleeding; mainly the left colon is involved; the small intestine is never involved. Clients often experience diarrhea, possibly 20 or more stools per day. Nausea, vomiting, anorexia, weight loss, and decreased serum potassium may occur with severe disease. The development of anemia depends on the degree of blood loss, severity of the illness, and dietary iron intake. Ankylosing spondylitis, anemia, and clubbing of the fingers are occasional findings.

Fever is present during acute disease. Nocturnal diarrhea is usually present when daytime diarrhea is prominent. Episodes of UC are precipitated by emotional stress, diet, ingestion of irritants such as laxatives or antibiotics, physical exertion, respiratory infections, and overfatigue.

Prognosis and Treatment. Permanent and complete cure with medical therapy is unusual, and life expectancy is shortened. The typical course of disease is characterized by remissions and exacerbations over a period of many years (Knauer, 1993a).

Cancer of the colon is more common among clients with UC than among the general population. The incidence is greatly increased among those who develop UC before the age of 16 years and those who have had the condition for more than 30 years.

As with CD, treatment attempts to terminate the acute attack, prevent recurrent attacks, and promote healing of the damaged mucosa. When medical management fails and complications such as perforation, hemorrhage, abscess, or obstruction de-

▼ Clinical Signs and Symptoms of
Ulcerative Colitis and Crohn's Disease

- Diarrhea
- Constipation
- Fever
- Abdominal pain
- Rectal bleeding
- Night sweats
- Decreased appetite, nausea, weight loss
- Skin lesions
- Uveitis (inflammation of the eye)
- Arthritis
- Migratory arthralgias

velop, surgical intervention is required.

Medical testing and diagnosis are required to differentiate between these inflammatory conditions. Most often, the physical therapist is faced with clients presenting complaints of pain located in the shoulder, back, or groin that may have a GI origin and not be true musculoskeletal dysfunction at all.

The client may have nonspecific symptoms common to chronic systemic disease:

- Depression
- Decreased appetite and resultant fatigue
- Overall muscular weakness from inactivity
- Irritability

Irritable Bowel Syndrome
(Schuster, 1993)

Irritable bowel syndrome (IBS) has been called the "common cold of the stomach"; it is a functional disorder of motility in the small and large intestines. It occurs as a result of the digestive tract's reaction to the stresses of daily life as well as to dietary patterns. There are no anatomic abnormalities, and no progressive organic diseases are in progress. Other descriptive names for this condition are spastic colon, irritable colon, nervous indigestion, functional dyspepsia, pylorospasm, spastic colitis, intestinal neuroses, and laxative or cathartic colitis (Ruder and Matassarin-Jacobs, 1993).

IBS is the most common gastrointestinal disorder in Western society and accounts for 50 per cent of subspecialty referrals. Although most common in women in early adulthood, IBS can begin after the age of 45 years. Symptoms of IBS occur in up to 25 per cent of otherwise healthy individuals and are intermittent with variable periods of remission. Episodes of emotional stress, fatigue, alcohol intake or eating—especially a large meal with a high fat content, roughage, or fruit —aggravate or precipitate symptoms (Ruder and Matassarin-Jacobs, 1993; Snape, 1992).

Clinical Signs and Symptoms. There is a highly variable complex of gastrointestinal symptoms, including nausea and vomiting, anorexia, foul breath, sour stomach, flatulence, cramps, and constipation or diarrhea. Nocturnal diarrhea, awakening the client from a sound sleep, is more often a result of organic disease of the bowel and is less likely to occur in IBS. Hysteria and depression are the most prevalent psychologic problems (Knauer, 1993a).

Pain may be steady or intermittent, and there may be a dull deep discomfort with sharp cramps in the morning or after eating. The typical pain pattern consists of lower left quadrant abdominal pain, constipation, and diarrhea (Ruder and Matassarin-Jacobs, 1993).

These primary symptoms occur when the natural motility of the bowel (rhythmic peristalsis) is disrupted by stress, smoking, eating, and drinking alcohol. Rapid alterations in the speed of bowel movement create an obstruction to the natural flow of stool and gas. The resultant pressure build-up in the bowel produces pain and spasm.

Prognosis and Treatment. Irritable bowel syndrome is not a life-threatening disorder, and prognosis is good for controlling symptoms through diet, medication, regular physical activity, and stress management. Physical therapists must be alert to clients who have developed breath-holding patterns or hyperventilation in response to stress. Teaching proper breathing techniques during exercise and daily relaxation techniques is important.

Clinical Signs and Symptoms of
Irritable Bowel Syndrome

- Painful abdominal cramps
- Constipation
- Diarrhea
- Nausea and vomiting
- Anorexia
- Flatulence
- Foul breath

Overview GASTROINTESTINAL PAIN PATTERNS

ESOPHAGEAL PAIN (Fig. 6–10)

Location:

Substernal discomfort at the level of the lesion

Lesion of upper esophagus: pain in the (anterior) neck

Lesion of lower esophagus: pain originating from the xiphoid process, radiating around the thorax

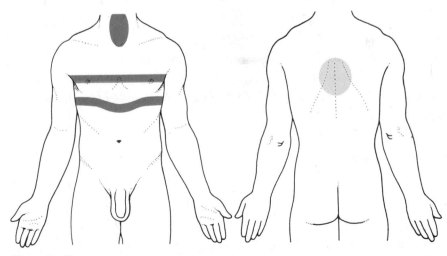

Figure 6–10
Esophageal pain may be projected around the chest at any level corresponding to the esophageal lesion. Only two of the possible bands of pain around the chest are shown here.

Referral: Severe esophageal pain: pain referred to the middle of the back

Back pain may be the only symptom or may be the earliest symptom of esophageal cancer

Description: Sharp, sticking, knifelike, stabbing

Strong burning pain (esophagitis)

Intensity: Varies from mild discomfort to severe pain

Duration: May be constant; associated with meals

Associated Signs and Symptoms: Dysphagia, odynophagia, melena

Possible Etiology: Obstruction of the esophagus (neoplasm)

Esophageal stricture secondary to acid reflux (peptic esophagitis)

Esophageal stricture of unknown cause

Achalasia

Esophagitis or esophageal spasm

Esophageal varices (usually asymptomatic except bleeding)

■ ■ ■ ■ ■ ■ ■ ■ ■ ■ ■

STOMACH AND DUODENAL PAIN (see Fig. 6–6)

Location: Pain in the midline of the epigastrium

Upper abdomen just below the xiphoid process

Referral: Common referral pattern to the back at the level of the lesion (T6–T10)

Right shoulder/upper trapezius

Lateral border of the right scapula

Description: Aching, burning, gnawing, cramplike pain (true visceral pain)

Intensity: Can be mild or severe

Duration: Comes in waves

Associated Signs and Symptoms: Early satiety

Melena

Symptoms may be associated with meals

Possible Etiology: Peptic ulcers: gastric, pyloric, duodenal

Stomach carcinoma

Kaposi's sarcoma (most common malignancy associated with acquired immunodeficiency syndrome [AIDS])

■ ■ ■ ■ ■ ■ ■ ■ ■ ■ ■

SMALL INTESTINE PAIN (Fig. 6–11)

Location: Midabdominal pain (about the umbilicus)

Referral: Pain referred to the back if the stimulus is sufficiently intense or if the individual's pain threshold is low

Description: Cramping pain

Intensity: Moderate to severe

Duration: Intermittent (pain comes and goes)

Associated Signs
and Symptoms: Nausea, fever, diarrhea

                     Pain relief may not occur after passing stool or gas

Possible
Etiology: Obstruction (neoplasm)

                     Increased bowel motility

                     Crohn's disease (regional enteritis)

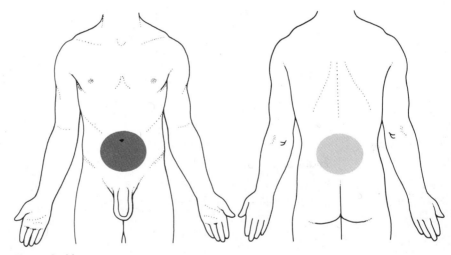

Figure 6–11

Midabdominal pain *(dark red)* caused by disturbances of the small intestine is centered around the umbilicus and may be referred *(light red)* to the low back area at the same level.

■ ■ ■ ■ ■ ■ ■ ■ ■ ■ ■

LARGE INTESTINE AND COLON PAIN (Fig. 6–12)

Location: Lower midabdomen (across either or both quadrants)
                    Poorly localized
Referral: Pain may be referred to the sacrum when the rectum is stimulated
Description: Cramping
Intensity: Dull
Duration: Steady
Associated Signs
and Symptoms: Bloody diarrhea, urgency
                    Constipation
                    Pain relief may occur after defecation or passing gas
Possible
Etiology: Ulcerative colitis
                    Crohn's disease (regional enteritis)
                    Carcinoma of the colon
                    Long-term use of antibiotics
                    Irritable bowel syndrome (IBS)

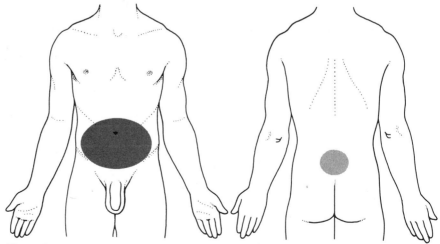

Figure 6–12

Pain associated with the large intestine and colon (dark red) may occur in the lower midabdomen across either or both abdominal quadrants. Pain may be referred to the sacrum (light red) when the rectum is stimulated.

■ ■ ■ ■ ■ ■ ■ ■ ■ ■

PANCREATIC PAIN (Fig. 6–13)

Location:	Midline or to the left of the epigastrium, just below the xiphoid process
Referral:	Referred pain in the middle or lower back is typical with pancreatic disease
	Somatic pain felt in the left shoulder may result from activation of pain fibers in the left diaphragm by an adjacent inflammatory process in the tail of the pancreas (Ridge and Way, 1993)
Description:	Terrifying, burning, or gnawing abdominal pain
Intensity:	Severe
Duration:	Constant pain, sudden onset

Associated Signs
and Symptoms:

Sudden weight loss

Jaundice

Nausea and vomiting

Light-colored stools (carcinoma)

Weakness

Fever

Malaise

Constipation

Flatulence

Tachycardia

Symptoms may be unrelated to digestive activities (carcinoma)

Symptoms may be related to digestive activities (pancreatitis)

Aggravating
Factors:

Walking and lying supine (pancreatitis)

Alcohol, large meals

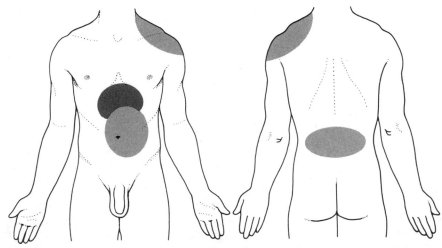

Figure 6–13

Pancreatic pain *(dark red)* occurs in the midline or left of the epigastrium, just below the xiphoid process, but may be referred *(light red)* to the left shoulder or to the middle or low back.

Relieving
Factors: Sitting and leaning forward (pancreatitis, pancreatic carcinoma)

Possible
Etiology: Pancreatitis

Pancreatic carcinoma (primarily disease of men, occurs during the 6th to 7th decade)

■ ■ ■ ■ ■ ■ ■ ■ ■ ■ ■ ■

APPENDICEAL PAIN (see Fig. 6–7)

Location: Right lower quadrant pain

Well localized

Referral: First referred to epigastric or periumbilical area

Referred pain pattern to the right hip and/or right testicle

Description: Aching, comes in waves

Intensity: Moderate to severe

Duration: Steadily progresses over time (usually 12 hours with acute appendicitis)

Associated Signs
and Symptoms: Positive McBurney's point for tenderness
Positive iliopsoas muscle test or positive obturator test

Anorexia, nausea, vomiting, low-grade fever

Coated tongue and bad breath

Dysuria (painful/difficult urination)

Iliopsoas abscess may occur; pain on movement and palpation of muscle

PHYSICIAN REFERRAL

A 67-year-old man is seeing you through home health care for a home program after discharge from the hospital 2 weeks ago for a total hip replacement. His recovery has been slowed by chronic diarrhea. A 25-year-old woman who is diagnosed as having a sacroiliac pain and joint dysfunction asks you what exercises she can do for constipation. A 44-year-old man with biceps tendinitis reports several episodes of fever and chills, diarrhea, and abdominal pain, which he contributes to "the stress of meeting deadlines on the job."

There are common examples of symptoms of a GI nature that are described by clients and are unrelated to current physical therapy treatment. These people may be seeking the physical therapist's advice as the only medical person with whom they have contact. Knowing the pain patterns associated with GI involvement and which follow-up questions to ask can assist the physical therapist in deciding when to suggest that the client return to a physician for a medical examination and treatment.

The client may not associate GI symptoms or already diagnosed GI disease with his or her musculoskeletal pain, which makes it necessary for the physical therapist to initiate questions to determine the presence of such GI involvement.

Taking the client's temperature and vital signs during the initial evaluation is recommended for any person who has musculoskeletal pain of unknown origin. Fever, low-grade fever over a long period (even if cyclic), or night sweats is indicative of systemic disease.

When appendicitis is suspected because of the client's symptoms, a physician should be notified immediately. The client should lie down and remain as quiet as possible. It is best to give her or him nothing by mouth because of the danger of aggravating the condition, possibly causing rupture of the appendix or in case surgery is needed. Applications of heat are contraindicated for the same reason (O'Toole, 1992).

On the other hand, the physical therapist may be evaluating a client who presents with shoulder, back, or groin pain and limitations that are not true musculoskeletal lesions but rather the result of GI involvement. The presence of associated GI symptoms in the absence of conclusive musculoskeletal findings will alert the physical therapist to the possible need for medical referral. Correlate the *history* with *pain patterns* and any *unusual findings* that may indicate systemic disease.

Systemic Signs and Symptoms Requiring Physician Referral

Bloody diarrhea
Boring, stabbing pain
Chills
Constant pain
Cutting, knifelike pain
Dark urine
Dysphagia
Early satiety
Fecal incontinence
Fever
Gnawing, burning pain
Iliopsoas muscle test (positive)
Jaundice
Kehr's sign (positive)
Light stools
McBurney's point (positive)
Melena
Migratory arthralgias
Night pain
Night sweats
Obturator test (positive)
Odynophagia
Skin lesions
Sudden weight loss
Uveitis
Vomiting

Key Points to Remember

- Gastrointestinal disorders can refer pain to the sternum, shoulder, scapula, low back, and hip.

- The membrane that envelops organs (visceral peritoneum) is insensitive to pain so that, except in the presence of inflammation/ischemia, it is possible to have extensive disease without pain.

- Clients may not relate known GI disorders to current (or new) musculoskeletal symptoms.

- Sudden and unaccountable changes in bowel habits, blood in the stool, or vomiting red blood or coffee-ground vomitus are red flag symptoms requiring medical follow-up.

- Antibiotics and NSAIDs are the drugs that most commonly induce GI symptoms.

- Kehr's sign (left shoulder pain) occurs as a result of free air or blood in the abdominal cavity causing distention (e.g., trauma, ruptured spleen).

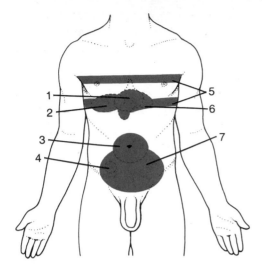

Figure 6–14

Full-figure **primary pain pattern:** (1) stomach/duodenum; (2) liver/gallbladder/common bile duct; (3) small intestine; (4) appendix; (5) esophagus; (6) pancreas; and (7) large intestine/colon.

- Epigastric pain radiating to the upper back or upper back pain alone can be the primary symptom of peptic ulcer, pancreatitis, or pancreatic carcinoma.
- Appendicitis and diseases of the intestines such as Crohn's disease and ulcerative colitis can cause abscess of the iliopsoas muscle, resulting in hip, thigh, or groin pain.

- Arthritis and migratory arthalgias occur in 25 per cent of Crohn's disease cases.

Figures 6–14 and 6–15 provide a summary of all the GI pain patterns described that can mimic the pain and dysfunction usually associated with musculoskeletal lesions.

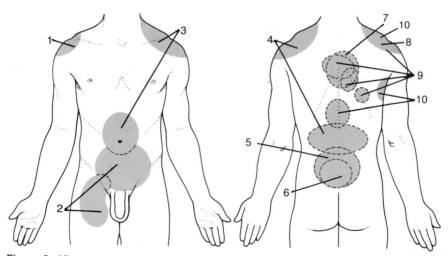

Figure 6–15

Full-figure **referred pain patterns:** (1) liver/gallbladder/common bile duct; (2) appendix; (3) pancreas; (4) pancreas; (5) small intestine; (6) colon; (7) esophagus; (8) stomach/duodenum; (9) liver/gallbladder/common bile duct; and (10) stomach/duodenum.

| SUBJECTIVE EXAMINATION | *Special Questions to Ask* |

After completing the initial intake interview, if there is cause to suspect GI involvement include the following additional questions:

- Do you have any problems chewing or swallowing food? Do you have any pain when swallowing food or liquids? **(Dysphagia, odynophagia)**
- Do you vomit frequently? **(Esophageal varices, ulcers)**
  - If so, how often?
  - Describe the vomitus.
  - Have you ever vomited blood?
  - Is your vomitus ever dark brown or black?
  - Do you ever take any medication for vomiting? If so, what?
  - Do you ever spit up blood?
- Have you seen a physician recently for abdominal or intestinal problems?
- Have you experienced any loss of appetite?
- Have you ever been treated for an ulcer?
  - If so, when?
  - Have you ever been x-rayed for an ulcer? If so, when?
  - Do you still have any pain from your ulcer?
- Does eating relieve your symptoms? **(Duodenal or pyloric ulcer)**
  - How soon after eating?
  - Does eating aggravate your symptoms? **(Gastric ulcer, gallbladder inflammation)**
- Does your pain occur 1 to 3 hours after eating or between meals? **(Duodenal or pyloric ulcers, gallstones, pancreatitis)**
  - Have you ever had gallstones?
- Have you noticed any change in your symptoms after drinking alcohol? **(Alcohol-associated pancreatitis)**
- Are you ever awakened at night with pain? **(Duodenal ulcer, cancer)**
  - Approximately what time does this occur? **(12 midnight to 3:00 a.m.: ulcer)**
  - Can you relieve the pain in any way and get back to sleep? If yes, how? **(Ulcer: eating and antacids relieve/Cancer: nothing relieves)**
- Do you have a feeling of fullness after only one or two bites of food? **(Early satiety: stomach and duodenum or gallbladder)**
- Have you had a sudden weight loss in the last month (i.e., 10 to 15 pounds in 2 weeks without trying)? **(Cancer)**

- Have you had a sudden change in your bowel movements? **(Constipation/bowel obstruction: normal frequency varies from three times a day to once every 3 or more days)**

- Do you have diarrhea? **(Ulcerative colitis, Crohn's disease, long-term use of antibiotics, colonic obstruction, amebic colitis, angiodysplasia)**

- Do you have more than two loose stools a day? If so, do you take medication for this problem? What kind of medication do you use?

- Do you have a sense of urgency: Do you have to find a bathroom immediately without waiting?

- Have you traveled outside of the United States within the last 6 months to 1 year? **(Amebic colitis associated with bloody diarrhea)**

■ Do you ever have any blood in your stool?

  - If so, how often?

  - Is the blood mixed in with the stool or does it coat the surface? **(Distal colon or rectum versus melena)**

  - Is the blood bright red or are your stools black or tarry? **(Distal colon or rectum versus melena)**

■ Do you have hemorrhoids?

  - If yes, have you ever had surgery for your hemorrhoids? **(Most common cause of bright red blood coating stools/check for fecal incontinence)**

■ Do you ever have bowel smears on your undergarments? **(Fecal incontinence)**

■ Do you ever have gray (clay)-colored stools? **(Lack of bile or caused by biliary obstruction: hepatitis, gallstones, cirrhosis, pancreatic carcinoma, hepatotoxic drugs)**

■ Are your stools ever pencil thin? **(Indicates bowel obstruction)**

■ Is your pain relieved after passing stool or gas? **(Yes: Large intestine and colon; No: small intestine)**

■ **Have you ever had your colon x-rayed?**

  - If so, when?

  - Have you ever undergone a colonoscopy or proctoscopy? If so, why and how long ago?

■ Have you ever had abdominal surgery?

  - If so, when? What type was it?

■ Have you sustained any injuries in the last week during a sports activity, fall, automobile accident, or assault? **(Ruptured spleen associated with pain in the left shoulder: positive Kehr's sign)**

■ Do you ever have episodes of fever and night sweats? **(Hallmark sign of systemic disease)**

■ Medications: Follow the usual line of questions provided in the subjective examina-

■ tion: Look for long-term use of antibiotics or hepatotoxic drugs. See Table 6–2 for a list of medications that cause constipation.

  ■ Do you use laxatives or stool softeners? How often?

  ■ Do you take iron pills?

■ Do you have any other medical or health-related problems?

CASE STUDY

REFERRAL

A 21-year-old woman comes to you with complaints of pain on hip flexion when she lifts her right foot off the brake in the car. There are no other aggravating factors, and she is unaware of any way to relieve the pain when she is driving her car. Before the onset of symptoms, she jogged 5 to 6 miles/day, but could not recall any injury or trauma that might contribute to this pain. The Family/Personal History form indicates no personal illness but shows a complex, positive family history for heart disease, diabetes, ulcerative colitis, stomach ulcers, stomach cancer, and alcoholism.

PHYSICAL THERAPY INTERVIEW

It is suggested that the physical therapist use the physical therapy interview to assess the client's complaints today and follow up with appropriate additional questions, such as those noted here.

Introduction to Patient

From your family history form, I notice that a number of your family members have reportedly been diagnosed with various diseases.

Do you have any other medical or health-related problems?

Have you sustained any injuries to the lower back, side, or abdomen in the last week—for example, during a sports activity, fall, automobile accident, or assault of any kind?

Although the symptoms that you have described appear to be a musculoskeletal problem, I would like to check out the possibility of a urologic, abdominal, or gynecologic source of this irritation. I will ask you some additional questions that may seem to be unrelated to the problem with your hip, but which will help me to put together the whole picture of the history, symptoms, and actual physical results from my examination today.

General Systemic

What other symptoms have you had with this problem? (After allowing the client to answer, you may prompt her by asking: For example, have you had any . . .)

  ■ Numbness

  ■ Fatigue

- Legs giving out from under you
- Burning, tingling
- Weakness

Gastrointestinal

- Nausea
- Diarrhea
- Loss of appetite
- Feeling of fullness after only one or two bites of a meal
- Unexpected weight gain or loss (10 to 15 pounds without trying)
- Vomiting
- Constipation
- Blood in your stool

If yes to any of these, follow-up with *Special Questions to Ask* from this chapter.

Have you noticed any association between when you eat and your symptoms? (After allowing the client to respond you may want to prompt her by asking whether eating relieves the pain or aggravates the pain.)

Is your pain relieved or aggravated during or after you have a bowel movement?

Gynecologic

Since your hip/groin/thigh symptoms started, have you been examined by a gynecologist to rule out any gynecologic causes of this problem?
If no:

- Have you ever been told that you have ovarian cysts, uterine fibroids, retroverted uterus, endometriosis, an ectopic pregnancy, or any other gynecologic problem?
- Are you pregnant or have you recently terminated a pregnancy either by miscarriage or abortion?
- Are you using an intrauterine device (IUD)?
- Are you having any unusual vaginal discharge?

If yes to any of these questions, see the follow-up questions for women in Chapter 2.

Urologic

Have you had any problems with your kidneys or bladder? If yes, please describe.

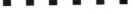

Have you noticed any changes in your ability to urinate since your pain or symptoms started? If no, it may be necessary to provide examples of what changes you are referring to; for example, difficulty in starting or continuing the flow of urine, numbness or tingling in the groin or pelvis, painful urination, urinary incontinence.

Have you had burning with urination during the last 1 to 3 weeks?

Have you noticed any blood in your urine?

OBJECTIVE EXAMINATION

Your objective examination reveals tenderness on palpation over the right anterior upper thigh muscles into the groin, with reproduction of the pain on resisted trunk flexion only. This woman attends daily ballet classes, stretches daily, and seems to be very active physically. All tests for flexibility were negative for tightness, including the Thomas' test for tight hip flexors. Other special tests for hip and a neurologic screen had negative results. The client's temperature was normal when it was taken today during the intake screen of vital signs, but during the physical therapy interview, when specifically asked about fevers and night sweats, she indicated several recurrent episodes of night sweats during the last 3 months.

RESULTS

Although the client's complaints are primarily musculoskeletal, the absence of trauma, positive family history for systemic disease, limited musculoskeletal findings, and the client's remark concerning the presence of night sweats will alert the physical therapist to the need for a medical referral to rule out the possibility of a systemic origin of symptoms.

The client's condition gradually worsened during a 3-week period and reexamination by the physician led to an eventual diagnosis of Crohn's disease (regional gastroenteritis). The client was treated with medications that reduced abdominal inflammation and eliminated subjective reports of pain on active hip flexion.

References

Allison, M.C., Howatson, A.G., and Torrance, C.J.: Gastrointestinal damage associated with the use of nonsteroidal anti-inflammatory drugs. New England Journal of Medicine *327*:749–754, 1992.

Babb, R.R.: Gastrointestinal complications of nonsteroidal anti-inflammatory drugs. Western Journal of Medicine *157*:444–447, 1992.

Bauwens, D.B., and Pain, R.: Thoracic pain. *In* Blacklow, R.S. (ed.): MacBryde's Signs and Symptoms, 6th ed. New York, J.B. Lippincott, 1983, pp. 139–164.

Butera, E.: Nursing care of clients with renal disorders. *In* Black, J., and Matassarin-Jacobs, E. (eds.): Luckmann and Sorensen's Medical-Surgical Nursing; A Psychophysiologic Approach, 4th ed. Philadelphia, W.B. Saunders, 1993, pp. 1487–1542.

Darlington, R.C.: O.T.C. laxatives. Journal of the American Pharmaceutical Association *6*:470, 1966.

DeVroede, G.: Constipation. *In* Sleisenger, M.H., and Fordtran, J.S. (eds.): Gastrointestinal Disease, 5th ed. Philadelphia, W.B. Saunders, 1993, pp. 837–887.

DiMagno, E.P.: Carcinoma of the pancreas. *In* Wyngaarden, J.B., Smith, L.H., and Bennett, J.C. (eds.): Cecil Textbook of Medicine, 19th ed. Philadelphia, W.B. Saunders, 1992, pp. 727–730.

Dugdale, D.C., Ramsey, P.G., Larson, E.B.: General medical care. *In* Ramsey, P.G., and Larson, E.B.

(eds.): Medical Therapeutics, 2nd ed. Philadelphia, W.B. Saunders, 1993, pp. 2–45.

Fine, K.D., Krejs, G.J., and Fordtran, J.S.: Diarrhea. *In* Sleisenger, M.H., and Fordtran, J.S. (eds.): Gastrointestinal Disease, 5th ed. Philadelphia, W.B. Saunders, 1993, pp. 1043–1071.

Fries, J.F., Williams, C.A., Bloch, D.A., and Michel, B.A.: Nonsteroidal anti-inflammatory drug-associated gastropathy: Incidence and risk factor models. American Journal of Medicine *91*:213–222, 1991.

Given, B.A., and Simmons, S.J.: Gastroenterology in Clinical Nursing. St. Louis, C.V. Mosby, 1979.

Guyton, A.: Human Physiology and Mechanisms of Disease. Philadelphia, W.B. Saunders, 1992.

Hanauer, S.B.: Inflammatory bowel disease. *In* Wyngaarden, J.B., Smith, L.H., and Bennett, J.C. (eds.): Cecil Textbook of Medicine, 19th ed. Philadelphia, W.B. Saunders, 1992, pp. 699–708.

Jaszewski, R.: Frequency of gastroduodenal lesions in asymptomatic patients on chronic aspirin or nonsteroidal anti-inflammatory drug therapy. Journal of Clinical Gastroenterology *12*:10–13, 1990.

Jewell, D.P.: Ulcerative Colitis. *In* Sleisenger, M.H., and Fordtran, J.S. (eds.): Gastrointestinal Disease, 5th ed. Philadelphia, W.B. Saunders, 1993, pp. 1305–1330.

Kallsen C.: Nursing care of clients with biliary and exocrine pancreatic disorders. *In* Black, J., and Matassarin-Jacobs, E. (eds.): Luckmann and Sorensen's Medical-Surgical Nursing; A Psychophysiologic Approach, 4th ed. Philadelphia, W.B. Saunders, 1993, pp. 1731–1754.

Knauer, C.M.: Alimentary tract. *In* Tierney, L.M., McPhee, S.J., Papadakis, M.A., and Schroeder, S.A.: Current Medical Diagnosis and Treatment. Norwalk, Connecticut, Appleton and Lange, 1993a, pp. 451–502.

Knauer, C.M.: Liver, biliary tract, and pancreas. *In* Tierney, L.M., McPhee, S.J., Papadakis, M.A., and Schroeder, S.A.: Current Medical Diagnosis and Treatment. Norwalk, Connecticut, Appleton and Lange, 1993b, pp. 503–537.

Kodner, I.J., and Fry, R.D.: Inflammatory bowel disease. Clinical Symposia *34*:1, 1982.

Long, B.C.: Assessment of the gastrointestinal system. *In* Phipps, W.J., Long, B.C., and Woods, N.: Medical-Surgical Nursing: Concepts and Clinical Practice. St. Louis, C.V. Mosby, 1991, pp. 1233–1248.

Matassarin-Jacobs, E., and Strasburg, K.: Nursing care of clients with hepatic disorders. *In* Black, J., and Matassarin-Jacobs, E. (eds.): Luckmann and Sorensen's Medical-Surgical Nursing; A Psychophysiologic Approach, 4th ed. Philadelphia, W.B. Saunders, 1993, pp. 1697–1730.

Ockner, R.K.: Introduction to gastrointestinal diseases. *In* Wyngaarden, J.B., Smith, L.H., and Bennett, J.C. (eds.): Cecil Textbook of Medicine, 19th ed. Philadelphia, W.B. Saunders, 1992, pp. 620–625.

O'Toole, M. (ed.): Miller-Keane Encyclopedia and Dictionary of Medicine, Nursing, and Allied Health, 5th ed. Philadelphia, W.B. Saunders, 1992.

Peterson, M.L.: Constipation and diarrhea. *In* Blacklow, R.S. (ed.): MacBryde's Signs and Symptoms, 6th ed. Philadelphia, J.B. Lippincott, 1983, pp. 375–392.

Pharmacology 44 (Suppl. 1):36–40, 1992. Laxative abuse.

Product Management Drugs Cosmetics: What the public spent for drugs, cosmetics, toiletries in 1974. Product Management Drugs Cosmetics *4*:37, 1975.

Richardson, C.T.: Peptic ulcer. *In* Wyngaarden, J.B., Smith, L.H., and Bennett, J.C. (eds.): Cecil Textbook of Medicine, 19th ed. Philadelphia, W.B. Saunders, 1992, pp. 652–656.

Ridge, J.A., and Way, L.W.: Abdominal pain. *In* Sleisenger, M.H., and Fordtran, J.S. (eds.): Gastrointestinal Disease, 5th ed. Philadelphia, W.B. Saunders, 1993, pp. 150–161.

Rose, S.J., and Rothstein, J.M.: Muscle mutability: General concepts and adaptations to altered patterns of use. Physical Therapy *62*:1773, 1982.

Ruder, S.: Nursing care of clients with ingestive disorders. *In* Black, J., and Matassarin-Jacobs, E. (eds.): Luckmann and Sorensen's Medical-Surgical Nursing; A Psychophysiologic Approach, 4th ed. Philadelphia, W.B. Saunders, 1993a, pp. 1571–1598.

Ruder, S.: Nursing care of clients with gastric disorders. *In* Black, J., and Matassarin-Jacobs, E. (eds.): Luckmann and Sorensen's Medical-Surgical Nursing; A Psychophysiologic Approach, 4th ed. Philadelphia, W.B. Saunders, 1993b, pp. 1599–1626.

Ruder, S., and Matassarin-Jacobs, E.: Nursing care of clients with intestinal disorders. *In* Black, J., and Matassarin-Jacobs, E. (eds.): Luckmann and Sorensen's Medical-Surgical Nursing; A Psychophysiologic Approach, 4th ed. Philadelphia, W.B. Saunders, 1993, pp. 1627–1674.

Scarpelli, D.G.: The pancreas. *In* Rubin, E., and Farber, J.L. (eds.): Pathology, 2nd ed. Philadelphia, J.B. Lippincott, 1994, pp. 787–803.

Schuster, M.M.: Irritable bowel syndrome. *In* Sleisenger, M.H., and Fordtran, J.S. (eds.): Gastrointestinal Disease, 5th ed. Philadelphia, W.B. Saunders, 1993, pp. 917–929.

Silverstein, F.: Nonsteroidal anti-inflammatory drugs and peptic ulcer disease. Postgraduate Medicine *89*:33–38, 1991.

Sleisenger, M.H.: Miscellaneous inflammatory diseases of the intestine. *In* Wyngaarden, J.B., Smith, L.H., and Bennett, J.C. (eds.): Cecil Textbook of Medicine, 19th ed. Philadelphia, W.B. Saunders, 1992, pp. 746–749.

Smeltzer, S., and Bare, B.: Brunner and Suddarth's Textbook of Medical-Surgical Nursing, 7th ed. Philadelphia, J.B. Lippincott, 1992.

Snape, W.J.: Disorders of gastrointestinal motility. *In* Wyngaarden, J.B., Smith, L.H., and Bennett, J.C. (eds.): Cecil Textbook of Medicine, 19th ed. Philadelphia, W.B. Saunders, 1992, pp. 671–680.

Soll, A.H.: Nonsteroidal anti-inflammatory drugs and

ulcers (editorial). Western Journal of Medicine *157*:465–468, 1992.

Steinberg, W.M.: Pancreatitis. *In* Wyngaarden, J.B., Smith, L.H., and Bennett, J.C. (eds.): Cecil Textbook of Medicine, 19th ed. Philadelphia, W.B. Saunders, 1992, pp. 721–727.

Travell, J.G., and Simons, D.G.: Myofascial Pain and Dysfunction: The Trigger Point Manual. Baltimore, Williams and Wilkins, 1983.

Tucker, D.M., Sandstead, H.H., Logan, G.M., Jr., et al.: Dietary fiber and personality factors as determinants of stool output. Gastroenterology *81*:879, 1981.

7

Overview of Renal and Urologic Signs and Symptoms

■ ■ ■ ■ ■ ■ ■ ■ ■ ■ ■ ■

Clinical Signs and Symptoms of:

Upper Urinary Tract Infections
Cystitis and Urethritis
Obstruction of the Upper Urinary Tract

Obstruction of the Lower Urinary Tract
Prostatitis

A 40-year-old athletic man comes to your clinic for an evaluation of back pain that he attributes to a very hard fall on his back while he was alpine skiing 3 days ago. His chief complaint is a dull, aching costovertebral pain on the left side, which is unrelieved by a change in position or by treatment with ice, heat, or aspirin. He stated that "even the skin on my back hurts." He has no previous history of any medical problems.

After further questioning, the client reveals that inspiratory movements do not aggravate the pain, and he has not noticed any change in color, odor, or volume of urine output. However, percussion of the costovertebral angle results in the reproduction of the symptoms. This type of symptomatology may suggest renal involvement even without obvious changes in urine.

Whether secondary to trauma or of insidious onset, a client's complaints of flank pain, low back pain, or pelvic pain may be of renal or urologic origin and should be screened carefully through the subjective and objective examinations. Medical referral may be necessary.

The urinary tract, consisting of kidneys, ureters, bladder, and urethra, is an integral component of human functioning that disposes of the body's toxic waste products and unnecessary fluid and expertly regulates extremely complicated metabolic processes. Disruption within this system can result in severe dysfunction of physiologic homeostasis. An understanding of the basic anatomy, physiology, and pathophysiology of the urinary tract will help the therapist determine more clearly whether the client's symptoms are musculoskeletal in origin or are related to disorders of the urinary system.

This chapter is intended to guide the physical therapist in understanding the origins and relationships of renal, ureteral, bladder, and urethral symptoms. It includes basic urinary tract anatomy and physiology and focuses on the major categories of urinary tract disease, related diagnostic procedures, and resultant clinical signs and symptoms, including pain patterns. In addi-

tion, a general discussion of renal failure and its related symptoms, medical consequences, and treatment options is presented.

UPPER URINARY TRACT

Structure

The upper urinary tract consists of the kidneys and ureters. The kidneys are located in the posterior upper abdominal cavity in a space behind the peritoneum (retroperitoneal space) (Fig. 7–1). Their position is in front of and on both sides of the vertebral column at the level of T12 to L2. The upper portion of the kidney is in contact with the diaphragm and moves with respiration. The kidneys are protected by the rib cage and abdominal organs ante-

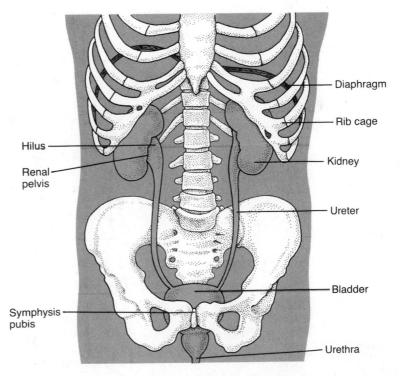

Figure 7–1

Urinary tract structures. The upper portion of each kidney is protected by the rib cage, and the bladder is partially protected by the symphysis pubis.

riorly and by large back muscles and ribs posteriorly. The lower portions of the kidney and the ureters extend below the ribs and are separated from the abdominal cavity by the peritoneal membrane.

Each kidney is approximately 4 to 6 oz (180 g) in weight; approximately 5 inches in length (11.5 cm); 3 inches wide (7.5 cm); and 1 inch (2.5 cm) thick. The central notch or hilus of each kidney supplies the organ with blood and nerves and contains the renal pelvis, which is the opening into the ureter (see Fig. 7–1). From the ureter, urine flows into the bladder, where it is stored until it is excreted through the urethra (a tubular structure connected to the bladder).

Function

The functional unit of the kidney is the nephron. Each kidney contains about one million nephrons. The nephron consists of several structures that form urine and maintain critical physiologic functions. The glomerulus, which is a cluster of capillaries, and Bowman's capsule are the structures that filter blood. The proximal convoluted tubule, the loop of Henle, and the distal convoluted tubule are the urine formation structures, which reabsorb the substances that the body needs and excrete the waste materials. Urine is collected in and transported out of the body through the collecting ducts (Fig. 7–2).

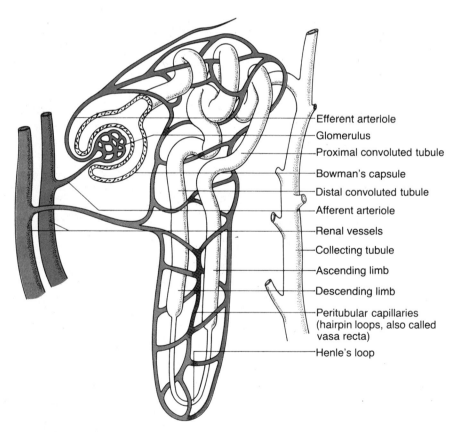

Efferent arteriole
Glomerulus
Proximal convoluted tubule
Bowman's capsule
Distal convoluted tubule
Afferent arteriole
Renal vessels
Collecting tubule
Ascending limb
Descending limb
Peritubular capillaries (hairpin loops, also called vasa recta)
Henle's loop

Figure 7–2

Components of the nephron. The afferent arteriole carries blood to the glomerulus for filtration through Bowman's capsule and the renal tubular system. (From Foster, R.L., Hunsberger, M.M., and Anderson, J.J.: Family-Centered Nursing Care of Children. Philadelphia, W.B. Saunders, 1989.)

Formation and excretion of urine by the nephrons is the major activity of the kidney. Through this process, the kidney is able to maintain a homeostatic environment in the body. Besides the excretory function of the kidney, which includes formation of urine and removal of wastes and excessive fluid, the kidney also plays an integral role in the balance of various essential body functions, including

- Acid-base balance
- Electrolyte balance
- Control of blood pressure with renin
- Formation of red blood cells (RBCs)
- Activation of vitamin D and calcium balance

The failure of the kidney to perform any of these functions results in severe alteration and disruption of the body's homeostasis.

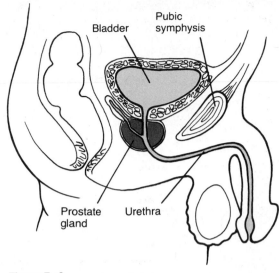

Figure 7–3

The prostate is located at the base of the bladder surrounding a part of the urethra. As the prostate enlarges, the urethra can become obstructed, interfering with the normal flow of urine.

LOWER URINARY TRACT

Structure and Function

The lower urinary tract consists of the bladder and urethra. From the renal pelvis, urine is moved by peristalsis to the ureters and into the bladder. The bladder, which is a muscular, membranous sac, is located directly behind the symphysis pubis and is used for storage and excretion of urine. The urethra is connected to the bladder and serves as a channel through which urine is passed from the bladder to the outside of the body.

Voluntary control of urinary excretion is based on learned inhibition of reflex pathways from the walls of the bladder. Release of urine from the bladder occurs under voluntary control of the urethral sphincter (Farley, 1991a).

In males the posterior portion of the urethra is surrounded by the prostate gland, a gland approximately 3.5 cm long by 3 cm wide (about the size of two almonds) (Fig. 7–3). The prostate gland is commonly di-

vided into five lobes. This gland can cause severe urethral obstruction if it enlarges. Prostate carcinoma usually affects the posterior lobe of the gland; the middle and lateral lobes typically are associated with the nonmalignant process called benign prostatic hypertrophy (Swartz, 1989).

Urine Formation

Urine is a complex body fluid that consists of 95 per cent water and approximately 5 per cent solids. It represents many biologic functions and is the end-product of vast numbers of metabolizing cells. There is a great quantity of blood flow through the kidneys, because about 20 per cent to 25 per cent of the blood from each heart beat flows through the kidney (Fischbach, 1992). Blood enters the glomerulus of each nephron through the afferent arteriole. Urine formation begins in the glomerular capillaries, with dissolved substances and fluid passing into the tubular system of

Table 7–1
URINE ANALYSIS (URINALYSIS)

	Test	Normal Result
General Measurements	Color	Yellow-amber
	Turbidity	Clear
	pH	4.6–8.0
	Specific gravity	1.01–1.025
Other Components	Glucose	Negative
	Ketones	Negative
	Blood	Negative
	Protein	Negative
	Bilirubin	Negative
Sediment	RBCs	Negative
	WBCs	Negative
	Casts	Occasional
	Mucous threads	Occasional
	Crystals	Occasional

Normal values are taken from Kee, J.: Laboratory and Diagnostic Tests with Nursing Implications, 3rd ed. Norwalk, Connecticut, Appleton & Lange, 1991.

the nephron. As this "filtrate" (water and dissolved substances) passes along the tubular system, more solutes may be added to the filtrate from the blood in capillaries that surround the tubular system and renal tubular tissue. Some solutes that were originally filtered and some water are then reabsorbed back into the blood from the tubules. This process depends on the needs of the body and the influence of hormones, such as aldosterone and antidiuretic hormone (ADH). For example, ADH increases the permeability of water-absorbing structures, such as tubule and renal duct walls, as part of urine formation. Fluid regulation, sodium regulation, blood chemistry, blood pressure, and nutrient intake also influence the character of urine formation (Guyton, 1992).

Elements of Urine (Table 7–1)

The primary elements contained in large quantities in the urine are urea, creatinine, metabolic acids, and sodium chloride. Many other dissolved substances are also present, and the composition of urine depends mainly on the amount and type of waste material produced by the body. Certain chemical elements of the blood, such as glucose, have a threshold level—a certain level of the substance must be reached in the blood before it is excreted by the kidney into the urine. All substances excreted in the urine are also present in some amount in the blood. By monitoring both urine and blood components of these elements, one can calculate a description of renal function, or "clearance," a valuable indicator of normal or abnormal renal function.

Protein and cellular components of the blood, such as red blood cells (RBCs) and white blood cells (WBCs), should not usually be present in the urine. These cells are typically too large to pass through the glomerular capillary membrane and, if present in the urine, may indicate renal damage or other problems within the urinary tract.

For example, in the condition known as *nephrotic syndrome,* damage to the glomerular basement membrane results in severe loss of protein in the urine. This heavy protein loss causes a decline in the serum albumin level (less than 2.5 g/dl), low

Table 7–2
URINARY TRACT INFECTIONS

Upper Urinary Tract Infection	Lower Urinary Tract Infection
Renal infections, such as pyelonephritis (renal parenchyma, i.e., kidney tissue) Acute or chronic glomerulonephritis (glomeruli) Renal papillary necrosis Renal tuberculosis	Cystitis (bladder infection) Urethritis (urethra infection)

plasma oncotic pressure, and subsequent development of severe peripheral edema (Butera, 1993).

Normal urine does, however, contain small numbers of cells and other components from the entire length of the urinary tract. These elements include casts (substances formed in the renal tubules by precipitation and jelling of urinary mucoproteins), crystals (vary with the pH of urine, but usually normal even in large quantity), and mucus threads (mixture of mucus, pus, and epithelial cells). Along with bacteria, these elements are examined through the use of a microscope (Fischbach, 1992). Abnormalities exist with the presence of certain types of casts (e.g., those formed from the presence of RBCs, WBCs, or protein in the urinary tract) and specific types of crystals (those formed from abnormal body metabolism, such as gout, not just urinary pH-related). Mucus threads in large quantities can indicate urinary tract irritation.

RENAL AND URINARY TRACT PROBLEMS

Pathologic conditions of the upper and lower urinary tracts can be categorized according to primary causative factors. Three general categories—inflammatory/infectious, obstructive, and mechanical (neuromuscular)—are used for discussion and classification of clinical symptoms in this text.

Inflammatory/Infectious Disorders

Inflammatory disorders of the kidney and urinary tract can be caused by bacterial infection, by changes in immune response, and by toxic agents such as drugs and radiation. Common infections of the urinary tract develop in either the upper or lower urinary tract (Table 7–2). Lower urinary tract infections include cystitis (bladder infection) or urethritis (urethra). Symptoms of urinary tract infection (UTI) depend on the location of the infection in either the upper or lower urinary tract (although rarely, infection could occur in both simultaneously).

Disorders of the Upper Urinary Tract

Infections or inflammations of the upper urinary tract (kidney and ureters) are considered to be more serious because these lesions can be a direct threat to renal tissue itself.

Pyelonephritis. Pyelonephritis, or inflammation of the renal parenchyma, is a relatively common renal infection and is associated directly with bacteria that enter through the urethra and ascend through the bladder and ureter to the kidney. It is usually sudden in onset and is associated with chills, fever, and dull pain in the flank over one or both kidneys. Palpation of the kidney elicits pain or tenderness. If the diaphragm is irritated, shoulder pain may

Table 7–3
**CLINICAL SYMPTOMS OF INFECTIOUS/INFLAMMATORY URINARY TRACT
PROBLEMS**

Upper Urinary Tract	Lower Urinary Tract	Renal Impairment
Costovertebral tenderness	Urinary frequency	Decreased urinary output
Flank pain	Urinary urgency	Hypertension
Fever and chills	Dysuria	Dependent edema
Hyperesthesia of dermatomes	Hematuria	Weakness
Hematuria	Pyuria	Anorexia
Pyuria	Bacteriuria	Shortness of breath
Bacteriuria	Low back pain	Mild headache
	Pelvic/lower abdominal pain	Proteinuria
	Dyspareunia	Abnormal blood serum values

occur. In many cases, there are also signs of bladder or urethral infection, such as urgency, burning, and frequency of urination. It is most commonly associated with pregnancy, obstruction, or trauma of the urinary tract and chronic health problems (e.g., diabetes mellitus).

Glomerulonephritis. Glomerulonephritis is an inflammatory problem of the glomeruli of both kidneys. Many causative factors

▼ *Clinical Signs and Symptoms of*
Upper Urinary Tract Infections (Table 7–3)

Symptoms of upper urinary tract infection, particularly renal infection, can be categorized according to urinary tract manifestations or systemic manifestations due to renal impairment. Clinical signs and symptoms of urinary tract involvement can include

- Unilateral costovertebral tenderness
- Flank pain
- Fever and chills
- Skin hypersensitivity
- Hematuria (blood in urine)
- Pyuria (pus in urine)
- Bacteriuria (presence of bacteria in urine)

are related to this disorder, including immunologic reactions, streptococcal infections, vascular injuries, and diabetes mellitus (Farley, 1991b). Glomerulonephritis can be *acute* (occurring 2 to 3 weeks after skin or strep throat infection), with school-aged children at highest risk, or *chronic* (causing slow, progressive destruction of glomeruli with gradual loss of renal function). There may be little or no evidence of renal infection or predisposing infection with chronic glomerulonephritis.

Renal Papillary Necrosis. This condition is characterized by the destruction (necrosis) of tissue in the renal medulla (inner portion of kidney containing collecting structures). It usually affects both kidneys and is associated with various underlying problems, such as pyelonephritis, diabetes mellitus, urinary tract obstruction, sickle cell disease, and analgesic abuse. The cause of this problem is thought to involve an alteration in renal blood flow, which results in ischemia to the renal medullary tissue and subsequent necrosis.

People with renal papillary necrosis become ill rapidly and suddenly and are not likely to seek medical attention from a physical therapist. However, because of its association with other problems such as diabetes, the physical therapist may be treating a client who develops papillary necrosis.

The condition is characterized by high

▼ *Clinical Signs and Symptoms of*
Renal Impairment (see Table 7–3)

- Hypertension
- Decreased urinary output
- Dependent edema
- Weakness
- Anorexia (loss of appetite)
- Dyspnea
- Mild headache
- Proteinuria (protein in urine, urine may be foamy)
- Abnormal blood serum level, such as elevated blood urea nitrogen (BUN) and creatinine

fever, chills, kidney tenderness, severe abdominal tenderness, and rebound abdominal pain (pain felt on release of pressure). The urine contains RBCs, WBCs without bacteria, and occasional fragments of medullary tissue. This sloughing of tissue produces ureteral obstruction and destruction of nephrons, leading to renal failure (LaValle, 1986).

Renal Tuberculosis. This condition is caused by the organism responsible for pulmonary tuberculosis *(Mycobacterium tuberculosis)*. It is a blood-borne infection secondary to an infection in another site (pulmonary tuberculosis). It is most common in men between 20 and 40 years of age. Signs and symptoms are usually mild and include loss of appetite, weight loss, and intermittent fever. RBCs may also be present in the urine; *M. tuberculosis* is present in the urine (Farley, 1991b).

Whether symptoms are systemic or involve the urinary tract, or both, renal and ureteral infections are extremely serious conditions and, if not treated promptly and properly, can result in permanent kidney damage.

Disorders of the Lower Urinary Tract

Both the bladder and urine have a number of defenses against bacterial invasion. These defenses are mechanisms such as voiding, urine acidity, osmolality, and the bladder mucosa itself, which is thought to have antibacterial properties (LaValle, 1986). Urine in the bladder and kidney is normally sterile, but urine itself is a good medium for bacterial growth. Interferences in the defense mechanisms of the bladder, such as the presence of residual or stagnant urine, changes in urinary pH or concentration, or obstruction of urinary excretion, can promote bacterial growth.

Routes of entry of bacteria into the urinary tract can be *ascending* (most commonly up the urethra into the bladder and then into the ureters and kidney), *blood-borne* (bacterial invasion through the bloodstream), or *lymphatic* (bacterial invasion through the lymph system, the least common route).

A lower UTI occurs most commonly in women because of the short female urethra and the proximity of the urethra to the vagina and rectum. The rate of occurrence increases with age and sexual activity. Chronic health problems, such as diabetes mellitus, gout, hypertension, and obstructive urinary tract problems, are also predisposing risk factors for the development of these infections.

Cystitis, or inflammation of the bladder, usually is caused by ascending UTIs. This condition may be acute or chronic. Structural and functional abnormalities of the lower urinary tract, obstruction of urine flow, and impaired bladder innervation all promote this problem.

In addition, there is a type of cystitis that is noninfectious. The disorder of *interstitial cystitis* (IC), also known as painful bladder disease, can be caused by chemical agents, radiation therapy, and possibly autoimmune responses. This disorder is poorly understood from a pathophysiologic standpoint. It occurs primarily in women; the factor that differentiates its symptoms from

▼ *Clinical Signs and Symptoms of*

Cystitis and Urethritis (see Table 7-3)

Lower urinary tract symptoms are directly related to irritation of the bladder and urethra. The intensity of symptoms depends on the severity of the infection. These symptoms include

- Urinary frequency
- Urinary urgency
- Dysuria (discomfort, such as pain or burning during urination)
- Hematuria (presence of RBCs in the urine: may be gross to slight)
- Pyuria (presence of WBCs in the urine)
- Bacteriuria
- Low back pain
- Pelvic/lower abdominal pain
- Pain during intercourse (dyspareunia)

those of bacterial cystitis is that urine is sterile when cultured from a client with IC. The symptoms of abdominal/pelvic pain, urinary urgency and frequency, and nocturia are the same for both infectious and noninfectious cystitis (Matassarin-Jacobs, 1993a).

Urethritis is an inflammation of the urethra that can be due to several different organisms, including those that are sexually transmitted (gonococcus, *Chlamydia trachomatis*). Inflammation of the urethra occurs most commonly along its anterior portion, although posterior and external meatal involvement is possible.

Clients presenting with any of these symptoms should be referred promptly to a physician for further diagnostic work-up and possible treatment. Infections of the lower urinary tract are potentially very dangerous due to the possibility of upward spread and resultant damage to renal tissue. Some people, however, are asymptomatic, and routine urine culture and microscopic examination are the most reliable methods of detection and diagnosis.

Case Example. A 55-year-old woman came to the clinic with back pain associated with paraspinal muscle spasms. Pain was of unknown cause (insidious onset), and the client reported that she was "just getting out of bed" when the pain started. The pain was described as a dull aching that was aggravated by movement and relieved by rest (musculoskeletal pattern). No numbness, tingling, or saddle anesthesia was reported, and the neurologic screening examination was negative. Sacroiliac (SI) testing was negative. Spinal movements were slow and guarded, with muscle spasms noted throughout movement and at rest. Because of her age and the insidious onset of symptoms, further questions were initiated to screen for medical disease.

This client was midmenopausal and taking no estrogen replacement hormones. She had had a bladder infection a month ago that was treated with antibiotics; tests for this were negative when she was evaluated and referred by her physician for back pain. Two weeks ago, she had had an upper respiratory infection (a "cold") and had been "coughing a lot." There was no previous history of cancer.

Local treatment to reduce paraspinal muscle spasms was initiated, but the client did not respond as expected over the course of five treatment sessions. Because of her recent history of upper respiratory and bladder infections, questions related to the presence of constitutional symptoms and changes in bladder function/urine color, force of stream, burning on urination, and so on were repeated. Occasional "sweats" (present sometimes during the day, sometimes at night) was the only red flag present. The combination of recent infection, failure to respond to treatment, and the presence of sweats suggested referral to the physician for early reevaluation.

The client did not return to the clinic for further treatment, and a follow-up telephone call indicated that she did indeed have a recurrent bladder infection that was treated successfully with antibiotics. Her back pain and muscle spasm were eliminated after only 24 hours on a different antibiotic.

Obstructive Disorders

Urinary tract obstruction can occur at any point in the urinary tract and can be the result of *primary* urinary tract obstructions (obstructions occurring within the urinary tract) or *secondary* urinary tract obstructions (obstructions resulting from disease processes outside the urinary tract). A primary obstruction might include problems such as acquired or congenital malformations, strictures, renal or ureteral calculi (stones), polycystic kidney disease, or neoplasms of the urinary tract (e.g., bladder, kidney).

Secondary obstructions produce pressure on the urinary tract from outside and might be related to conditions such as prostatic enlargement (benign or malignant), abdominal aortic aneurysm, gynecologic conditions such as pregnancy, pelvic inflammatory disease, and endometriosis, or neoplasms of the pelvic or abdominal structures.

Obstruction of any portion of the urinary tract results in a backup or collection of urine behind the obstruction. The result is dilatation or stretching of the urinary tract structures that are positioned behind the point of blockage. Muscles near the affected area contract in an attempt to push urine around the obstruction. Pressure accumulates above the point of obstruction and can result eventually in severe dilatation of the renal collecting system (hydronephrosis) and in renal failure. The greater the intensity and duration of the pressure, the greater the destruction of renal tissue.

Because urine flow is decreased with obstruction, urinary stagnation and infection or stone formation can result. Stones are formed because urine stasis permits clumping or precipitation of organic matter and minerals. Lower urinary tract obstruction can also result in constant bladder distention, hypertrophy of bladder muscle fibers, and formation of herniated sacs of bladder mucosa. These herniated sacs result in a large, flaccid bladder that cannot empty completely. In addition, these sacs retain stagnant urine, which causes infection and stone formation.

Disorders of the Upper Urinary Tract

Obstruction of the upper urinary tract may be sudden (acute) or slow in development. Tumors of the kidney or ureters may develop slowly enough that symptoms are totally absent or very mild initially, with eventual progression to pain and signs of impairment. *Acute* ureteral or renal blockage by a stone (calculus consisting of mineral salts), for example, may result in excruciating, spasmodic, and radiating pain accompanied by severe nausea and vomiting.

Calculi form primarily in the kidney. This process is called *nephrolithiasis*. The stones can remain in the kidney (renal pelvis) or travel down the urinary tract and lodge at any point in the tract. The most characteristic symptom of renal or ureteral stones is sudden, sharp, severe pain. If the pain originates deep in the lumbar area and radiates around the side and down toward the testi-

Clinical Signs and Symptoms of
Obstruction of the Upper Urinary Tract

- Pain (depends on the rapidity of onset and on the location)
  - Acute, spasmodic, radiating
  - Mild and dull flank pain
  - Lumbar discomfort with some renal diseases or renal back pain with ureteral obstruction
- Hyperesthesia of dermatomes (T10–L1)
- Nausea and vomiting
- Palpable flank mass
- Hematuria
- Fever and chills
- Abdominal muscle spasms
- Renal impairment indicators (Table 7–4; see also Table 7–3)

Table 7–4
RENAL BLOOD STUDIES*

Test	Normal Result	Renal Impairment
Creatinine	0.6–1.2mg/dl†	Increased
BUN	8.0–25.0 mg/dl	Increased
Uric acid	2.8–7.8 mg/dl	Increased
Potassium	3.5–5.0 mEq/L‡	Increased
Sodium	135–145 mEq/L	Depends on the type of impairment
Calcium	9.0–10.6 mg/dl	Decreased
Phosphorus	2.5–4.5 mg/dl	Increased
RBCs	Male: 4.6–6.0 (ml/mm³)§	Decreased
	Female: 4.0–5.0	
Hematocrit	Male: 40–54%	Decreased
	Female: 36–46%	
Hemoglobin	Male: 13.5–18 g/dl	Decreased
	Female: 12–16 g/dl	

* Normal values are taken from Kee, J.: Laboratory and Diagnostic Tests with Nursing Implications, 3rd ed. Norwalk, Connecticut, Appleton & Lange, 1991.
† mg/dl = milligrams per deciliter.
‡ mEq/L = milliequivalent per liter.
§ ml/mm³ = milliliter per cubic millimeter.
Reference values for laboratory tests vary from one laboratory to another. Always refer to the normal values used in each hospital or laboratory as being the appropriate reference for normal.

cle in the male and the bladder in the female, it is termed *renal colic. Ureteral colic* occurs if the stone becomes trapped in the ureter. Ureteral colic is characterized by radiation of painful symptoms toward the genitalia and thighs (Matassarin-Jacobs, 1993b).

Recent studies have suggested that 10 per cent to 25 per cent of the population may have symptomatic nephrolithiasis. These statistics represent an increase in incidence of this disorder (Fang, 1993).

Renal tumors may also be detected as a flank mass combined with unexplained weight loss, fever, pain, and hematuria. The presence of any amount of blood in the urine is always grounds for referral to a physician for further diagnostic evaluation, because this is a primary symptom of urinary tract neoplasm.

Disorders of the Lower Urinary Tract

Common conditions of obstruction of the lower urinary tract are bladder tumors (bladder cancer is the most common site of urinary tract cancer) and prostatic enlargement, either benign (benign prostatic hypertrophy [BPH]) or malignant (cancer of the prostate). An enlarged prostate gland can occlude the urethra partially or completely.

Benign prostatic hypertrophy is a common complaint in men over 50 years of age. Because of the prostate's position around the urethra, enlargement of the prostate quickly interferes with the normal passage of urine from the bladder. Urination becomes increasingly difficult, and the bladder never feels completely empty. If left untreated, continued enlargement of the prostate eventually obstructs the bladder completely, and emergency measures become necessary to empty the bladder. If the prostate is greatly enlarged, chronic constipation may result. The usual remedy is prostatectomy. Prostatitis is a relatively common inflammation of the prostate and may be acute or chronic (O'Toole, 1992). (See the case study at the end of this chapter.)

Clinical Signs and Symptoms of

Obstruction of the Lower Urinary Tract

Lower urinary tract symptoms of blockage are related most commonly to bladder or urethral pressure. This pressure results in bladder distention and subsequent pain. Common symptoms of lower urinary tract obstruction include

- Bladder palpable above the symphysis pubis
- Suprapubic or pelvic pain
- Difficulty in voiding
- Hesitancy: difficulty in initiating urination or an interrupted flow of urine
- Small amounts of urine with voiding
- Lower abdominal discomfort with a feeling of the need to void
- Nocturia (unusual voiding during the night)
- Hematuria (RBCs in the urine)
- Low back, pelvic, and/or femur pain

Clinical Signs and Symptoms of

Prostatitis

- Sudden moderate-to-high fever
- Chills
- Low back and perineal pain
- Urinary frequency and urgency
- Nocturia
- Dysuria
- General malaise
- Arthralgia
- Myalgia

Cancer of the prostate may occur in men over 50 years of age. It is the third leading cause of death in men in the United States and is the most common cancer among men. Most men with prostate cancer are over the age of 50 years, with risk increasing as age increases. Younger men who are diagnosed with prostate cancer appear to have more aggressive disease and have a higher incidence of metastasis at the time of diagnosis (Matassarin-Jacobs, 1993c). Prostate cancer is often diagnosed when the man seeks medical assistance because of symptoms of urinary obstruction or low back, hip, or leg pain. These symptoms can be caused by metastasis of the cancer to the bones of the pelvis, lumbar spine, or femur.

Mechanical (Neuromuscular) Disorders

Mechanical problems of the urinary tract relate specifically to difficulty with emptying urine from the bladder. Improper emptying of the bladder results in urinary retention and in impairment of voluntary bladder control (incontinence). Several possible causes of mechanical bladder dysfunction include mechanical stress (stress incontinence), spinal cord injury, central nervous system disease (e.g., multiple sclerosis and Guillain-Barré syndrome), UTI, partial urethral obstruction, trauma, and removal of the prostate gland (Farley and Roberts, 1991).

Incontinence (Dunbar, 1991)

To better promote the study and treatment of urinary incontinence, the International Continence Society Standardization Committee established general definitions for four types of incontinence: stress, urge, reflex, and overflow (Bates et al., 1979). Causes of incontinence can range from urologic/gynecologic to neurologic, psychologic, or environmental. Disruptions in the cycle of micturition (urination) may occur for two different physiologic reasons: passive incontinence occurs secondary to muscular weakness of the pelvic floor and sphincters; active incontinence occurs owing to inappropriate bladder contractions known as detrusor malfunction (Willington, 1980). Only stress and urge incontinence are included in this discussion for physical therapists.

Stress incontinence occurs when pressure applied to the bladder from coughing, sneezing, laughing, lifting, exercising, or other physical exertion increases abdominal pressure and when the pelvic floor musculature cannot counteract the urethral/bladder pressure. This type of incontinence causes 75 per cent to 80 per cent of all cases of urinary incontinence in women and is primarily related to urethral sphincter weakness, pelvic floor weakness, and laxity (Burgio et al., 1985; Burgio et al., 1988; Wall and Davidson, 1992). *Urge incontinence* is the involuntary loss of urine associated with a strong desire to void (urgency). The bladder involuntarily contracts or is unstable. Biofeedback testing to assess pelvic floor function and subsequent pelvic floor strengthening has been a successful treatment for stress incontinence for a large number of women (Fall and Lindstrom, 1991; Perry et al., 1988).

NEUROGENIC PROBLEMS CAUSING INCONTINENCE

Other types of bladder problems are neurogenic and may require bladder retraining or artificial drainage, such as urinary catheterization. There are three primary categories of neurogenic bladder dysfunction—flaccid (hypotonic), spastic (hypertonic), and uninhibited (Tanagho and Schmidt, 1992).

Flaccid Bladder. Flaccid bladder can be the consequence of smooth muscle denervation of the bladder wall. This is a lower motor neuron dysfunction of the spinal cord involving the region of the cord where the spinal reflex for micturition is located (parasympathetic nervous system via S2, S3, and S4) (Perkash, 1990). Most spinal cord lesions are both sensory and motor lesions and result in a limp, flaccid bladder with a greatly increased capacity. The person has no urgency to void and must empty the bladder mechanically by using some form of massage or internal pressure, such as the Valsalva or Credé maneuver. This type of bladder dysfunction can result in urinary back-up, ureteral and renal parenchymal dilatation, and eventual impairment.

Spastic Bladder. A spastic bladder preserves reflex bladder activity, but the detrusor muscle contracts with very small amounts of urine present (20 to 50 ml). This is considered to be an upper motor neuron problem, with the presence of a lesion above the spinal reflex centers, and results in urinary incontinence. A high-pressure system occurs because of the continual spastic activity as the bladder and sphincter alternately experience spasms, resulting in a high rate of bladder destruction. This condition of noncongruent bladder/sphincter spasming is known as the *detrusor sphincter dyssynergism*. The spastic bladder can respond to minimal stimuli, such as touching or stroking the genitalia or thighs. UTI causes further, more severe spasm (Perkash, 1990).

Treatment may include the use of anticholinergic drugs to decrease the bladder spasm, intermittent urinary catheterization, and possible surgical destruction of the sphincter muscles (McGuire, 1986).

Uninhibited Bladder. The uninhibited bladder is neither flaccid nor spastic. The client has a lack of control or sensation of bladder activity and becomes incontinent. This problem most commonly originates from a cerebral lesion, such as a stroke, head injury, or impaired cerebral function. Control can sometimes be established through the use of a persistent retraining schedule. However, if loss of control is a result of unconsciousness, treatment may be limited to external or indwelling urinary drainage or use of waterproof or absorbent pads.

Mechanical bladder dysfunctions of any kind predispose the person to various additional urinary tract problems, including infection, obstruction, or kidney damage. Such clients need to be assessed carefully for any symptoms relating to further urinary tract impairment and need immediate medical referral if a problem is suspected.

Renal Failure

A person is unlikely to seek treatment for renal problems from the physical therapist. However, renal patients/clients may receive treatment for primary musculoskeletal lesions in both inpatient and outpatient clinics. An understanding of the basic physiologic problems associated with renal failure (acute or chronic) is necessary to appropriately evaluate the client's complaints and to treat musculoskeletal conditions in these individuals.

Etiologies

Renal failure exists when the kidneys can no longer maintain the homeostatic balances within the body that are necessary for life. Renal failure is classified as acute or chronic in origin and progression.

Acute renal failure refers to the abrupt cessation of kidney activity, usually occurring over a period of hours to a few days. Acute renal failure is often reversible, with return of kidney function in 3 to 12 months (Butera, 1993).

The numerous causes for acute renal failure are organized into three categories depending on the physiologic location of the problem (Ulrich, 1989). *Prerenal causes* include insults that affect blood supply to the kidney, such as hypovolemic shock, severe hypertension, or vascular obstruction.

Renal (intrarenal) causes are specific to the problems that involve direct damage to the kidney tissue itself, such as acute renal infection, chemical and radiation toxicity, or sudden intrarenal vascular lesions. *Postrenal causes* develop from conditions that block or obstruct the normal flow of urine through the urinary tract. These obstructions can occur from the renal pelvis to the urethral meatus. Common causes of obstruction include prostatic enlargement, nephrolithiasis (renal stones), tumors of the urinary tract or surrounding structures, or a neurogenic bladder causing bladder overfill and urinary backup (Butera, 1993; Ulrich, 1989) (see Causes of Urinary Tract Obstruction).

Chronic renal failure, or irreversible renal failure, is defined as a state of progressive reduction of renal functioning resulting in eventual permanent loss of kidney function. It can develop slowly over a period of years or can result from an episode of acute renal failure that does not resolve. Common causes of chronic renal failure (end-stage renal disease) include

- Unresolved acute renal failure
- Genetic disorders (e.g., polycystic kidney disease)
- Vascular disorders (e.g., hypertension)
- Collagen diseases (e.g., systemic lupus erythematosus)
- Diabetes mellitus

Diabetes mellitus and hypertension are the most common causes of chronic renal failure (Butera, 1993).

Clinical Signs and Symptoms

Failure of the filtering and regulating mechanisms of the kidney can be either acute (sudden in onset and potentially reversible) or chronic (called uremia, which develops gradually and is usually irreversible). People with either type of renal failure develop signs and symptoms charac-

CAUSES OF URINARY TRACT OBSTRUCTION

URETHRA AND BLADDER NECK

- Benign prostatic hypertrophy
- Urethral stricture
- Urethral valves
- Meatal stenosis
- Phimosis

BLADDER

- Neurogenic bladder
- Blood clot
- Calculus
- Carcinoma of bladder

URETER

- Intrinsic obstruction (calculus, blood clot, renal papilla, carcinoma of ureter)
- Extrinsic obstruction (retroperitoneal or pelvic tumors, strictures, retroperitoneal fibrosis, uterine prolapse, ureterocele)
- Reflux (vesicoureteral reflux, megaloureter)

URETEROPELVIC JUNCTION

- Intrinsic obstruction (calculus, blood clot, renal papilla)
- Extrinsic obstruction (stricture, aberrant vessels, fibrous band)

RENAL PELVIS

- Calculus
- Blood clot
- Papilla
- Carcinoma of renal pelvis, carcinoma of kidney
- Tuberculosis

From Fang, L.S.T.: Renal diseases. *In* Ramsey, P.G., and Larson, E.B.: Medical Therapeutics. Philadelphia, W.B. Saunders, 1993.

teristic of impaired fluid and waste excretion and altered renal regulation of other body metabolic processes, such as pH regulation, RBC production, and calcium-phosphorus balance.

Blood serum abnormalities typical of the failing kidney include elevated BUN, creatinine, and uric acid levels, elevated phosphorus levels combined with decreased calcium levels (imbalance results in bone deterioration), and decreased bicarbonate levels (imbalance results in metabolic acidosis). Normal blood serum results are shown in Table 7–4.

Urine volume is frequently decreased (oliguria) or is totally absent (anuria). This insufficiency in the excretion of urine causes an accumulation of fluid in both the vascular system and in body tissues, which in turn causes hypertension and edema. Some clients with renal failure have a normal output of urine, but the urine's content of waste product is greatly decreased and it may contain abnormal constituents, such as glucose, protein, and blood cells.

Due to the limited ability of the impaired kidney to produce erythropoietin (a hormone essential for RBC production in the bone marrow), many renal clients are severely anemic. The anemia is usually associated with extreme fatigue and intolerance to even normal daily activities. A pale skin color is also characteristic of the decrease in RBCs.

In addition, the continuous presence of toxic waste products in the bloodstream (urea, creatinine, uric acid) results in damage to many other body systems, including the central nervous system, peripheral nervous system, eyes, GI tract, integumentary system, endocrine system, and cardiopulmonary system (Table 7–5).

Treatment

Treatment of renal failure involves several elements that are designed to replace the lost excretory and metabolic functions of this organ. Treatment options include

- Dialysis (removal of wastes and fluid; and balance of electrolytes through the use of an artificial kidney or the client's peritoneal membrane)
- Diet (restricted in sodium, potassium, fluid, and some protein)
- Drug therapy (used to assist in regulation of lost metabolic processes)
  - Antihypertensives
  - RBC production stimulants, such as testosterone derivatives
  - Vitamin replacements, especially active vitamin D
  - Phosphate binders (usually antacids) used to remove phosphate through the gastrointestinal (GI tract)
- Renal transplantation (completely *replaces* lost functions; clients need immunosuppressants and antirejection drugs for a period of time)

The choice of treatment options, such as dialysis, transplantation, or no treatment, depends on many factors, including the person's age, underlying physical problems, and availability of compatible organs for transplantation. Untreated or chronic renal failure results eventually in death.

RENAL AND UROLOGIC PAIN

Upper Urinary Tract (Renal/Ureteral)

The kidneys and ureters are innervated by both sympathetic and parasympathetic fibers. The kidneys receive sympathetic innervation from the lesser splanchnic nerves through the renal plexus, which is located next to the renal arteries. Renal vasoconstriction and increased renin release are associated with sympathetic stimulation. Parasympathetic innervation is derived from the vagus nerve, and the function of this innervation is not known (Perlmutter and Blacklow, 1983).

Renal sensory innervation is not completely understood even though the cap-

Table 7–5

SYSTEMIC MANIFESTATIONS OF RENAL FAILURE

Systemic Symptoms	Probable Causes
Urinary System	
Decreased urinary output	Damaged renal tissue
Abnormal urinary constituents (blood cells, protein, casts)	
Cardiopulmonary	
Hypertension	Fluid overload
Congestive heart failure	
Pulmonary edema	
Pericarditis	Uremic toxins irritate pericordial sac
Gastrointestinal Tract	
Bleeding	Irritation of gastric mucosa by uremic toxins combined with platelet changes
Nausea and vomiting	
Uremic breath	Uremic toxins change saliva
Anorexia	
Nervous System	
Central (CNS)	
Irritability	Effect of uremic toxins on brain cells (usually resolve with dialysis treatment)
Impaired judgment	
Inability to concentrate	
Seizures	
Lethargy/coma	
Sleep disturbances	
Peripheral (PNS)	
Loss of vibratory sense and deep tendon reflexes	Effect of uremic toxins on peripheral nerves
Impairment of motor nerve conduction velocity	
Burning, tingling, paresthesias	
Tremors	Electrolyte imbalances (calcium, sodium, potassium)
Muscle cramps, muscle twitching	
Foot drop	
Weakness	
Integumentary (Skin)	
Pruritus (itching)/excoriation (scratching)	Skin calcifications related to calcium/phosphorus imbalances
Hyperpigmentation	Retained uremic pigments
Pallor	Anemia
Bruising	Platelet dysfunction
Eyes	
Band keratopathy	Corneal calcifications related to calcium/phosphorus imbalance
Visual blurring	
Red eyes	Conjunctival calcifications related to calcium/phosphorus imbalance
Endocrine	
Fertility and sexual dysfunction	Effect of uremic toxins on menstrual cycles, ovulation, and sperm production
Hyperparathyroidism	Result of calcium/phosphorus imbalance

Table 7–5
SYSTEMIC MANIFESTATIONS OF RENAL FAILURE *Continued*

Systemic Symptoms	Probable Causes
Hematopoietic	
Anemia	Decreased production of erythropoietin by kidney
	Destruction of RBCs by dialysis
Platelet dysfunction	Uremic toxins interfere with platelet aggregation
Skeletal	
Renal osteodystrophy (demineralization of bones)	Related to decreased calcium absorption and resultant calcium/phosphorus imbalance
Joint pain	Joint calcifications

sule (covering of the kidney) and the lower portions of the collecting system seem to cause pain with stretching (distention) or puncture. Information transmitted by renal and ureteral pain receptors is transmitted by sympathetic nerves that enter the spinal cord at T10 to L1 (Richard, 1986).

Because visceral and cutaneous sensory fibers enter the spinal cord in close proximity and actually converge on some of the *same* neurons, when visceral pain fibers are stimulated, concurrent stimulation of cutaneous fibers also occurs. The visceral pain is then felt as though it is skin pain (hyperesthesia), similar to the condition of the alpine skier who stated that "even the skin on my back hurts." Renal and urethral pain can be felt throughout the T10 to L1 dermatomes.

Renal pain (Fig. 7–4) is felt typically in the posterior subcostal and costovertebral regions. To assess the kidney, the test for costovertebral angle tenderness can be included in the objective examination (Fig. 7–5). Ureteral pain is felt in the groin and genital area (Fig. 7–6). With either renal pain or ureteral pain, radiation forward around the flank into the lower abdominal quadrant and abdominal muscle spasm with rebound tenderness can occur on the same side as the source of pain.

The pain can also be generalized throughout the abdomen. Nausea, vomiting, and impaired intestinal motility (progressing to intestinal paralysis) can occur with severe, acute pain (Perlmutter and Blacklow, 1983). Nerve fibers from the renal plexus are also in direct communication with the spermatic plexus, and because of this close relationship, testicular pain may also accompany renal pain (Richard, 1986). Neither renal nor urethral pain is altered by changing body position.

The typical renal pain sensation is aching and dull in nature but can occasionally be a severe, boring type of pain. The constant dull and aching pain usually accompanies distention or stretching of the renal capsule, pelvis, or collecting system. This stretching can result from intrarenal fluid accumulation, such as inflammatory edema, inflamed or bleeding cysts, and bleeding or neoplastic growths. Whenever the renal capsule is punctured, a dull pain can also be felt by the client. Ischemia of renal tissue caused by blockage of blood flow to the kidneys results in a *constant* dull or a *constant* sharp pain.

Pseudorenal pain (McAninch, 1992) may occur secondary to radiculitis or irritation of the costal nerves caused by mechanical derangements of the costovertebral or costotransverse joints. Disorders of this sort

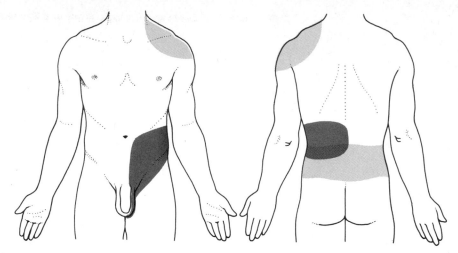

Figure 7–4

Renal pain is felt typically in the posterior subcostal and costovertebral region *(dark red)*. It can radiate across the low back *(light red)* and/or forward around the flank into the lower abdominal quadrant. Ipsilateral testicular pain may also accompany renal pain. Pressure from the kidney on the diaphragm may cause ipsilateral shoulder pain.

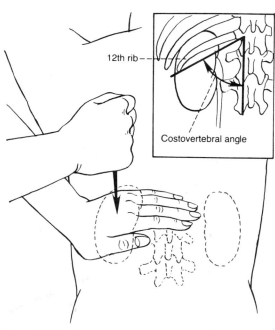

12th rib

Costovertebral angle

Figure 7–5

Costovertebral angle tenderness. Indirect fist percussion causes the tissues to vibrate. To assess the kidney, position the client prone or sitting and place one hand over the rib at the costovertebral angle on the back. Thump that hand with the ulnar edge of your other fist. The person normally feels a thud but no pain. (From Black, J.M., and Matassarin-Jacobs, E. [eds.]: Luckmann and Sorensen's Medical-Surgical Nursing, 4th ed. Philadelphia, W.B. Saunders, 1993.)

are common in the cervical and thoracic areas, but the most common sites are T10 and T12 (Smith and Raney, 1976). Irritation of these nerves causes costovertebral pain that often radiates into the ipsilateral lower abdominal quadrant.

The onset is usually acute with some type of traumatic history, such as lifting a heavy object, sustaining a blow to the costovertebral area, or falling from a height onto the buttocks. The pain is affected by body position, and although the client may be awakened at night when assuming a certain position (e.g., sidelying on the affected side), it is usually absent on awakening and increases gradually during the day. The pain is also aggravated by prolonged periods of sitting, especially when driving on rough roads in the car, and again is relieved by changing to another position.

Radiculitis may mimic ureteral colic or renal pain, but true renal pain is seldom affected by movements of the spine. Exerting pressure over the costovertebral angle (CVA) with the thumb may elicit local tenderness of the involved peripheral nerve at its point of emergence, whereas gentle percussion over the angle may be necessary to elicit renal pain, indicating a deeper, more visceral sensation (Matassarin-

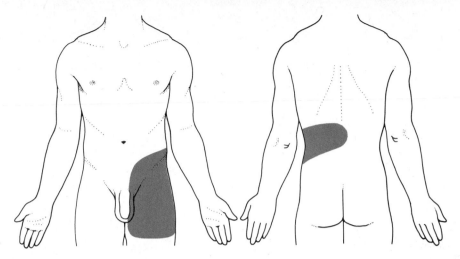

Figure 7–6
Ureteral pain may begin posteriorly in the costovertebral angle and may then radiate anteriorly to the ipsilateral lower abdomen, upper thigh, testes, or labium.

Jacobs, 1993b). Figure 7–5 illustrates percussion over the CVA (Murphy's percussion).

Ureteral obstruction (e.g., from a urinary calculus or "stone" consisting of mineral salts) results in distention of the ureter and causes spasm that produces intermittent or constant severe colicky pain until the stone is passed. Pain of this origin usually starts in the costovertebral angle and radiates to the ipsilateral lower abdomen, upper thigh, testis, or labium (see Fig. 7–6). Movement of a stone down a ureter can cause *renal colic,* an excruciating pain that radiates to the region just described and usually increases in intensity in waves of colic or spasm.

Chronic ureteral pain and renal pain tend to be vague, poorly localized, and easily confused with many other problems of abdominal or pelvic origin. There are also areas of *referred pain* related to renal or ureteral lesions. For example, if the diaphragm becomes irritated owing to pressure from a renal lesion, shoulder pain may be felt. If a lesion of the ureter occurs *outside* the ureter, pain may occur on movement of the adjacent iliopsoas muscle. Abdominal rebound tenderness results when the adjacent peritoneum becomes inflamed (Perlmutter and Blacklow, 1983). Active trigger points along the upper rim of the pubis and the lateral half of the inguinal ligament may lie in the lower internal oblique muscle and possibly in the lower rectus abdominis. These trigger points can cause increased irritation and spasm of the detrusor and urinary sphincter muscles, producing urinary frequency, retention of urine, and groin pain (Travell and Simons, 1983).

Lower Urinary Tract (Bladder/Urethra)

Bladder innervation occurs through sympathetic, parasympathetic, and sensory nerve pathways. Sympathetic bladder innervation assists in the closure of the bladder neck during seminal emission. Afferent sympathetic fibers also assist in providing awareness of bladder distention, pain, and abdominal distention caused by bladder distention. This input reaches the cord at T9 or higher. Parasympathetic bladder innervation is at S2, S3, and S4 and provides motor coordination for the act of voiding.

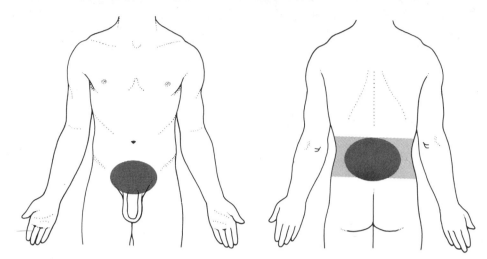

Figure 7-7

Left, Bladder or urethral pain is usually felt suprapubically or ipsilaterally in the lower abdomen. *Right,* Bladder or urethral pain may also be perceived in the low back area (*dark red:* primary pain center; *light red:* referred pain). Low back pain may occur as the first and only symptom associated with bladder/urethral pain, or it may occur along with suprapubic or abdominal pain or both.

Afferent parasympathetic fibers assist in sensation of the desire to void, proprioception (position sensation), and perception of pain (Perlmutter and Blacklow, 1983).

Sensory receptors are present in the mucosa of the bladder and in the muscular bladder walls. These fibers are more plentiful near the bladder neck and the junctional area between the ureters and bladder.

Urethral innervation, also at the S2, S3, and S4 level, occurs through the pudendal nerve. This is a mixed innervation of both sensory and motor nerve fibers. This innervation controls the opening of the external urethral sphincter (motor) and an awareness of the imminence of voiding and heat (thermal) sensation in the urethra (McGuire, 1986).

Bladder or urethral pain is felt above the pubis (suprapubic) or low in the abdomen. The sensation is usually characterized as one of urinary urgency, a sensation to void, and dysuria (painful urination). Irritation of the neck of the bladder or of the urethra can result in a burning sensation localized to these areas, probably owing to the urethral thermal receptors (Fig. 7-7).

Other causes of pain similar to upper or lower urinary tract pain of either an acute or chronic nature may include

- Perforated viscus (any large internal organ)
- Intestinal obstruction
- Cholecystitis (inflammation of the gallbladder)
- Pelvic inflammatory disease
- Tuboovarian abscess
- Ruptured ectopic pregnancy
- Twisted ovarian cyst

Overview RENAL AND UROLOGIC PAIN PATTERNS

KIDNEY (see Fig. 7–4)

Location	Posterior subcostal and costovertebral region
	Usually unilateral
Referral:	Radiates forward, around the flank or the side into the lower abdominal quadrant (T11 to T12)
	Pressure from the kidney on the diaphragm may cause ipsilateral shoulder pain
Description:	Dull aching, boring
Intensity:	Acute: severe, intense
	Chronic: vague and poorly localized
Duration:	Constant
Associated Signs and Symptoms:	Hyperesthesia of associated dermatomes (T9 and T10)
	Ipsilateral or generalized abdominal pain
	Spasm of abdominal muscles
	Nausea and vomiting when severely acute
	Testicular pain may occur in men
	Unrelieved by a change in position

■ ■ ■ ■ ■ ■ ■ ■ ■ ■ ■

URETER* (see Fig. 7–6)

Location:	Costovertebral angle
	Unilateral or bilateral
Referral:	Radiates to the lower abdomen, upper thigh, testis, or labium on the same side (groin and genital area)
Description:	Described as crescendo waves of colic
Intensity:	Excruciating, severe
Duration:	Ureteral pain caused by calculus is intermittent or constant without relief until treated or until the stone is passed
Associated Signs and Symptoms:	Rectal tenesmus (painful spasm of anal sphincter with urgent desire to evacuate the bowel/bladder; involuntary straining with little passage of urine or feces)
	Nausea, abdominal distention, vomiting

*Note: Ureteral pain is usually acute and caused by a calculus (kidney stone). Lesions outside the ureter are usually painless until advanced progression of the disease occurs.

Hyperesthesia of associated dermatomes (T10 and L1)
Tenderness over the kidney or ureter
Unrelieved by a change in position
Movement of iliopsoas may aggravate symptoms associated with a lesion outside the ureter

■ ■ ■ ■ ■ ■ ■ ■ ■ ■ ■ ■

BLADDER/URETHRA (see Fig. 7–7)

Location:	Suprapubic or low abdomen, low back
Referral:	Pelvis
	Can be confused with gas
Description:	Sharp, localized
Intensity:	Moderate to severe
Duration:	Intermittent; may be relieved by emptying the bladder
Associated Signs and Symptoms:	Great urinary urgency
	Tenesmus
	Dysuria
	Hot or burning sensation during urination

DIAGNOSTIC TESTING

Urinalysis

Screening of the composition of the urine is called urinalysis (UA), and UA is the commonly used method of determining various properties of urine. This analysis is actually a series of several tests of urinary components and is a valuable aid in the diagnosis of urinary tract or metabolic disorders. Normal urinary constituents are shown in Table 7–1. A more detailed examination of the chemical, electrolyte, and cellular composition of urine can also be done to assist in the identification of disease processes. Urine cultures are also very important studies in the diagnosis of UTIs.

Blood Studies

A blood sample can be separated (by centrifuge) into two primary constituents: serum (plasma) and cellular elements (RBCs, WBCs, and platelets). Studies of the serum portion of the blood are usually labeled "blood chemistry" or "serum panel" evaluations. These studies measure many of the chemicals that are present in the blood serum. The examination and description of the cellular elements of the blood are called hematology and include counting of various cellular types as well as defining important cellular characteristics (e.g., size, shape, and amount of hemoglobin).

Various blood studies can be done to assess renal function (see Table 7–4). These studies examine both the serum and cellular components of the blood for specific changes characteristic of renal performance. Substances that must be examined in the serum are those that are a *direct* reflection of renal function, such as creatinine, and others that are more *indirect* in renal evaluation, such as BUN, pH-related substances, uric acid, various ions, electrolytes, and cellular components (RBCs).

Creatinine is a byproduct of normal muscle metabolism and is regulated and excreted almost solely by the kidney. Very few factors, other than renal function changes, will affect or influence the presence of creatinine in the blood serum. Creatinine is present in very small amounts in the blood serum and in very large amounts in the urine. It can rise in the serum with only mild renal impairment.

Urea is formed in the liver and consists of the primary nonprotein nitrogenous end-product of dietary protein breakdown in the body. It is excreted in the urine as a waste product. A rise in the BUN level usually indicates an impairment of excretion by the renal tubules, but other metabolic factors, such as shock, dehydration, GI hemorrhage, or excessive protein intake, also can cause an increase in this value. Another component affected by metabolic processes, but reflective of renal function, is *uric acid* (increases also occur in gout, malignancies, starvation, and shock). Substances related to pH, such as bicarbonate, certain ions, and electrolytes, are also measured to assist in the determination of renal performance, but these substances are influenced greatly by other body processes (Richard, 1986). Potassium, a critical ion that is very plentiful within body cells, must be balanced meticulously by the kidney because its accumulation in the bloodstream can result in abnormalities of cardiac muscle contraction and potentially can lead to lethal arrhythmias.

RBCs (erythrocytes) also need to be assessed carefully, because erythropoiesis (RBC production) is influenced greatly by the functioning kidney. The total RBC count and hematocrit (percentage of RBCs per plasma volume) are valuable indicators of the kidney's ability to produce erythropoietin.

PHYSICIAN REFERRAL

Pain related to urinary tract pathology is often similar to pain felt from an injury to the back, flank, abdomen, or upper thigh. Further diagnostic testing and medical examination must be performed by the physician to differentiate urinary tract conditions from musculoskeletal problems. The proximity of the kidneys, ureters, bladder, and urethra to the ribs, vertebrae, diaphragm, and accompanying muscles and tendinous insertions often can make it difficult to identify the client's problems accurately.

The physical therapist must be able to recognize the systemic origin of urinary tract symptoms that mimic musculoskeletal pain. Many conditions that produce urinary tract pain also include an elevation in temperature and abnormal urinary constituents, and also changes in color, odor, or amount of urine. The presence of any amount of blood in the urine always requires a referral to a physician. However, the presence of abnormalities in the urine may not be obvious, and thus a thorough diagnostic analysis of the urine may need to be done. Careful questioning of the client regarding urinary tract history, urinary patterns, urinary characteristics, and pain patterns may elicit valuable information relating to potential urinary tract symptoms.

Referral by a physical therapist to the physician is recommended when the client presents with any combination of systemic signs and symptoms presented in this chapter. Damage to urinary tract structures can occur concurrently with trauma and damage to musculoskeletal structures, which are in the same anatomic location. For example, the alpine skier discussed at the beginning of the chapter had a dull, aching costovertebral pain on the left side, which was unrelieved by a change of position or by ice, heat, or aspirin. His pain is related directly to a traumatic episode, and musculoskeletal injury is a definite possibility in his case. He has no medical history of urinary tract problems and denies any urine changes. Because the pain is constant and is unrelieved by usual measures, and the location of the pain is approximate to the renal structures, a medical follow-up and urinalysis would be recommended.

The physical therapist should review the

signs and symptoms listed in the next section when making a medical referral and also the findings of the objective examination combined with the medical history and present symptomatology.

Systemic Signs and Symptoms Requiring Physician Referral

The physical therapist is advised to question the client further whenever any of the following signs and symptoms are reported or observed because they may indicate systemic disease, and the client should therefore be referred to a physician for further evaluation (see Common Symptoms of Genitourinary Disease).

Abdominal muscle spasms

Anorexia

Anuria (totally absent urine)

Decreased urinary output

Dependent edema

Dyspnea

Dysuria

Fever and chills

Flank pain

Foul odor to urine

Headache

Hematuria (change in color: black, brown, gray, or red)

Hesitancy

Hypertension

Incontinence

Low back and perineal pain

Nausea and vomiting

Proteinuria

Pyuria (cloudy)

Shoulder pain (result of pressure from the kidney on the diaphragm)

Skin hyperesthesia (T10–L1)

Small amounts of urine with voiding

Spasmodic, radiating pain to the testis, labia, thigh, suprapubic or pelvic area

Unilateral costovertebral tenderness

Unusual nocturia

Urinary frequency

Urinary urgency

Weakness

COMMON SYMPTOMS OF GENITOURINARY DISEASE

WOMEN

- Abnormal vaginal bleeding
- Painful menstruation (dysmenorrhea)
- Pelvic masses or lesions
- Vaginal itching or discharge
- Abdominal, low back, or pelvic pain
- Pain during intercourse (dyspareunia)
- Changes in urinary pattern
- Pain with urination
- Changes in menstrual pattern
- Infertility

MEN

- Urinary tract, pelvic, low back, or leg pain
- Painful burning on urination
- Changes in urinary pattern or urine flow
- Red urine
- Discharge
- Penile lesions
- Enlargement of scrotal contents
- Swelling or mass in groin
- Impotence
- Infertility

Adapted from Swartz, M.: Textbook of Physical Diagnosis. Philadelphia, W.B. Saunders, 1989.

 Key Points to Remember

- Renal and urologic pain can be referred to the shoulder or low back.
- Lesions outside the ureter can cause pain on movement of the adjacent iliopsoas muscle.
- Radiculitis can mimic ureteral colic or renal pain, but true renal pain is seldom affected by movements of the spine.

- Low back, pelvic, or femur pain may be the first symptom of prostate cancer.
- Inflammatory pain may be relieved by a change in position. Renal colic remains unchanged by a change in position.
- All the possible pain patterns discussed in this chapter are presented as follows:

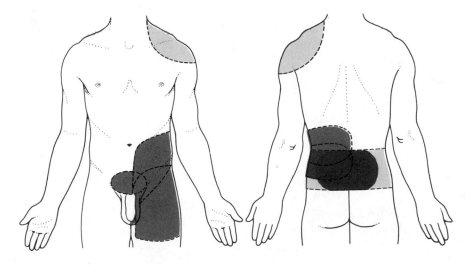

SUBJECTIVE EXAMINATION	*Special Questions to Ask*

Clients may be reluctant to answer the physical therapist's questions concerning bladder and urinary function. The physical therapist is advised to explain the need to rule out possible causes of pain related to the kidneys and bladder and to give the client time to respond if answers seem to be uncertain. For example, the physical therapist may ask the client to observe urinary function over the next 2 days. These questions should be reviewed again at the next appointment.

■ Do you have any problems with your kidneys or bladder? If so, can you describe them?

■ Have you ever had kidney or bladder stones? If so, how were these stones treated?

■ Have you had an injury to your bladder or to your kidneys? If so, how was this injury treated? **(Be aware of unreported domestic abuse/assault.)**

■ Have you had any kidney or bladder infections? How were these infections treated?

  ■ Were they related to any specific circumstances **(e.g., pregnancy, intercourse, after strep throat or strep skin infections)?**

■ Have you ever had surgery on your bladder or kidneys? If so, what kind of surgery and how long ago did it occur?

■ Have you had side (flank) pain **(kidney or ureter)** or pain just above the pubic area **(suprapubic: bladder or urethra)?**

  ■ If so, what relieves this pain?

  ■ Does a change of position affect it? **(Inflammatory pain** may be relieved by a change in position. **Renal colic** remains unchanged by a change in position.)

  ■ **For women:** Have you noticed any unusual vaginal discharge during the time that you had pain just above the pubic area (suprapubic pain)? **(Infection)**

  ■ **For men:** Have you noticed any unusual discharge from your penis during the time you had pain above the pubic area (suprapubic pain)? **(Infection)**

  ■ Have you had any problems with your prostate?

  ■ Have you had any hernias?

■ Have you noticed a change in the amount or number of times that you urinate in the last 2 to 3 weeks? **(Infection)**

■ How much fluid do you usually drink on an average day (excluding alcohol)?

■ When you urinate, do you have trouble starting or continuing the flow of urine? **(Urethral obstruction)**

■ Do you urinate in a steady stream or do you start and stop the flow of urination? **(Urethral obstruction)**

■ Has your urine stream changed in size? If so, please describe. **(Urethral obstruction;** early symptoms of enlarging prostate may be ignored)

- When you are finished urinating, do you feel like your bladder is completely empty? **(Bladder dysfunction)**

- Do you ever have a pain or burning sensation when you urinate? **(Lower urinary tract irritation)**

- Have you ever had or been treated for a venereal disease? (May cause a burning sensation on urination or urgency)

- Have you had a need to urinate during the night that is unusual for you during the last 2 to 3 weeks?

  - Does this happen every night or just when you drink a large amount of fluid before bedtime? **(Diminished bladder capacity, inability to empty the bladder completely)**

- Do you ever have urinary dribbling, leaking, or trouble holding your urine?

  - Do you accidentally leak when you sneeze, laugh, cough, or bear down? **(Stress incontinence;** may be caused by weakness or medications, such as antihistamines, antispasmodics, sedatives, diuretics, and psychotropic drugs)

- Does your urine look brown, red, or black? **(Hematuria** or may be normal with some medications and foods such as beets or rhubarb)

- Is your urine clear? If not, please describe how it looks. How frequently does this happen? (could indicate **upper or lower UTI)**

- Have you noticed a foul or unusual odor coming from your urine? **(Infection, secondary to medication;** may be normal after eating asparagus)

  - **For men:** Have you ever been treated for a prostate problem? If so, how long ago did it occur and what was the treatment?

■ ■ ■ ■ ■ ■   ■ ■ ■ ■ ■   ■

CASE STUDY

REFERRAL

The client is self-referred and states that he has been to your hospital-based outpatient clinic in the past. He has a very extensive chart containing his entire medical history for the last 20 years.

BACKGROUND INFORMATION

He is a 44-year-old man who describes his current occupation as "errand boy/gopher," which requires minimal lifting, bending, or strenuous physical activity. His chief complaint today is pain in the lower back, which comes and goes and seems to be aggravated by sitting. The pain is poorly described, and the client is unable to specify any kind of descriptive words for the type of pain, intensity, or duration.

■ ■ ■ ■ ■ ■ ■ ■ ■ ■ ■

SPECIAL QUESTIONS TO ASK

See Chapter 12 for *Special Questions to Ask* about the back. The client's answer to any questions related to bowel and bladder functions is either "I don't know" or "Well, you know," which makes a complete interview impossible.

SUBJECTIVE/OBJECTIVE FINDINGS

There are radiating symptoms of numbness down the left leg to the foot. The client denies any saddle anesthesia. Deep tendon reflexes are intact bilaterally, and the client stands with an obvious scoliotic list to one side. He is unable to tell you whether his symptoms are relieved or alleviated on performing a lateral shift to correct the curve. There are no other positive neuromuscular findings or associated systemic symptoms.

RESULT

After 3 days of treatment over the course of 1 week, the client has had no subjective improvement in symptoms. Objectively, the scoliotic shift has not changed. A second opinion is sought from two other staff members, and the consensus is to refer the client to his physician. The physician performs a rectal examination and confirms a positive diagnosis of prostatitis based on the results of laboratory tests. These test results were consistent with the client's physical findings and previous history of prostate problems 1 year ago. The client was reluctant to discuss bowel or bladder function with the female therapist but readily suggested to his physician that his current symptoms mimicked an earlier episode of prostatitis.

It is not always possible to elicit thorough responses from clients concerning matters of genitourinary function. If the client hesitates or is unable to answer questions satisfactorily, it may be necessary to present the questions again at a later time (e.g., next treatment session), to ask a colleague of the same sex to confer with the client, or to refer the client to his or her physician for further evaluation. Occasionally, the client will answer negatively to any questions regarding observed changes in urinary function and will then report back at the next session that there was some pathology that was not noted earlier.

In this case, a close review of the extensive medical records may have alerted the physical therapist to the client's previous treatment for the same problem, which he was reluctant to discuss.

References

Bates, P., et al.: The standardization of terminology of lower urinary tract function. Journal of Urology *121*:551–554, 1979.

Burgio, K., Robinson, J., and Engel, B.: The role of biofeedback in Kegel exercise training for stress urinary incontinence. American Journal of Obstetrics and Gynecology *95*:1049–1053, 1988.

Burgio, K.L., Whitehead, W.E., and Engel, B.T.: Urinary incontinence in the elderly. Annals of Internal Medicine *104*:507–515, 1985.

Butera, E.: Nursing care of clients with renal disorders. *In* Black, J.M., and Matassarin-Jacobs, E.: Luckmann and Sorensen's Medical-Surgical Nursing, 4th ed. Philadelphia, W.B. Saunders, 1993, pp. 1487–1542.

Dunbar, A.: The Silent Problem: Taking the Patient History One Step Further. Journal of Obstetric and Gynecologic Physical Therapy *15*(2):4–5, 1991.

Fall, M., and Lindstrom, I.: Electrical stimulation: A physiologic approach to the treatment of urinary incontinence. Urologic Clinics of North America 18(2):393–407, 1991.

Fang, L.S.: Renal diseases. In Ramsey, P.G., and Larson, E.B. (eds.): Medical Therapeutics, 2nd ed. Philadelphia, W.B. Saunders, 1993, pp. 192–237.

Farley, F.: Assessment of urinary function. In Phipps, W., Long, B., Woods, N., and Cassmeyer, V. (eds.): Medical-Surgical Nursing: Concepts and Clinical Practice, 4th ed. St. Louis, C.V. Mosby, 1991a, pp. 1385–1402.

Farley, F.: Management of persons with urinary tract problems. In Phipps, W., Long, B., Woods, N., and Cassmeyer, V. (eds.): Medical-Surgical Nursing: Concepts and Clinical Practice, 4th ed. St. Louis, C.V. Mosby, 1991b, pp. 1403–1440.

Farley, F., and Roberts, R.: Common interventions for urinary problems. In Phipps, W., Long, B., Woods, N., and Cassmeyer, V. (eds.): Medical-Surgical Nursing: Concepts and Clinical Practice, 4th ed. St. Louis, C.V. Mosby, 1991, pp. 1441–1460.

Fischbach, F.: A Manual of Laboratory and Diagnostic Tests, 4th ed. Philadelphia, J.B. Lippincott, 1992.

Guyton, A.: Human Physiology and Mechanisms of Disease, 8th ed. Philadelphia, W.B. Saunders, 1992.

LaValle, S.: Infections and obstructive diseases of the kidney. In Richard, C. (ed.): Comprehensive Nephrology Nursing. Boston, Little, Brown, 1986, pp. 86–97.

Linker, C.A.: Blood. In Tierney, L.M., McPhee, S.J., Papadakis, M.A., Schroeder, S.A. (eds.): Current Medical Diagnosis and Treatment. Norwalk, Connecticut, Appleton and Lange, 1993, pp. 399–450.

Matassarin-Jacobs, E.: Nursing care of clients with disorders of the ureters, bladder and urethra. In Black, J.M., and Matassarin-Jacobs, E. (eds.): Luckmann and Sorensen's Medical-Surgical Nursing, 4th ed. Philadelphia, W.B. Saunders, 1993a, pp. 1443–1486.

Matassarin-Jacobs, E.: Assessment of clients with urinary disorders. In Black, J.M., and Matassarin-Jacobs, E. (eds.): Luckmann and Sorensen's Medical-Surgical Nursing, 4th ed. Philadelphia, W.B. Saunders, 1993b, pp. 1419–1442.

Matassarin-Jacobs, E.: Nursing care of men with reproductive urinary disorders. In Black, J.M., and Matassarin-Jacobs, E. (eds.): Luckmann and Sorensen's Medical-Surgical Nursing, 4th ed. Philadelphia, W.B. Saunders, 1993c, pp. 2087–2118.

McAninch, J.W. (ed.): Symptoms of disorders of the genitourinary tract. In General Urology, 13th ed. Los Altos, California, Lange Medical Publications, 1992, pp. 30–39.

McGuire, E.: Neuromuscular dysfunction of the lower urinary tract. In Walsh, P., Perlmutter, A., Gittes, T., and Stamey, T. (eds.): Campbell's Urology, 5th ed. Philadelphia, W.B. Saunders, 1986, pp. 616–638.

O'Toole, M. (ed.): Miller-Keane Encyclopedia and Dictionary of Medicine, Nursing and Allied Health, 5th ed. Philadelphia, W.B. Saunders, 1992.

Perkash, I.: Management of neurogenic dysfunction of the bladder and bowel. In Kottke, F.I., Stillwell, K., and Lehmann, J. (eds.): Krusen's Handbook of Physical Medicine and Rehabilitation, 4th ed. Philadelphia, W.B. Saunders, 1990, pp. 724–745.

Perlmutter, A., and Blacklow, R.: Urinary tract pain, hematuria and pyuria. In Blacklow, R.S. (ed.): MacBryde's Signs and Symptoms. Philadelphia, J.B. Lippincott, 1983, pp. 181–192.

Perry, J.D., Hullett, L.T., Bollinger, J.R.: EMG feedback: Treatment of incontinence (abstract). Paper presented at meeting of Biofeedback Society of America, Colorado Springs, Colorado, March 26, 1988.

Richard, C.: Renal assessment with nursing implications. In Richard, C. (ed.): Comprehensive Nephrology Nursing. Boston, Little, Brown, 1986.

Smith, D.R., and Raney, F.L., Jr.: Radiculitis distress as a mimic of renal pain. Journal of Urology 116:269, 1976.

Swartz, M.H.: Textbook of Physical Diagnosis. Philadelphia, W.B. Saunders, 1989.

Tanagho, E., and Schmidt, R.A.: Neuropathic bladder disorders. In Tanagho, E.A., and McAninch, J.W. (eds.): General Urology, 13th ed. Los Altos, California, Lange Medical Publications, 1992, pp. 454–472.

Travell, J.G., and Simons, D.G.: Myofascial pain and dysfunction. In The Trigger Point Manual. Baltimore, Williams & Wilkins, 1983.

Ulrich, B.: Nephrology Nursing; Concepts and Strategies. Norwalk, Connecticut, Appleton and Lange, 1989.

Wall, L.L., and Davidson, T.G.: The role of muscular re-education by physical therapy in the treatment of genuine stress urinary incontinence. Obstetrical and Gynecological Survey 47(5):322–331, 1992.

Willington, F.: Incontinence: A practical approach. Geriatrics 35:41–48, 1980.

8

Overview of Hepatic and Biliary Signs and Symptoms

According to the American Liver Foundation, 27,000 Americans die each year from one of more than 100 varieties of liver and/or biliary tract diseases. Medical understanding of these diseases has increased in the last decade owing to the advances in diagnostic techniques, including ultrasonography and computed tomography (CT). The increased knowledge in the field of viral hepatitis and advances made in the basic sciences that pertain to liver structure and function have also contributed to a better understanding of the pathogenesis and, therefore, treatment of liver diseases.

As with many of the organ systems in the human body, the hepatic and biliary organs (liver, gallbladder, and common bile duct) can develop diseases that mimic primary musculoskeletal lesions. The musculoskeletal symptoms associated with hepatic and biliary pathology are generally confined to the midback, scapular, and right shoulder regions. These musculoskeletal symptoms can occur alone (as the only presenting symptom) or in combination with other systemic signs and symptoms discussed in this chapter.

HEPATIC AND BILIARY PHYSIOLOGY

Liver

Structure

The liver is the largest internal organ in the human body, averaging 2.5 per cent of the body weight in a normal adult and weighing slightly more than 3 pounds (1200 to 1600 g).

Located above the right kidney, stomach, pancreas, and intestines and immediately below the diaphragm, the liver divides into a left and a right lobe (the right lobe is six times larger than the left); these lobes are separated by the falciform ligament. Glisson's capsule, a network of connective tissue, covers the entire organ and extends into the parenchyma along blood vessels and bile ducts (Fig. 8–1).

Within the parenchyma, cylindrical lobules are the basic functional units of the liver, consisting of cellular plates that radi-ate from a central vein, like spokes in a wheel (Fig. 8–2). Small bile canaliculi (extremely narrow tubular passages or channels) fit between the cells in the plates and empty into terminal bile ducts. These ducts join two larger ones, which merge into a single hepatic duct after leaving the liver. The hepatic duct then joins the cystic duct to form the common bile duct (see Fig. 8–1).

The liver receives blood from two major sources: the hepatic artery and the portal vein (see Fig. 8–2). These two vessels carry approximately 1500 ml/min of blood to the liver, almost 75 per cent of which is supplied by the portal vein. Sinusoids (offshoots of both the hepatic artery and the portal vein) run between each row of hepatic cells. Phagocytic Kupffer's cells (Fig. 8–3), part of the reticuloendothelial system, line the sinusoids, destroying old or defective red blood cells (RBCs) and detoxifying harmful substances, such as metabolizing and inactivating many drugs. The liver has a large lymphatic supply, and

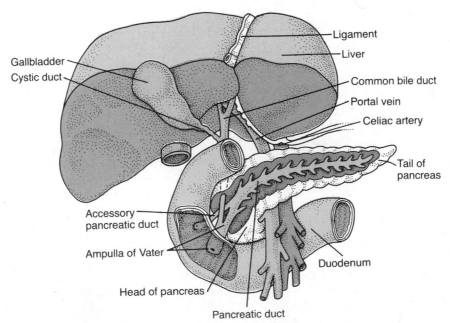

Figure 8–1.
Anatomy of the liver, gallbladder, common bile duct, and pancreas.

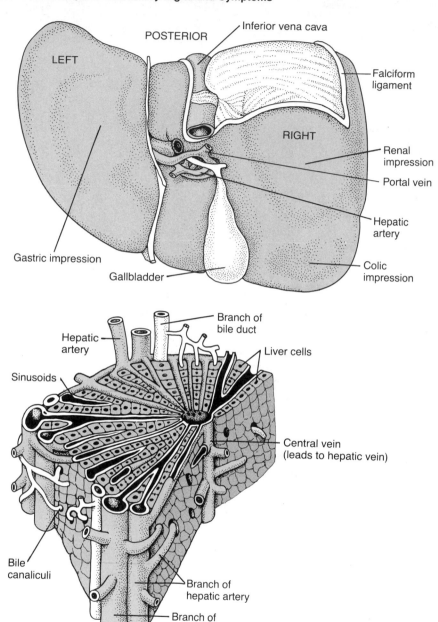

Figure 8–2

The liver receives blood from the hepatic artery and the portal vein. Most of the blood supply arriving in the portal vein has already passed through the intestine. The cylindrical plates radiating from the central vein are visualized. (Modified from Jackson, G.: Digestion: Fueling the system. New York, Torstar Books, 1984, p. 101).

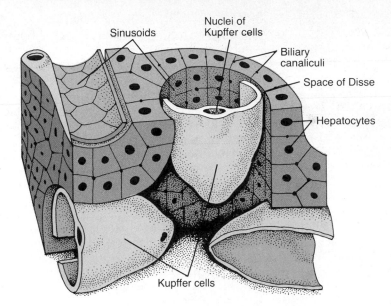

Sinusoids

Nuclei of
Kupffer cells

Biliary
canaliculi

Space of Disse

Hepatocytes

Kupffer cells

Figure 8–3
Kupffer cells lining the hepatic sinusoid.

consequently, cancer frequently metastasizes to the liver (Wilson and Lester, 1992).

Functions

The liver performs more than 500 separate functions, including the formation and secretion of bile; detoxification of harmful substances; production of clotting factors; storage of vitamins; and metabolism of carbohydrates, fats, and proteins. The liver has a large reserve capacity. As little as 10 per cent to 20 per cent of functioning liver tissue is required to maintain life (Wilson and Lester, 1992).

Bilirubin Metabolism. One of the liver's most important functions is to convert bilirubin into bile. Bilirubin (red bile pigment) is the end-product of RBCs (heme) and comes from hemoglobin, myoglobin, and respiratory enzymes. When hemoglobin (an oxygen-carrying blood protein) breaks down, it produces a compound called biliverdin. This substance then converts to bilirubin, which is taken up by the liver and excreted into bile. Six grams of hemoglobin are broken down daily, forming 250

to 350 mg of bilirubin. However, if the amount of hemoglobin being broken down increases significantly, such as occurs in hemolytic blood diseases (diseases that cause increased destruction of red blood cells), excess bilirubin production and resulting jaundice (yellow skin and yellow mucous membranes) occur. Because the normal liver has the capacity to excrete two to three times the normal amount of bilirubin without difficulty, jaundice may not occur until the bilirubin levels are severely elevated.

Eighty per cent of this bilirubin metabolism takes place in the reticuloendothelial cells* in the liver and spleen. Twenty per cent of this process occurs within RBCs in the spleen and bone marrow. Microsomal heme oxygenase, an enzyme, actually converts the heme to bilirubin. The bilirubin is then transported in the plasma tightly bound to albumin, a transport protein that carries large organic anions, such as fatty acids, bilirubin, hormones such as cortisol

---

* The reticuloendothelial cells are a system of macrophages within the network of cells in the liver and spleen.

and thyroxine, and many drugs and antibiotics. The bilirubin must compete with these other substances for albumin (Guyton, 1992).

During the albumin-bound transport time, the bilirubin is not water soluble and is called *unconjugated bilirubin*. The subsequent excretion of bilirubin depends on its transfer from the blood plasma to the liver cell, its conjugation (joining) to the acid glucuronide, and its secretion into the bile channels as water-soluble conjugated bilirubin. After being secreted into the bile channels, the conjugated bilirubin is then secreted into the duodenum. In the gastrointestinal tract, the conjugated bilirubin is then metabolized to urobilinogen, which is excreted in the feces or is reabsorbed. Reabsorbed urobilinogen is either recycled by the liver and re-excreted in bile or excreted in the urine (Strasburg and Matassarin-Jacobs, 1993).

Bilirubin is readily bound to elastic tissue (skin, blood vessels, sclerae, synovium), which in turn becomes easily icteric (jaundiced or yellow).

Gallbladder

Structure

The gallbladder is a pear-shaped organ that lies in the fossa on the underside of the liver (see Fig. 8–2) and is capable of holding approximately 50 ml (2 oz) of bile.

Attached to the liver above, to the peritoneum, and to blood vessels, the gallbladder is divided into four parts: the fundus (broad inferior end), the body (funnel-shaped and bound to the duodenum), the neck (which empties into the cystic duct), and the infundibulum (which lies between the body and the neck and sags to form Hartmann's pouch) (Fig. 8–4).

The hepatic artery supplies both the cystic and hepatic ducts with blood; the blood then drains out of the gallbladder through the cystic vein. Lymph vessels in the submucosal layer also drain the gallbladder and the head of the pancreas.

Functions

The principal function of the gallbladder is the concentration and storage of bile, which it receives continuously from the liver (Wilson and Lester, 1992). The biliary duct system provides a passage for bile from the liver to the intestine and regulates the bile flow. The gallbladder collects, concentrates, and stores bile. In the normally functioning gallbladder, the lymphatic vessels and blood vessels absorb water and inorganic salts, so that gallbladder bile is about ten times as concentrated as bile formed in the liver (Wilson and Lester, 1992).

After the ingestion of fats, the gallbladder empties its contents into the common bile duct, which leads into the duodenum by contraction of the gallbladder muscle coat and relaxation of the sphincter of Oddi (muscle fibers that surround the common bile duct and pancreatic duct as they open into the duodenum).

Bile helps digestion by alkalinizing the intestinal contents and plays a role in the emulsification, absorption, and digestion of fat. Its chief constituents are conjugated bile salts, cholesterol, phospholipid, bilirubin, and electrolytes. The bile salts emulsify fats by breaking large fat globules into smaller ones so that they can be acted on by the fat-splitting enzymes of the intestine and pancreas. A healthy liver produces bile according to the body's needs and does not require stimulation by drugs. Infection or disease of the liver, inflammation of the gallbladder, or any obstruction such as gallstones can interfere with the flow of bile into the duodenum (O'Toole, 1992).

Abnormal composition or function of bile can occur in gallbladder and liver diseases, affecting the digestion and absorption of fats. The client often has an intolerance to fatty foods, anorexia, nausea, vomiting,

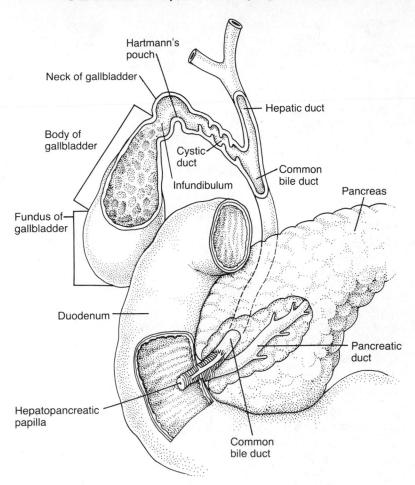

Figure 8-4

The gallbladder and its divisions: fundus, body, infundibulum, and neck. Obstruction of either the hepatic or common bile duct by stone or spasm blocks the exit of bile from the liver, where it is formed, and prevents bile from ejecting into the duodenum.

flatulence (excess gas in the stomach or intestines), and diarrhea or constipation (Elrod, 1992).

HEPATIC AND BILIARY PATHOPHYSIOLOGY

The major causes of acute hepatocellular injury include viral hepatitis, drug-induced hepatitis, and ingestion of toxins (Carithers, 1993). Taking a careful history and making close observations of the client's physical condition and appearance can detect telltale signs of hepatic disease.

Referred Shoulder Pain

Referred shoulder pain may be the only presenting symptom of hepatic or biliary disease. Sympathetic fibers from the biliary system are connected through the celiac and splanchnic plexuses to the hepatic fibers in the region of the dorsal spine. These connections account for the intercostal and radiating interscapular pain that accompanies gallbladder disease (Fig. 8-5). Although the innervation is bilateral, most of the biliary fibers reach the cord through the right splanchnic nerves, producing pain in the right shoulder (Ridge and Way, 1993).

▼ *Clinical Signs and Symptoms of*

Liver Disease (Wilson and Lester, 1992)

- Sense of fullness of the abdomen
- Anorexia, nausea, and vomiting
- Jaundice (a result of increased serum bilirubin levels)
- Ascites (abnormal accumulation of serous fluid in the peritoneal cavity)
- Edema and oliguria (reduced urine secretion in relation to fluid intake)
- Right upper quadrant (RUQ) abdominal pain
- Right shoulder pain
- Neurologic symptoms
  - Confusion
  - Muscle tremors
  - Asterixis (motor disturbance resembling body or extremity flapping)*
- Pallor (often linked to cirrhosis or carcinoma)
- Bleeding disorders
  - Purpura (blood under the skin and through the mucous membranes that appears deep red or purple)
  - Ecchymosis (bruises)
- Spider angiomas (branched dilatation of the superficial capillaries resembling a spider)†
- Palmar erythema (redness of the skin over the palms)
- Light-colored or clay-colored feces
- Gynecomastia (enlargement of breast tissue in men)

---

* To test for asterixis (flapping tremor called liver flap), ask the client to dorsiflex the hand with the rest of the arm resting on the bed (supported). Watch for quick, irregular extensions and flexions of the wrist and fingers.

† Both spider angiomas and palmar erythema occur as a result of increased estrogen levels normally detoxified by the liver.

▼ *Clinical Signs and Symptoms of*

Gallbladder Disease

- Right upper abdominal and epigastric pain
- Jaundice (result of blockage of the common bile duct)
- Fever, chills
- Indigestion
- Nausea
- Intolerance of fatty foods
- Sudden, excruciating pain in the midepigastrium with referral to the back and right shoulder (acute cholecystitis)

Diagnosis of liver or gallbladder disease is made by x-ray or ultrasonic scan of the gallbladder and CT scan of the abdomen, including the liver. Gallstones (choleliths) located in the gallbladder or in the bile ducts consist of cholesterol crystals, fragments of bacteria,* and calcium and can be related to an increased serum cholesterol and high dietary fat intake. Inflammatory debris can also form a point of origin for stone growth. Laboratory tests useful in the diagnosis and treatment of liver and biliary tract disease are listed in Table 8–1.

Jaundice (O'Toole, 1992)

Jaundice (icterus) is not a disease. It is a symptom of a number of different diseases and disorders of the liver and gallbladder that causes yellowness of skin, sclerae, mucous membranes, and excretions. The change in color is due to staining by the bile pigment bilirubin (hyperbilirubinemia). Normally, the liver cells absorb the biliru-

---

* *Escherichia coli (E. coli),* a bacterium found in the large intestine, increases the amount of bilirubin available for pigment stones (Kallsen, 1993).

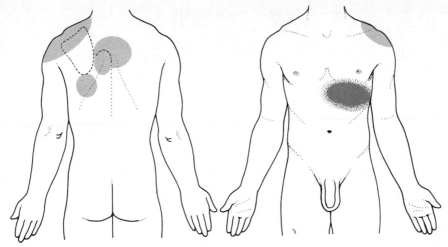

Figure 8–5

Pain from the liver, gallbladder, and common bile duct *(dark red)* occur typically in the midepigastrium or right upper quadrant of the abdomen, with referred pain *(light red)* to the right shoulder, interscapular, or subscapular area.

Table 8–1

LABORATORY TESTS FOR LIVER AND BILIARY TRACT DISEASE

Serum Bilirubin	
Direct (conjugated)	0.1–0.3 mg/dl
Indirect (unconjugated)	0.2–0.8 mg/dl
Total amount	0.1–1.0 mg/dl
Urine Bilirubin	0
Serum Cholesterol	150–250 mg/dl; elevated when its excretion is blocked by bile duct obstruction; reduced when severe liver damage prevents its synthesis
Total Protein	6–8 g/dl; decreased when liver is damaged—synthesis is impaired
Serum Albumin	3.5–5.5 g/dl; decreased in liver damage
Blood Ammonia	<75 μg/dl; increased in severe liver damage; liver unable to break down ammonia
Serum Enzymes	
AST (aspartate aminotransferase)	5–40 U/L; increased in liver damage; released by liver when damage occurs to liver cells
ALT (alanine aminotransferase)	5–35 U/L (same as above)
LDH (lactic dehydrogenase)	45–90 U/L (same as above)
GGTP (gamma glutamyl transpeptidase)	<65 U/L; elevated with significant liver disorder
Alkaline phosphatase	30–85 U/L; increased in biliary obstruction
Cancer-Associated Antigen	
AFP (alpha-fetoprotein)	<10 ng/dl; made by fetus but not by healthy adult; value >1000 ng/mg indicates likely hepatocellular carcinoma
Coagulation Functions	
Prothrombin time (PT)	12–15 seconds; prolonged with liver damage
Platelets	150,000–400,000/mm^3; may drop when spleen is enlarged from portal hypertension

bin and secrete it along with other bile constituents. If the liver is diseased, if the flow of bile is obstructed, or if destruction of erythrocytes is excessive, the bilirubin accumulates in the blood and eventually produces jaundice.

In some situations jaundice may be the first and only manifestation of disease. Jaundice is usually first noticeable in the eyes when the concentration of serum bilirubin exceeds 2 mg/dl (N = 0.1 to 1 mg/dl), although it may come on so gradually that it is not immediately noticed by those in daily contact with the jaundiced person.

Dark urine and light stools associated with jaundice occur when the bilirubin level increases from normal to a value of 2 or 3 mg/dl. When bilirubin reaches this level, the sclera of the eye takes on a yellow hue. When the bilirubin level reaches 5 to 6 mg/dl, the skin becomes yellow. The liver's function to metabolize bilirubin from the blood is impaired by any damage to the liver. Impairment of liver function caused by cirrhosis (chronic disease of the liver), liver cancer, or infection/inflammation of the liver results in jaundice. Normally, bile causes the stool to assume a brown color. Light-colored (almost white) stools and urine the color of tea or cola indicate an inability of the liver or biliary system to excrete bilirubin properly. These changes in urine, stool, or skin color may be caused by hepatitis, gallstones, or pancreatic cancer blocking the bile duct, cirrhosis, or hepatotoxic medications.

Causes

Jaundice may be caused by a wide range of disorders that result in the excessive accumulation of bilirubin in the blood serum. The causes of jaundice are numerous and are classified according to the location of the pathologic events that cause its development.

Classifications (Matassarin-Jacobs and Strasburg, 1993)

Prehepatic. In the prehepatic state, bilirubin increases *before it reaches the liver* as a result of its overproduction, usually secondary to hemolysis (destruction) of red blood cells. Causes of prehepatic jaundice can include

- Hemolytic blood transfusion reaction
- Blood incompatibility between mother and infant
- Autoimmune hemolytic anemias

Hepatic. The hepatic state of jaundice results in a bilirubin increase because of pathology *within the liver itself,* causing an inability to excrete bilirubin adequately. Causes of hepatic jaundice can include

- Hepatocellular diseases (e.g., viral or drug/alcohol-induced hepatitis)
- Metabolic and infiltrative disorders (e.g., anorexia or metastatic tumors)
- Immaturity of the liver conjugating system (e.g., physiologic jaundice of the newborn)
- Disorders of the intrahepatic biliary system (e.g., primary biliary cirrhosis)

Posthepatic. Posthepatic jaundice occurs when bilirubin increases because of a problem occurring after the bilirubin *leaves the liver.* This may occur owing to large bile duct obstructions, which can include

- Bile duct strictures
- Gallstones
- Pancreatic stones
- Pancreatitis
- Tumors that affect the ducts themselves or important adjacent structures

Conjugated or Unconjugated. In addition, jaundice can also be categorized according to whether the bilirubin is primarily conjugated or unconjugated. Those pathologies that develop owing to excessive bilirubin or to defective conjugation of bilirubin in the liver result in *unconjugated hyperbilirubinemia*. The pathologies related to improper excretion of bilirubin from the liver or to obstructed flow of bile from outside the liver result in *conjugated hyperbilirubinemia*. Thus, a logical first step in the physician's diagnosis of a jaundiced client is to determine whether the bilirubin is predominantly conjugated or unconjugated. This determination can be done by both urine and blood serum testing (Wilson and Lester, 1992). It is interesting to note that there are situations in which more than one mechanism may be responsible for jaundice in the same person.

Clinical History and Observations

A careful history and close observation of the client are important in determining whether a person may need a medical referral for possible jaundice. Jaundice in the postoperative client is not uncommon but may be a potentially serious complication of surgery and anesthesia. Clinical management of jaundice is complicated by anything capable of damaging the liver, including stress, hypoxemia, blood loss, infection, and administration of multiple drugs. The following factors are considered when evaluating the clinical history and observations (Sherlock and Dooley, 1993):

- *Occupation:* employment involving alcohol consumption; contact with rats carrying Weil's disease (a type of Mediterranean jaundice)
- *Place of origin:* Mediterranean, Africa, Far East (may suggest carriage of hepatitis B antigen)
- *Personal/family history:* history of jaundice, hepatitis, anemia, splenectomy, cholecystectomy
- *Contact with jaundiced persons:* dialysis patients, drug abusers, homosexuals, prostitutes

- *Injections* within the last 6 months: blood tests, drug abuse, tuberculosis testing, dental treatment, tattoo (receiving or removal), blood or plasma transfusion
- *Consumption of shellfish*
- *Previous travel* to areas where hepatitis is endemic (present in a community at all times)
- *Onset* is important in determining the type:
  Viral hepatitis
    Nausea
    Anorexia
    Aversion to smoking in smokers
    Sudden onset (develops in a matter of hours)
  Cholestatic hepatitis
    Slow onset
    Persistent pruritus (itching)
    Dark urine and light stools preceding illness
- *Age and sex:*
  Incidence of type A hepatitis decreases with age (most commonly seen in children)
  No age is exempt from hepatitis B and hepatitis C
  Probability of occurrence of cancerous biliary obstruction increases with age
- *Skin color:*
  Mild yellow—hemolytic jaundice (rupture of RBCs with the release of hemoglobin into the blood plasma)
  Orange—hepatocellular jaundice (involving liver directly)
  Green hue—Prolonged biliary obstruction
- *Mental state:* hepatocellular jaundice
  Slight intellectual deterioration
  Mild personality change
  Flapping tremor (liver flap) may indicate developing hepatic coma

Treatment

The goal of treatment for jaundice is to resolve the underlying disease (e.g., hemolytic anemia). Rest and time are the major components of treatment of jaundice caused by hepatitis. Surgical exploration and removal of biliary obstructions and carcinomas are the primary surgical interventions related to treatment for posthepatic (obstructive) jaundice (Matassarin-Jacobs and Strasburg, 1993). Anyone with jaundice has a significant liver, biliary, or hematologic problem. If a client presents with jaundice, he or she needs immediate referral to a physician. Active, intense exercise should be avoided when the liver is compromised (i.e., during jaundice or any other active disease), because the cornerstone of treatment and promotion of healing of the liver is rest.

Physiologic Jaundice of the Newborn

A mild, unconjugated hyperbilirubinemia that can develop between the second and fifth neonatal days is called *physiologic jaundice of the newborn.* This results from immaturity of bilirubin conjugation enzymes. The unconjugated bilirubin cannot be excreted into the intestine, and build-up of bilirubin in the bloodstream causes the characteristic yellow skin of jaundice. This is especially true with premature infants, who have an even less developed liver. The maximal serum bilirubin concentration (less than 13 mg/dl) occurs at 3 to 4 days of age, at which time a mild condition of jaundice may occur in approximately 50 per cent of all healthy full-term neonates. The incidence of jaundice is usually much higher with premature neonates.

Treatment. The activity of the needed enzyme normally increases within 2 weeks after birth, and the jaundice resolves spontaneously and without treatment (Wilson and Lester, 1992). However, if serum bilirubin levels increase to greater than 13 mg/dl, phototherapy is initiated to prevent neurologic damage associated with high bilirubin levels. Phototherapy, or the exposure to prolonged irradiation with visible blue light, modifies bilirubin into a water-soluble form that helps the reabsorption process and facilitates excretion of bilirubin (Andrews and Huether, 1990).

Kernicterus

Kernicterus (bilirubin encephalopathy) is a *severe* condition of unconjugated hyperbilirubinemia in the newborn. Bilirubin levels exceed 13 mg/dl and often exceed 20 mg/dl. Kernicterus results from the deposition of unconjugated bilirubin in the basal ganglia of the brain. If it is untreated, serious neurologic damage or death can occur (Andrews and Huether, 1990).

Factors that can precipitate this severe form of hyperbilirubinemia include the usual cause of physiologic jaundice on which is superimposed other conditions that increase the unconjugated bilirubin level, such as accelerated RBC breakdown (Wilson and Lester, 1992). One cause of an acceleration in RBC breakdown is blood group incompatibility between mother and fetus. For example, if the mother has A+ blood type and the neonate has O+, the neonate carries the mother's antibodies to the neonate's O+ blood. These antibodies break down the neonate's RBCs (hemolysis), releasing into the blood large amounts of bilirubin that the immature liver of the neonate cannot handle.

Another well-documented cause of increases in unconjugated bilirubin in infants is the use of oxytocin (Pitocin) during labor and delivery. It is generally accepted that the use of oxytocin approximately doubles the incidence of neonatal hyperbilirubinemia and increases its severity in a dose-related manner. Studies have shown that infants born after oxytocin-induced labor exhibit enhanced osmotic fragility of RBCs (Singh and Singh, 1979). The antidiuretic effects of oxytocin, along with the large amounts of the electrolyte-free dextrose solutions used to administer it, cause osmotic swelling of RBCs and thus more rapid destruction of the cells, with resultant hyperbilirubinemia (Buchan, 1979).

Treatment. Treatment of kernicterus includes phototherapy for levels of bilirubin greater than 13 mg/dl and exchange transfusion (mechanical removal of the baby's blood and replacement with fresh blood) for levels greater than 20 mg/dl (Andrews and Huether, 1990).

Liver Diseases

Hepatitis

Hepatitis is an acute or chronic inflammation of the liver. It can be caused by a virus, a chemical, a drug reaction, or alcohol abuse. In addition, hepatitis can be secondary to disease conditions, such as an infection with other viruses like Epstein-Barr virus or cytomegalovirus (Marx, 1993).

VIRAL HEPATITIS

Viral hepatitis is an acute infectious inflammation of the liver caused by one of five identified viruses: A, B, C, D, and E. Hepatitis is a major uncontrolled public health problem for several reasons: not all the causative agents have been identified, there are no specific drugs for its treatment, its incidence has increased in relation to illicit drug use, and it can be communicated before the appearance of observable clinical symptoms. It is spread easily to others and usually results in an extended period of convalescence with loss of time from school or work. It is estimated that 60 per cent to 90 per cent of viral hepatitis cases are unreported because many cases are subclinical or involve mild symptoms (Smeltzer and Bare, 1992).

Hepatitis affects people in three stages: the initial or preicteric stage, the icteric or jaundiced stage, and the recovery period. During the *initial* or *preicteric stage,* which lasts for 1 to 3 weeks, the person experiences vague gastrointestinal (GI) and general body symptoms. Fatigue, malaise, lassitude, weight loss, and anorexia are common. Many people develop an aversion to food, alcohol, and cigarette smoke. Nausea, vomiting, diarrhea, arthralgias, and influenza-like symptoms may occur. The liver becomes enlarged and tender, and intermittent itching (pruritus) may develop. One to fourteen days before the icteric stage, the urine darkens and the stool lightens as less bilirubin is conjugated and excreted (Cassmeyer, 1991a).

The *icteric stage* is characterized by the appearance of jaundice, which peaks in 1 to 2 weeks and persists for 6 to 8 weeks. During this stage, the acuteness of the inflammation subsides. The GI symptoms begin to disappear, and after 1 to 2 weeks of jaundice the liver decreases in size and becomes less tender. During the icteric stage, the postcervical lymph nodes and spleen are enlarged. Persons who have been treated with human immune serum globulin (ISG) may not develop jaundice (Cassmeyer, 1991a).

The *recovery stage* lasts for 3 to 4 months, during which time the person generally feels well but fatigues easily (Cassmeyer, 1991a).

People with mild-to-moderate acute hepatitis rarely require hospitalization. The emphasis is on preventing the spread of infectious agents and avoiding further liver damage when the underlying cause is drug-induced or toxic hepatitis. People with fulminant (severe, sudden intensity, sometimes fatal) hepatitis require special management because of the rapid progression of their disease and the potential need for urgent liver transplantation (Carithers, 1993).

Acute Hepatitis A Virus. Hepatitis A virus (HAV), formerly known as infectious hepatitis, is caused by a virus of the enterovirus family. The primary mode of transmission of this disease is the oral-fecal route,* usually by intake of food or water

---

* The oral-fecal route of transmission is primarily from poor or improper handwashing and personal hygiene, particularly after using the lavatory and then handling food for public consumption. This route of transmission may also occur through the shared use of oral utensils, such as straws, silverware, and toothbrushes.

▼ *Clinical Signs and Symptoms of*
Hepatitis A

Hepatitis A is often acquired in childhood as a mild infection with symptoms similar to the "flu" and may be misdiagnosed or ignored. It does not usually cause lasting damage to the liver, although the following symptoms may persist for weeks:

- Extreme fatigue
- Anorexia
- Fever
- Arthralgias and myalgias (generalized aching)
- Right upper abdominal pain
- Clay-colored stools
- Dark urine
- Icterus (jaundice)
- Headache
- Pharyngitis
- Alterations in the senses of taste and smell
- Loss of desire to smoke cigarettes or drink alcohol
- Low-grade fever
- Indigestion (varying degrees of nausea, heartburn, flatulence)

contaminated with feces that has been infected with the virus. Hepatitis A is commonly found in environments of poor sanitation and overcrowding, such as day care centers and schools, and is prevalent in underdeveloped countries. An infected food handler can spread HAV, and major outbreaks of HAV often occur when people consume water or shellfish from sewage-contaminated waters.

The incubation period for HAV is estimated to be from 15 to 50 days (2 to 7 weeks), with an average incubation of 30 days. Hepatitis A is highly contagious, with the peak time of viral excretion and contamination occurring during the 2-week period *before* the onset of symptoms of jaundice. Thus, the greatest danger of infection is during the incubation period, when the person is probably unaware that the virus is present. The illness can last from 4 to 8 weeks; it generally lasts longer and is more severe in people over the age of 40 years (Smeltzer and Bare, 1992).

The antibody to hepatitis A (anti-HAV) appears in serum soon after the onset of symptoms and disappears after 3 to 12 months. IgM antibody to HAV also indicates recent infection with HAV and remains positive up to 6 months after infection.

Preventive measures include universal and enteric precautions and the administration of ISG therapy, also referred to as gamma globulin therapy, during the period of incubation. If the ISG therapy is administered within 2 weeks of exposure to the HAV infection, it bolsters the person's own antibody production and provides 6 to 8 weeks of passive immunity. ISG is also recommended for household members and sexual partners of persons with HAV. A vaccine for HAV is currently under investigation (Smeltzer and Bare, 1992).

Treatment. Treatment is primarily symptomatic, and bed rest is recommended for people who are jaundiced to avoid complications from liver damage. Hospitalization may be required for anyone who has excessive vomiting and subsequent fluid and electrolyte imbalance. During the period of anorexia, the client should receive nutritional supplements and possibly intravenous glucose infusions. Hepatitis A virus is rarely fatal and does not lead to chronic hepatitis or cirrhosis. Most people recover fully from the hepatitis A virus and become immune to it. The fatal form of hepatitis, fulminant hepatitis, develops in only about 0.1 per cent of people with HAV (Marx, 1993).

Acute Hepatitis B Virus. Hepatitis B virus

(HBV), formerly called serum hepatitis, is transmitted through needle sticks, sexual relations, intravenous drug use and shared needles, dialysis, blood transfusions, and 6perinatal transmission from mother to child. The major source of this infection is blood serum or body secretions (saliva, urine, feces, semen, vaginal secretions including menstrual blood, and breast milk) of an infected person. Blood serum is the most common route or source of contact. HBV can survive on environmental surfaces such as countertops or other objects for at least a week, making it difficult to determine the source of viral transmission. In addition, because this disease can be transmitted through heterosexual or homosexual intercourse, it is also considered to be a sexually transmitted disease.

Even though approximately 300,000 new cases of hepatitis B are reported yearly in the United States, HBV is considered one of the most underreported diseases in this country (Marx, 1993). Persons at high risk for contact with HBV include

- Persons who have received multiple blood transfusions
- Dialysis patients
- Morticians
- Persons tattooed
- Parenteral drug users
- Homosexually active men
- Health care workers in high-risk areas (areas of work in which body fluid or blood contact is likely)

Health care workers are at risk for contact with HBV owing to their close contact with the blood or body fluids of carriers. According to the Centers for Disease Control and Prevention (CDC), approximately 12,000 health care workers contract HBV every year. Of those, 200 to 300 die of the disease. Therapists at risk should receive active immunization against HBV and should follow universal precautions meticu-

lously to protect themselves (see Appenc at the end of this chapter).

The incubation period for HBV is 45 to 180 days (6 to 26 weeks). The period of infectivity begins *before* symptoms appear and may continue for a lifetime if the person becomes a carrier. As discussed earlier, hepatitis A usually has been eliminated from the body by the time jaundice appears, but the body is not always able to rid itself of HBV and the virus can persist in body fluids indefinitely. Nurses, physicians, laboratory technicians, blood bank workers, and dentists are frequent victims of HBV, often as a result of not wearing gloves or wearing defective gloves while working. Persons who are carriers of the disease are a continual threat to others.

Hepatitis B surface antigen (HBsAg), formerly called the Australia antigen, is the first marker to appear in the blood serum of infected clients. This antigen is positive for about 2 weeks before the onset of clinical symptoms and usually disappears as the infection is resolving. However, this surface antigen can remain as long as 6 months in some people.

The presence of HBsAg means that the person is contagious and can transmit HBV to others. Other antigens appear concurrently or shortly after HBsAg disappears (HBeAg; HBcAg). In addition, antibodies to these antigens become detectable in blood serum after the appearance of clinical hepatitis, and these antibodies persist indefinitely. The presence of the anti-HBc antibody is the best and clearest marker of

Clinical Signs and Symptoms of
Hepatitis B

Hepatitis B may be asymptomatic but can include
- Jaundice
- Arthralgias
- Rash

Table 8–2
HEPATITIS

	Hepatitis A (HAV)	Hepatitis B (HBV)	Hepatitis C (HCV)	Hepatitis D (HCV)	Hepatitis E (HEV)
Source	Fecal-oral; contaminated water and food	Parenteral or sexual; blood and body fluids	Parenteral; blood and blood products	Same as B (coinfection with hepatitis B)	Fecal-oral (same as hepatitis A)
Incubation Period	2–7 weeks (15–50 days)	6–26 weeks (45–180 days)	2–26 weeks (14–180 days)	2–9 weeks (15–64 days)	2–7 weeks (15–50 days)
Diagnostic Tests	Anti-HAV; IgM	HBsAg; HBeAg; HbcAg (and several others)	Anti-HCV	Anti-HDV	No test available
Preventive Measures	Universal and enteric precautions; no vaccine yet available	Universal precautions; hepatitis B vaccine (Heptavax)	Universal precautions; no vaccine available	Same as hepatitis B	Universal and enteric precautions, no vaccine available
	Immunoglobulin for postexposure prophylaxis	Hepatitis B immunoglobulin for postexposure prophylaxis	Screening of blood donors	Avoid exposure to Hepatitis B	
Prognosis	Rarely fatal; no carrier or chronic state; lifetime immunity	High mortality; can develop lifetime immunity or carrier state; can become chronic; associated with liver cancer	Can progress to chronic state; can become carrier or immune; possibly associated with liver cancer	Immunity to hepatitis B confers immunity to D; prognosis same as for hepatitis B	10% mortality in pregnant women; does not progress to chronic state and is not fatal in nonpregnant person

Table 8–3

ASSOCIATION OF ARTHRALGIA WITH AGE IN HBsAg-NEGATIVE PATIENTS

Age (yr)	No Arthralgia	Arthralgia	Total	% Suffering from Arthralgia
0–14	95	21	116	18
15–29	96	41	137	30
>30	56	45	101	45
Total	247	107	354	30

From Stewart, J.S., Farrow, L.J., Clifford, R.E., et al.: A three-year survey of viral hepatitis in West London. Quarterly Journal of Medicine *187*:365, 1978.

immunity owing to actual HBV infection (Wilson and Lester, 1992).

Hepatitis B follows a course similar to that of hepatitis A. The onset, however, is usually insidious (hepatitis A has an abrupt onset). Hepatitis B differs from hepatitis A in the degree and severity of symptoms, but the general symptoms are similar (Table 8–2).

Studies dealing with the natural history of acute hepatitis have provided perspective on the frequency of skin and joint manifestations in these infections (Stewart et al., 1978). More than one third of the adults studied had joint pains during the course of their illness. There was no difference in the incidence of these symptoms between HBsAg-positive and HBsAg-negative clients, although the duration of joint symptoms was slightly longer (more than 2 weeks) in clients who were HBsAg positive. Examination of the antigen-negative clients showed a strong association between arthralgia and the age of the person (Table 8–3); the frequency of this symptom increases with age. Joint pains affected only 18 per cent of children, compared with 45 per cent of adults over 30 years of age (Gocke, 1982).

Prevention of HBV includes meticulous use of universal precautions in all encounters with infected persons, carriers, and suspected carriers (high-risk persons). Careful screening of donor blood products and use of volunteer rather than paid donors has helped prevent HBV transmission through the transfused blood supply. Clients with HBV should not share with others razors, toothbrushes, washcloths, cigarettes, or other personal items.

Hepatitis B vaccine (active immunization) may provide permanent immunity to HBV prior to exposure. This vaccine is recommended for persons in the high-risk categories for HBV (including health care workers who have a high chance of body fluid contact with clients). Standard immunoglobulin (IgG) may contain antibodies against HBV, but another preparation called specific hepatitis B immunoglobulin contains much higher levels of HBV antibodies. The hepatitis B immunoglobulin is not a vaccine, so it does not confer permanent immunity to HBV. It is instead a measure that is prescribed *after* a nonimmune person is exposed to percutaneous (needle stick) HBV. This immunoglobulin provides passive immunity (temporary) protection in a person who is not already immune to the virus (Matassarin-Jacobs and Strasburg, 1993).

Hepatitis B has a high mortality rate and is a very serious, potentially fatal illness. It can progress to cirrhosis, chronic hepatitis (5 to 10 per cent of clients), hepatocellular carcinoma, and death (Marx, 1993). In addition, approximately 10 per cent of infected persons become lifetime *carriers* of HBV.

Acute Hepatitis C. Hepatitis C (HCV), formerly posttransfusion non-A, non-B hepatitis, is another prevalent and underreported disease in the United States, with approximately 170,000 new cases per year (Marx, 1993). Hepatitis C accounts for 60 to 90 per cent of posttransfusion hepatitis and also occurs among users of illicit drugs, individuals with hemophilia receiving blood-derived factor replacement, dialysis patients, and health care personnel.

The primary transmission of HCV is parenteral, spread by blood and blood products. In past years, HCV was easily transmitted through blood products because the virus had not been identified and there was no way to detect it in donor screening procedures. However, the recent development and approval of a blood-screening test for HCV is expected to reduce drastically the numbers of blood transfusion–related cases of this virus (Lab Tech Bulletin, 1990; Marx, 1993).

The incubation period of hepatitis C is 14 to 180 days (2 to 26 weeks). The period of infectivity begins before onset of symptoms and may continue for a lifetime if the infected person becomes a carrier. Clinically, HCV is very similar to HBV; significant symptoms include malaise, fever, headache, general muscle fatigue, loss of appetite, nausea, abdominal and joint pain, jaundice, and dark urine.

An anti-HCV antibody is detectable in client serum 2 to 6 months after exposure to hepatitis C virus. Appearance of this antibody indicates *past infection* with HCV. However, this antibody may not appear until over 1 year after infection, and its presence has been detected up to 12 years after recovery from infection (Kuo et al., 1989).

Universal precautions are indicated as a preventive measure. Currently no vaccine is available to prevent this virus, and no immunoglobulin is effective in treating exposure.

The person infected with this virus can become a chronic carrier; 50 per cent of all cases progress to chronic hepatitis, and 20 percent of chronic cases progress to cirrhosis. In addition, there is a suggested association between the presence of HCV and the development of liver cancer (Marx, 1993).

Case Example. A 43-year-old man, 1 year following traumatic injury to the right forearm, underwent surgery to transplant his great toe to function as a thumb. The surgery took place in another state, and the man, who had been a client in our facility before surgery, returned for postoperative rehabilitation. Complaints of hives of the involved forearm, fatigue, depression, and increased perspiration were documented but attributed by his physician to recovery from the traumatic injury and the multiple operations. Medical records from the hospital consisted of therapy notes only. Eventually, the client developed a yellowing of the sclerae (white outer coat of the eyeballs). Medical referral was requested, and the client was evaluated by an internal medicine specialist. Hepatitis C was diagnosed, and full medical records then obtained revealed that although the man had donated his own blood in advance for the surgery, he was short by one unit of blood, which he received through a blood bank.

Acute Hepatitis D. Hepatitis D (delta virus) occurs in some cases of hepatitis B as a coinfection. Because the virus requires hepatitis B surface antigen for its replication, only individuals with hepatitis B are at risk for hepatitis D. Hepatitis D (HDV) is transmitted the same way as hepatitis B. Its incubation is 15 to 64 days (2 to 10 weeks), and the infectivity period is not known.

Persons at risk for hepatitis D are the same group at risk for hepatitis B. The symptoms of hepatitis D are similar to those of hepatitis B except that clients are more likely to have fulminant hepatitis and to develop chronic active hepatitis and cirrhosis (Smeltzer and Bare, 1992). Hepatitis D has a high mortality rate.

An anti-HDV antibody indicates past or present infection with hepatitis D, and it appears after symptoms develop. Its presence is often short-lived (Marx, 1993).

Universal precautions are indicated for prevention of this infection. Hepatitis B vaccination is recommended for preexposure immunization, and hepatitis B immunoglobulin therapy is indicated for postexposure prophylaxis. Immunity to hepatitis B also confers immunity to hepatitis D.

Acute Hepatitis E. Hepatitis E, also called enteric non-A, non-B hepatitis, is believed to be nonfatal except in pregnant women (10 per cent mortality rate). This virus is transmitted through fecal contamination of water, primarily in developing countries, and is very rare in the United States. Clients experience an acute infection that does not progress to chronic hepatitis.

Its incubation is 15 to 50 days (2 to 7 weeks), but the infectivity period is not known. No test is yet available to indicate the presence of this virus in the blood serum. Universal and enteric precautions are the preventive measures indicated. No vaccine and no postexposure prophylaxis are available at this time. Hepatitis E is not yet a reportable disease in the United States, and it is diagnosed by ruling out all other forms of viral hepatitis (Marx, 1993).

CHRONIC HEPATITIS (O'Toole, 1992)

Chronic hepatitis is the term used to describe an illness associated with prolonged inflammation of the liver after unresolved viral hepatitis or associated with *chronic active hepatitis* (CAH) of unknown etiology. "Chronic" is defined as inflammation of the liver for 6 months or more. The symptoms and biochemical abnormalities may continue for months or years. It is divided by findings on liver biopsy into CAH and *chronic persistent hepatitis* (CPH).

Chronic Active Hepatitis. This type of hepatitis refers to seriously destructive liver disease that can result in cirrhosis. CAH is often a result of viral infection (HBV, HCV, and HDV) but can also be secondary to drug sensitivity (e.g., methyldopa [Aldomet], an antihypertensive medication, and isoniazid [INH], an antitubercular drug). Steroid therapy is sometimes

Clinical Signs and Symptoms of
Chronic Active Hepatitis

The clinical signs and symptoms of chronic active hepatitis may range from asymptomatic to the person who is bedridden with cirrhosis and advanced hepatocellular failure. In the latter, the prominent signs and symptoms may reflect multisystem involvement, including

- Fatigue
- Jaundice
- Abdominal pain
- Anorexia
- Arthralgia
- Fever
- Splenomegaly and hepatomegaly
- Weakness
- Ascites
- Hepatic encephalopathy

recommended for clients with evidence of aggressive liver inflammation and necrosis (identified by liver biopsy) as a result of these drugs.

Prognosis and Treatment. If CAH is left untreated, its course is unpredictable and may range from progressive deterioration of liver function to spontaneous remissions and exacerbations (Wilson and Lester, 1992). In untreated cases, the mortality from CAH can be as high as 50 per cent within 3 to 5 years.

Steroids may be used to treat CAH. They are usually prescribed for a period of 3 to 5 years. In addition, recombinant interferon-alpha-2b injections in low doses over a 6-month period have been shown to improve hepatic function in people with CAH (Marx, 1993).

Chronic Persistent Hepatitis. This type of hepatitis occurs most commonly secondary to a viral infection (usually HBV,

▼ *Clinical Signs and Symptoms of*
Chronic Persistent Hepatitis

- Right upper quadrant pain
- Anorexia
- Mild fatigue
- Malaise

HCV, or HDV). Many clients with CPH are asymptomatic and appear to be healthy or have only minor complaints. Episodes of acute illness are infrequent, and the prognosis for recovery is good (Wilson and Lester, 1992). No treatment is necessary because the condition slowly resolves on its own. CPH is generally considered benign, usually asymptomatic, anicteric (without jaundice), and without progression to cirrhosis.

Metabolic Disease. The most common metabolic diseases that can cause chronic hepatitis of interest to a physical therapist are Wilson's disease and hematochromatosis, also termed hemochromatosis. Both these diseases are dealt with in greater detail as metabolic disorders in Chapter 9.

Wilson's disease is an autosomal recessive disorder in which biliary excretion of copper is impaired, and as a consequence, total body copper is progressively increased (Deiss, 1992). There may be mild-to-severe neurologic dysfunction, depending on the rate of hepatocyte injury.

Hemochromatosis is the most common genetic disorder (autosomal recessive defect in iron absorption) causing liver failure. Excessive iron is stored in various parenchymal organs with subsequent development of fibrosis. Arthralgias and arthropathy may develop and are often confused with rheumatoid arthritis or osteoarthritis. The second and third metacarpophalangeal joints are usually involved first. Knees, hips, shoulders, and lower back may be affected. Acute synovitis with pseudogout of the knees has been observed (Motulsky, 1992).

NONVIRAL HEPATITIS

Nonviral hepatitis is a form of liver inflammation that occurs secondary to exposure to certain chemicals or drugs. It is considered to be a toxic or drug-induced hepatitis from which most people recover without serious complications. Specific chemical hepatotoxins may include carbon tetrachloride, trichloroethylene, poisonous mushrooms (*Amanita phalloides* and related species, rare in the United States but more common in Europe), alcohol (most common in the United States), and vinyl chloride. Careful questioning regarding occupational exposure to these toxins is important.

Drug-induced hepatitis occurs after the administration of one of various drugs to clients who demonstrate a hypersensitivity reaction.

Toxic hepatitis causes liver alterations, with liver responses being dose-related and predictable or idiosyncratic and unpredictable depending on the chemical nature of the hepatotoxin or the genetic makeup of the person (Matassarin-Jacobs and Strasburg, 1993). A reaction that is termed idio-

▼ *Clinical Signs and Symptoms of*
Toxic and Drug-Induced Hepatitis

These vary with the severity of liver damage and the causative agent. In most individuals, symptoms resemble those of acute viral hepatitis:

- Anorexia, nausea, vomiting
- Fatigue and malaise
- Jaundice
- Dark urine
- Clay-colored stools
- Headache, dizziness, drowsiness (carbon tetrachloride poisoning)
- Fever, rash, arthralgias, epigastric or right upper quadrant pain (halothane anesthetic)

Table 8–4
COMMON HEPATOTOXIC DRUGS

Drug or Drug Type	Clinical Uses
Phenytoin (Dilantin)	Anticonvulsant
Tetracyclines	Antibiotic
Cytotoxic drugs	Antineoplastic
Acetaminophen	Analgesic/antipyretic
Tannic acid	Astringent
Aspirin	Antiinflammatory/analgesic/antipyretic
Monoamine oxidase inhibitors	Antidepressant
Chlorpromazine and other phenothiazines	Antipsychotic
Oxacillin sodium	Antibiotic
Halothane	Gas anesthetic
Isoniazid	Antitubercular
Aminosalicylic acid	Antitubercular
Rifampin	Antibiotic
Erythromycin estolate	Antibiotic
Oral contraceptives	Contraceptive
Anabolic steroids	Anticatabolic/increase hemoglobin
Novobiocin	Antibiotic
Chloramphenicol	Antibiotic
Radiographic contrast agents	Diagnostic testing

syncratic is often due to hypersensitivity (immune response) to the agent involved. Necrosis of the liver usually occurs within 2 or 3 days after acute exposure to a dose-related toxic drug. Several weeks may pass before clinical manifestations of idiosyncratic reactions appear, however. Repeated exposure to some hepatotoxins in small or minimal amounts over long periods of time may also cause severe damage to liver tissue (Matassarin-Jacobs and Strasburg, 1993).

The following list of the most common substances that act as hepatotoxins is categorized according to whether the hepatotoxic reaction is dose-related and predictable or idiosyncratic (Matassarin-Jacobs and Strasburg, 1993).

Dose-Related

- Acetaminophen* (Tylenol) (analgesic; suicide attempt)
- *Amanita phalloides* (poisonous mushroom)

* Acetaminophen is Tylenol and is not an NSAID. It has no antiinflammatory properties, only analgesic and antipyretic uses. It has no relationship to ibuprofen.

- Aspirin
- Benzene
- Carbon tetrachloride
- Chloroform (anesthetic)
- Methotrexate (antineoplastic agent)
- Tetracyclines (antibiotic)

Idiosyncratic

- Alpha-methyldopa (antihypertensive)
- Halothane (anesthetic)
- Isoniazid (antituberculin)
- Nitrofurantoin
- Phenytoin (Dilantin) (anticonvulsant)
- Quinidine (antiarrhythmic)
- Sulfasalazine (antibiotic)

A number of other antiinflammatory and minor analgesic agents have caused hepatic injury (Table 8–4). Again, the mechanism by which these agents induce overt injury is clearly unusual susceptibility of individuals (i.e., the adverse effects are idiosyncratic reactions). Some drugs (e.g., oral contraceptives) may impair liver function and produce jaundice without causing necrosis, fatty infiltration of liver cells, or a hypersensitivity reaction.

Cirrhosis

Cirrhosis is a chronic hepatic disease characterized by the destruction of liver cells and by the replacement of connective tissue by fibrous bands. As the liver becomes more and more scarred (fibrosed), blood and lymph flow becomes impaired, causing hepatic insufficiency and increased clinical manifestations. The causes of cirrhosis can be varied, although alcohol is the most common cause of liver disease in the United States. The following list describes the primary causes of cirrhosis:

- Alcoholic cirrhosis (Laennec's cirrhosis)
- Biliary cirrhosis (caused by any bile duct disease that suppresses bile flow)
- Posthepatic cirrhosis
- Cardiac cirrhosis (rare form resulting from right ventricular failure)
- Pigment cirrhosis (as a result of hemochromatosis, a disorder of iron metabolism)
- Idiopathic cirrhosis (unknown causes account for approximately 10 per cent of people)

The activity level of the client with cirrhosis is determined by the symptoms. Because hepatic blood flow diminishes with moderate exercise, rest periods are advised and are adjusted according to the level of fatigue experienced by the client both during the exercise and afterward at home. The person may return to work with medical approval but is advised to avoid straining, such as lifting heavy objects, if portal hypertension and esophageal varices are a problem. Because stress decreases hepatic blood flow, any reduction of stress at

▼ *Early Clinical Signs and Symptoms of* **Cirrhosis**

- Mild right upper quadrant pain (progressive)
- GI symptoms
  - Anorexia
  - Indigestion
  - Weight loss
  - Nausea and vomiting
  - Diarrhea or constipation
- Dull abdominal ache
- Ease of fatigue (with mild exertion)
- Weakness
- Fever

home, at work, or during treatment is therapeutic (Matassarin-Jacobs and Strasburg, 1993).

Prognosis and Treatment. These can vary dramatically in the client with alcoholic liver disease. People with liver disease have high short-term mortality, whereas the prognosis for those with mild disease depends on the degree and number of complications and whether they can abstain from alcohol (Carithers, 1993).

PORTAL HYPERTENSION

As the cirrhosis progresses and hepatic insufficiency and portal hypertension occur, late symptoms that affect the entire body develop (Table 8–5). Portal hypertension is the elevated pressure in the portal vein (through which blood passes from the GI tract and spleen to the liver). As the blood meets increased resistance from fibrotic tissue, portal pressure rises and the blood backs up into the spleen. The blood then bypasses the liver through collateral vessels.

Table 8–5
CLINICAL MANIFESTATIONS OF CIRRHOSIS

Body System	Clinical Manifestations
Respiratory	Limited thoracic expansion (due to ascites) Hypoxia 　Dyspnea 　Cyanosis 　Clubbing
Central nervous system (CNS) (progressive to hepatic coma)	Subtle changes in mental acuity (progressive) Mild memory loss Poor reasoning ability Irritability Paranoia and hallucinations Slurred speech Asterixis (tremor of outstretched hands) Peripheral neuritis Peripheral muscle atrophy
Hematologic	Impaired coagulation/bleeding tendencies 　Nosebleeds 　Easy bruising 　Bleeding gums Anemia (usually caused by GI blood loss from esophageal varices)
Endocrine (due to liver's inability to metabolize hormones)	Testicular atrophy Menstrual irregularities Gynecomastia (excessive development of breasts in men) Loss of chest and axillary hair
Integument (cutaneous and skin)	Severe pruritus (itching) Extreme dryness Poor tissue turgor Abnormal pigmentation Prominent spider angiomas (benign tumor made up of blood vessels) Palmar erythema (redness caused by extensive collection of arteriovenous anastomoses) Jaundice
Hepatic	Hepatomegaly (enlargement of the liver) Ascites Edema of the legs Hepatic encephalopathy
Gastrointestinal (GI)	Anorexia Nausea Vomiting Diarrhea

ASCITES

Ascites is an abnormal accumulation of serous (edematous) fluid within the peritoneal cavity. In portal and venous hepatic hypertension, there is increased pressure within the sinusoids and hepatic veins (see Fig. 8–2). As the pressure increases, there is movement of protein-rich plasma filtrate into the hepatic lymphatics. Some fluid enters the thoracic duct, but if the pressure is high enough, the excess fluid will ooze from the surface of the liver into the peritoneal cavity.

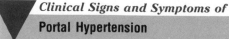

Clinical Signs and Symptoms of
Portal Hypertension

- Ascites (abnormal collection of fluid in the peritoneal cavity)
- Dilated collateral veins
  - Esophageal varices (upper GI)
  - Hemorrhoids (lower GI)
- Splenomegaly (enlargement of the spleen)
- Thrombocytopenia (decreased number of blood platelets for clotting)

Clinical Signs and Symptoms of
Hemorrhage Associated with Esophageal Varices

- Restlessness
- Pallor
- Tachycardia
- Cooling of the skin
- Hypotension

The liver is the only organ that synthesizes albumin, a plasma protein. Albumin maintains colloid osmotic pressure in the vasculature. With decreased albumin, the plasma colloid osmotic pressure is decreased, allowing fluid to escape to the interstitial fluid spaces. Likewise, because this fluid had a high colloidal osmotic pressure owing to its high protein content, it is not readily reabsorbed from the peritoneal cavity (O'Toole, 1992). This shift of fluid is noticeable as edema in dependent locations, such as the ankles, and fluid accumulates in the abdomen (ascites) (Guyton, 1992).

For the physical therapist, abdominal hernias and lumbar lordosis observed in clients with ascites may present symptoms mimicking musculoskeletal involvement, such as groin or low back pain.

Treatment. Treatment includes diuresis through dietary sodium restriction, diuretic therapy (medications), and paracentesis (surgical puncture of the abdomen for removal of fluid).

ESOPHAGEAL VARICES

Esophageal varices are dilated veins of the lower esophagus that develop when hepatic fibrosis compresses hepatic veins, impeding outflow through the vena cava and increasing portal pressure. These thin-walled vessels accommodate portal circulation poorly and become dilated, causing rupture with subsequent hemorrhaging. The hemorrhage occurs because of two underlying pathophysiologic processes: the diseased liver fails to produce blood-clotting factors, and the increased portal hypertension predisposes the person to peptic ulceration and hemorrhage. Additionally, alcohol is toxic to gastric mucosa and can induce hemorrhagic gastritis (Purtilo and Purtilo, 1989). Esophageal varices are, in terms of hospitalization and ultimate mortality, the single most significant complication of cirrhosis (Matassarin-Jacobs and Strasburg, 1993). Hemorrhage from esophageal varices almost always occurs in cirrhotic individuals with ascites and often occurs when the abdomen is tightly distended.

Treatment. Beta-blockers are effective in reducing the risk of variceal hemorrhage (Pascal and Cales, 1987). Sclerotherapy (injection of sclerosing solutions) is effective in controlling bleeding in 75 per cent of cases (Larson et al., 1986). Hospitalization and possible surgery may be required for recurrent, uncontrolled bleeding (Carithers, 1993).

Hepatic Encephalopathy (Hepatic Coma)

Hepatic encephalopathy leading to coma is a neuropsychiatric syndrome that occurs secondary to acute or chronic liver disease. Any disease of the liver that becomes destructive of liver parenchyma or results in abnormal shunting of blood around functioning liver tissue may predispose the client to hepatic encephalopathy (Wilson and Lester, 1992).

Ammonia from the intestine (produced by protein breakdown) is normally transformed by the liver to urea, glutamine, and asparagine. Increased serum ammonia levels are directly toxic to central and peripheral nervous system function. Flapping tremors (asterixis) and numbness/tingling (misinterpreted as carpal tunnel syndrome) are common resultant symptoms of this ammonia abnormality.

> **Case Example.** A 45-year-old truck driver was diagnosed by a hand surgeon as having bilateral carpal tunnel syndrome (CTS) and was referred to physical therapy. During the course of treatment, the client commented that he was seeing an acupuncturist who had told him that liver disease was the cause of his bilateral CTS. Further questioning at that time indicated the absence of any other associated symptoms to suggest liver or hepatic involvement. However, because his symptoms were bilateral and there is a known correlation between liver disease and CTS, the referring physician was notified of these findings. The client was referred for evaluation, and a diagnosis of liver cancer was confirmed. Physical therapy for CTS was appropriately discontinued.

When portal blood shunts past the liver, ammonia directly enters the systemic circulation and is carried to the brain. The excess ammonia reaches the brain as a result of reduced hepatic function or of the bypass of blood around the liver parenchyma. Other factors that predispose to rising ammonia levels include

- Excessive protein intake
- Excessive accumulation of nitrogenous body wastes (constipation, GI hemorrhage)
- Bacterial action on protein and urea to form ammonia

- Fluid and electrolyte abnormalities
- Sedatives, tranquilizers, narcotic analgesics
- Severe infection (bacterial pneumonia, pyelonephritis, septicemia [blood poisoning], spontaneous bacterial peritonitis)

Clinical manifestations of hepatic encephalopathy vary, depending on the severity of neurologic involvement, and develop in four stages as the ammonia level increases in the serum with the following accompanying clinical features.

Prodromal Stage (Stage I) (subtle symptoms that may be overlooked)

- Slight personality changes
  - Disorientation, confusion
  - Euphoria or depression
  - Forgetfulness
  - Slurred speech
- Slight tremor
- Muscular incoordination
- Impaired handwriting

Impending Stage (Stage II)

- Tremor progresses to asterixis
- Resistance to passive movement (increased muscle tone)
- Lethargy
- Aberrant behavior
- Apraxia*
- Ataxia
- Facial grimacing and blinking

Stuporous Stage (Stage III) (patient can still be aroused)

- Hyperventilation
- Marked confusion
- Abusive and violent
- Noisy, incoherent speech
- Asterixis (liver flap)

---

* This type of motor apraxia can be best observed by keeping a record of the client's handwriting and drawings of simple shapes, such as a circle, square, triangle, rectangle. Check for progressive deterioration.

- Muscle rigidity
- Positive Babinski reflex*
- Hyperactive deep tendon reflexes

    Comatose Stage (Stage IV) (patient cannot be aroused, responds only to painful stimuli)

- No asterixis
- Positive Babinski reflex
- Hepatic fetor (musty, sweet odor to the breath due to the liver's inability to metabolize the amino acid methionine)

For the physical therapist, the inpatient with impending hepatic coma has difficulty in ambulating and is unsteady. Protection from falling and seizure precautions must be taken. Skin breakdown in a client who is malnourished due to liver disease, immobile, jaundiced, and edematous can occur in less than 24 hours. Careful attention to skin care, passive exercise, and frequent changes in position are required.

Treatment. Treatment involves a variety of possible measures including dietary management to reduce protein in the intestine. If no other precipitating factors are present, this alone may eliminate symptoms. Neomycin, an antibacterial substance, is administered orally or by enema to reduce bacterial production of ammonia. (Matassarin-Jacobs and Strasburg, 1993).

Liver Abscess

A liver abscess occurs when bacteria or protozoa destroy hepatic tissue and produce a cavity that fills with infectious organisms, liquefied liver cells, and leukocytes.

---

* A reflex action of the toes that is normal during infancy but abnormal after 12 to 18 months. It is elicited by a firm stimulus (usually scraping with the handle of a reflex hammer) on the sole of the foot from the heel along the lateral border of the sole to the little toe, across the ball of the foot to the big toe. Normally such a stimulus causes all the toes to flex downward. A positive Babinski reflex occurs when the great toe flexes upward and the smaller toes fan outward (O'Toole, 1992).

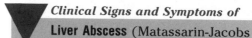

Clinical Signs and Symptoms of

Liver Abscess (Matassarin-Jacobs and Strasburg, 1993)

Clinical signs and symptoms of liver abscess depend on the degree of involvement; some people are acutely ill, others are asymptomatic. Depending on the type of abscess, the onset may be sudden or insidious. The most common signs include

- Right abdominal pain
- Right shoulder pain
- Weight loss
- Fever, chills
- Diaphoresis
- Nausea and vomiting
- Anemia

Necrotic tissue then isolates the cavity from the rest of the liver.

Even though liver abscess is relatively uncommon, it carries a mortality of 30 per cent to 50 per cent. This rate rises to more than 80 per cent with multiple abscesses and to more than 90 per cent with complications such as rupture into the peritoneum, pleura, or pericardium.

Signs of right pleural effusion, such as dyspnea and pleural pain, develop if the abscess extends through the diaphragm. Extensive damage to the liver may cause jaundice.

Treatment. Treatment consists of long-term antibiotic therapy.

Liver Cancer

Metastatic tumors occur 20 times more often than primary liver tumors because the liver is one of the most common sites of metastasis from other primary cancers (e.g., colorectal, stomach, pancreas, esophagus, lung, breast). Although various sarcomas as well as lymphomas may originate in the liver, more than 98 per cent of primary cancers of the liver are hepatomas, cholangiocellular carcinomas, or mixed types (Cassmeyer, 1991a). Persons with occupational exposure to vinyl chloride over a long period may develop liver angiosarcoma, a malignant tumor.

Primary liver tumors (hepatocellular carcinoma [HCC]) are usually associated with cirrhosis but can be linked to other predisposing factors (Matassarin-Jacobs and Strasburg, 1993):

■ Fungal infection (common in moldy foods of Africa)

■ Viral hepatitis

■ Excessive use of anabolic steroids

■ Trauma

■ Nutritional deficiencies

■ Exposure to hepatotoxins

Several types of benign and malignant hepatic neoplasms can result from the administration of chemical agents. For example, adenoma (a benign tumor) can occur in recipients of oral contraceptives. Regression of the tumor occurs after withdrawal of the drug.

Interference with liver function does not occur until approximately 80 per cent to 90 per cent of the liver is replaced by metastatic carcinoma or primary carcinoma. Cholangiocarcinoma is a primary cancer that develops in bile ducts within the liver. Cholangiocarcinoma is not associated with cirrhosis, but both hepatocarcinoma and cholangiocarcinoma are fatal despite treatment with chemotherapy (Purtilo and Purtilo, 1989).

Metastatic tumors to the liver originating in some organs (stomach, lung) never give rise to hepatic symptoms, whereas others produce hepatic symptoms or jaundice with less than 60 per cent replacement of the liver. Certain tumors (colon, breast,

Clinical Signs and Symptoms of
Liver Neoplasm

If clinical signs and symptoms of liver neoplasm do occur (whether of primary or metastatic origin), these may include

■ Jaundice (icterus)

■ Progressive failure of health

■ Anorexia and weight loss

■ Overall muscular weakness

■ Epigastric fullness and pain or discomfort

■ Constant ache in the epigastrium or midback

■ Early satiety (cystic tumors)

melanoma) typically replace the 90 per cent of liver mentioned before jaundice develops.

Melanomas are associated with such minimal tissue reaction that almost complete hepatic replacement is required before hepatic symptoms develop. Following the diagnosis of liver cancer and if intervention fails to terminate the tumor process, the individual usually dies of hepatic failure within 4 to 6 months (Matassarin-Jacobs and Strasburg, 1993).

Gallbladder and Duct Diseases

Cholelithiasis

Gallstones are stonelike masses called calculi (singular: calculus) that form in the gallbladder possibly as a result of changes in the normal components of bile.

Although there are two types of stones, pigment and cholesterol stones, most types of gallstone disease in the United States, Europe, and Africa are from cholesterol stones (Wilson and Lester, 1992). Most cholesterol stones are not pure cholesterol but a mixture of cholesterol, calcium salts, bile acids, fatty acids, protein, and phospholipids, with some fraction of bile pigment at the center.

Cholelithiasis, the presence or formation of gallstones, is the fifth leading cause of hospitalization among adults and accounts for 90 per cent of all gallbladder and duct diseases. The incidence of gallstones increases with age, occurring in more than 40 per cent of people over 70 years of age (Steinberg, 1983).

The risk factors to look for in a client's history that correlate with the incidence of gallstones include the following:

- Age: incidence increases with age
- Sex: women affected more than men
- Elevated estrogen levels
  - Pregnancy
  - Oral contraceptives
  - Postmenopausal therapy
  - Multiparity (woman who has had two or more pregnancies resulting in viable offspring)
- Obesity
- Diet: high cholesterol, low fiber
- Diabetes mellitus
- Liver disease

Although the formation of gallstones is not well understood, three specific factors appear to contribute: metabolic factors, stasis, and inflammation (Cassmeyer, 1991b).

An increased content of any one of the three bile constituents (bile acids, bile pigments, and cholesterol) can result in precipitation of these substances, causing stone formation. An increased serum cholesterol level is an example of a *metabolic disorder* and occurs in situations such as diabetes mellitus, pregnancy, and obesity. Approximately 75 per cent of gallstones in Western cultures are cholesterol stones (Cassmeyer, 1991b).

Biliary stasis leads to stagnation of bile, excessive resorption of water by the gallbladder, and subsequent mixed stone formation. Situations of delayed gallbladder emptying, such as obstructions caused by liver pathology, hormonal influences, and pregnancy, can facilitate biliary stasis.

Inflammation of the biliary system causes the bile constituents to become altered, with stone formation occurring from these changes (Cassmeyer, 1991b).

Clients with gallstones may be asymptomatic or may present with symptoms of a gallbladder attack described in the next section. The prognosis is usually good with medical treatment, depending on the severity of disease, presence of infection, and response to antibiotics.

Cholecystitis

Cholecystitis, or inflammation of the gallbladder, may be acute or chronic and occurs as a result of impaction of gallstones in the cystic duct (see Fig. 8–1), causing painful distention of the gallbladder. Other causes of acute cholecystitis

Clinical Signs and Symptoms of
Acute Cholecystitis

- Chills, low-grade fever
- Jaundice
- GI symptoms
  - Nausea
  - Anorexia
  - Vomiting
- Tenderness over the gallbladder
- Severe pain in the right upper quadrant and epigastrium (increases on inspiration and movement)
- Pain radiating into the right shoulder and between the scapulae

▼ *Clinical Signs and Symptoms of*

Chronic Cholecystitis

These may be vague or a sense of indigestion and abdominal discomfort after eating, unless a stone leaves the gallbladder and causes obstruction of the common duct (called choledocholithiasis), causing

- Biliary colic: severe, steady pain for 3 to 4 hours in the right upper quadrant
- Pain: may radiate to the midback between the scapulae (due to splanchnic fibers synapsing with phrenic nerve fibers)
- Nausea (intolerance of fatty foods: decreased bile production results in decreased fat digestion)
- Abdominal fullness
- Heartburn
- Excessive belching
- Constipation and diarrhea

may be typhoid fever or a malignant tumor obstructing the biliary tract. Whatever the cause of the obstruction, the normal flow of bile is interrupted and the gallbladder becomes distended and ischemic. The acute form is most common during middle age; the chronic form, among the elderly (Kallsen, 1993).

Gallstones may also cause chronic cholecystitis (persistent gallbladder inflammation) in which the gallbladder atrophies and becomes fibrotic, adhering to adjacent organs. It is not unusual for clients to have repeated episodes before seeking medical attention (O'Toole, 1992).

Prognosis and Treatment. Prognosis for both acute and chronic cholecystitis is good with medical intervention, which may include controlling the symptoms with dietary measures (e.g., restriction of fat and alcohol intake, eating smaller meals more often) or surgical removal of the gallbladder (cholecystectomy).

Case Example. A 48-year-old schoolteacher was admitted to the hospital following an episode of intense, sharp pain that started in the epigastric region and radiated around her thorax to the interscapular area. Her gallbladder had been removed 2 years ago, but she remarked that her current symptoms were "exactly like a gallbladder attack." The client was referred to physical therapy for "back care/education" on the day of discharge.

On examination, the client was in acute distress, unable to tolerate a full examination. She had not been able to transfer or ambulate independently. She was instructed in relaxation and breathing techniques to reduce her extreme level of anxiety associated with pain and given supportive reassurance. Instruction and assistance was provided in all transfers to minimize pain and maximize independent function. Given her discharge status, outpatient physical therapy was recommended for follow-up.

She returned to physical therapy as planned and was provided with a back care program. She was also treated locally for scar tissue adhesion at the site of the gallbladder removal. Symptomatic relief was obtained in the first two sessions without recurrence of symptoms. This case example is included to demonstrate how scar tissue associated with organ removal can reproduce visceral symptoms that are actually of musculoskeletal origin—the opposite concept of what we are presenting in this text.

Primary Biliary Cirrhosis

Primary biliary cirrhosis (PBC) is a chronic, progressive, inflammatory disease of the liver that involves primarily the intrahepatic bile ducts and results in impairment of bile secretion. The disease, which often affects middle-aged women, begins with pruritus or biochemical evidence of

▼ *Clinical Signs and Symptoms of*
Primary Biliary Cirrhosis

- Pruritus
- Jaundice
- GI bleeding
- Ascites
- Fatigue
- Right upper quadrant pain (posterior)
- Sensory neuropathy of hands/feet (rare)
- Osteoporosis (decreased bone mass)
- Osteomalacia (softening of the bones)
- Burning, pins and needles, prickling of the eyes
- Muscle cramping

cholestasis and progresses at a variable rate to jaundice, portal hypertension, and liver failure. The cause of PBC is unknown, although various factors are being investigated (Wilson and Lester, 1992).

Many clients have associated autoimmune features, particularly Sjögren's syndrome, autoimmune thyroiditis, and renal tubular acidosis. The most significant clinical problem for PBC clients is bone disease characterized by impaired osteoblastic activity and accelerated osteoclastic activity. Calcium and vitamin D should be carefully monitored and appropriate replacement instituted. Physical activity following an osteoporosis protocol should be encouraged (Carithers, 1993).

No specific treatment has been established yet for PBC other than liver transplantation or supportive measures for the clinical symptoms described.

Overview LIVER/BILIARY PAIN PATTERNS

LIVER PAIN (see Fig. 8–5)

Location:
Pain in the midepigastrium or right upper quadrant (RUQ) of abdomen
Pain over the liver, especially after exercise (hepatitis)

Referral:
Right upper quadrant pain may be associated with right shoulder pain
Both right upper quadrant and epigastrium pain may be associated with back pain between the scapulae
Pain may be referred to the right side of the midline in the interscapular or subscapular area

Description:
Dull abdominal aching
Sense of fullness of the abdomen or epigastrium

Intensity:
Mild at first, then increases steadily

Duration:
Constant

Associated Signs and Symptoms:
Nausea, anorexia (viral hepatitis)
Early satiety (cystic tumors)
Aversion to smoking for smokers (viral hepatitis)
Aversion to alcohol (hepatitis)
Arthralgias and myalgias (hepatitis A or B)

Headaches (hepatitis A, drug-induced hepatitis)

Dizziness/drowsiness (drug-induced hepatitis)

Low-grade fever (hepatitis A)

Pharyngitis (hepatitis A)

Extreme fatigue (hepatitis A, cirrhosis)

Alterations in the sense of taste and smell (hepatitis A)

Rash (hepatitis B)

Jaundice

Dark urine, light or clay-colored stools

Ascites

Edema and oliguria

Neurologic symptoms (hepatic encephalopathy)
  Confusion, forgetfulness
  Muscle tremors
  Asterixis
  Slurred speech
  Impaired handwriting

Pallor (often linked with cirrhosis or carcinoma)

Bleeding disorders
  Purpura
  Ecchymosis

Spider angiomas

Palmar erythema

Diaphoresis (liver abscess)

Overall muscular weakness (cirrhosis, liver carcinoma)

Peripheral neuropathy (chronic liver disease)

Possible Etiology:	Any liver disease
	Hepatitis
	Cirrhosis
	Metastatic tumors
	Pancreatic carcinoma
	Liver abscess
	Medications: use of hepatotoxic drugs

■ ■ ■ ■ ■ ■ ■ ■ ■ ■ ■

GALLBLADDER PAIN (see Fig. 8–5)

Location:	Pain in the midepigastrium (heartburn)
	Right upper quadrant of abdomen
Referral:	Right upper quadrant pain may be associated with right shoulder pain
	Both may be associated with back pain between the scapulae

	Pain may be referred to the right side of the midline in the interscapular or subscapular area
Description:	Dull aching
	Deep visceral pain (gallbladder suddenly distends)
	Biliary carcinoma is more persistent and boring
Intensity:	Mild at first, then increases steadily to become severe
Duration:	2 to 3 hours
Aggravating Factors:	
	Respiratory inspiration
	Upper body movement
	Lying down
Associated Signs and Symptoms:	
	Dark urine, light stools
	Jaundice
	Skin: green hue (prolonged biliary obstruction)
	Persistent pruritus (cholestatic jaundice)
	Pain and nausea occur 1 to 3 hours after eating (gallstones)
	Pain immediately after eating (gallbladder inflammation)
	Intolerance of fatty foods or heavy meals
	Indigestion, nausea
	Excessive belching
	Flatulence (excessive intestinal gas)
	Anorexia
	Weight loss (gallbladder cancer)
	Bleeding from skin and mucous membranes (late sign of gallbladder cancer)
	Vomiting
	Feeling of fullness
	Low-grade fever, chills
Possible Etiology:	
	Gallstones (cholelithiasis)
	Gallbladder inflammation (cholecystitis)
	Neoplasm
	Medications: use of hepatotoxic drugs

■ ■ ■ ■ ■ ■ ■ ■ ■ ■ ■ ■

COMMON BILE DUCT PAIN (see Fig. 8–5)

Location:	Pain in midepigastrium or right upper quadrant of abdomen
Referral:	Epigastrium: heartburn (choledocholithiasis)

Right upper quadrant pain may be associated with right shoulder pain

Both may be associated with back pain between the scapulae

Pain may be referred to the right side of the midline in the interscapular or subscapular area

Description:	Dull aching
	Vague discomfort (pressure within common bile duct increasing)
	Severe, steady pain in right upper quadrant (choledocholithiasis)
	Biliary carcinoma is more persistent and boring
Intensity:	Mild at first, increases steadily
Duration:	Constant
	3 to 4 hours (choledocholithiasis)
Associated Signs and Symptoms:	Dark urine, light stools
	Jaundice
	Nausea after eating
	Intolerance of fatty foods or heavy meals
	Feeling of abdominal fullness
	Skin: green hue (prolonged biliary obstruction)
	Low-grade fever, chills
	Excessive belching (choledocholithiasis)
	Constipation and diarrhea (choledocholithiasis)
	Sensory neuropathy (primary biliary cirrhosis)
	Osteomalacia (primary biliary cirrhosis)
	Osteoporosis (primary biliary cirrhosis)
Possible Etiology:	Common duct stones
	Common duct stricture (previous gallbladder surgery)
	Pancreatic carcinoma (blocking the bile duct)
	Medications: use of hepatotoxic drugs
	Neoplasm
	Primary biliary cirrhosis
	Choledocholithiasis (obstruction of common duct)

PHYSICIAN REFERRAL

A careful history and close observation of the client are important in determining whether a person may need a medical referral for possible hepatic or biliary involvement. Any client presenting with mid-back, scapular, or right shoulder pain without a history of trauma (including forceful movement of the spine, repetitive movements of the shoulder or back, or easy lifting) (Table 8–6) should be screened for possible systemic origin of symptoms.

For the physical therapist treating the in-

Table 8–6

REFERRED PAIN PATTERNS: LIVER, GALLBLADDER, COMMON BILE DUCT

Systemic Causes	Location
Thorax/Scapulae Area	
Gallbladder	Midback between scapulae; right upper trapezius
Acute cholecystitis	Right subscapular area, between scapulae
Biliary colic	Right upper back, midback between scapulae; right interscapular or subscapular areas
Shoulder Area	
Liver disease (abscess, cirrhosis, tumors, hepatitis)	Right shoulder, right subscapular
Ruptured spleen	Left shoulder
Gallbladder disease	Right upper trapezius
Acute cholecystitis irritating diaphragm	Right shoulder; between scapulae; right subscapular area

patient population, jaundice in the postoperative individual is not uncommon and may be a potentially serious complication of surgery and anesthesia. Clinical management of jaundice is complicated by anything capable of damaging the liver, including stress (emotional or physical), hypoxemia, blood loss, infection, and administration of multiple drugs.

When making the referral, it is important to report to the physician the results of your objective findings, especially when there is a lack of physical evidence to support a musculoskeletal lesion. The *Special Questions to Ask* may assist in assessing the client's overall health status.

Systemic Signs and Symptoms Requiring Physician Referral

Whenever the client reports any of the following accompanying systemic signs or symptoms that have not been evaluated or treated, the physician should be notified.

Alterations in sense of smell/taste
Anorexia
Arthralgias
Ascites
Asterixis
Aversion to cigarettes, alcohol
Changes in skin color (yellow, green)
Chills, fever
Constipation
Dark urine
Diaphoresis
Diarrhea
Dizziness
Drowsiness
Early satiety
Ecchymosis
Edema

Excessive belching
Fatigue
Feeling of abdominal fullness
Fever, chills
Flatulence
Headaches
Heartburn
Intolerance to fatty foods
Jaundice
Light-colored stools
Malaise
Mental confusion
Muscle tremors
Myalgias
Nausea, especially after eating
Oliguria (reduced urine secretion)
Pallor
Palmar erythema

Pharyngitis	Restlessness	Tachycardia
Pruritus (itching)	Skin rash	Vomiting
Purpura (subcutaneous bleeding)	Slurred speech	Weakness
	Spider angiomas	*See also* Table 8–5

Key Points to Remember

- Primary signs and symptoms of liver diseases vary and can include GI symptoms, edema/ascites, dark urine, light-colored or clay-colored feces, and right upper abdominal pain.

- Neurologic symptoms such as confusion, muscle tremors, and asterixis may occur.

- Skin changes associated with the hepatic system include jaundice, pallor, orange or green skin, bruising, spider angiomas, and palmar erythema.

- Active, intense exercise should be avoided when the liver is compromised (jaundice or other active disease).

- Antiinflammatory and minor analgesic agents can cause drug-induced hepatitis. Nonviral hepatitis may occur postoperatively.

- When liver dysfunction results in increased serum ammonia and urea levels, peripheral nerve function is impaired. Flapping tremors (asterixis) and numbness/tingling (carpal tunnel syndrome) can occur.

- Musculoskeletal locations of pain associated with the hepatic and biliary systems include thoracic spine between scapulae, right shoulder, right upper trapezius, right interscapular, right subscapular areas.

- Referred shoulder pain may be the only presenting symptom of hepatic or biliary disease.

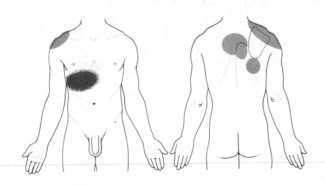

SUBJECTIVE EXAMINATION	*Special Questions to Ask*

Have you ever had an ulcer, anemia, gallbladder disease, your spleen removed **(splenectomy),** or hepatitis/jaundice?

- If yes to hepatitis or jaundice: Do you remember how you got this? or How did you get this?

- Do you have any contact with rodents or exposure to toxins (carbon tetrachloride, beryllium, or vinyl chloride)? (Predispose to hepatic disease)

- Do you work in a clinical laboratory or with dialysis patients? **(Hepatitis)**

- Have you been out of the United States in the last 6 to 12 months? **(Parasitic infection, country where hepatitis is endemic)**

- Have you had any recent contact with hepatitis or with a jaundiced person?

- Have you eaten any raw shellfish recently? **(Jaundice)**

- Have you had any recent blood or plasma transfusion, blood tests, acupuncture, ear piercing, tattoos, or dental work done? **(Viral hepatitis)**

- Have you had any kind of injury or trauma to your abdomen? **(Possible damage to the liver)**

- Do you bruise or bleed easily? **(Liver disease)**

- Have you noticed any change in the color of your stools or urine? **(Dark urine, light or clay-colored stools associated with jaundice)**

- Has your weight fluctuated 10 to 15 pounds or more recently without a change in diet? **(Cancer, cirrhosis, ascites)**

- Have you noticed your clothes fitting tighter around the waist from abdominal swelling or bloating? **(Ascites)**

- Do you have a feeling of fullness after only one or two bites of food? **(Early satiety: stomach and duodenum, cystic tumors, or gallbladder)**

- Does your stomach feel swollen or bloated after eating? **(Abdominal fullness)**

- Do you have any abdominal pain? (Abdominal pain may be *visceral* from an internal organ [dull, general, poorly localized], *parietal* from inflammation of overlying peritoneum [sharp, precisely localized, aggravated by movement], or *referred* from a disorder in another site) (Jarvis, 1992).

- Does eating relieve your pain? **(Duodenal or pyloric ulcer)**

  - How soon after eating?

- Does eating aggravate your pain? **(Gastric ulcer, gallbladder inflammation)**

- Are there any particular foods you have noticed that aggravate your symptoms?

  - If yes, which ones? **(Intolerance to fatty foods)**

■ **For clients with only shoulder or back pain:** Have you noticed any association between when you eat and when your symptoms increase or decrease?

■ Has anyone in your family ever been diagnosed with Wilson's disease **(excessive copper retention)** or hemochromatosis **(excessive iron absorption)? (Hereditary)**

■ When asking about drug history, keep in mind that oral contraceptives may cause cholestasis (suppression of bile flow) or liver tumors. Some common over-the-counter drugs (e.g., acetaminophen) may have hepatotoxic effects.

■ **For women:** Are you currently using oral contraceptives? **(Hepatitis, adenoma)**

■ Use questions to determine possible consumption of alcohol as a hepatotoxin.

■ Have you noticed any unusual aversion to odors, food alcohol, or (for people who smoke) smoking? **(Jaundice)**

CASE STUDY

REFFERAL

A 29-year-old male law student has come to you (self-referral) with whiplash injury with headaches; the accident occurred 18 months ago.

The headaches occur two to three times each week, starting at the base of the occiput and progressing up the back of his head to localize in the forehead, bilaterally. The client has a sedentary life style with no regular exercise, and he describes his stress level as being 6 on a scale from 0 to 10. The Family/Personal History form indicates that he has had hepatitis.

PHYSICAL THERAPY INTERVIEW

What follow-up questions will you ask this client related to the hepatitis?

Introductory remarks: I see from your History form that you have had hepatitis.

When did you have hepatitis?

(Remember the three stages when trying to determine whether this person may still be contagious, requiring handwashing and hygiene precautions, including avoidance of any body fluids on your part through the use of protective gloves. This is especially true when treating a person with diabetes requiring fingerstick blood testing while in the physical therapy department.)

Do you know how you initially came in contact with hepatitis?

(In this person's case, the only possible cause he can postulate is a shot he received for influenza when he was travelling with a singing group in a rural area of the United States. This information is inconclusive in assisting the physician to establish a direct causative factor.) Other considerations requiring further questioning may include:

- Illicit or recreational drug use
- Poor sanitation in close quarters with travel companion
- Ingestion of contaminated food, water, milk, or seafood
- Recent blood transfusion or contact with blood/blood products
- For type B: modes of sexual transmission

What type of hepatitis did you have?

Give the client a chance to respond, but you may have to prompt with "type A," "type B," or "types C or D." (Remember that hepatitis A is communicable before the appearance of any observable clinical symptoms [i.e., during the initial and icteric stages that usually last from 1 to 6 weeks]. Hepatitis B can persist in body fluids indefinitely, requiring necessary precautions by you.)

MEDICAL TREATMENT

Did you receive any medical treatment? (In this case, the client and the members of his travelling group received gamma globulin shots.)

How soon after you were diagnosed did you receive the gamma globulin shots?

(Gamma globulin shots are considered most effective in producing passive immunity for 3 to 4 months when administered as soon as possible after exposure to the hepatitis virus, but within 2 weeks after the onset of jaundice.)

Are you currently receiving follow-up care for your hepatitis through a local physician?

(This information will assist you in determining the appropriate medical source for further information if you need it and, in a case like this, assist you in choosing further follow-up questions that may help you determine whether this person requires additional medical follow-up. If the client is receiving no further medical follow-up [especially if no gamma globulin was administered initially*], consider these follow-up questions):

ASSOCIATED SYMPTOMS

What symptoms did you have with hepatitis?

Do you have any of those symptoms now?

Are you experiencing any unusual fatigue or muscle or joint aches and pains?

Have you noticed any unusual aversion to foods, alcohol, or cigarettes/smoke that you did not have before?

Have you had any problems with diarrhea, vomiting, or nausea?

---

* Persons who have been treated with human immune serum globulin (ISG) may not develop jaundice, but those who have not received the gamma globulin usually develop jaundice.

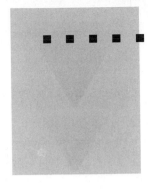

■ Have you noticed any change in the color of your stools or urine?
(One to 4 days before the icteric stage, the urine darkens and the stool lightens.)

■ Have you noticed any unusual skin rash developing recently?

■ When did you notice the headaches developing?
(Try to correlate this with the onset of hepatitis, because headaches can be persistent symptoms of hepatitis A.)

References

Andrews, M., and Huether, S.: Alteration of digestive function in children. *In* McCance, K., and Huether, S. (eds.): Pathophysiology; The Biologic Basis for Disease in Adults and Children. St. Louis, C.V. Mosby, 1990, pp. 1267–1292.

Buchan, P.C.: Pathogenesis of neonatal hyperbilirubinemia after induction of labour with oxytocin. British Medical Journal *2*:1255, 1979.

Carithers, R.L.: Liver diseases. *In* Ramsey, P.G., and Larson, E.B.: Medical Therapeutics, 2nd ed. Philadelphia, W.B. Saunders, 1993, pp. 330–373.

Cassmeyer, V.: Management of persons with liver problems. *In* Phipps, W., Long, B., Woods, N., and Cassmeyer, V. (eds.): Medical-Surgical Nursing; Concepts and Clinical Practice, 4th ed. St. Louis, Mosby–Year Book, 1991a, pp. 1139–1150.

Cassmeyer, V.: Management of persons with problems of the gallbladder and exocrine pancreas. *In* Phipps, W., Long, B., Woods, N., and Cassmeyer, V. (eds.): Medical-Surgical Nursing; Concepts and Clinical Practice, 4th ed. St. Louis, Mosby–Year Book, 1991b, pp. 1363–1384

Deiss, A.: Wilson's disease. *In* Wyngaarden, J.B., Smith, L.H., and Bennett, J.C. (eds.): Cecil's Textbook of Medicine, 19th ed. Philadelphia, W.B. Saunders, 1992, pp. 1132–1133.

Elrod, R.: Nursing role in management problems of the liver, biliary tract and pancreas. *In* Lewis, S., and Collier, I. (eds.): Medical-Surgical Nursing; Assessment and Management of Clinical Problems, 3rd ed. St. Louis, C.V. Mosby, 1992, pp. 1121–1168.

Gocke, D.J.: Systemic manifestations of viral liver disease. *In* Gitnick, G.L. (ed.): Current Hepatology. Vol. 2. New York, John Wiley and Sons, 1982, pp. 273–288.

Guyton, A.: Human Physiology and Mechanisms of Disease, 5th ed. Philadelphia, W.B. Saunders, 1992.

Jarvis, C.: Physical Examination and Health Assessment. Philadelphia, W.B. Saunders, 1992.

Kallsen, C.: Nursing care of clients with biliary and exocrine pancreatic disorders. *In* Black, J., and Matassarin-Jacobs, E. (eds.): Luckmann and Sorensen's Medical-Surgical Nursing; A Pathophysiologic Approach, 4th ed. Philadelphia, W.B. Saunders, 1993, pp. 1731–1754.

Kuo, G., Choo, Q.L., and Alter, H.J.: An assay for circulating antibodies to a major etiologic virus of human non-A, non-B hepatitis. Science *244*:362–364, 1989.

Lab Tech/Med Tech Bulletin: Detection of antibody to Hepatitis C virus. August 1990, pp. 1–2.

Larson, A.W., Cohen, H., Zweiban, B., et al.: Acute esophageal variceal sclerotherapy. Results of a prospective randomized controlled trial. Journal of the American Medical Association *255*:497–500, 1986.

Marx, J.: Viral hepatitis: Unscrambling the alphabet. Nursing 93, *23*(1): 34–41, 1993.

Matassarin-Jacobs, E., and Strasburg, K.: Nursing care of clients with hepatic disorders. *In* Black, J., and Matassarin-Jacobs, E. (eds.): Luckmann and Sorensen's Medical-Surgical Nursing; A Pathophysiologic Approach, 4th ed. Philadelphia, W.B. Saunders, 1993, pp. 1697–1730.

Motulsky, A.G.: Hemochromatosis (iron storage disease). *In* Wyngaarden, J.B., Smith, L.H., and Bennett, J.C. (eds.): Cecil's Textbook of Medicine, 19th ed. Philadelphia, W.B. Saunders, 1992, pp. 1133–1136.

O'Toole, M. (ed.): Miller-Keane Encyclopedia and Dictionary of Medicine, Nursing, and Allied Health, 5th ed. Philadelphia, W.B. Saunders, 1992.

Pascal, J.-P., and Cales, P.: Multicenter Study Group: Propranolol in the prevention of first upper gastrointestinal tract hemorrhage in patients with cirrhosis of the liver and esophageal varices. New England Journal of Medicine *317*:856–861, 1987.

Purtilo, D.T., and Purtilo, R.B.: A Survey of Human Diseases, 2nd ed. Boston, Little, Brown, 1989.

Ridge, J.A., and Way, L.W.: Abdominal pain. *In* Sleisenger, M.H. (ed.): Gastrointestinal Disease, 5th ed. Philadelphia, J.B. Lippincott, 1993, pp. 150–161.

Sherlock, S., and Dooley, J.: Diseases of the Liver and Biliary System, 9th ed. Oxford, England, Blackwell Scientific Publications, 1993.

Singh, S., and Singh, M.: Pathogenesis of oxytocin-induced neonatal hyperbilirubinemia. Archives of Disease in Childhood *54*:400, 1979.

Smeltzer, S., and Bare, B.: Brunner and Suddarth's

Medical-Surgical Nursing, 7th ed. New York, J.B. Lippincott, 1992, pp. 971–1021.

Steinberg, F.U.: Care of the Geriatric Patient. St. Louis, C.V. Mosby, 1983.

Stewart, J.S., Farrow, J.L., Clifford, R.E., et al.: A three-year survey of viral hepatitis in West London. Quarterly Journal of Medicine *187*:365, 1978.

Strasburg, K., and Matassarin-Jacobs, E.: Structure and function of the liver, biliary system, and exocrine pancreas. *In* Black, J., and Matassarin-Jacobs, E. (eds.): Luckmann and Sorensen's Medical-Surgical Nursing; A Pathophysiologic Approach, 4th ed. Philadelphia, W.B. Saunders, 1993, pp. 1677–1684.

Wilson, L., and Lester, L.: Liver, biliary tract and pancreas. *In* Price, S., and Wilson, L. (eds.): Pathophysiology; Clinical Concepts of Disease Processes, 4th ed. St. Louis, Mosby–Year Book, 1992, pp. 337–368.

Appendix

Universal Precautions to Prevent Occupational Transmission of HIV and Hepatitis B Virus

The increasing prevalence of HIV increases the risk that health care workers will be exposed to blood from clients infected with HIV or Hepatitis B, especially when blood and body fluid precautions are not followed for all clients. The Centers for Disease Control and Prevention emphasize the need for health care workers to consider *all* clients as being potentially infected with HIV or other blood-borne pathogens and to adhere rigorously to infection control precautions for minimizing the risk of exposure to blood and body fluids of all clients.

Therapists at greatest risk include those who perform electromyographic (EMG) studies and those who provide decubitus or pressure ulcer care, treat open wounds, handle bandages and dressings, and provide temporomandibular joint (TMJ) treatment. Any therapist who assists in patient toiletting or changing diapers (adults or children) is at increased risk. Other risk factors include human bites, contact with sputum and pleural fluid tinged with blood, and exposure to blood-borne pathogens when working with hospice clients who have AIDS.

Although the potential for HBV transmission in the workplace is greater than that for HIV, the modes of transmission for these two viruses are similar. Both have been transmitted in occupational settings **only** by percutaneous inoculation or contact with an open wound, nonintact (e.g., chapped, abraded, weeping, or dermatitic) skin, or mucous membranes with blood, blood-contaminated body fluids, or concentrated virus. **Blood is the single most important source of HIV and HBV in the workplace.**

In the hospital and other health care settings, universal precautions should be followed when workers are exposed to blood, certain other body fluids (amniotic fluid, pericardial fluid, peritoneal fluid, pleural fluid, synovial fluid, cerebrospinal fluid, semen, and vaginal secretions), or any body fluid visibly contaminated with blood. The hepatitis B vaccine substantially reduces the risk of infection and should be available to all employees who have occupational exposure to the virus.

Because HIV and HBV transmission has not been documented from exposure to other body fluids (feces, nasal secretions, sputum, sweat, tears, urine, and vomitus), universal precautions do not apply to these fluids. Universal precautions also do not apply to saliva, except in the dental setting, where saliva is likely to be contaminated with blood.

Adapted from Centers for Disease Control: Guidelines for Prevention of HIV and Hepatitis B Virus Transmission to Health Care and Public Safety Workers. Morbidity and Mortality Weekly Report *38*:S-6, June 23, 1989.

- All health care workers should routinely use appropriate barrier precautions to prevent skin and mucous membrane exposure when contact with blood or other body fluids of any person is anticipated. Gloves should be worn for touching
  - Blood and body fluids
  - Mucous membranes
  - Nonintact skin of all patients/clients
  - Items or surfaces soiled with blood or body fluids
- Gloves should be changed after contact with each client.
- Masks and protective eyewear or face shields should be worn during procedures that are likely to generate droplets of blood or other body fluids, to prevent exposure of mucous membranes of the mouth, nose, and eyes.
- Gowns or aprons should be worn during procedures that are likely to generate splashes of blood or other body fluids.
- Hands and other skin surfaces should be washed immediately and thoroughly if contaminated with blood or other body fluids. Hands should be washed immediately after gloves are removed.
- All health care workers should take precautions to prevent injuries
  - Caused by sharp instruments, such as scissors or scalpels during procedures

  - When handling sharp instruments after procedures
  - When cleaning used instruments
  - During disposal of used needles. Dispose of needles and sharp instruments in a puncture-resistant container
- Although saliva has not been implicated in the transmission of HIV or Hepatitis B, to minimize the need for emergency mouth-to-mouth resuscitation, mouthpieces, resuscitation bags, or other ventilation devices should be available for use in areas in which the need for resuscitation is predictable.
- Health care workers who have exudative lesions or weeping dermatitis should refrain from all direct client care and from handling patient-care equipment until the condition resolves.
- Pregnant health care workers are not known to be at a greater risk of contracting HIV infection than health care workers who are not pregnant; however, if a health care worker develops HIV infection during pregnancy, the infant is at risk of infection resulting from perinatal transmission. Because of this risk, pregnant health care workers should be especially familiar with and strictly adhere to precautions to minimize the risk of HIV transmission.

9

Overview of Endocrine and Metabolic Signs and Symptoms

■ ■ ■ ■ ■ ■ ■ ■ ■ ■ ■ ■

Clinical Signs and Symptoms of:

Diabetes Insipidus
Syndrome of Inappropriate Secretion
  of Antidiuretic Hormone
Acromegaly
Adrenal Insufficiency
Cushing's Syndrome
Goiter
Thyroiditis
Thyroid Carcinoma
Untreated or Uncontrolled Diabetes
  Mellitus
Diabetic Ketoacidosis
Hyperglycemic, Hyperosmolar,
  Nonketotic Coma

Hypoglycemia
Dehydration or Fluid Loss
Water Intoxication
Edema
Metabolic Alkalosis
Metabolic Acidosis
Gout
Hemochromatosis
Osteoporosis
Osteomalacia
Paget's Disease
Ochronosis

The musculoskeletal system is composed of a variety of connective tissue structures in which normal growth and development are influenced strongly and sometimes controlled by various hormones and metabolic processes.

Alterations in these control systems can result in structural changes and altered function of various connective tissues, producing musculoskeletal signs and symptoms including muscle weakness, fatigue, and pain; carpal tunnel syndrome; crystal deposition and other findings in synovial fluid; periarthritis; chondrocalcinosis; spondyloarthropathy; and hand stiffness (Louthrenoo and Schumacher, 1990).

Muscle weakness, myalgia, and fatigue may be early manifestations of thyroid or parathyroid disease, acromegaly, diabetes, Cushing's syndrome, and osteomalacia. In endocrine disease, most proximal muscle weakness is usually painless and unrelated to either the severity or the duration of the underlying disease.

Bilateral carpal tunnel syndrome (CTS) resulting from median nerve compression at the wrist is a common finding in people with certain endocrine and metabolic disorders (Beard et al., 1985; Bluestone et al., 1971), including

- Myxedema associated with hypothyroidism
- Diabetes mellitus
- Graves' disease
- Rheumatoid arthritis
- Acromegaly (abnormal enlargement of the skeleton)
- Benign tumors (e.g., lipomata, hemangiomata, ganglia)
- Deposits of gouty tophi and calcium
- Multiple myeloma (amyloidosis)

Thickening of the transverse carpal ligament itself may be sufficient to compress the median nerve in certain systemic disorders (e.g., acromegaly, myxedema), and any condition that increases the volume of the contents of the carpal tunnel compresses the median nerve (e.g., neoplasm, calcium, and gouty tophi deposits). The fact that the majority of people with CTS are women at or near menopause suggests that the soft tissues about the wrist may be affected in some way by hormones (Grossman et al., 1961; Phalen, 1966). Bilateral median nerve neuritis has long been recognized as the first symptom of multiple myeloma, rheumatoid arthritis, and amyloid disease, both primary and secondary (Grokoest and Demartini, 1954).

Periarthritis (inflammation of periarticular structures, including the tendons, liga-

Table 9–1

ENDOCRINE AND METABOLIC DISORDERS ASSOCIATED WITH CHONDROCALCINOSIS

Endocrine	Metabolic
Hypothyroidism	Hemochromatosis
Hyperparathyroidism	Hypomagnesemia
Acromegaly	Hypophosphatasia
	Ochronosis
	Oxalosis
	Wilson's disease

Adapted from Louthrenoo, W., and Schumacher, H.R.: Musculoskeletal clues to endocrine or metabolic disease. Journal of Musculoskeletal Medicine, 7(9):41, 1990.

ments, and joint capsule) and *calcific tendinitis* occur most often in the shoulders of people who have endocrine disease. *Chondrocalcinosis* (deposition of calcium salts in the cartilage of joints; when accompanied by attacks of goutlike symptoms, it is called *pseudogout*) is commonly seen on x-ray films as calcified hyaline or fibrous cartilage. In 5 per cent to 10 per cent of people with chondrocalcinosis, there is an associated underlying endocrine or metabolic disease, such as hypothyroidism, hyperparathyroidism, and acromegaly (Table 9–1) (Louthrenoo and Schumacher, 1990).

Spondyloarthropathy (disease of joints of the spine) and *osteoarthritis* occur in individuals with various metabolic or endocrine diseases, including hemochromatosis (disorder of iron metabolism with excess deposition of iron in the tissues; also known as bronze diabetes and iron storage disease), ochronosis (metabolic disorder resulting in discoloration of body tissues caused by deposits of alkapton bodies), acromegaly, and diabetes mellitus.

Hand stiffness and hand pain, as well as arthralgias of the small joints of the hand, can occur with endocrine and metabolic diseases. In persons with hypothyroidism, flexor tenosynovitis with stiffness is a common finding. This condition often accompanies CTS (Louthrenoo and Schumacher, 1990).

In the healthy person, bone growth and development are influenced by various hormones, especially the parathyroid hormone. Disorder of that hormone can produce bone pain. One cause of bone pain is fracture, a common complication of osteoporosis that is discussed later in this chapter (Hahn, 1989).

Endocrinology is the study of ductless (endocrine) glands that produce hormones. These hormones are released directly into the bloodstream, thus permitting effects at distant sites called target glands (Table 9–2). A hormone acts as a chemical agent that is transported by the bloodstream to target tissues, where it regulates or modifies the activity of the target cell.

The pituitary (hypophysis), thyroid, parathyroids, adrenals, and pineal are glands of the endocrine system whose functions are solely endocrine. Other glands in the body have dual functions. For example, the pancreas produces the hormone insulin from its islet cells, but it also produces digestive enzymes, which are carried by ducts and are thus exocrine.

The endocrine system cannot be understood fully without consideration of the nervous system's effects on the endocrine system. The hypothalamus can synthesize and release hormones from its axon terminals into the blood circulation. These *neurosecretory cells* are so called because the neurons have a hormone-secreting function (Marshall, 1986). Hormones that can stimulate the neural mechanism, resulting in the release of hormones and chemicals, such as acetylcholine (a neurotransmitter that is released at synapses to allow messages to pass along a nerve network), have been described as *neurohormones*. The interacting endocrine and neural systems can be considered to constitute the neuroendocrine system (Marshall, 1986).

Table 9–2
ENDOCRINE GLANDS: SECRETION, TARGET, AND ACTIONS*

Gland	Hormone	Target	Basic Action
Pituitary Gland			
ANTERIOR LOBE	Somatotropin (growth hormone [GH])	Bones, muscles, organs	Retention of nitrogen to promote protein anabolism
	Thyroid-stimulating hormone (TSH)	Thyroid	Promotes secretory activity
	Follicle-stimulating hormone (FSH)	Ovaries, seminiferous tubules	Promotes development of ovarian follicle, secretion of estrogen, and maturation of sperm
	Luteinizing hormone	Follicle, interstitial cell	Promotes ovulation and formation of corpus luteum, secretion of progesterone, and secretion of testosterone
	Prolactin (luteotropic hormone)	Corpus luteum, breast	Maintains corpus luteum and progesterone secretion; stimulates milk secretion
	Adrenocorticotropic hormone (ACTH)	Adrenal cortex	Stimulates secretory activity

*When reading a patient's chart, it is important to know basic hormone functions or effects that may have an impact on physical therapy treatment. At least 30 different hormones have been identified, but only those most common to physical therapy patients are included here.

Table continued on following page

Table 9–2
ENDOCRINE GLANDS: SECRETION, TARGET, AND ACTIONS* *Continued*

Gland	Hormone	Target	Basic Action
POSTERIOR LOBE	Antidiuretic hormone (ADH) Oxytocin	Distal tubules of kidney Uterus	Resorption of water Stimulates contraction
Thyroid	Thyroxine (T_4) Triiodothyronine (T_3)	Widespread	Regulates oxidation rate of body cells and growth and metabolism; influences gluconeogenesis, mobilization of fats, and exchange of water, electrolytes, and protein
	Calcitonin	Skeleton	Calcium and phosphorus metabolism
Parathyroids	Parathyroid hormone (PTH)	Bone, kidney, intestinal tract	Essential for calcium and phosphorus metabolism and calcification of bone
Adrenal Gland			
CORTEX	Mineralocorticoid (aldosterone)	Widespread, primarily kidney	Maintains fluid/electrolyte balance; resorbs sodium chloride; excretes potassium
	Glucocorticoids (cortisol)	Widespread	Concerned with food metabolism and body response to stress; preserves carbohydrates and mobilizes amino acids; promotes gluconeogenesis; suppresses inflammation
	Sex hormones (testosterone, estrogen, progesterone)	Gonads	Ability to influence secondary sex
MEDULLA	Epinephrine	Widespread	Vasoconstriction with increased blood pressure; increases blood sugar via glycolysis; stimulates ACTH production
	Norepinephrine	Widespread	Vasoconstriction
Pancreas	Insulin	Widespread	Increases utilization of carbohydrate, decreases lipolysis and protein catabolism; decreases blood sugar
	Glucagon	Widespread	Hyperglycemic factor; increases blood sugar via glycogenolysis
Gonads			
OVARIES	Estrogen	Widespread	Secondary sex characteristics; maturation and sexual function
	Progesterone	Uterus, breast	Preparation for and maintenance of pregnancy; development of mammary gland secretory tissue
TESTES	Testosterone	Widespread	Secondary sex characteristics; maturation and normal sex function

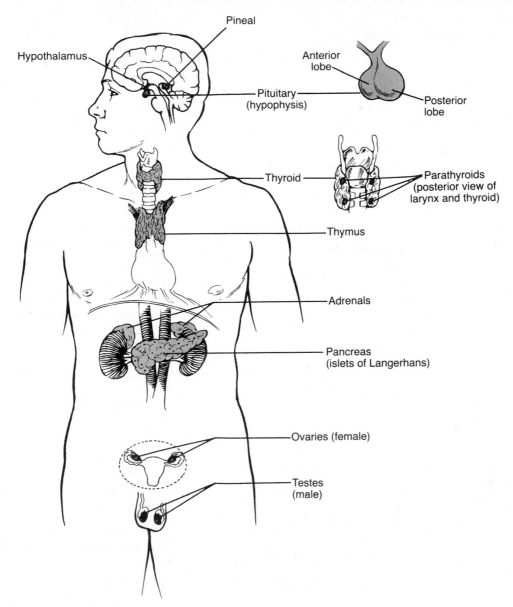

Figure 9–1

Location of the nine endocrine glands. (From Butts-Krakoff, D.: Structure and function: Assessment of clients with metabolic disorders. *In* Black, J.M., and Matassarin-Jacobs, E. [eds.]: Luckmann and Sorensen's Medical-Surgical Nursing, 4th ed. Philadelphia, W.B. Saunders, 1993, p. 1759.)

ENDOCRINE PHYSIOLOGY

The endocrine system works with the nervous system to regulate metabolism, water and salt balance, blood pressure, response to stress, and sexual reproduction. The endocrine system is slower in response and takes longer to act than the nervous system when transferring biochemical information. The glands shown in Figure 9–1 are part of the endocrine system and secrete essential hormones (see Table 9–2) into the bloodstream. The pituitary gland has been called the master gland, because its anterior lobe has direct control over the thyroid gland (thyroid-stimulating hormone [TSH]), adrenal cortex (adrenocorticotropic hormone [ACTH]), and the gonads (luteinizing hormone [LH] and follicle-stimulating hormone [FSH]). The hypothalamus controls pituitary function and thus has an important, indirect influence on the other glands of the endocrine system. Feedback mechanisms exist to keep hormones at normal levels.

Hypothalamus

The endocrine system meets the nervous system at the hypothalamic-pituitary interface. The hypothalamus and pituitary form an integrated axis that maintains control over much of the endocrine system. The hypothalamus exerts *direct* control over both the anterior and posterior portions of the pituitary gland. Disorders of the hypothalamic-pituitary axis are usually clinically manifested either by syndromes of hormone excess or deficiency or by visual impairment from optic nerve compression (Benson and Rosenthal, 1993).

The hypothalamus regulates pituitary activity through two pathways: a neural and a portal venous pathway. *Neural pathways* extend from the hypothalamus (Fig. 9–2), where two hormones—antidiuretic hormone (ADH) (also called vasopressin) and oxytocin—are synthesized, to the posterior pituitary lobe, where the hormones are stored and secreted. *Portal venous pathways,* which connect the hypothalamus to the anterior pituitary lobe, carry releasing and inhibiting hormones (Schteingart, 1992a).

Pituitary Gland

The pituitary is an oval gland measuring approximately 1 cm in diameter. It is lo-

cated at the base of the skull in an indentation of the sphenoid bone. The pituitary is joined to the hypothalamus by the pituitary stalk (neurohypophyseal tract). The pituitary gland consists of two parts: the anterior pituitary and the posterior pituitary. The anterior pituitary secretes six different hormones (see Table 9–2).

The posterior pituitary is a downward offshoot of the hypothalamus and contains many nerve fibers. The posterior pituitary produces no hormones of its own. The hormones ADH (vasopressin) and oxytocin are produced in the hypothalamus and then stored and released by the posterior pituitary. These hormones pass down nerve fibers from the hypothalamus through the pituitary stalk to nerve endings in the posterior pituitary. These two hormones accumulate in the posterior pituitary during less active periods of the body. Transmitter substances, such as acetylcholine and norepinephrine, are thought to activate the release of these substances by the posterior pituitary gland when they are stimulated by nerve impulses from the hypothalamus (Schteingart, 1992a).

Adrenal Glands

The adrenals are two small glands located on the upper part of each kidney. Each adrenal gland consists of two relatively discrete parts: an outer cortex and an inner medulla. The outer cortex is responsible for the secretion of mineralocorticoids (steroid hormones that regulate fluid and mineral balance), glucocorticoids (steroid hormones responsible for controlling the metabolism of glucose), and androgens (sex hormones). The centrally located adrenal medulla is derived from neural tissue and secretes epinephrine and norepinephrine, which exert widespread effects on vascular tone, the heart, and the nervous system, as well as affecting glucose metabolism. Together, the adrenal cortex and medulla are major factors in the body's response to stress (Marshall, 1986).

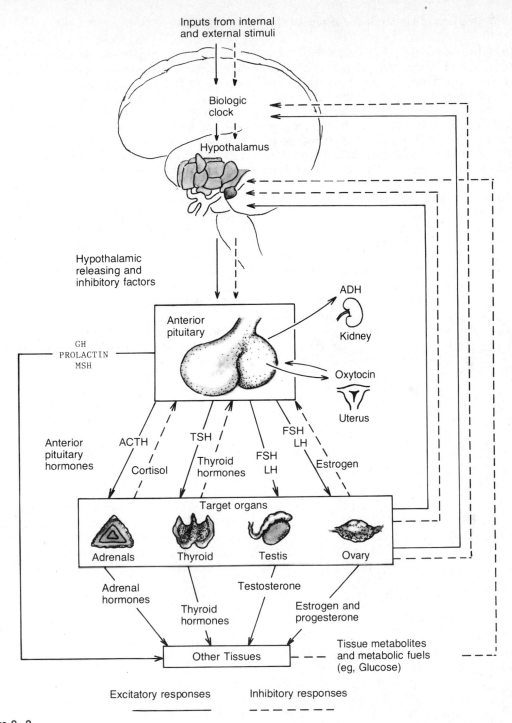

Figure 9–2

Control of the endocrine system by the nervous system. Note that the hypothalamus controls the pituitary gland through releasing and inhibiting factors. The anterior lobe of the pituitary gland then releases trophic (stimulating) hormones that act on target glands (thyroid, adrenals, and gonads). (From Purtilo, D.T., and Purtilo, R.B.: A Survey of Human Diseases, 2nd ed. Boston, Little, Brown, 1989.)

Thyroid Gland

The thyroid gland is located in the anterior portion of the lower neck below the larynx, on both sides of and anterior to the trachea. The chief hormones produced by the thyroid are thyroxine (T_4), triiodothyronine (T_3), and calcitonin. Both T_3 and T_4 regulate the metabolic rate of the body and increase protein synthesis (Marshall, 1986). Calcitonin has a weak physiologic effect on calcium and phosphorus balance in the body. Thyroid function is regulated by the hypothalamus and pituitary feedback controls, as well as by an intrinsic regulator mechanism within the gland itself (Guyton, 1992).

Thyroid disorders affect women more often than men and develop from functional or structural changes of the thyroid gland, or both. Changes in the thyroid's ability to function normally result in excessive or deficient levels of thyroid hormone. Thyroid gland enlargement may or may not be associated with abnormal thyroid hormone secretion. An enlarged thyroid gland can be the result of iodine deficiency, inflammation, or benign or malignant tumors (Birch, 1993).

Basic thyroid disorders of significance to physical therapy practice include goiter, hyperthyroidism, hypothyroidism, and cancer. Alterations in thyroid function produce changes in hair, nails, skin, eyes, gastrointestinal (GI) tract, respiratory tract, heart and blood vessels, nervous tissue, bone, and muscle (Guyton, 1992).

Parathyroid Glands

Two parathyroid glands are located on the posterior surface of each lobe of the thyroid gland. These glands secrete parathyroid hormone (PTH), which regulates calcium and phosphorus metabolism. Parathyroid disorders include hyperparathyroidism and hypoparathyroidism (Guyton, 1992).

Variations in location and color as well as the minute size of parathyroid glands make identification very difficult and may result in glandular damage or accidental removal during thyroid surgery. If damage or removal of these glands occurs, the resulting hypoparathyroidism (temporary or permanent) causes hypocalcemia, which can result in cardiac arrhythmias and neuromuscular irritability (tetany) (Birch, 1993).

The physical therapist will see clients with parathyroid disorders in acute care settings and postoperatively, because these disorders can result from diseases and operations.

Pancreas

The pancreas is a fish-shaped organ that lies behind the stomach. Its head and neck are located in the curve of the duodenum, and its body extends horizontally across the posterior abdominal wall. The pancreas is usually 6 to 9 inches long and 1 to 1.5 inches wide. It varies in size, depending on the individual, and is larger in men.

The pancreas has dual functions. It acts as both an *endocrine gland,* secreting the hormones insulin and glucagon, and an *exocrine gland,* producing digestive enzymes. The cells of the pancreas that function in the endocrine capacity are the islets of Langerhans. These cells comprise approximately 1 per cent to 2 per cent of the pancreatic mass.

Hormonal Action

Glucagon is a polypeptide hormone secreted by the alpha cells of the islets of Langerhans in response to decreased blood glucose levels, increased amino acid levels, or stimulation by growth hormone (O'Toole, 1992). The primary function of glucagon hormone is to increase the circulating blood glucose level. When stimulated, glucagon converts stored glucose (primarily in the liver) to circulating glucose. When the need for glucose is greater than the amount that can be mobilized from the liver, glucagon promotes glucose formation, using both fat and protein. Glucagon is a counterregulatory hormone to insulin, as are epinephrine (adrenal medulla), growth hormones (anterior pituitary), and glucocorticoids (adrenal cortex). These hormones function together to restore low blood sugar to a normal level (Schteingart, 1992b).

Insulin is a protein substance that affects the metabolism of glucose and fats by mobilizing circulating glucose to storage and use in the liver, fat cells, and muscle cells. Insulin, therefore, decreases the circulating blood glucose level. The effect of insulin on blood glucose level and the utilization of glucose in the cells of the body is thought to be the result of insulin's ability to change the permeability of cell membranes, thus allowing easier entry by glucose and promoting the use of glucose in those cells. The primary stimulus for insulin secretion is glucose, but intake of amino acids can also result in release of insulin. In the nondiabetic person, insulin has an unstimulated continuous secretion that affects metabolism between meals (Cassmeyer, 1991a).

ENDOCRINE PATHOPHYSIOLOGY

Disorders of the endocrine glands can be classified as primary or secondary diseases and are a result of either an excess (hyperfunction) or insufficiency (hypofunction) of hormonal secretions. *Primary dysfunction* of the endocrine system associated with excessive hormone production by a gland may be caused by a tumor or by another abnormal stimulus (e.g., antibodies mimicking hormonal stimulators). Endocrine hypofunction can result from congenital abnormalities, neoplasms, infarctions, infections, and autoimmune disorders affecting the gland itself.

Secondary dysfunction occurs when an abnormal stimulus causes excessive or insufficient hormone production by a target gland (i.e., a gland specifically affected by a pituitary hormone). For example, in chronic renal failure, abnormal levels of phosphate and calcium may cause secondary hyperparathyroidism, or chronic liver disease can affect both the pituitary gland and the testes, leading to decreased testosterone production and increased estrogen levels. Secondary dysfunction may also occur (iatrogenically) as a result of chemotherapy, surgical removal of glands, therapy for a nonendocrine disorder such as the use of large doses of corticosteroids resulting in Cushing's syndrome (see p. 337), or excessive therapy for an endocrine disorder (Butts-Krakoff, 1993).

Pituitary Gland

Diabetes Insipidus

Pathogenesis. Vasopressin, also known as antidiuretic hormone is secreted by the posterior pituitary gland. This hormone stimulates the distal tubules of the kidney to resorb water. Without ADH, water moving through the kidney is not resorbed but is lost through the urine. Uncontrolled diuresis (increased urine excretion) and polyuria (excessive excretion of urine) occur. Deficiency of this hormone is called *diabetes insipidus* and can be a result of injury or loss of function of the hypothalamus, the neurohypophyseal tract, or the posterior pituitary gland.

▼ ***Clinical Signs and Symptoms of***
Diabetes Insipidus

- Polyuria (increased urination)
- Polydipsia (increased thirst, which occurs subsequent to polyuria in response to the loss of fluid)
- Dehydration

Central or neurogenic diabetes insipidus, which is the most common type, can be familial or idiopathic (primary), or it can be related to other causes (secondary), such as pituitary trauma, head injury, infections like meningitis or encephalitis, pituitary neoplasm, and vascular lesions like aneurysms (Alspach, 1991).

Inadequate resorption of water by the kidney can result in a loss of as much as 10 L/day of urine and a specific gravity as low as 1.001 to 1.005 (normal: 1.01 to 1.03). If the person is conscious and is able to respond appropriately to the thirst mechanism, hydration can be maintained. However, if the person is unconscious or confused and is unable to take in necessary fluids to replace those fluids lost, rapid dehydration, shock, and death can occur. Because sleep is interrupted by the persistent need to void (nocturia), fatigue and irritability result. The onset of symptoms may be rapid and abrupt, and individuals often can remember the exact time that the symptoms began. In addition, people usually prefer water for fluid replacement (Schteingart, 1992c).

Treatment. Treatment is usually replacement of the ADH by the use of exogenous (administered from an external source) vasopressin or a synthetic derivative (e.g., aqueous Pitressin). Side effects of any type of ADH administration are very serious. ADH stimulates smooth muscle contraction of the vascular system, causing increased blood pressure; of the GI tract, causing diarrhea; and of the coronary arteries, causing angina or myocardial infarction (Degland and Vallerand, 1993). Increases in blood pressure can cause additional serious problems in some people, particularly those with hypertension or coronary artery disease (CAD) and cerebrovascular disease (CVD).

Syndrome of Inappropriate Secretion of Antidiuretic Hormone

Syndrome of inappropriate secretion of ADH (SIADH) is an excess or inappropriate secretion of vasopressin that results in marked *retention* of water in excess of sodium in the body. Urine output decreases dramatically as the body retains large amounts of water. Almost all the excess water is distributed within body cells, causing intracellular water gain and cellular swelling (water intoxication) (Gray and Lugwig-Beymer, 1990).

Pathogenesis. Causative factors for the development of SIADH include pituitary damage due to infection, trauma, or neoplasm; secretion of vasopressin-like substances from some types of malignant tumors (particularly pulmonary malignancies); and thoracic pressure changes from compression of pulmonary or cardiac pressure receptors, or both. Compression of thoracic pressure receptors, caused by conditions such as tuberculosis or by the inappropriate use of mechanical ventilation, signals the pituitary gland to secrete vasopressin, resulting in water retention. Certain medications such as oral hypoglycemic agents (e.g., Diabenese) and some antineoplastic drugs also stimulate release of ADH (Alspach, 1991).

Clinical Signs and Symptoms. Symptoms of SIADH are the clinical opposite of symptoms of diabetes insipidus. Symptoms are the result of water retention and the subsequent dilution of sodium in the blood serum and body cells. Neurologic and neuromuscular signs and symptoms predominate and are directly related to the swell-

▼ *Clinical Signs and Symptoms of*

Syndrome of Inappropriate Secretion of Antidiuretic Hormone (Alspach, 1991)

- Headache, confusion, lethargy (most significant, early indicators)
- Decreased urine output
- Weight gain without visible edema
- Seizures
- Muscle cramps
- Vomiting, diarrhea

ing of brain tissue and sodium changes within neuromuscular tissues.

In addition, urine specific gravity is increased to greater than 1.030 (normal is 1.010 to 1.030), and serum sodium is decreased to below 130 mEq/L (normal is 135 to 145 mEq/L) owing to the severe serum dilution from retained water.

Treatment. Treatment is based on the severity of the diluted serum sodium. If the serum sodium is below 125 mEq/L, treatment includes absolute restriction of water, fluid restriction in varying degrees, and the use of the diuretic furosemide (Lasix). Medications that suppress or block the activity of vasopressin, such as demeclocycline (tetracycline), also may be used (Alspach, 1991).

Acromegaly (Louthrenoo and Schumacher, 1990)

Pathogenesis. Acromegaly is an abnormal enlargement of the extremities of the skeleton resulting from hypersecretion of growth hormone (GH) from the pituitary gland. This condition is relatively rare and occurs in adults, most often owing to a tumor of the pituitary gland. In children, overproduction of GH stimulates growth of long bones and results in gigantism, in which the child grows to exaggerated heights. With adults, growth of the long bones has already stopped, so the bones most affected are those of the face, jaw, hands, and feet. Other signs and symptoms include amenorrhea, diabetes mellitus, profuse sweating, and hypertension (O'Toole, 1992).

Clinical Signs and Symptoms. Degenerative arthropathy may be seen in the peripheral joints of a client with acromegaly, most frequently attacking the large joints (Khaleeli et al., 1984; Layton et al., 1988). On x-ray studies, osteophyte formation may be seen, along with widening of the joint space because of increased cartilage thickness. In late-stage disease, joint spaces become narrowed, and occasionally chondrocalcinosis may be present.

Stiffness of the hand, typically of both hands, is associated with a broad enlargement of the fingers from bony overgrowth and with thickening of the soft tissue. X-ray findings of soft tissue thickening and widening of the phalangeal tufts are typical. In clients with these x-ray findings, much of the pain and stiffness is believed to be due to premature osteoarthritis.

Carpal tunnel syndrome is seen in up to 50 per cent of people with acromegaly (Bluestone et al., 1971). The CTS that occurs with this growth disorder is thought to be caused by compression of the median nerve at the wrist from soft tissue hypertrophy or bony overgrowth, or by hypertrophy of the median nerve itself.

About half the individuals with acromegaly have back pain (Bluestone et al., 1971; Layton et al., 1988). X-ray studies demonstrate increased intervertebral disc spaces and large osteophytes along the anterior longitudinal ligament (ALL), mimicking diffuse idiopathic skeletal hyperostosis (DISH). DISH is characterized by abnormal ossification of the ALL, resulting in an x-ray image of large osteophytes seemingly "flowing" along the anterior border of the spine (Sartoris, 1990). DISH is particularly common in the thoracic spine and has been reported to be more prevalent among persons with diabetes than among the non-diabetic population.

▼
Clinical Signs and Symptoms of
Acromegaly

- Bony enlargement (face, jaw, hands, feet)
- Amenorrhea
- Diabetes mellitus
- Profuse sweating (diaphoresis)
- Hypertension
- Carpal tunnel syndrome
- Hand pain and stiffness
- Back pain (thoracic and/or lumbar)

Treatment. Treatment for acromegaly is determined by the underlying cause. Pituitary tumors can be irradiated to destroy the tumor. Pharmacologic management is used in reducing the levels of growth hormone and decreasing tumor size. Surgical removal (partial or complete) of the pituitary gland is usually followed with permanent cortisone replacement (Loriaux, 1993).

Adrenal Glands

Adrenal Insufficiency

Primary Adrenal Insufficiency. Chronic adrenocortical insufficiency (hyposecretion by the adrenal glands) may be primary or secondary. *Primary adrenal insufficiency* is also referred to as Addison's disease (hypofunction), named after the physician who first studied and described the associated symptoms. It can be treated by the administration of exogenous cortisol (one of the adrenocortical hormones). Primary adrenal insufficiency occurs when a disorder exists within the adrenal gland itself. This adrenal gland disorder results in decreased production of cortisol and aldosterone, two of the primary adrenocortical hormones (Schteingart, 1992d).

The most frequent cause of primary adrenal insufficiency is an autoimmune process that causes destruction of the adrenal cortex. Less frequent causes of primary insufficiency (Alspach, 1991; Marshall, 1986) include

- Tuberculosis
- Bilateral adrenalectomy
- Adrenal hemorrhage or infarction
- Radiation to the adrenal glands
- Malignant adrenal neoplasm
- Destruction of the adrenal glands by chemical agents

The most striking physical finding in the person with primary adrenal insufficiency is the increased pigmentation of the skin and mucous membranes. This may vary in the white population from a slight tan or a few black freckles to an intense generalized pigmentation, which has resulted in persons being mistakenly considered to be of a darker-skinned race.

Melanin, the major product of the melanocyte, is largely responsible for the coloring of skin. In primary adrenal insufficiency, the increase in pigmentation is initiated by the excessive secretion of melanocyte-stimulating hormone (MSH) that occurs in association with increased secretion of ACTH. ACTH is increased in an attempt to stimulate the diseased adrenal glands to produce and release more cortisol (Wilson and Foster, 1985). Most commonly, pigmentation is visible over extensor surfaces, such as the backs of the hands, elbows, knees, creases of the hands, lips, and mouth. Increased pigmentation of scars formed after the onset of the disease is common. However, it is possible for the person with primary adrenal insufficiency to demonstrate no significant increase in pigmentation (Nelson, 1989).

Members of darker-skinned races may develop a slate-gray color that is obvious only to family members. Determining the presence of such changes in skin coloration requires that additional questions be asked of members of the client's family.

Secondary Adrenal Insufficiency. *Secondary adrenal insufficiency* refers to a dysfunction of the gland because of insufficient stimulation of the cortex owing to a lack of pituitary ACTH. Causes of secondary disease include tumors of the hypothalamus or pituitary, removal of the pituitary, or rapid withdrawal of corticosteroid drugs (Loriaux, 1993).

Clinical manifestations of secondary disease do not occur until the adrenals are almost completely nonfunctional and are somewhat different from symptoms for primary disease. Whereas most symptoms of primary adrenal insufficiency arise from cortisol and aldosterone deficiency, symptoms of secondary disease are related to

▼ *Clinical Signs and Symptoms of*
Adrenal Insufficiency

- Dark pigmentation of the skin, especially mouth and scars (primary only: Addison's disease)
- Hypotension (low blood pressure causing orthostatic symptoms)
- Progressive fatigue (improves with rest)
- Hyperkalemia (generalized weakness and muscle flaccidity)
- GI disturbances
  - Anorexia and weight loss
  - Nausea and vomiting
- Arthralgias, myalgias (secondary only)
- Tendon calcification
- Hypoglycemia

cortisol deficiency only. Because the gland is still intact, aldosterone is secreted normally, but the lack of stimulation from ACTH results in deficient cortisol secretion (Loriaux, 1993).

Treatment. Treatment of adrenal insufficiency includes replacement of ACTH and dietary measures to replace the lost sodium and fluid and to decrease intake of potassium. Too much ACTH replacement can result in the development of Cushing's syndrome (Fitzgerald, 1994).

Cushing's Syndrome

Cushing's syndrome (hyperfunction of the adrenal gland) is a general term for increased secretion of cortisol by the adrenal cortex. When corticosteroids are administered externally, a condition of hypercortisolism called *Cushing's syndrome* occurs, producing a group of associated signs and symptoms. Hypercortisolism caused by excess secretion of ACTH (e.g.,

from pituitary stimulation) is called *Cushing's disease,* and symptoms are the same as those associated with Cushing's syndrome. Physical therapists often treat people who have developed Cushing's syndrome after these clients have received large doses of cortisol (also known as hydrocortisone) or cortisol derivatives (e.g., dexamethasone) for a number of inflammatory disorders.

It is important to remember that whenever corticosteroids are administered externally, the increase in serum cortisol levels triggers a negative feedback signal to the anterior pituitary gland to stop its secretion of ACTH. This decrease in ACTH stimulation of the adrenal cortex results in adrenal cortical atrophy during the period of external corticosteroid administration. If external corticosteroids are stopped suddenly rather than reduced gradually, the atrophied adrenal gland will not be able to provide the cortisol necessary for physiologic needs. A life-threatening situation known as *acute adrenal insufficiency* will ensue, requiring emergency cortisol replacement.

All clients receiving long-term or high-dose external corticosteroid therapy should be identified as such by a medical bracelet or tag so that doses are not missed in illness or emergency situations (Loriaux, 1993). Gradual reduction of cortisol use returns the person's adrenal function to normal (Purtilo and Purtilo, 1989).

Because cortisol suppresses the inflammatory response of the body, it can mask early signs of infection. *Any unexplained fever without other symptoms should be a warning to the physical therapist of the need for medical follow-up.*

Effects of Cortisol on Connective Tissue. Overproduction of cortisol or closely related glucocorticoids by abnormal adrenocortical tissue leads to a protein catabolic state. This overproduction causes liberation of amino acids from muscle tissue. The resultant weakened protein structures (muscle and elastic tissue) cause a protuberant abdomen; poor wound healing; gen-

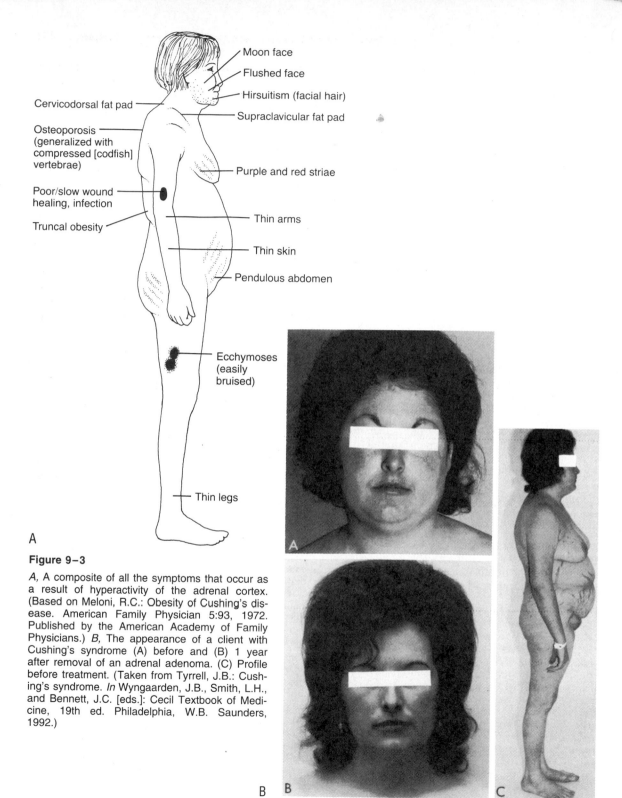

A

Figure 9–3

A, A composite of all the symptoms that occur as a result of hyperactivity of the adrenal cortex. (Based on Meloni, R.C.: Obesity of Cushing's disease. American Family Physician 5:93, 1972. Published by the American Academy of Family Physicians.) *B,* The appearance of a client with Cushing's syndrome (A) before and (B) 1 year after removal of an adrenal adenoma. (C) Profile before treatment. (Taken from Tyrrell, J.B.: Cushing's syndrome. *In* Wyngaarden, J.B., Smith, L.H., and Bennett, J.C. [eds.]: Cecil Textbook of Medicine, 19th ed. Philadelphia, W.B. Saunders, 1992.)

Labels in figure A:
- Moon face
- Flushed face
- Hirsuitism (facial hair)
- Supraclavicular fat pad
- Cervicodorsal fat pad
- Osteoporosis (generalized with compressed [codfish] vertebrae)
- Purple and red striae
- Poor/slow wound healing, infection
- Thin arms
- Truncal obesity
- Thin skin
- Pendulous abdomen
- Ecchymoses (easily bruised)
- Thin legs

B

> ▼ *Clinical Signs and Symptoms of*
>
> ## Cushing's Syndrome (Fig. 9-3)
>
> - "Moon" face (very round)
> - Buffalo hump at the neck (fatty deposits)
> - Protuberant abdomen with accumulation of fatty tissue and stretch marks
> - Muscle wasting and weakness
> - Decreased density of bones (especially spine)
> - Kyphosis and back pain (secondary to bone loss)
> - Easy bruising
> - Psychiatric or emotional disturbances
> - Impaired reproductive function (e.g., decreased libido and changes in menstrual cycle)
> - Diabetes mellitus
> - Slow wound healing
> - For women: masculinizing effects (e.g., hair growth, breast atrophy, voice changes)

eralized muscle weakness; and marked osteoporosis (demineralization of bone causing reduced bone mass), which is made worse by an excessive loss of calcium in the urine (Forsham, 1984).

Excessive glucose resulting from this protein catabolic state is transformed mainly into fat and appears in characteristic sites, such as the abdomen, supraclavicular fat pads, and facial cheeks (Forsham, 1984). The change in facial appearance may not be readily apparent to the client or to the physical therapist, but pictures of the client taken over a period of years may provide a visual record of those changes.

The effect of increased circulating levels of cortisol on the muscles of clients varies from slight to very marked. There may be so much muscle wasting that the condi-

tion simulates muscular dystrophy. Marked weakness of the quadriceps femoris muscle often prevents affected clients from rising out of a chair unassisted. Those with Cushing's syndrome of long duration almost always demonstrate demineralization of bone. In severe cases, this condition may lead to pathologic fractures but results more commonly in wedging of the vertebrae, kyphosis, bone pain, and back pain.

Poor wound healing characteristic of this syndrome becomes a problem when any surgical procedures are required. Inhibition of collagen formation with corticosteroid therapy is responsible for the frequency of wound breakdown in postsurgical clients.

Thyroid Gland

Goiter

Goiter, an enlargement of the thyroid gland, occurs in areas of the world where iodine (necessary for the production of thyroid hormone) is deficient in the diet. It is believed that when factors (e.g., a lack of iodine) inhibit normal thyroid hormone production, hypersecretion of TSH occurs because of a lack of a negative feedback loop. The TSH increase results in an increase in thyroid mass (Cassmeyer, 1991b).

Pressure on the trachea and esophagus causes difficulty in breathing, dysphagia, and hoarseness. With the use of iodized salt, this problem has almost been elimi-

> ▼ *Clinical Signs and Symptoms of*
>
> ## Goiter
>
> - Increased neck size
> - Pressure on adjacent tissue (e.g., trachea and esophagus)
> - Difficulty in breathing
> - Dysphagia
> - Hoarseness

nated in the United States. Although the younger population in the United States may be goiter-free, elderly people may have developed goiter during their childhood or adolescent years and may still have clinical manifestations of this disorder.

Thyroiditis

Thyroiditis is an inflammation of the thyroid gland. Causes can include infection and autoimmune processes. The most common form of this problem is a chronic thyroiditis called Hashimoto's thyroiditis. This condition affects women more frequently than men and is most often seen in the 30- to 50-year-old age group (Cassmeyer, 1991b).

Hashimoto's thyroiditis causes destruction of the thyroid gland because of the infiltration of the gland by lymphocytes and antithyroid antibodies. This infiltration results in decreased serum levels of T_3 and T_4 and thus stimulates the pituitary gland to increase the production of TSH. The increased TSH causes hyperfunction of the tissue, and goiter (enlargement of the gland) formation results.

Because some of the thyroid tissue has been destroyed, this increase in function helps maintain a normal hormonal level for a period of time. Eventually, however, when enough of the gland is destroyed, hypothyroidism develops.

Usually, both sides of the gland are enlarged, although one side may be larger than the other. Other symptoms are related to the functional state of the gland itself. Early involvement may cause mild symptoms of hyperthyroidism, whereas later symptoms cause hypothyroidism.

Rheumatoid arthritis, systemic lupus erythematosus, seronegative arthritis, and other inflammatory polyarthritides and autoimmune disorders have been associated with Hashimoto's thyroiditis (Becker et al., 1963). The mechanisms for these relationships are unclear; however, some investigators believe that cellular immunity may play a role in the pathogenesis of both Hashimoto's thyroiditis and inflammatory arthritis (Louthrenoo and Schumacher, 1990).

Treatment. Treatment can include administration of thyroid hormone or surgery, depending on the severity of the problem. The goiter may become so large that it is disfiguring or pressing on adjacent structures, and surgery may be needed to correct this problem. No treatment is administered if the person is asymptomatic and the disease is mild.

Hyperthyroidism

Hyperthyroidism (hyperfunction), or thyrotoxicosis, refers to those disorders in which the thyroid gland secretes excessive amounts of thyroid hormone. Excessive thyroid hormone creates a generalized elevation in body metabolism. The effects of thyrotoxicosis occur gradually and are manifested in almost every system (Fig. 9–4; Table 9–3) (Schteingart, 1992e).

Graves' disease is a type of excessive thyroid activity characterized by a generalized enlargement of the gland (or goiter leading to a swollen neck) and, often, protruding eyes caused by retraction of the eyelids and inflammation of the ocular muscles (Marshall, 1986). Graves' disease accounts for more than 85 per cent of cases of thyrotoxicosis. The cause of Graves' disease is unknown. Theoretically, the immune system may produce abnormal thyroid-stimulating antibodies, which in turn direct the thyroid gland to produce an excess of thyroid hormone (Schteingart, 1992e).

▼ **Clinical Signs and Symptoms of**
Thyroiditis

■ Painless thyroid enlargement
■ Dysphagia or choking

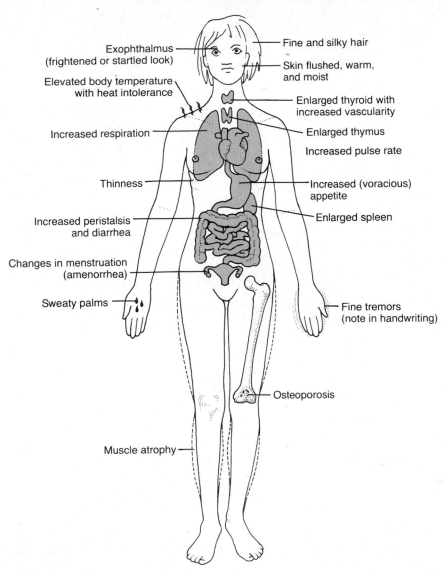

Figure 9-4
Various parts of the body are affected by the symptoms and pathophysiology of hyperthyroidism. (Adapted from Muthe, N.C.: Endocrinology: A Nursing Approach. Boston, Little, Brown, 1981, p. 93.)

Chronic periarthritis is also associated with hyperthyroidism. Inflammation that involves the periarticular structures, including the tendons, ligaments, and joint capsule, is termed periarthritis. The syndrome is associated with pain and reduced range of motion. Calcification, whether periarticular or tendinous, may be seen on x-ray studies. Both periarthritis and calcific tendinitis occur most often in the shoulder, and both are common findings in clients who have endocrine disease (Louthrenoo and Schumacher, 1990).

Clinical Signs and Symptoms. Painful re-

Table 9–3

SYSTEMIC MANIFESTATIONS OF HYPERTHYROIDISM

CNS Effects	Cardiovascular and Pulmonary Effects	Joint and Integumentary Effects	Ocular Effects	GI Effects	GU Effects
Tremors Hyperkinesis (abnormally increased motor function or activity) Nervousness Emotional lability Weakness and muscle atrophy Increased deep tendon reflexes	Increased pulse rate/tachycardia/palpitations Dysrhythmias (palpitations) Weakness of respiratory muscles (breathlessness, hypoventilation) Increased respiratory rate	Chronic periarthritis Capillary dilatation (warm, flushed, moist skin) Heat intolerance Oncholysis (separation of the fingernail from the nail bed) Easily broken hair and increased hair loss Hard, purple area over the anterior surface of the tibia with itching, erythema, and occasionally pain	Weakness of the extraocular muscles (poor convergence, poor upward gaze) Sensitivity to light Visual loss Spasm and retraction of the upper eyelids, lid tremor	Hypermetabolism (increased appetite with weight loss) Diarrhea, nausea, and vomiting Dysphagia	Polyuria (frequent urination) Amenorrhea (absence of menses) Female infertility

striction of shoulder motion associated with periarthritis has been widely described among clients with hyperthyroidism (Wohlgethan, 1987). The involvement can be unilateral or bilateral and can worsen progressively to become adhesive capsulitis, or frozen shoulder. Acute calcific tendinitis of the wrist also has been described in such clients. While antiinflammatory agents may be needed for the acute symptoms, chronic periarthritis usually responds to treatment of the underlying hyperthyroidism.

Proximal muscle weakness (most marked in the pelvic girdle and thigh muscles), accompanied by muscle atrophy known as myopathy, has been described in up to 70 per cent of people with hyperthyroidism (Ramsey, 1965; 1966; 1974). The pathogenesis of the weakness is still a subject of controversy (Feibel and Campa, 1976; McComas et al., 1974). Studies by Ramsey (1966) showed that muscle strength returned to normal in about 2 months after medical treatment, whereas muscle wasting resolved more slowly. In severe cases, normal strength may not be restored for months.

The incidence of myasthenia gravis is increased in clients with hyperthyroidism, which in turn can aggravate muscle weakness. If the hyperthyroidism is corrected, improvement of myasthenia gravis follows in about two thirds of clients (Louthrenoo and Schumacher, 1990; Ramsey, 1966).

Treatment. The goals of care for clients with Graves' disease and hyperthyroidism are to curtail the excessive secretion of thyroid hormone and to prevent and treat complications. Choice of intervention is based on age, goiter size, and whether other health problems exist. The three major forms of therapy are antithyroid medication, radioiodine treatment, and surgery (Birch,1993).

Table 9–4
SYSTEMIC MANIFESTATIONS OF HYPOTHYROIDISM

CNS Effects	Musculoskeletal Effects	Cardiovascular Effects	Integumentary Effects	GI Effects
Slowed speech and hoarseness Slow mental function (loss of interest in daily activities, poor short-term memory) Fatigue and increased sleep Headache	Proximal muscle weakness Myalgias Stiffness Carpal tunnel syndrome Prolonged deep tendon reflexes (especially Achilles) Subjective report of paresthesias without supportive objective findings Muscular and joint edema Back pain	Bradycardia Congestive heart failure Poor peripheral circulation (pallor, cold skin, intolerance to cold, hypertension) Severe atherosclerosis Angina	Myxedema (periorbital and peripheral) Thickened, cool, and dry skin Scaly skin (especially elbows and knees) Carotenosis (yellowing of the skin) Coarse, thinning hair Intolerance to cold Nonpitting edema of hands and feet Poor wound healing Thin, brittle nails	Anorexia Constipation Weight gain disproportionate to caloric intake

Hypothyroidism

Hypothyroidism (hypofunction) results from insufficient thyroid hormone and creates a generalized depression of body metabolism. The condition may be classified as either primary or secondary. *Primary hypothyroidism* results from reduced functional thyroid tissue mass or impaired hormonal synthesis or release. Congenital defects, loss of thyroid tissue following treatment of hyperthyroidism with radioiodine, and defective hormone synthesis resulting from autoimmune thyroiditis, iodine deficiency, or antithyroid drugs are causes of primary thyroid disease. Hypothyroidism in fetal development and infants is usually a result of absent thyroid tissue and hereditary defects in thyroid hormone synthesis. Untreated congenital hypothyroidism is referred to as *cretinism* (Gray and Lugwig-Beymer, 1990).

Secondary hypothyroidism (which accounts for a small percentage of all cases of hypothyroidism) occurs as a result of inadequate stimulation of the gland because of pituitary disease (e.g., pituitary tumor, pituitary insufficiency, postpartum necrosis of the pituitary) (Gray and Lugwig-Beymer, 1990).

Clinical Signs and Symptoms. As with all disorders affecting the thyroid and parathyroid glands, clinical signs and symptoms affect many systems of the body (Table 9–4) (Utiger, 1988).

The characteristic sign of hypothyroidism is *myxedema* (often used synonymously with hypothyroidism). Myxedema is a result of an alteration in the composition of the dermis and other tissues, causing connective tissues to be separated by increased amounts of mucopolysaccharides and proteins. This mucopolysaccharide-protein complex binds with water, causing a nonpitting, boggy edema especially around the eyes, hands, and feet and in the supraclavicular fossae. In addition, the binding of this protein-mucopolysaccharide complex causes thickening of the tongue and the laryngeal and pharyngeal mucous membranes. This results in hoarseness and thick, slurred speech, which are also characteristic of hypothyroidism (Gray and Lugwig-Beymer, 1990).

Because the thyroid hormones play such an important role in the body's metabolism, lack of these hormones seriously upsets the balance of body processes. Among the primary symptoms associated with hypothyroidism are intolerance to cold, excessive fatigue and drowsiness, headaches, weight gain, dryness of the skin, and increasing thinness and brittleness of the nails. In women, menstrual bleeding may become irregular. Medical tests reveal slow tendon reflexes, low blood iodine, below-normal metabolic rate, and abnormal uptake of radioiodine by the thyroid gland (O'Toole, 1992).

In addition, persons who have myxedematous hypothyroidism demonstrate synovial fluid that is highly distinctive. The white blood cell count is usually less than 1000 μ/L (normal is 0 to 200 μ/L [Chernecky et al., 1993]), and the fluid's high viscosity results in a slow fluid wave that creates a sluggish "bulge" sign visible at the knee joint. Often the fluid contains calcium pyrophosphate dihydrate (CPPD) crystal deposits that may be associated with chondrocalcinosis (deposit of calcium salts in joint cartilage). Thus, a finding of a highly viscous, "noninflammatory" joint effusion containing CPPD crystals may suggest to the physician possible underlying hypothyroidism (Louthrenoo and Schumacher, 1990).

When these hypothyroid clients have been treated with thyroid replacement, some have experienced attacks of acute pseudogout, caused by CPPD crystals remaining in the synovial fluid (Dorwart and Schumacher, 1975).

In hypothyroidism, the body's defenses against infection are weakened. If the person has heart disease, it is likely to worsen owing to bradycardia (slowed heart rate) and difficulty in mobilizing retained fluids. In addition, progressive mental deterioration, including extreme fatigue, somnolence, and eventual coma, can occur. Other conditions such as psychosis and paranoid delusions have been associated with severe hypothyroidism (Alspach, 1991).

Pronounced atherosclerosis is also a problem in the severely hypothyroid client. This increased atherosclerosis results from abnormal lipid metabolism and causes angina and other symptoms of coronary artery disease. Treatment of hypothyroidism-induced angina can be a difficult problem, because thyroid hormone replacement increases the heart's need for oxygen by increasing body metabolism. This increase in metabolism then precipitates angina and aggravates the anginal condition (Isley, 1988).

Neuromuscular symptoms are among the most frequent manifestations of hypothyroidism (Layzer, 1985). Flexor tenosynovitis with stiffness often accompanies carpal tunnel syndrome in people with hypothyroidism (Louthrenoo and Schumacher, 1990). Carpal tunnel syndrome (CTS) can develop before other signs of hypothyroidism become evident. It is thought that this CTS arises from deposition of myxedematous tissue in the carpal tunnel area. Acroparesthesias may occur owing to median nerve compression at the wrist. The paresthesias are almost always located bilaterally in the hands. Most clients do not require surgical treatment because the symptoms respond to thyroid replacement. However, in long-standing cases, the presence of fat and fibrosis may require surgical treatment (Layzer, 1985).

Proximal muscle weakness is common in clients who have hypothyroidism and is sometimes accompanied by pain (Golding, 1970). As mentioned earlier, muscle weakness is not always related to either the severity or the duration of hypothyroidism and can be present several months before the diagnosis of hypothyroidism is made. Muscle bulk is usually normal; muscle hypertrophy is rare (Norris and Panner, 1966). Deep tendon reflexes are characterized by slowed muscle contraction and relaxation.

Characteristically, the muscular complaints of the client with hypothyroidism are aches and pains and cramps or stiffness. Involved muscles are particularly likely to develop persistent myofascial trigger points (TPs). Of particular interest to the physical therapist is the concept that, clinically, any compromise of the energy metabolism of muscle aggravates and perpetuates trigger points.

The correlation between hypothyroidism and *fibromyalgia syndrome* (FMS) is now being investigated (Carette and LeFrançois, 1988). People with FMS may have a blunted response to thyrotropin, a hypothalamic-releasing hormone that stimulates the anterior pituitary to secrete thyroid-stimulating hormone (Ferraccioli, 1990). Chronic fatigue that may approach lethargy is noticeable on arising in the morning and is usually worse during midafternoon. These clients are "weather conscious," with muscular pain increasing with the onset of cold, rainy weather (Layzer, 1985; Travell and Simons, 1983).

Treatment. Hypothyroidism is treated by administration of thyroid extract or similar synthetic preparations. If treatment is begun soon after the symptoms appear, recovery may be complete. Delayed or interrupted treatment may mean permanent deterioration. In most instances, treatment with thyroid hormones or synthetics must be continued through the client's lifetime (O'Toole, 1992).

Persons with hypothyroidism experience only temporary pain relief with specific myofascial therapy until it is supplemented by thyroid hormone (Travell and Simons, 1983). People with FMS and clients with undiagnosed myofascial symptoms should be referred to a physician for evaluation of hypothyroidism.

Neoplasms* (Ingbar and Woeber, 1981)

Cancer of the thyroid is not uncommon and is often the incidental finding in persons being treated for other disorders (e.g.,

---

* Primary cancers of other endocrine organs are rare and are unlikely to be encountered by the clinical therapist.

▼ *Clinical Signs and Symptoms of*
Thyroid Carcinoma

- Presence of asymptomatic nodule or mass in thyroid tissue
- Nodule is firm, irregular, painless
- Hoarseness
- Dyspnea

musculoskeletal disorders involving the head and neck). Thyroid tumors are generally slow-growing and are readily treated by surgery, administration of radioiodine, or suppression of tumor growth with thyroid hormone.

Thyroid cancers seldom metastasize beyond regional lymph nodes of the neck; thus, the prognosis is good for all clients except those with the most aggressive types of cancer (Marshall, 1986). Benign neoplasms of the thyroid gland are called adenomas. Almost all malignant neoplasms of the thyroid are epithelial in origin and are therefore considered carcinomas.

Parathyroid Glands

Disorders of the parathyroid glands may produce periarthritis and tendinitis. Both types of inflammation may be crystal-induced and can be associated with periarticular or tendinous calcification (Moskowitz et al., 1969). Cases of ruptured tendons due to bone resorption at the insertions have been reported in clients with primary hyperparathyroidism (Preston, 1972).

Hyperparathyroidism

Hyperparathyroidism (hyperfunction), or the excessive secretion of parathyroid hormone (PTH), disrupts calcium, phosphate, and bone metabolism. The primary func-

Table 9–5

SYSTEMIC MANIFESTATIONS OF HYPERPARATHYROIDISM

Early CNS Symptoms	Musculoskeletal Effects	GI Effects	GU Effects
Lethargy, drowsiness, paresthesia Slow mentation, poor memory Easily fatigued Hyperactive deep tendon reflexes Occasionally glove-and-stocking distribution sensory loss	Mild-to-severe proximal muscle weakness of the extremities Muscle atrophy Bone decalcification (bone pain, especially spine; pathologic fractures; bone cysts) Gout and pseudogout Arthralgias involving the hands Myalgia and sensation of heaviness in the lower extremities Joint hypermobility	Peptic ulcers Pancreatitis Nausea, vomiting, anorexia Constipation	Renal colic associated with kidney stones Hypercalcemia (polyuria, polydipsia, constipation) Kidney infections

tion of PTH is to maintain a normal serum calcium level. Elevated PTH causes release of calcium by the bone and accumulation of calcium in the bloodstream. Symptoms of hyperparathyroidism are related to this release of bone calcium into the bloodstream. This causes demineralization of bone and subsequent loss of bone strength and density. At the same time, the increase of calcium in the bloodstream can cause many other problems within the body (Schteingart, 1992f).

Classification. Hyperparathyroidism may be classified as primary, secondary, tertiary, or ectopic. The major cause of primary hyperparathyroidism is adenoma of a parathyroid gland, which results in the autonomous secretion of PTH without the usual feedback control mechanisms. Secondary hyperparathyroidism is a compensatory response of the parathyroid glands to chronic hypocalcemia, such as that which occurs from decreased renal activation of vitamin D in renal failure. Hyperplasia of the gland occurs as it attempts to raise serum calcium levels. Also in secondary hyperparathyroidism, vascular calcification may lead to an ischemic muscular necrosis with pain and swelling (Louthrenoo and Schumacher, 1990).

Tertiary hyperparathyroidism may occur after chronic parathyroid stimulation in renal failure; ectopic hyperparathyroidism occurs most commonly with lung or kidney carcinomas.

Clinical Signs and Symptoms. Many systems of the body are affected by hyperparathyroidism (Table 9–5) (Aurbach et al., 1985a). Proximal muscle weakness and fatigability are common findings and may be secondary to a peripheral neuropathic process (Mallette et al., 1975; Patten et al., 1974).

Inflammatory erosive polyarthritis may be associated with chondrocalcinosis and CPPD deposits in the synovial fluid (Weinstein et al., 1968). This erosion is described as *osteogenic synovitis,* which emphasizes the role played by bony destruction in this acquired polyarthritis. Concurrent illness and surgery (most often parathyroidectomy) are recognized inducers of acute arthritic episodes (Louthrenoo and Schumacher, 1990).

Hyperparathyroidism can also cause gastrointestinal (GI) problems, pancreatitis, bone decalcification, and psychotic paranoia (Fig. 9–5). A chief concern in hyperparathyroidism is damage to the kidneys from calcium deposits, which can result

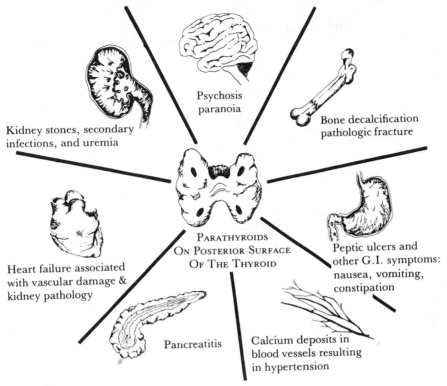

Psychosis
paranoia

Bone decalcification
pathologic fracture

Kidney stones, secondary
infections, and uremia

Peptic ulcers and
other G.I. symptoms:
nausea, vomiting,
constipation

Heart failure associated
with vascular damage &
kidney pathology

PARATHYROIDS
ON POSTERIOR SURFACE
OF THE THYROID

Pancreatitis

Calcium deposits in
blood vessels resulting
in hypertension

Figure 9–5

The pathologic processes of body structures as a result of excess parathyroid hormone. (From Muthe, N.C.: Endocrinology: A Nursing Approach. Boston, Little, Brown, 1981, p. 115.)

eventually in extensive renal damage. This condition may produce hypertension and possibly death from heart failure or uremia (renal failure). In the type of hyperparathyroidism that is secondary to renal failure, osteogenic synovitis (erosion) has been described as affecting the hands, wrists, shoulder, knees, clavicle, and axial skeleton (Rubin et al., 1984).

The classic bone disease affecting people with hyperparathyroidism is *osteitis fibrosa cystica.* It is characterized by demineralization, subperiosteal bone resorption, bone pain, fracture, and cystlike bone lesions called brown tumors (Hahn, 1989). Bone resorption occurs in 5 per cent to 10 per cent of people with hyperparathyroidism and most often affects the middle phalanx

and the clavicle (Louthrenoo and Schumacher, 1990).

Treatment. Treatment for primary hyperparathyroidism is surgical removal (parathyroidectomy). Regression of the osteitis fibrosis cystica may follow surgery, but an acute arthritic episode may be triggered. The prognosis for treatment is good if the condition is identified and treated early. If present, kidney pathology is irreversible, and it tends to progress even with treatment for excess PTH.

Hypoparathyroidism

Hypoparathyroidism (hypofunction), or insufficient secretion of PTH, most com-

Table 9–6

SYSTEMIC MANIFESTATIONS OF HYPOPARATHYROIDISM

CNS Effects	Musculoskeletal Effects*	Cardiovascular Effects*	Integumentary Effects	GI Effects
Personality changes (irritability, agitation, anxiety, depression)	Hypocalcemia (neuromuscular excitability and muscular tetany, especially involving flexion of the upper extremity) Spasm of intercostal muscles and diaphragm compromising breathing Positive Chvostek's sign (twitching of facial muscles with tapping of the facial nerve in front of the ear)	Cardiac arrhythmias Eventual heart failure	Dry, scaly, coarse, pigmented skin Tendency to have skin infections Thinning of hair, including eyebrows and eyelashes Fingernails and toenails become brittle and form ridges	Nausea and vomiting Constipation or diarrhea Neuromuscular stimulation of the intestine (abdominal pain)

* Musculoskeletal and cardiovascular effects are the most common and important for the physical therapist to be aware of.

monly results from accidental removal or injury of the parathyroid gland during thyroid or anterior neck surgery. A less common form of the disease can occur from a genetic autoimmune destruction of the gland. Hypofunction of the parathyroid gland results in insufficient secretion of PTH and subsequent hypocalcemia, hyperphosphatemia, and pronounced neuromuscular and cardiac irritability (Birch, 1993).

Any factor that limits the availability of vitamin D without compensatory treatment (e.g., GI surgery, pancreatitis, hepatic or renal disease, or drugs such as phenobarbital and phenytoin) may cause hypoparathyroidism.

Clinical Signs and Symptoms. Muscle weakness and pain have been reported along with hypocalcemia in clients with hypoparathyroidism (Kruse et al., 1982).

Hypocalcemia occurs when the parathyroids become inactive. The resultant deficiency of calcium in the blood alters the function of many tissues in the body. These altered functions are described by the systemic manifestations of signs and symptoms associated with hypoparathyroidism (Table 9–6). The most significant clinical consequence of hypocalcemia is neuromuscular irritability. This irritability results in muscle spasms, paresthesias, tetany, and life-threatening cardiac arrhythmias (Birch, 1993).

Treatment. Acute hypoparathyroidism with its major manifestation of acute tetany is a life-threatening disorder. The three goals of emergency care are to elevate serum calcium levels as rapidly as possible, prevent or treat convulsions, and control laryngeal spasm and subsequent respiratory obstruction. The goal of intervention for clients with chronic hypoparathyroidism is to restore the serum calcium level to normal concentrations. This is done more gradually than with acute hypoparathyroidism. Treatment is primarily through pharmacologic management (IV calcium gluconate, oral calcium salts, and vitamin D) (Birch, 1993).

Pancreas

Diabetes Mellitus

Diabetes mellitus (DM) is a chronic, multifaceted disorder caused by deficient insulin or defective insulin action in the body. It is characterized by hyperglycemia (excess glucose in the blood) and disruption of the metabolism of carbohydrates, fats, and proteins. Over time, it results in serious small and large vessel vascular complications and neuropathies.

According to the American Diabetes Association, more than 12 million Americans are known diabetics, and approximately 7 million more have undiagnosed DM. If left untreated, diabetes can lead to crippling or fatal complications, including heart disease, stroke, kidney disease, blindness, and amputation of the lower limbs.

Diabetes, with its severe complications, is ranked third as the cause of death from disease in the United States; it is the leading cause of blindness and renal failure in adults (Butts-Krakoff and Black, 1993). Risk factors include

- Being African-American, Hispanic, Native American (highest rate of noninsulin-dependent diabetes mellitus [NIDDM]/Type II DM in the world)
- Being over 40 years of age
- Being obese
- Having given birth to a baby weighing more than 9 pounds
- Family history of DM (sibling or parent)

DM is currently classified according to the various types of glucose abnormalities. This classification system not only provides for the insulin-dependent diabetic (IDDM/Type I DM) and the NIDDM/Type II DM but also includes persons with impaired glucose tolerance or a previous history of glucose abnormalities and persons with potential for glucose abnormalities (Cassmeyer, 1991a). IDDM, in which little or no insulin is produced, accounts for about

10 per cent of all cases and occurs usually in children and young adults. NIDDM, in which insulin is produced but not utilized properly, accounts for 90 per cent of cases occurring after age 40 years.

This text focuses primarily on the IDDM and NIDDM classifications, because these types of DM are more common and more likely to be encountered by the physical therapist in the clinical setting. Table 9–7 depicts the major differences between IDDM and NIDDM in presentation and treatment.

Pathology. In DM, insulin is either insufficient in amount or ineffective in action. There is a difference in the pathology related to insulin response and secretion in IDDM and NIDDM. Some form of true deficiency in insulin secretion occurs with IDDM and results from a lack of, or destruction of, the pancreatic beta cells. In NIDDM, insulin levels may be depressed, normal, or increased, but the available insulin is ineffective in some way. Many factors may contribute to the problem of ineffective insulin (Cassmeyer, 1991a):

- Islet cell defects, resulting in slowed or delayed insulin response
- Abnormalities or changes in insulin receptor sites
- Cellular resistance to insulin action

A defect in the alpha-cell function of the pancreas is also present in the individual with DM, so that glucagon function is impaired. Glucagon does not respond normally to changes in blood glucose levels. This results in a chronically increased glucagon level, which in turn contributes to hyperglycemia (Cassmeyer, 1991a).

Specific physiologic changes occur when insulin is lacking or ineffective. Normally, after a meal, the blood glucose level rises. A large amount of this glucose is taken up by the liver for storage or for use by other tissues, such as skeletal muscle and fat. When insulin function is impaired, the glucose in the general circulation is not taken

Table 9-7

PRIMARY DIFFERENCES BETWEEN IDDM AND NIDDM

Factors	IDDM (Type I)	NIDDM (Type II)
Age of onset	Usually 30 years	Usually over 35 years
Type of onset	Abrupt	Gradual
Endogenous (own) insulin production	Little or none	Below normal or above normal
Incidence	10%	90%
Ketoacidosis	May occur	Unlikely
Insulin injections	Required	Needed in 20%–30% of clients
Body weight at onset	Normal or thin	80% are obese
Management	Diet, exercise, insulin	Diet, exercise, oral hypoglycemic agents or insulin
Etiology	Possible viral/autoimmune, resulting in destruction of islet cells	Obesity-associated insulin receptor resistance
Hereditary	Yes	Yes

Adapted from Butts-Krakoff, D., and Black, J.M.: Nursing care of clients with endocrine disorders of the pancreas. *In* Black, J.M., and Matassarin-Jacobs, E. (eds.): Luckmann and Sorensen's Medical-Surgical Nursing, 4th ed., Philadelphia, W.B. Saunders, 1993, p. 1776.

up or removed by these tissues; thus, it continues to accumulate in the blood. Because new glucose has not been "deposited" into the liver, the liver synthesizes more glucose and releases it into the general circulation, which increases the already elevated blood glucose level (Cassmeyer, 1991a).

Protein synthesis is also impaired because amino acid transport into cells requires insulin. The metabolism of fats and fatty acids is altered, and instead of fat formation, fat breakdown begins in an attempt to liberate more glucose. The oxidation of these fats causes the formation of ketone bodies. Because the formation of these ketones can be rapid, they can build quickly and reach very high levels in the bloodstream. When the renal threshold for ketones is exceeded, the ketones appear in the urine as acetone (ketonuria) (Schteingart, 1992b).

The accumulation of high levels of glucose in the blood creates a hyperosmotic condition in the blood serum. This highly concentrated blood serum then "pulls" fluid from the interstitial areas, and fluid is lost through the kidneys (osmotic diuresis). Because large quantities of urine are excreted (polyuria), serious fluid losses occur, and the conscious individual becomes extremely thirsty and drinks large amounts of water (polydipsia). In addition, the kidney is unable to resorb all the glucose, so glucose begins to be excreted in the urine (glycosuria).

Certain medications can cause or contribute to hyperglycemia. Corticosteroids taken orally have the greatest glucogenic effect. Any diabetic person taking corticosteroid medications needs to be monitored for changes in blood glucose levels. In addition, antihypertensive diuretics, such as furosemide, thiazides, and ethacrynic acid, and oral contraceptives can affect blood glucose levels in already compromised clients (Lumley, 1988).

Other hormones produced by the body also affect blood glucose levels and can have a direct influence on the severity of

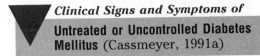

Clinical Signs and Symptoms of

Untreated or Uncontrolled Diabetes Mellitus (Cassmeyer, 1991a)

The classic clinical signs and symptoms of untreated or uncontrolled diabetes mellitus usually include one or more of the following:

- Polyuria: increased urination due to osmotic diuresis
- Polydipsia: increased thirst in response to polyuria
- Polyphagia: increased appetite and ingestion of food (usually only in IDDM)
- Weight loss in the presence of polyphagia: weight loss due to improper fat metabolism and breakdown of fat stores (usually only in IDDM)
- Hyperglycemia: increased blood glucose level (fasting level greater than 140 mg/dl)
- Glycosuria: presence of glucose in the urine
- Ketonuria: presence of ketone bodies in the urine (byproduct of fat catabolism)
- Fatigue and weakness
- Blurred vision

diabetic symptoms. Epinephrine, glucocorticoids, and growth hormone can cause significant elevations in blood glucose levels by mobilizing stored glucose to blood glucose during times of physical or psychologic *stress.*

When diabetic persons are under stress, such as during surgery, trauma, pregnancy, puberty, or infectious states, blood glucose levels can rise and result in the need for increased amounts of insulin. If these insulin needs cannot be met, a hyperglycemic emergency such diabetic ketoacidosis can result (Butts-Krakoff and Black, 1993).

It is essential to remember that diabetic clients *under stress* will have increased insulin requirements and may become symptomatic even though their disease is usually well-controlled in normal circumstances.

Physical Complications of Diabetes Mellitus. The client with DM may present with a variety of serious physical problems. Infection and atherosclerosis are the two primary long-term complications of this disease and are the usual causes of severe illness and death in the diabetic person.

Blood vessels and nerves sustain major pathologic changes in the diabetic person. Atherosclerosis in both large vessels (macrovascular changes) and small vessels (microvascular changes) develops at a much earlier age and progresses much faster in the diabetic person. The precise mechanism underlying the development of these fatty plaques is unknown at this time, but it may involve the interaction of several factors, such as abnormal lipid metabolism, hormonal imbalances, hyperglycemia, and abnormal platelet function. The blood vessel changes result in decreased blood vessel lumen size, compromised blood flow, and resultant tissue ischemia. The pathologic end-products are cerebrovascular disease (CVD), coronary artery disease (CAD), renal artery stenosis, and peripheral vascular disease (Donahue and Orchard, 1992).

Microvascular changes, characterized by the thickening of capillaries and damage to the basement membrane, result in *diabetic nephropathy* (kidney disease) and *diabetic retinopathy* (disease of the retina). Again, the exact mechanism of pathology is unknown, but these changes are considered to be due to uncontrolled diabetes (Strowig and Raskin, 1992).

Poorly controlled DM can lead to various tissue changes that result in impaired wound healing. Loss of fat deposits under the skin, loss of glycogen, and catabolism of body proteins can diminish the ability of tissue to repair itself. Catabolism of body proteins and resultant protein loss hamper the inflammatory process. Phagocytosis, migration of leukocytes, and bacterial killing are also impaired in the diabetic person and result in increased susceptibility to tissue infections. In addition, decreased circulation to the skin can further delay or diminish healing (Cassmeyer, 1991a).

Diabetic Neuropathy. Neuropathy is the most common chronic complication of long-term DM. Neuropathy in the diabetic client is thought to be related to the accumulation in the nerve cells of sorbitol, a byproduct of improper glucose metabolism. This accumulation then results in abnormal fluid and electrolyte shifts and nerve-cell dysfunction (Strowig and Raskin, 1992). The combination of this metabolic derangement and the diminished vascular perfusion to nerve tissues contributes to the severe problem of diabetic neuropathy (Leon, 1993).

Neuropathy may affect the central nervous system, peripheral nervous system, or autonomic nervous system. The most common form of diabetic neuropathy is polyneuropathy, which affects peripheral nerves in distal lower extremities, causing burning and numbness in the feet. It can result in muscle weakness, atrophy, and foot drop.

Diabetic neuropathy can produce a syndrome of bilateral but asymmetric proximal muscle weakness called *diabetic amyotrophy.* Although the muscle enzyme levels are usually normal, muscle biopsy reveals atrophy of type II muscle fibers (Locke et al., 1963; Louthrenoo and Schumacher, 1990).

Carpal tunnel syndrome is also a common finding in people with diabetes mellitus; it represents one form of diabetic neuropathy. As many as 5 per cent to 16 per cent of people with CTS have underlying diabetes (Pastan and Cohen, 1978). The mechanism is thought to be ischemia of the median nerve resulting from diabetes-related microvascular damage. This ischemia then causes increased sensitivity to even minor pressure exerted in the carpal tunnel area (Louthrenoo and Schumacher, 1990).

Charcot's joint, or neuropathic arthropathy, is a well-known complication of diabetes mellitus. This condition is due, at least in part, to the loss of proprioceptive sensation that marks diabetic neuropathy. Severe degenerative arthritis similar to Charcot's joint has been noted in clients with CPPD crystal deposition disease (Louthrenoo and Schumacher, 1990).

The large- and small-vessel changes that occur with DM contribute to the changes in the feet of diabetic persons. Sensory neuropathy, which may lead to painless trauma and ulceration, can progress to infection. Neuropathy can result in drying and cracking of the skin, which creates more openings for bacteria to enter. The combination of all these factors can lead ultimately to gangrene and eventually require amputation. Prevention of these problems by meticulous care of the diabetic foot can reduce the need for amputation by 50 per cent to 75 per cent (Cassmeyer, 1991a).

Whether a poorly controlled blood glucose level is a causative factor in the development of the long-term physical complications of diabetes is still controversial, but it does seem clear that these complications increase with the duration of the disease (Strowig and Raskin, 1992).

Periarthritis (Louthrenoo and Schumacher, 1990). Periarthritis of the shoulder has been reported in as many as 11 per cent of persons with DM (Bridgman, 1972); it is five times as common in this group as among nondiabetic persons. The condition most often affects insulin-dependent people, and involvement is typically bilateral.

The mechanism of this association is unclear, but it is believed to be related to fibroblast proliferation in the connective tissue structures around joints or to micro-angiopathy (disorder involving small blood vessels) involving the tendon sheaths (Pastan and Cohen, 1978). This periarthritic condition can behave unpredictably: it may regress spontaneously, remain stable, or progress to adhesive capsulitis.

Hand Stiffness (Louthrenoo and Schumacher, 1990). Diabetic stiff hand, limited joint mobility (LJM) syndrome, cheirarthritis (inflammation of the hand and finger joints), and diabetic contractures are common in DM. Limited joint mobility occurs in up to 55 per cent of insulin-dependent diabetic persons and in 76 per cent of those who are not insulin-dependent. It seems to increase in direct relation to the presence and duration of microvascular complications (Kapoor and Sibbitt, 1989; Starkman et al., 1986).

Flexor tenosynovitis, caused by accumulation of excessive dermal collagen in the fingers, results in thickening and induration of the skin around the joints. This condition can lead to sclerodactyly (hardening and shrinking of fingers and toes), which in turn can mimic scleroderma. Nonenzymatic glycosylation of collagen and other proteins, along with an increase in sugar alcohol (sorbitol) in the connective tissue, is thought to be the mechanism.

Dupuytren's contracture has a strong association with diabetes. The syndrome is characterized by nodular thickening of the palmar fascia and flexion contracture of the digits. Clients usually have pain in the palm and digits, with decreased mobility and contracture of the fingers. In clients with diabetes, Dupuytren's contracture must be differentiated from LJM, which may involve the entire hand and is frequently bilateral, and from flexor tenosynovitis, which is marked by trigger finger (Kapoor and Sibbitt, 1989).

People with DM may develop reflex sympathetic dystrophy (RSD) syndrome, which is characterized by pain, hyperesthesia, vasomotor and dystrophic skin changes, and tenderness and swelling around the hands and feet. To aid in making the diagnosis, the physician may employ x-ray films and bone scanning to show increased uptake of the radioisotope.

Diagnosis and Monitoring. Diagnosis of DM occurs through a variety of laboratory tests that measure blood glucose levels either at random or during a fasting state. The glucose tolerance test (GTT) is the most significant diagnostic test to determine levels of glucose intolerance. Frequent self-monitoring of glucose levels is also important in the long-term management of DM. This is most often accomplished by using a direct blood sampling by fingerstick technique.

Treatment. Medical management of the diabetic client is directed primarily toward maintenance of blood glucose values within the normal range of 70 to 120 mg/dl. The three primary treatment modalities used in the management of DM are diet, exercise, and medication (insulin and oral hypoglycemic agents) (Table 9–8).

Insulin. Insulin is a replacement hormone derived from beef or pork pancreas or produced from human insulin (recombinant DNA techniques). All clients with IDDM must inject insulin daily, and some people with NIDDM may require insulin if blood glucose levels cannot be effectively controlled with diet, exercise, and oral hypoglycemic agents. Insulin is usually injected by the subcutaneous route in any area of the body containing fatty subcutaneous tissue, such as the backs of the arms, the thighs, buttocks, or abdomen, and between the shoulder blades. In emergency situations, insulin is commonly administered intravenously. It is rarely given intramuscularly because of inconsistent absorption rates, and it cannot be given orally because of digestive enzyme inactivation. Insulin lowers blood glucose levels by assisting in the transport of glucose into body cells and by inhibiting the conversion of stored glucose to blood glucose (Butts-Krakoff and Black, 1993).

There are three primary groups of insulin. These insulins are categorized based on their rapidity and length of action in the body: (1) short acting; (2) intermediate acting; and (3) long acting (Table 9–8). The primary and most significant side effect of insulin therapy is *hypoglycemia,* or decreased blood sugar levels (see section on

Table 9-8
INSULIN ACTION (AVERAGE FOR CLASSIFICATIONS)

Type	Onset (Hrs)	Peak (Hrs)	Duration (Hrs)
Rapid-acting (e.g., regular insulin, Semilente)	0.5–1	2–6	5–12
Intermediate-acting (e.g., NPH, Lente)	1–3	6–12	16–24
Long-acting (e.g., Ultralente, protamine zinc)	4–8	16–18	36+

Hypoglycemia Associated with Diabetes Mellitus).

In addition to potential hypoglycemia, other problems can occur with insulin administration (Butts-Krakoff and Black, 1993):

■ Tissue changes (lipodystrophy) due to repeated injection of insulin in any one site (injection sites should be carefully rotated among appropriate body areas).

■ Erratic insulin action related to irregular dietary, exercise, and rest habits; poor injection technique; effects of counteractive drugs such as corticosteroids.

■ Insulin allergy usually caused by sensitivity to the beef- or pork-derived insulin preparations. Humulin (human insulin) is nonallergenic.

■ Insulin resistance caused by insulin antagonistic medications or by circulating antibodies that bind insulin in the serum and make it unavailable for use.

Oral Hypoglycemic Agents. These are used only for the person with NIDDM. Oral hypoglycemic agents function by stimulating islet cells to increase endogenous insulin secretion and enhance insulin receptor binding. Clients with NIDDM may have their condition controlled by diet and exercise alone and need oral hypoglycemic agents only in stressful situations. Other NIDDM clients may require small doses of insulin in addition to the diet and oral medication regimen, or they may need insulin only when under additional stress (Schteingart, 1992b).

Dietary Management. Dietary management of diabetes mellitus is directed toward controlling the number of calories and carbohydrates consumed daily. The recommended number of calories varies depending on weight-reduction needs. The carbohydrate allowance must be distributed in such a way that the intake matches the client's needs throughout the day. When exercise is added to the treatment regimen, carbohydrate intake needs to be increased because exercise facilitates the transport of glucose into the cells. The client who takes insulin, exercises, and does not concomitantly increase carbohydrate intake could have a hypoglycemic reaction from a significant drop in blood glucose level (Schteingart, 1992b).

Exercise. Exercise as a planned program, including all the elements of fitness (flexibility, muscle strength, cardiovascular endurance), has been shown to be of great benefit to the diabetic person (Butts-Krakoff and Black, 1993). Exercise to increase cardiovascular endurance is usually recommended 4 to 7 days a week at 50 per cent to 70 per cent VO_{2max}, for 20 to 60 minutes per session (Leon, 1993). Benefits of exercise for the diabetic client include the following (Leon, 1993):

■ Improvement of blood glucose control

■ Enhancement of insulin sensitivity to tissue receptors

■ Reduction of insulin requirements

■ Management of atherogenic risk factors (including blood lipid disorders, hypertension, and hypercoagulability of the blood)

■ Prevention of obesity/weight management

■ Improvement of quality of life

Exercise for the diabetic person must be planned and instituted cautiously and monitored carefully because significant complications can result from strenuous exercise.

Physiologic complications can include the following (Leon, 1993):

■ **Hyperglycemia** leading to diabetic ketoacidosis in the person with poor glucose control—i.e., glucose levels greater than 250 mg/dl (occurs due to release of epinephrine during strenuous exercise)

■ **Hypoglycemia** due to decreased insulin needs

■ **Cardiovascular complications** related to underlying coronary artery disease

■ **Musculoskeletal and foot problems** due to poor circulation and peripheral neuropathy

■ **Aggravation of retinopathy or nephropathy** or both, due to increased blood pressure during exercise

Prior to initiating any program of exercise, the diabetic client must have a thorough medical evaluation so that retinal, cardiac, and renal function can be carefully evaluated (Leon, 1993). Clients with active retinopathy and nephropathy should avoid high-intensity exercise that causes significant increases in blood pressure because such increases can cause further damage to the retinas and kidneys. Any exercise that places the head below the waist also can aggravate retinal problems (Leon, 1993).

Exercise-related complications can be prevented by careful monitoring of the client's blood glucose level before, during, and after strenuous exercise sessions (safe levels are 100 to 250 mg/dl). If the blood glucose level is greater than 250 mg/dl, the session should be postponed until the blood glucose level is under better control. If the blood glucose level is less than 100 mg/dl, a 10- to 15-g carbohydrate snack should be given and the glucose retested in 15 minutes to ensure an appropriate level.

In addition, it is very important to have the client avoid insulin injection to active extremities within 1 hour of exercise because insulin is absorbed much more quickly in an active extremity. It is important to know the type, dose, and time of the client's insulin injections so that exercise is not planned for the peak activity times of the insulin (Leon, 1993).

Clients with IDDM may have to reduce the insulin dose or increase food intake when initiating an exercise program. During prolonged activities, a 10- to 15-g carbohydrate snack is recommended for each 30 minutes of activity. Activities should be promptly stopped with the development of any symptoms of hypoglycemia, and blood glucose should be tested. In addition, diabetic clients should not exercise alone. Partners, teammates, and coaches must be educated regarding the possibility of hypoglycemia and the way to manage it (Leon, 1993).

Prevention of musculoskeletal injuries and foot problems includes appropriate selection of activities, slow and gradual progress, and warm-up/cool-down periods. Foot hygiene and proper footwear are essential for the exercising diabetic client.

Exercise can be a very valuable part of the care and rehabilitation of the diabetic client. With use of proper precautionary measures, it can provide a goal-oriented, positive activity.

Severe Hyperglycemic States

The two primary life-threatening metabolic conditions that can develop if uncontrolled or untreated DM progresses to a state of severe hyperglycemia (>400 mg/dl)

Table 9–9
CLINICAL SYMPTOMS OF LIFE-THREATENING GLYCEMIC STATES

Hyperglycemia		Hypoglycemia
Diabetic Ketoacidosis (DKA) *Gradual Onset*	*Hyperglycemic, Hyperosmolar, Nonketotic Coma (HHNC)* *Gradual Onset*	*Insulin Shock* *Sudden Onset*
Headache	Thirst	Pallor
Thirst	Polyuria leading quickly to decreased urine output	Perspiration
Hyperventilation	Volume loss from polyuria leading quickly to renal insufficiency	Piloerection
Fruity odor to breath	Severe dehydration	Increased heart rate
Lethargy/confusion/coma	Lethargy/confusion	Palpitation
Coma	Seizures	Irritability/nervousness
Abdominal pain and distention	Coma	Weakness
Dehydration	Abdominal pain and distention	Hunger
Polyuria	Blood glucose level >300 mg/dl	Shakiness
Flushed face		Headache
Elevated temperature		Double/blurred vision
Blood glucose level >300 mg/dl		Slurred speech
Serum pH <7.30		Fatigue
		Numbness of lips/tongue
		Confusion
		Convulsion/coma
		Blood glucose level <70 mg/dl

▼ *Clinical Signs and Symptoms of*
Diabetic Ketoacidosis

- Dry mouth
- Hot, dry skin
- Elevated body temperature from a fluid deficit
- Fruity (acetone) odor to the breath
- Overall weakness
- Confusion/lethargy/coma
- Deep, rapid respirations (Kussmaul's respirations, a compensatory response of the lungs to neutralize acidosis)*
- Muscle and abdominal cramps (due to a loss of electrolytes)

---

* Dyspnea characterized by increased respiratory rate (above 20/min), increased depth of respiration, panting, and labored respiration typical of air hunger (O'Toole, 1992).

are diabetic ketoacidosis and hyperglycemic, hyperosmolar, nonketotic coma (HHNC) (Table 9–9).

Diabetic ketoacidosis (DKA) occurs with severe insulin deficiency caused either by undiagnosed DM or by a situation in which the insulin needs of the person become greater than usual (e.g., infection, trauma, emotional upsets). It is most often seen in the client with IDDM but can, in rare situations, occur in the client with NIDDM (Cassmeyer, 1991a). Medical treatment is most often intravenous (IV) insulin, IV bicarbonate for buffering, and fluid and electrolyte replacement.

Hyperglycemic, hyperosmolar, nonketotic coma occurs most commonly in the elderly person with NIDDM. This complication is extremely serious and, in many cases, is fatal. Factors that can precipitate this crisis are

- Infections (e.g., pneumonia, pyelonephritis)

▼ *Clinical Signs and Symptoms of*

Hyperglycemic, Hyperosmolar, Nonketotic Coma (HHNC)

- Severe polyuria (usually combined with poor fluid intake)
- Decreased temperature
- Signs of severe dehydration
- Lethargy/confusion/coma
- Seizures
- Gastric distention (paralysis of the intestine due to severe electrolyte losses)

- Medications that elevate the blood glucose level (e.g., corticosteroids)
- Procedures, such as dialysis, surgery, or total parenteral nutrition (TPN)

There are specific clinical features that identify HHNC. Some of these are similar to those of DKA, such as severe hyperglycemia (1000 to 2000 mg/dl) and dehydration. The major differentiating feature between DKA and HHNC, however, is the absence of ketosis in HHNC. Treatment of this problem includes insulin therapy and fluid and electrolyte replacement (Cassmeyer, 1991a).

Because it is likely that the physical therapist will work with diabetic clients in the clinical setting, it is imperative that the clinical symptoms of DM and its potentially life-threatening metabolic states be understood. *If any diabetic client arrives for a clinical appointment in a confused or lethargic state or exhibiting changes in mental function, fingerstick glucose testing should be performed. Immediate physician referral is necessary.*

Hypoglycemia

Hypoglycemia (blood glucose of <70 mg/dl) is a major complication of the use of insulin or oral hypoglycemic agents. Hypoglycemia is usually the result of a decrease in food intake or an increase in physical activity in relation to insulin administration. It is a potentially lethal problem. The hypoglycemic state interrupts the oxygen consumption of nervous system tissue. Repeated or prolonged attacks can result in irreversible brain damage and death (Cassmeyer, 1991a).

HYPOGLYCEMIA ASSOCIATED WITH DIABETES MELLITUS

Hypoglycemia during or after exercise can be a problem for any diabetic person. When the circulating insulin level is high (which occurs during peak activity of the medication), the liver production of glucose induced by exercise is suppressed. Hypoglycemia results as glucose is utilized by the working muscles. The degree of hypoglycemia depends on such factors as

- Preexercise blood glucose levels
- Duration and intensity of exercise
- Blood insulin concentration

Clinical Signs and Symptoms. The severity and number of signs and symptoms depend on the individual client and the rapidity of the drop in blood glucose. The clinical manifestations of a rapid drop in blood glucose are primarily sympathetic in origin. A more gradual decrease in glucose can be a result of the use of longer-acting insulins and oral hypoglycemics. Symptoms in this situation are most often CNS related. If a rapid drop is allowed to continue, both sympathetic and CNS manifestations may develop (Cassmeyer, 1991a).

It is important to note that clients can exhibit signs and symptoms of hypoglycemia when their elevated blood glucose level drops rapidly to a level that is still elevated (e.g., 400 to 200 mg/dl). The *rapidity* of the drop is the stimulus for sympathetic activity; even though a blood glucose level appears elevated, clients may still have hypoglycemia (Cassmeyer, 1991a).

▼ *Clinical Signs and Symptoms of*

Hypoglycemia (Cassmeyer, 1991a)

The signs and symptoms of hypoglycemia are related to two body responses: increased sympathetic activity and deprivation of CNS glucose supply.

- Sympathetic activity
  - Pallor
  - Perspiration
  - Piloerection (erection of the hair)
  - Increased heart rate
  - Heart palpitation
  - Nervousness and irritability
  - Weakness
  - Shakiness/trembling
  - Hunger
- CNS activity
  - Headache
  - Blurred vision
  - Slurred speech
  - Numbness of the lips and tongue
  - Confusion
  - Euphoria
  - Convulsion
  - Coma

Clients receiving beta-adrenergic–blockers (e.g., propranolol) can be at special risk for hypoglycemia by the actions of this medication. These beta-blockers inhibit the normal physiologic response of the body to the hypoglycemic state or block the appearance of the sympathetic manifestations of hypoglycemia (Lumley, 1988). Clients may also have hypoglycemia during nighttime sleep (most often related to the use of intermediate- and long-acting insulins given more than once a day) with the only symptoms being (Cassmeyer, 1991a)

- Nightmares
- Sweating
- Headache

Treatment. Hypoglycemia can be treated in the conscious client by immediate administration of sugar. It is always safer to give the sugar, even when in doubt concerning the origin of symptoms (DKA and HHNC can also present with similar CNS symptoms). Most often 10 to 15 g of carbohydrate are sufficient to reverse the episode of hypoglycemia. Some examples of immediate-acting glucose sources that should be kept in every physical therapy department include (Leon, 1993)

- 1/2 cup of fruit juice
- 1/2 cup of sugared cola
- 1/2 cup of gelatin dessert
- 4 cubes or 2 packets of sugar
- 2 to 3 pieces of hard candy
- 2-oz tube of cake-decorating gel

Most diabetic people carry a rapid-acting source of carbohydrate so that it is readily available for use if a hypoglycemic episode occurs. Intramuscular glucagon is also used by some diabetic individuals. If the client loses consciousness, emergency personnel will need to be notified, and glucose will be administered intravenously. Any episode or suspected episode of hypoglycemia must be treated promptly and must be reported to the client's physician. It is important to question each diabetic client regarding his or her individual response to hypoglycemia. Information regarding individual symptoms, frequency of episodes, and precipitating factors may be invaluable to the physical therapist in preventing or minimizing a hypoglycemic attack.

FASTING HYPOGLYCEMIA

This type of hypoglycemia is commonly manifested as a side effect of insulin or oral hypoglycemic medication. It can also be the result of pathologies that cause an underproduction of glucose (e.g., hormonal deficiencies of ACTH, cortisol, glucagon, catecholamines), or it can be the result of an overproduction of insulin or insulin-like material (e.g., tumors such as insulinomas, autoimmune disease) (Cassmeyer, 1991a).

REACTIVE HYPOGLYCEMIA

This type of hypoglycemia (functional hypoglycemia) occurs after the intake of a meal and occurs usually as a result of stomach or duodenal surgery. After certain types of gastric surgery (e.g., gastrectomy), food is emptied rapidly into the jejunum and does not undergo the usual dilutional changes that occur in the stomach. The blood glucose level rises rapidly as glucose is quickly absorbed into the bloodstream but then falls rapidly to below normal levels as an exaggerated response of insulin output develops. This rapid drop in the blood glucose level results in symptoms of hypoglycemia. The cause of reactive hypoglycemia unrelated to gastric surgery is unknown, and this condition is called *idiopathic reactive hypoglycemia*. Diagnosis in this situation is usually difficult, because the criteria for diagnosis are inconsistent among medical practitioners, and the condition is frequently overdiagnosed (Cassmeyer, 1991a).

Clinical Signs and Symptoms. Clinical signs and symptoms of both fasting and reactive hypoglycemia are the same as those described earlier for hypoglycemia related to DM.

Treatment. Treatment consists of glucose replacement for immediate symptom management and then treatment of the underlying cause, if applicable (e.g., surgery for tumors; correction of hormonal or hepatic problems; discontinuation of drugs that induce hypoglycemia, such as alcohol, salicylates). The client is warned to avoid fasting and simple sugars. Some dietary modifications, such as low-carbohydrate, high-protein diets, have been suggested, but the effectiveness of these measures is largely unproved (Cassmeyer, 1991a).

INTRODUCTION TO METABOLISM
(O'Toole, 1992)

As noted earlier, the endocrine system works with the nervous system to regulate and integrate the body's metabolic activities. Metabolism is the physical and chemical processes of the body broken down into two phases:

- Anabolic phase
- Catabolic phase

The anabolic, or constructive, phase is concerned with the conversion of simpler compounds derived from nutrients into living, organized substances that the body cells can use. In the catabolic, or destructive, phase these organized substances are reconverted into simpler compounds, with the release of energy necessary for the proper functioning of body cells (Guyton, 1992).

The rate of metabolism can be increased by exercise, by elevated body temperature (e.g., high fever), by hormonal activity (e.g., thyroxine, insulin, epinephrine), and by specific dynamic action that occurs after the ingestion of a meal.

Although acid-base metabolism is not in itself a sign or a symptom, the consequences of an acid-base metabolism disorder can result in many signs and symptoms. Physical therapists are unlikely to evaluate someone with a primary musculoskeletal lesion that reflects an underlying metabolic disorder. However, many inpatients in hospitals and some outpatients may be affected by disturbances in acid-base metabolism and other specific metabolic disorders. Only those conditions that are likely to be encountered by a physical therapist are included in this text.

Fluid Imbalances (Table 9–10)

Approximately 45 per cent to 60 per cent of the human body is water. The amount and distribution of body water varies with age, sex, and body fat content. About 75 per cent of the body of the newborn infant is water, whereas the body water of the adult female is 50 per cent and that of the adult male is 60 per cent. Body water also

Table 9–10
FLUID IMBALANCES

Imbalance	Symptoms
Fluid Deficit (Dehydration)	

INCREASED SOLUTES, DECREASED H_2O/ DECREASED SOLUTES, DECREASED H_2O	Thirst
	Weight loss
	Dryness of mouth, throat, face
	Poor skin turgor
	Decreased urine output
	Absence of sweat
	Postural changes from lying to standing
	   Increased pulse (10 beats/min)
	   Decreased blood pressure (10 mm Hg systolic when standing; 20 mm Hg systolic or diastolic when moving from supine to sitting)
	Dizziness when standing
	Confusion

Fluid Excess (Water Intoxication)	

INCREASED H_2O, DECREASED SOLUTES	Decreased mental alertness
	Sleepiness
	Anorexia
	Poor motor coordination
	Confusion
	Convulsions
	Sudden weight gain
	Hyperventilation
	Warm, moist skin
	Increased intracerebral pressure
	   Decreased pulse
	   Increased systolic blood pressure
	   Decreased diastolic blood pressure
	Mild peripheral edema

Fluid Excess (Edema)	

INCREASED H_2O, INCREASED SOLUTES	Weight gain
	Dependent edema
	Pitting edema
	Increased blood pressure
	Neck vein engorgement
	Effusions
	   Pulmonary
	   Pericardial
	   Peritoneal
	Congestive heart failure

decreases with increased body fat, because fat is free of water.

Body water contains the electrolytes that are essential to human life. This life-sustaining fluid is found within various body compartments, including the

■ Interstitial compartment

■ Intravascular compartment

■ Transcellular compartment

Fluid found inside cells (intracellular fluid [ICF]) comprises about 60 per cent of the total amount of body fluid, while the fluid found outside cells (extracellular fluid [ECF]) comprises the remaining 40 per cent. The ECF is contained in the interstitial compartment (space between cells) and in the intravascular compartment (vascular spaces). A third compartment, called the transcellular compartment, consists of fluid that is present in the body but is separated from body tissues by a layer of epithelial cells. This fluid includes digestive juices, water and solutes in the renal tubules and bladder, intraocular fluid, and cerebrospinal fluid (Lehman et al., 1991).

Because many situations in the body cause both normal and abnormal fluid shifts, it is important to have a clear understanding of fluid compartments. The recognition of pathologic conditions, such as edema, dehydration, ketoacidosis, and various types of shock, can depend on the understanding of these concepts.

Body fluids have many functions: digestion, gas and nutrient transport, elimination of wastes, temperature regulation, and chemical function within the cells. In the healthy body, fluids and electrolytes are constantly lost or exchanged between compartments. This balance must be maintained for the body to function properly. The amount of fluid used in these functions depends on such factors as humidity, temperature, physical activity, and metabolic rate. Fluids are lost daily from the GI tract, skin, respiratory tract, and renal system. Balance is achieved through fluid intake and dietary consumption.

Movement of fluid and solutes between body compartments occurs by one of three ways:

- Diffusion

- Osmosis

- Active transport

Diffusion. Diffusion is the movement of *solutes* or particles from an area of greater concentration to an area of lesser concentration (along the concentration gradient) through a semipermeable membrane. This action does not require any use of energy but may sometimes require a carrier substance to transport the solute across the cell membrane (e.g., insulin is a "carrier" for glucose transport into the cell).

Osmosis. Osmosis is the movement of *water* from an area of low solute concentration (high water concentration) to an area of high solute concentration (low water concentration) across a semipermeable membrane. A solution with a high water concentration and a low solute concentration is a *hypotonic* solution. A solution that consists of a large amount of solute and a small amount of water is called *hypertonic*. If a solution contains both water and solutes in the same concentration as that of the fluid in the body, it is called an *isotonic* solution (Lehman et al., 1991).

Active Transport. Active transport is a mechanism that moves *solutes* from an area of low concentration to one of high concentration (against the concentration gradient) and requires energy expenditure. This mechanism regulates the movement of sodium (Na^+) and potassium (K^+) into and out of the cell. It is the major factor in the maintenance of Na^+ and K^+ concentrations in the cells and is a primary factor in maintaining appropriate cellular electrical potential (Lehman et al., 1991).

Fluid Deficit

Fluid deficit can occur as a result of two primary types of imbalance. There is either a loss of water without loss of solutes or a loss of both water and solutes.

The loss of body water without solutes results in the excess concentration of body solutes within the interstitial and intravascular compartments. To preserve equilibrium, water will then be forced to shift by osmosis from inside cells to these outside compartments. If the hypertonic state persists, large amounts of body water will be shifted and excreted (osmotic diuresis), and severe cellular dehydration will result. This type of imbalance can occur as a result of several conditions:

■ Decreased water intake (e.g., unavailability, unconsciousness)

■ Water loss without proportionate solute loss (e.g., prolonged hyperventilation, diabetes insipidus)

■ Increased solute intake without proportionate water intake (tube feeding)

■ Excess accumulation of solutes (e.g., high glucose levels such as in DM)

The second type of fluid imbalance results from a loss of *both* water and solutes. This is called an isotonic or volume-related fluid loss. This loss is restricted to the extracellular compartment and does not cause fluid-shifting from the intracellular spaces.

Causes of the loss of both water and solutes include

■ Hemorrhage

■ Profuse perspiration (marathon runners)

■ Loss of GI tract secretions (vomiting, diarrhea, draining fistulas, ileostomy)

Severe losses of water and solutes can lead to hypovolemic shock. It is important for the physical therapist to be aware of possible fluid losses or water shifts in any client who is already compromised by advanced age or by a situation such as an ileostomy or tracheostomy that results in a continuous loss of fluid. Because the response to fluid loss is highly individual, it is important to recognize the early clinical symptoms of fluid loss and to carefully monitor clients who are at risk.

Athletes and normal adults may experience orthostatic hypotension when slightly dehydrated, especially when intense exercise increases the core body temperature. The normal vascular system can accommodate this effectively.

Laboratory tests reveal increased hematocrit measurements (blood becomes depleted of fluid, so the percentage of red

---

▼ *Clinical Signs and Symptoms of*
Dehydration or Fluid Loss

Early clinical signs and symptoms:

■ Thirst

■ Weight loss

As the condition worsens, other symptoms may include

■ Poor skin turgor

■ Dryness of the mouth, throat, and face

■ Absence of sweat

■ Increased body temperature

■ Low urine output

■ Postural changes (increased heart rate by 10 beats/min and decreased systolic or diastolic blood pressure by 20 mm Hg when moving from a supine to a sitting position)

■ Dizziness when standing

■ Confusion

---

blood cells [RBCs] to fluid appears to be higher).

Treatment. Treatment consists of water or solute replacement and correction of the underlying problem. The person under medical care is carefully assessed for hydration level, fluid intake, and urine output.

Fluid Excess

Fluid excess can occur in two major forms:

■ Water intoxication (excess of water without an excess of solutes)

■ Edema (excess of both solutes and water)

Because the etiology, symptoms, and outcomes related to these problems are substantially different, these fluid imbalances are discussed separately.

Water Intoxication. Water intoxication is an excess of extracellular water in relationship to solutes. The ECF becomes diluted and water must then move into cells to equalize solute concentration on both sides of the cell membrane. Water excess can be caused by an accumulation of solute-free fluid. An increase in solute-free fluid can occur for several possible reasons, which can include (Lehman et al., 1991)

- Psychogenic polydipsia (psychologic problem that involves the intake of large amounts of tap water)

- Intake of only tap water after vomiting (many people can tolerate water when experiencing vomiting and thus ingest water without solutes to replace lost fluid; this is an inadequate source of electrolytes)

- Excess secretion of ADH (vasopressin) (e.g., stress, anesthesia, tumors, endocrine disorders)

- Poor renal function (water resorbed inappropriately)

- Solute loss without water loss (e.g., GI or biliary drainage, severe dietary sodium restriction)

Laboratory results reveal low hematocrit measurements (blood serum diluted so that the percentage of RBCs appears to be less). Treatment is usually careful restriction of water with possible sodium and solute replacement.

Edema. An excess of solutes and water is called an isotonic volume excess. The excess fluid is retained in the extracellular compartment and results in fluid accumulation in the interstitial spaces *(edema)*. Edema can be produced by many different situations, including (Lehman et al., 1991)

- Vein obstruction (e.g., thrombophlebitis, varicose veins)

▼ *Clinical Signs and Symptoms of*
Water Intoxication

- Decreased mental alertness

Other accompanying symptoms:

- Sleepiness
- Anorexia
- Poor motor coordination
- Confusion

In a severe imbalance, other symptoms may include

- Convulsions
- Sudden weight gain
- Hyperventilation
- Warm, moist skin
- Signs of increased intracerebral pressure
  - Slow pulse
  - Increased systolic blood pressure (>10 mm Hg)
  - Decreased diastolic blood pressure (>10 mm Hg)
- Mild peripheral edema
- Low serum sodium

- Increased aldosterone (e.g., Cushing's disease, steroid therapy, renal impairment)

- Loss of serum protein (e.g., decreased dietary intake, burns, renal impairment, decreased production in the liver, allergic reactions)

- Decreased cardiac output (e.g., congestive heart failure [CHF])

Treatment. The treatment of volume excess depends on the condition that caused it to develop. For example, diuretics and cardiac medications may be used to treat congestive heart failure and to remove ex-

▼ *Clinical Signs and Symptoms of*
Edema

- Weight gain (primary symptom)
- Excess fluid (several liters may accumulate before edema is evident)
- Dependent edema (collection of fluid in lower parts of the body)
- Pitting edema (finger pressed into edematous area leaves a persistent indentation in tissues)

cess fluid. Some restriction of sodium intake may also be a part of the treatment for edema and prevention of further fluid gain. Malnutrition and protein losses are treated with increased protein intake (Lehman et al., 1991).

Diuretic medications are used frequently to treat isotonic volume excess. Various diuretic medications may be used depending on the underlying cause of the problem and the desired effect of the drug. The most commonly used are the thiazide diuretics (e.g., chlorothiazide, hydrochlorothiazide). These medications inhibit sodium and water resorption by the kidneys. Potassium is usually also lost with the sodium and water, so continuous replacement of potassium is a major concern for anyone receiving nonpotassium-sparing diuretics (Lehman et al., 1991).

It is essential to monitor clients who take diuretics for signs and symptoms of potassium depletion:

- Muscle weakness
- Fatigue
- Cardiac arrhythmias
- Abdominal distention
- Nausea and vomiting

It is also very important to check laboratory data for the potassium level in any client taking diuretics, particularly before

exercise. Any value below the normal range (<3.5 mEq/L) could be potentially dangerous and could result in a lethal cardiac arrhythmia even with moderate cardiovascular exercise. In addition, it is important to assess clients who take diuretic therapy for potential fluid loss and dehydration by observing for clinical symptoms of both. Questions concerning the correlation of potassium levels with exercise and possible appearance of symptoms consistent with dehydration should be discussed with a physician before physical therapy treatment.

METABOLIC DISORDERS

Metabolic Alkalosis

Metabolic alkalosis results from metabolic disturbances that cause either an increase in available bases or a loss of nonrespiratory body acids. Blood pH rises to a level greater than 7.45 (Table 9–11).

▼ *Clinical Signs and Symptoms of*
Metabolic Alkalosis

- Nausea
- Prolonged vomiting
- Diarrhea
- Confusion
- Irritability
- Agitation, restlessness
- Muscle twitching and muscle cramping
- Muscle weakness
- Paresthesias
- Convulsions
- Eventual coma
- Slow, shallow breathing

Table 9–11

LABORATORY VALUES: UNCOMPENSATED AND COMPENSATED METABOLIC ACIDOSIS AND ALKALOSIS

| | Arterial Blood | | | |
	pH (7.35–7.45)	PCO$_2$ (35–45 mm Hg)	HCO$_3$ (22–36 mEq/L)	Signs/Symptoms
METABOLIC ACIDOSIS				
Uncompensated	<7.35	Normal	<22	Headache
				Fatigue
				Nausea, vomiting
Compensated	Normal	<35	<22	Diarrhea
				Muscular twitching
				Convulsions, coma
				Hyperventilation
METABOLIC ALKALOSIS				
Uncompensated	>7.45	Normal	>26	Nausea
				Vomiting
				Diarrhea
Compensated	Normal	>45	>26	Confusion
				Irritability
				Agitation
				Muscle twitch
				Muscle cramp
				Muscle weakness
				Paresthesias
				Convulsions
				Slow breathing

Common causes of metabolic alkalosis include (Lehman, 1991)

- Excessive vomiting (loss of stomach acids)
- Ingestion of large quantities of base (sodium bicarbonate preparations used as stomach antacids)
- Upper GI tract intubation and suctioning (loss of stomach acids)
- Use of diuretics (loss of hydrogen and chloride ions)
- Prolonged hypercalcemia (relationship unknown)
- Cushing's syndrome

Decreased respirations may occur as the respiratory system attempts to compensate by buffering the basic environment. The lungs attempt to retain carbon dioxide (CO_2) and thus hydrogen ions (H^+).

Treatment. Treatment of alkalosis is correction of the underlying cause and neutralization of the increased pH. Potassium and chloride lost through the loss of the stomach acids or the use of diuretics should be replaced. The medication acetazolamide (Diamox) can be used to increase renal excretion of bicarbonate. Acidic solutions (e.g., ammonium chloride) can be given to add hydrogen ions and to decrease pH.

It is important for the physical therapist to ask clients about the use of antacids, because symptoms of alkalosis can affect muscular function by causing muscle fasciculation and cramping. Prevention of problems related to alkalosis may be accomplished by education of the client regarding antacid use.

Metabolic Acidosis

Metabolic or nonrespiratory acidosis is an accumulation of fixed (nonvolatile) acids or a deficit of bases. This condition is due primarily to an alteration in the utilization and metabolism of various nutrients and chemical compounds. Blood pH decreases to a level below 7.35 (see Table 9–11).

Common causes of metabolic acidosis include (Lehman, 1991)

- Ketoacidosis (diabetic or alcoholic)
- Renal failure
- Lactic acidosis
- Severe diarrhea
- Chemical intoxication (e.g., salicylate poisoning)

For example, ketoacidosis occurs because insufficiency of insulin for the proper use of glucose results in increased breakdown of fat. This accelerated fat breakdown produces ketones and other acids. These acids accumulate to high levels. While the body attempts to neutralize these increased acids, the plasma bicarbonate (HCO_3) is used up. Renal failure results in acidosis because the failing kidney not only is unable to rid the body of excess acids but also cannot produce necessary bicarbonate. Lactic acidosis occurs as excess lactic acid is produced during strenuous exercise or when oxygen is insufficient for proper use of carbohydrate (CHO), glucose, and water (H_2O). Intestinal and pancreatic secretions are highly alkaline so that severe diarrhea depletes the body of these necessary bases. Metabolic acidosis can also result from ingestion of large quantities of acetylsalicylic acid (salicylates), and symptoms of possible metabolic acidosis should be carefully assessed in clients on high-dose aspirin therapy (Lehman, 1991).

Hyperventilation may also occur as the respiratory system attempts to rid the body of excess acid by increasing the rate and depth of respiration. The result is an increase in the amount of carbon dioxide and hydrogen excreted through the respiratory system.

▼ *Clinical Signs and Symptoms of*
Metabolic Acidosis

- Headache
- Fatigue
- Drowsiness, lethargy
- Nausea, vomiting
- Diarrhea
- Muscular twitching
- Convulsions
- Coma (severe)
- Rapid, deep breathing (hyperventilation)

Treatment. Acidosis is usually treated by correction of the underlying cause of the condition. Sodium bicarbonate may also be used if the acidosis is severe and requires immediate treatment.

Gout

Primary gout is the manifestation of an inherited inborn error of purine metabolism characterized by an elevated serum uric acid (hyperuricemia). Gout is not hyperuricemia, and hyperuricemia is not necessarily gout. One fourth of all people with acute gout have no hyperuricemia, and the majority of people with hyperuricemia will not develop gout, even though having hyperuricemia places them at increased risk (Louthrenoo and Schumacher, 1990).

Hyperuricemia is defined technically as a serum uric acid level two standard deviations above the mean uric acid level for the population.* Uric acid is a waste product resulting from the breakdown of purines that are commonly found in certain foods (e.g., kidney, liver, sweetbreads, sardines, anchovies, meat extracts) (Hellmann, 1994).

---

* Most laboratories define an elevated serum uric acid level as a value greater than 6.5 mg/dl in men and greater than 5.5 mg/dl in women.

Table 9–12
CAUSES OF SECONDARY HYPERURICEMIA

Hematopoietic	**Renal**
Hemolytic anemia	Hemodialysis
Myeloproliferative disorders	Renal insufficiency
Polycythemia vera	**Drugs**
Myeloma	Low-dose aspirin
Neoplastic	Diuretics
Leukemia	Antineoplastic
Lymphoma	agents
Multiple myeloma	Alcohol
Endocrine	**Other**
Hypoparathyroidism	Chondrocalcinosis
Hyperparathyroidism	Psoriasis
Hypothyroidism	Sarcoidosis
Diabetes mellitus	Obesity
	Hyperlipidemia
	Starvation

From Wade, J.P., and Liang, M.H.: Avoiding common pitfalls in the diagnosis of gout. Journal of Musculoskeletal Medicine 5(8):16–27, 1988.

Increased serum uric acid levels are associated with middle age, obesity, white race, stress (including surgery, medical illness), and high dietary intake of purine-rich foods. A variety of medications may increase the serum uric acid level, as may a number of acute or chronic disorders (Wade and Liang, 1988).

Table 9–12 represents the causes of disorders associated with hyperuricemia other than gout. The serum uric acid level rises in people with hematologic disorders, characterized by increased cell turnover (polycythemia vera, myeloma, hemolytic anemia, myeloproliferative disorders). It can also rise in those with mild renal disease and decreased urinary uric acid clearance (Wade and Liang, 1988).

Uric acid is usually dissolved in the blood until it is passed into the urine through the kidneys. In individuals with gout, the uric acid changes into crystals (urate) that deposit in joints (causing gouty arthritis) and other tissues such as the kidneys, causing renal disease.

Gout may occur as a result of another disorder or of its therapy. This is referred to as *secondary gout*. Secondary gout may be associated with neoplasm, renal disease, or other metabolic disorders, such as DM and hyperlipidemia (excess serum lipids). Gout affects men predominantly, and the usual form of primary gout is uncommon before the third decade, with its peak incidence in the forties and fifties. After menopause, the frequency of gout in women approaches that in men (Gilliland and Gardner, 1993).

Pseudogout is an arthritic condition caused by calcium pyrophosphate dihydrate (CPPD) crystals. It occurs about one eighth as often as gout. Pseudogout is marked by attacks of goutlike symptoms, usually affecting a single joint (particularly the knee) and associated with chondrocalcinosis (deposition of calcium salts in joint cartilage). In persons with pseudogout, routine x-ray studies of the knee and wrist frequently demonstrate cartilage calcification, or chondrocalcinosis. Because these changes are found in up to 10 per cent of elderly people, diagnosis must be made through aspiration of synovial fluid to identify the crystals (Wade and Liang, 1988).

Pathogenesis. Attacks of gout may be precipitated by conditions that produce metabolic acidosis and a decrease in the excretion of uric acid in the urine. These conditions may include surgery, minor trauma, fatigue, emotional stress, infection, starvation (even the relative starvation resulting from crash diets), administration of drugs (e.g., penicillin, insulin, or thiazide diuretics), and dietary or alcoholic excesses (Hall, 1983). Low-dose aspirin and thiazide diuretics diminish urate excretion; alcohol increases serum urate levels by blocking urinary uric acid secretion (Wade and Liang, 1988).

Additionally, secondary gout may occur as a side effect of chemotherapy for tumors or impairment of clearance due to the use of hypertensive drugs (e.g., hydrochlorothiazide) (O'Toole, 1992).

Clinical Signs and Symptoms. Gouty arthritis results in periarticular and subcutaneous deposits of sodium urate (or urate salts), referred to as tophus (tophi). Before urate-lowering agents became available, 30 per cent to 50 per cent of people with acute gouty arthritis developed tophi. Today, chronic tophaceous gout is rarely seen. Tophi typically occur around the tendons, ears, olecranon bursae, and extensor surfaces of the forearms. The formation of tophi is directly related to the elevation of serum urate; the higher the client's serum urate concentration, the higher the rate of urate deposition in soft tissue (Wade and Liang, 1988).

The peripheral joints of the hands and feet are involved, with 90 per cent of gouty clients having attacks in the metatarsophalangeal joint of the great toe. Other typical sites of initial involvement (in order of frequency) are the instep, ankle, heel, knee, and wrist, although any joint in the body may be involved (Wyngaarden and Kelley, 1989).

These deposits produce an acute inflammatory response that then leads to acute arthritis and later to chronic arthritis (Purtilo and Purtilo, 1989; Salter, 1983). Enlarged tophi on the joints of the hands and feet may erupt and discharge chalky masses of urate crystals (Berkow and Fletcher, 1992).

Many diseases have a presentation similar to that of acute gouty arthritis. Gout and septic arthritis occasionally occur together. The diagnosis of gout must be based on the demonstration of monosodium urate crystals by synovial fluid analysis rather than on the clinical presentation alone (Wade and Liang, 1988).

Onset of pain is sudden and severe and increases in intensity in one or more joints. The pain usually reaches its maximal intensity within 12 hours after its onset. Exquisite tenderness is accompanied by swelling of the inflamed joint, and any pressure (even the touch of clothes or bedsheets) on the joint is intolerable. Untreated, the attack lasts from 10 days to 2 weeks.

Treatment. Nonsteroidal antiinflammatory drugs (NSAIDs) have become the treatment of choice for acute gout. However, active peptic ulcer disease, impaired renal function, and a history of allergic reaction to NSAIDs are contraindications to the use of these drugs. Corticosteroids are reserved for clients with acute gout who are unable to take NSAIDs. Treatment may also include analgesics, bed rest, and dietary management. Without treatment, the attacks tend to occur more and more frequently. In the early stages of the disease, the attacks are separated by asymptomatic periods that may last for months to years. In later stages, there is continual discomfort, and attacks are often polyarticular and more severe and may be accompanied by fever (Hellmann, 1994).

Hemochromatosis (Flexner, 1991)

Hemochromatosis, also termed *hematochromatosis,* is an inborn error of iron metabolism (Fairbanks and Baldus, 1990). It is an inherited disorder characterized by excessive gastrointestinal absorption and body retention of iron, with progressive tissue damage in parenchymal organs (Conrad, 1991). Hemochromatosis, like hypertension, has been labeled a "silent disease," occurring in 1 of 200 people.

Hemochromatosis is found five to ten times more often in men than in women, because women lose blood through menstruation and pregnancy (Ashinsky, 1992).

▼ **Clinical Signs and Symptoms of**
Gout

- Tophi: lumps under the skin or actual eruptions through the skin of chalky urate crystals
- Joint pain and swelling (especially first metatarsal joint)
- Fever and chills
- Malaise
- Redness

Men seldom have symptoms until after 50 years of age and are rarely symptomatic before 30 years of age. Because of menstrual blood loss, women display symptoms 10 years later than men (median age: 60 years).

Alcohol and ascorbic acid seem to accelerate the absorption of dietary iron. The high incidence of alcoholism among clients with hemochromatosis (40 per cent) supports this concept.

Pathogenesis. The cardinal defect in hemochromatosis is the lack of regulation of iron absorption, but the exact mechanism is unknown. The intestinal tract absorbs more iron than is required, thus producing an excess. Apparently the defect lies in proteins that transport or store mucosal iron. One theory is that the function of the mucosal transferrin (iron-transporting plasma protein) is also abnormal, or perhaps the mucosal cells fail to convert absorbed iron into ferritin (a soluble form of iron), thereby weakening the barriers to unwanted excess iron. A final theory is that there is an abnormal cycling of iron caused by macrophages in the spleen and liver that are not storing iron normally.

In its early stages, hemochromatosis produces no symptoms, because it takes many years of iron accumulation to produce warning signs or symptoms. Unfortunately, when the disease becomes evident, it is often too late because iron accumulation has caused irreversible tissue or end-organ damage in the heart, liver, endocrine glands, skin, joints, bone, and pancreas. About half the clients with hemochromatosis will develop arthritis (Dorfman et al., 1969; Dymock et al., 1970).

Clinical Signs and Symptoms. For many years, hemochromatosis was identified by a classic clinical triad of enlarged liver, skin hyperpigmentation, and diabetes. The term "bronze diabetes" was used to describe this presentation. However, hemochromatosis may present with many different signs and symptoms, confusing early diagnosis.

Hemochromatosis has a well-known association with chondrocalcinosis (deposition of calcium salts in the cartilage of joints). Joint damage occurs not from iron, but from deposition of calcium phosphate in the knees, shoulders, wrists, hips, and vertebral discs. Arthritic manifestations associated with calcium pyrophosphate dihydrate (CPPD) crystal deposition in metacarpophalangeal joints are characteristic and highly suggestive of chondrocalcinosis associated with hemochromatosis (Atkins et al., 1969; Axford et al., 1992; Dymock et al., 1970). A biopsy of synovial tissue reveals iron deposition in the cells of the synovial lining, which is noninflammatory (Louthrenoo and Schumacher, 1990).

Hyperpigmentation is caused by an increase in the number of melanocytes and a thinning of the epidermis. Iron deposits stimulate melanin production and alter epidermal thickness (Ashinsky, 1992; Holland and Spivack, 1989).

Diagnosis and Treatment. Serum iron level determinations are made to confirm saturation percentage, liver biopsy is done to assess tissue damage, and magnetic res-

▼ *Clinical Signs and Symptoms of*
Hemochromatosis

- Arthropathy (joint disease)
- Arthralgias
- Myalgias
- Progressive weakness
- Bilateral pitting edema (lower extremities)
- Vague abdominal pain
- Hypogonadism (lack of menstrual periods, impotence)
- Congestive heart failure
- Hyperpigmentation of the skin (gray/blue to yellow)
- Loss of body hair
- Diabetes mellitus

onance imaging (MRI) is done to detect tissue iron to establish the diagnosis of hemochromatosis. Once it is diagnosed, phlebotomy therapy (removing 500 ml, or 1 unit, of blood) takes place twice weekly until the client's body iron stores are returned to normal. To prevent reaccumulation, phlebotomy therapy must be continued throughout the client's life, even after normal iron stores return. This can be accomplished by performing four to six phlebotomies per year.

Prognosis. As iron leaves the storage organs, the evidence of injury subsides. The liver shrinks, and abnormal liver functions improve. In some cases, after prolonged therapy, cirrhosis (scarring of the liver) disappears. In one third of those with diabetes, insulin requirements are decreased. Unfortunately, even with removal of these excessive amounts of accumulated iron, arthritis, impotency, and sterility are usually not affected.

One study (Niederau, 1985) has confirmed that clients with hemochromatosis diagnosed in the precirrhotic stage and treated by venesection have a normal life expectancy, whereas cirrhotic clients have a shortened life span and a high risk of hepatocellular cancer, even when complete iron depletion has been achieved. The survival time of untreated persons is about 2 years (Ashinsky, 1992). Hepatoma (hepatocellular carcinoma), liver failure, and cardiac problems are the most common causes of death in hemochromatosis.

Metabolic Bone Disease

Connective tissue disorders represent a group of diseases with certain clinical and histologic features that are manifestations of connective tissue—that is, tissues that provide the supportive framework (musculoskeletal structures) and protective covering (skin, mucous membranes, and vessel linings) for the body (O'Toole, 1992). Of the metabolic disorders involving connective tissue, muscle, and bone, only the most commonly presented diseases in a physical therapy practice are presented.

Pathologic loss of bone mineral density is most often due to osteoporosis or osteomalacia. These two disorders differ in both their pathogenesis and their treatment. Osteoporosis, an age-related thinning of bone, is primarily a disease of postmenopausal women, 25 per cent of whom will experience wrist, vertebral, or hip fracture after age 65 years. Osteomalacia, a defect in calcification of bone osteoid, is associated with low levels of circulating vitamin D (Benson and Rosenthal, 1993).

Osteoporosis and osteomalacia are the histologic manifestations of deficient bone metabolism in chronic alcoholism, in which vitamin D deficiency plays a major role. Osteoporosis is the predominant bone condition in most clients with cirrhosis (Schapira, 1990).

Osteoporosis
(O'Toole, 1992)

Osteoporosis, meaning "porous bone" and defined as a decreased mass per unit volume of normally mineralized bone compared with age- and sex-matched controls, is the most prevalent bone disease in the world. After the age of 30 years, human bone tissue begins to diminish gradually, owing to an imbalance between bone resorption and formation during the remodeling cycle. The body excretes more calcium than it retains, resulting in reduction of bone mass. Intestinal absorption of calcium becomes less efficient with age; older persons need more rather than less dietary calcium to maintain a positive calcium balance.

Traditionally, osteoporosis has been considered a single disease entity, but according to Sinnett (1993), there are two osteoporotic syndromes: postmenopausal osteoporosis and senile osteoporosis. Within those two categories, others outline *diet-related bone loss, disuse osteoporosis, heritable osteoporosis, endocrine-mediated bone* loss, disease-related bone loss, and *idiopathic osteoporosis* (O'Toole, 1992; Aloia, 1986).

Postmenopausal osteoporosis is associated with accelerated bone loss in the perimenopausal period, accompanied by high fracture rates involving the vertebrae (Sinnett, 1993).

Bone mass maintenance is related to estrogen levels, as estrogen has a protective effect on the bone by suppressing resorption. Estrogen stimulates the production of calcitonin, which prevents removal of calcium from the bone (Richart and Lindsay, 1984; Whedon, 1981). Estrogen improves calcium absorption in the intestinal tract and decreases calcium losses in the urine (Heaney et al., 1978). After menopause, when estrogen secretion diminishes, bone becomes increasingly sensitive to parathyroid hormone, and bone resorption increases (MacKinnon, 1988).

More than half the women in the United States who are 50 years of age or older are likely to have radiologically detectable evidence of abnormally decreased bone mass (osteopenia) in the spine. More than a third of these women develop major orthopedic problems related to osteoporosis. Most fractures sustained by women over

the age of 50 years are secondary to osteoporosis (O'Toole, 1992).

Senile osteoporosis, or *age-related osteoporosis,* increases with advancing age; it is caused by the bone loss that normally accompanies aging. Men can be affected, especially those on dialysis or long-term steroid administration. Inactivity results in calcium excretion, which is a bone mineral loss. Osteoporosis associated with aging involves fractures of the proximal femur and vertebrae as well as the hip, pelvis, proximal humerus, distal radius, and tibia.

Many risk factors are associated with osteoporosis (see Osteoporosis Risk Factors), but osteoporosis is the most common bone disease in elderly, Caucasian women of northern European descent who have inadequate dietary calcium intakes and who lead sedentary life styles (Aisenbrey, 1987). The Appendix at the end of this chapter presents a questionnaire to assess risk factors in clients.

Additionally, researchers are beginning to examine the environmental influences associated with industrialized countries such as the United States (Gallagher et al., 1980). For example, although menopause is universal, and the resulting estrogen deficiency is presumably similar for all women,

---

OSTEOPOROSIS RISK FACTORS

- Caucasian with European, British, or Asian ancestry
- Gender: women more than men
- Age: postmenopausal (over 65 years)
- Fair skin
- Small frame
- Smoker
- Alcohol consumption
- Prolonged use of thyroid medications, antiinflammatories, or seizure medications.
- Excessive dietary intake of protein, salt, calcium, alcohol, or caffeine

- Surgical removal of ovaries
- Allergy to milk/milk products
- Stress
- Infrequent exercise
- Family history of osteoporosis
- Underweight/thin
- Vitamin D deficiency
- Previous history of hyperthyroidism, hyperparathyroidism, rheumatoid arthritis, liver or kidney disease

Table 9–13

ENDOCRINE AND METABOLIC CAUSES OF SECONDARY OSTEOPOROSIS

Diabetes mellitus
Glucocorticoid excess:
   Iatrogenic Cushing's syndrome
   Hyperadrenalism
Hyperparathyroidism
Hyperthyroidism
Hypocystinuria (inborn error of amino acid metabolism)
Hypogonadism
Marfan's syndrome
Premature ovarian failure
Testicular insufficiency

▼ *Clinical Signs and Symptoms of*
Osteoporosis

- Compression fracture of the spine
- Decrease in height (more than 1″ shorter than maximum adult height)
- Kyphosis
- Dowager's hump
- Episodic, acute low thoracic/high lumbar pain
- Decreased activity tolerance
- Early satiety

differences in the occurrence of osteoporosis among countries cannot be explained just on the basis of estrogen deficiency (Sinnett, 1993). Countries with the highest incidence of osteoporosis also have a high incidence of heart disease and the highest consumption of carbohydrates, fat, protein, salt, and caffeine (Gallagher et al., 1980; Sinnett, 1993).

Endocrine-mediated bone loss can produce osteoporosis because numerous endocrine hormones affect skeletal remodeling and hence skeletal mass. Secondary osteoporosis may accompany various endocrine and metabolic disorders that can produce associated osteopenia (Table 9–13).

Other hormone-related problems include posthysterectomy or oophorectomy (removal of ovaries) states and amenorrhea (absence of menses) as a result of heavy exercise by a woman with very low body fat (Cirullo, 1989). Lack of exercise is considered a risk factor, but because exercise-induced amenorrhea results in bone loss, the lack of estrogen appears to be a more important factor in developing osteoporosis than the lack of exercise (MacKinnon, 1988).

Early osteoporosis has no visible signs or symptoms. Mild-to-severe back pain and loss of height may be the only early signs observed. Changes in bone density do not show up on x-rays until they reach a 30 per cent loss (National Osteoporosis Foundation, 1991a).

To make the diagnosis of osteoporosis associated with endocrine or metabolic disorders, physicians look for hormonal abnormalities, x-ray findings of generalized osteopenia (reduced bone mass), and marked loss of trabecular bone (bone density studies). Serum levels of calcium, phosphorus, alkaline phosphatase, and parathyroid hormone are usually normal (Louthrenoo and Schumacher, 1990).

Treatment. The objective of all rehabilitation measures (diet, exercise, hormones, vitamins) is to preserve the skeletal integrity despite bone loss (Sinaki et al., 1990). Weight-bearing exercise against gravity and extension exercises are recommended, but the benefits of exercise last only as long as the person maintains the program (National Osteoporosis Foundation, 1991b).

Kyphotic posture is one of the most disfiguring effects of osteoporosis. A newly developed posture-training support has been evaluated as an alternative to other supportive measures when bracing cannot be tolerated or when extensive bracing is not indicated (Sinaki et al., 1990). Although rigid back supports have been advocated for years to prevent further compression and wedging, Sinaki et al. (1990) propose improvement of the natural anatomic support of the spine by strengthening the erector spinae muscles.

Getting enough calcium, whether through

diet or through supplements, is essential to maintaining bone strength and can play a vital role in preventing osteoporosis-related fractures. Vitamin D supplementation may be necessary to enhance calcium absorption.

Estrogen replacement therapy (ERT) for menopausal women may be indicated. The risk of increased uterine and breast cancer associated with ERT can be offset by the addition of progesterone. Excessive use of alcohol reduces estrogen levels in women and testosterone levels in men and is directly toxic to the cells that build bone. Moderating alcohol intake is recommended to reduce the risk of developing osteoporosis. Excessive alcohol use is also linked to greater susceptibility to falling and may cause malnutrition and reduced calcium absorption (National Osteoporosis Foundation, 1991b).

For both men and women already suffering from osteoporosis, calcitonin may be prescribed to prevent further bone loss by slowing bone removal. Calcitonin has also been reported to provide relief from the pain associated with osteoporosis (National Osteoporosis Foundation, 1992).

Osteomalacia (Louthrenoo and Schumacher, 1990; O'Toole, 1992)

Osteomalacia is a softening of the bones resulting from impaired mineralization in bone matrix. This failure in mineralization results in a reduced rate of bone formation (Mankin, 1974). Osteomalacia is caused by a vitamin D deficiency in adults. A similar condition in children, occurring before epiphyseal plate closure, is called rickets.

In children with rickets, x-ray findings include the well-known bowing of the long bones, in addition to widening, fraying, and clubbing of the areas of active bone growth. These areas especially include the metaphyseal ends of the long bones and the sternal ends of the ribs, the so-called rachitic rosary.

The deficiency may be due to lack of exposure to ultraviolet rays, inadequate intake of vitamin D in the diet, failure to absorb or utilize vitamin D, increased catabolism of vitamin D, a renal tubular defect, or a pathologically reduced number of vitamin D receptor sites in tissues.

The disease is characterized by decalcification of the bones, particularly those of the spine, pelvis, and lower extremities. X-ray examination reveals transverse, fracture-like lines in the affected bones and areas of demineralization in the matrix of the bone. These pseudofractures, known as Looser's transformation zones, are bilateral. The most common sites are the ribs, long bones, lateral scapular margin, upper femur, and pubic rami. As the bones soften, they become bent, flattened, or otherwise deformed. Looser's zones are believed to result from pressure on the softened bone by the nutrient arteries of its blood supply (Mankin, 1974).

Severe bone pain, skeletal deformities, fractures, and severe muscle weakness and pain are common in people with osteomalacia. Clients typically complain of muscle weakness and pain that sometimes mimic polymyositis or muscular dystrophy (Schott and Wills, 1976).

Other metabolic diseases that have been reported in people who have osteomalacia include chronic hypophosphatemia (deficiency of serum phosphates), renal tubular acidosis type I, and Fanconi's syndrome. The latter two disorders can progress to chronic hypophosphatemia as a result of chronic renal phosphate wasting.

Treatment. Treatment consists of administration of large daily doses of vitamin

▼ *Clinical Signs and Symptoms of*
Osteomalacia

- Bone pain
- Skeletal deformities
- Fractures
- Severe muscle weakness
- Myalgia

D and dietary measures to ensure adequate calcium and phosphorus intake.

Paget's Disease (Salter, 1983)

Paget's disease (osteitis deformans), named after Sir James Paget circa mid-1880s, is a relatively common disorder of bone remodeling that affects men more often than women (3:2 ratio). Although Paget's disease affects approximately 3 per cent of the population over 40 years of age, it is most commonly seen in the elderly population (10 per cent older than 70 years of age), most of whom are asymptomatic.

This metabolic bone disorder is characterized by slowly progressive enlargement and deformity of multiple bones, associated with unexplained acceleration of both deposition and resorption of bone. Although originally thought to be an inflammatory process, it is now considered to be caused by a slow virus that takes years to become symptomatic. During the early and more active phase, resorption exceeds deposition, and the bone, although enlarged, becomes spongelike, weakened, and deformed. This osteolytic phase is followed by an osteosclerotic phase in which the deposition of bone results in enlarged, thick, and dense bones.

The bones most commonly involved include (in decreasing order) pelvis, lumbar spine, sacrum, femur, tibia, skull, shoulders, thoracic spine, cervical spine, and ribs (Guyer, 1981). Inadequate tensile strength of involved bone may lead to deformities, typically bowing of the femur or tibia, which may impair walking (Aurbach et al., 1985b).

Complications of this disease process include progressive deformities due to the enlargement and bending of bones in the osteolytic phase, pathologic fractures, and occasionally malignant change in the hyperactive osteoblasts, resulting in osteogenic sarcoma (malignant and fatal). The femur and the humerus are the most common sites of malignant transformation,

---

▼ **Clinical Signs and Symptoms of**
Paget's Disease

These depend on the location and severity of the bone lesions and may include

- Pain and stiffness
- Fatigue
- Headaches and dizziness
- Deformity
  - Bowing of long bones
  - Increased size and abnormal contour of clavicles
  - Osteoarthritis of adjacent joints
- Periosteal tenderness
- Increased skin temperature over long bones*
- Decreased auditory acuity
- Compression neuropathy
  - Spinal stenosis
  - Paresis
  - Paraplegia
  - Muscle weakness

---

* Increased skin temperature over affected long bones is a typical finding and is explained by soft tissue vascularity surrounding the bones (Singer, 1987).

---

which may be signaled by increased pain and rapid soft tissue swelling.

Clinical Signs and Symptoms. Although this disorder is often asymptomatic, when symptoms do develop they occur insidiously (gradually). Bone pain is described as aching, deep, and occasionally severe. The person may have pain at night, awaken with pain, and be unable to go back to sleep despite all efforts. This night pain occurs especially in the person who has developed an osteogenic sarcoma associated with Paget's disease.

Treatment. No specific medical treatment for Paget's disease exists, although therapeutic agents (e.g., calcitonin, diphospho-

Table 9-14
OSTEOGENESIS IMPERFECTA

Type	Inheritance	Fractures	Sclerae	Dentinogenesis Imperfecta	Special Features
IA	Autosomal dominant	+	Blue	−	Birth/perinatal fractures are rare Joint hypermobility Easy bruising
IB	Autosomal dominant	+	Blue	+	Same as IA
II	Autosomal recessive	+++	Blue		Intrauterine or early infant death Intrauterine growth retardation Marked tissue fragility Beaded ribs Poor cranial calcification
III	Autosomal recessive	++	Blue at birth but less blue with age	+	Congenital fractures Postnatal growth retardation Kyphoscoliosis
IVA	Autosomal dominant	+	White	−	Kyphoscoliosis Postnatal growth retardation
IVB	Autosomal dominant	+	White	+	Same as IVA

Adapted from Stanbury, J.B., Wyngaarden, J.B., Fredrickson, D.S., et al.: The Metabolic Basis of Inherited Disease, 5th ed. New York, McGraw-Hill, 1983.

nates, mithramycin) have been shown to reduce both bone resorption and bone formation and thus reduce the associated bone pain. The primary indication for treatment is pain. Analgesics such as aspirin, indomethacin, or ibuprofen may decrease bone pain. Physical therapy and orthopedic treatment may be indicated for severe disabling arthritis, severe bowing deformities of the femur or tibia, muscle atrophy, deconditioning, and pathologic fractures. Calcitonin and etidronate may be administered to retard bone resorption (Rauscher, 1993).

Osteogenesis Imperfecta (Pinnell and Murad, 1989; Salter, 1983)

Osteogenesis imperfecta (OI) is an inherited condition (occurring 1 in 20,000) char-acterized by abnormally brittle and fragile bones that are subject to gross pathologic fracture.

Pathogenesis. This disorder is transmitted by an autosomal dominant gene. The underlying defect is an abnormality in collagen synthesis that leads to increased bone fragility and a variable incidence of extraskeletal manifestations (Aurbach et al., 1985b). Salter (1983) attributes the cause to a failure of periosteal and endosteal intramembranous ossification of unknown origin. As a result of an imbalance between bone deposition and bone resorption, the cortical bone and the trabeculae of cancellous bone are extremely thin.

There are six types of OI described by clinical and genetic features (Table 9-14). The severity of the defect, which varies considerably, is indicated by the age at which the fractures occur. The most common OI is the mild-to-moderate form (type I, or infantile type). The affected infant has many gross fractures during early childhood (often at the time of standing and walking), which affect weight-bearing bones. The infant develops severe limb deformities from bending of bones and may be stunted in growth.

In the most severe form (type II, or fetal type), multiple fractures have already occurred in utero, and more fractures occur during the birth process. Type II is rare and is generally lethal, and associated mortality is high during early infancy. Although this disorder affects bones primarily, other connective tissue can be affected, including tendons, ligaments, fascia, sclerae, and dentin.

Clinical Signs and Symptoms. Extraskeletal manifestations of osteogenesis imperfecta may include

- Blue sclerae (whites of the eyes)
- Hearing loss or deafness
- Thin skin
- Cardiac abnormalities (e.g., aortic or mitral valve insufficiency)

These extraskeletal features may be related to abnormal collagen synthesis. For example, the hearing loss may be due to abnormalities of bone conduction (as a result of ligamentous laxity) as well as abnormalities of nerve conduction. The extraskeletal anomalies listed occur more frequently in the milder type I form of OI. Abnormal, discolored, brittle teeth due to abnormal dentin synthesis, called dentinogenesis imperfecta, occur in subgroups within the various types of OI (see Table 9–14). Lax ligaments and joints are additional features. Short stature is probably secondary to repeated fracture and deformity (Aurbach et al., 1985b).

Frequency of fractures diminishes after puberty. This reduction is attributed to the hormonal influence on connective tissue metabolism.

Treatment. No medical treatment is currently effective, although surgery (multiple osteotomies of the long bones and internal fixation) to prevent deformity may be appropriate in selected cases. Physical therapists often treat those clients receiving protective long leg braces, provide care directed toward fracture prevention, and give mobility training after a fracture.

Ochronosis (Louthrenoo and Schumacher, 1990)

This rare genetic metabolic disorder results from a deficiency of homogentisic acid oxidase. It results in the accumulation and deposition in the joints and connective tissues of a dark-pigmented polymer of homogentisic acid. If this substance is deposited in the articular cartilage, it brings about premature cartilaginous degeneration. In people with this disorder, the synovial fluid is "noninflammatory:" clear, yellow, and viscous, with mononuclear cells predominating (Schumacher and Holdsworth, 1977). CPPD crystals may be present.

Spondylopathy (disease of the vertebrae) is one of the most common musculoskeletal complications of ochronosis. The affected client, who is likely to be more than 30 years old, has back stiffness and discomfort. The spinal changes, which result from the accumulation of homogentisic acid polymer in the cartilaginous tissue, usually begin in the lumbosacral spine. The client's stooped posture can resemble that of an individual with ankylosing spondylitis.

A peripheral arthropathy (joint disease) that is clinically indistinguishable from osteoarthritis may occur. The most commonly affected joints are knees, hips, and shoulders. Because the shoulder is an unusual site for primary osteoarthritis, its presence in a client's shoulder may suggest an underlying ochronosis as a possible cause (if occupational factors can be ruled out).

The diagnosis of ochronosis is suggested by the dark urine and is established by

Clinical Signs and Symptoms of
Ochronosis

- Spondylopathy
- Stooped posture
- Peripheral arthropathy (knees, hips, shoulders)
- Dark urine

measurement of the homogentisic acid level in the urine. An x-ray study will demonstrate calcification and ossification of the intervertebral disc. Blue-black pigment deposits may be found in the sclerae, tip of the nose, skin, and ear cartilage.

PHYSICIAN REFERRAL

Disorders of the endocrine and metabolic systems may present with recognizable clinical signs and symptoms but almost always require a combination of clinical and laboratory findings for accurate identification. The physical therapist is encouraged to complete a thorough Family/Personal History form, augmented by the interview with the client and careful clinical observations, in order to provide the physician with as much information as possible when making a referral. When appropriate, the Osteoporosis Screening Evaluation in the Appendix may be helpful.

In most cases, the client who has suffered from an endocrine disorder has already been diagnosed and may have been referred for physical therapy for some other musculoskeletal complaint. These clients may have musculoskeletal problems that can be affected by symptoms associated with hormone imbalances (see Tables 9–3 through 9–6).

Any diabetic client demonstrating signs of confusion, lethargy, or changes in mental alertness and function should undergo an immediate fingerstick glucose test with a follow-up visit to the physician on the same day. Likewise, any episode or suspected episode of hypoglycemia must be treated promptly and reported to the diabetic client's physician.

It is important to monitor any client taking diuretics for signs or symptoms of potassium depletion or fluid dehydration before exercising the individual. Consultation with the physician is advised.

Systemic Signs and Symptoms Requiring Physician Referral

Diseases of the endocrine-metabolic system account for some of the most common disorders encountered in human beings—diabetes, obesity, and thyroid abnormalities. In recent years, new laboratory techniques have greatly enhanced the physician's ability to diagnose these diseases. Nevertheless, in many cases, the disorder remains unrecognized until relatively late in its course; signs and symptoms may be attributed to some other disease process or musculoskeletal disorder (e.g., weakness may be the major complaint in Addison's disease) (Frohman et al., 1987). Thus, any client who has any of the following generalized signs and symptoms without obvious or already known cause should be further evaluated by a physician.

Abdominal cramps	Coarse, dry skin
Abdominal distention	Confusion/lethargy
Absence of sweat	Constipation
Acroparesthesias	Deep, rapid respirations
Arthralgias	Dependent edema
Buffalo hump	Diarrhea
Carpal tunnel syndrome	Dizziness
Changes in appetite	Dry mouth, throat, face
Changes in body or skin temperature	Dysphagia
	Dyspnea
Changes in skin pigmentation	Ecchymosis
	Excessive sweating

Fatigue
Fever and chills
Fruity breath odor
Headaches
Heart palpitations
Hoarseness
Low urine output
Myalgias
Myoedema

Myokymia
Nausea
Night sweats
Nightmares
Nocturia
Numbness (lips, tongue)
Peripheral neuropathy

Pitting edema
Polydipsia
Polyphagia
Polyuria
Postural hypotension
Prolonged reflexes
Proximal muscle weakness

Shakiness/trembling
Striae
Tachycardia/ palpitations
Trigger points
Weakness
Weight loss or gain

Key Points to Remember

- Clients with a variety of endocrine and metabolic disorders commonly complain of fatigue, muscle weakness, and occasionally muscle or bone pain (Louthrenoo and Schumacher, 1990).

- Muscle weakness associated with endocrine and metabolic disorders usually involves proximal muscle groups.

- Periarthritis and calcific tendinitis of the shoulder is common in endocrine clients. Symptoms usually respond to treatment of underlying endocrine pathology.

- Carpal tunnel syndrome (CTS), hand stiffness, and hand pain can occur with endocrine and metabolic diseases.

- There is a correlation between hypothyroidism and fibromyalgia syndrome (FMS), which is being investigated. Any compromise of muscle energy metabolism aggravates and perpetuates trigger points (TPs).

- Exercise for the diabetic client must be carefully planned, because significant complications can result from strenuous exercise.

- Exercise with the insulin-dependent diabetic client should be coordinated to avoid peak insulin dosage whenever possible. Any diabetic client who appears confused or lethargic must be tested immediately by fingerstick for glucose level. Other precautions for the physical therapist are covered in the text.

- When it is impossible to differentiate between ketoacidosis and hyperglycemia, administration of some source of sugar (glucose) is the immediate action to take.

- Early osteoporosis has no visible signs and symptoms. History and risk factors are important clues.

- Cortisol suppresses the body's inflammatory response, masking early signs of infection. Any unexplained fever without other symptoms should be a warning to the physical therapist of the need for medical follow-up.

SUBJECTIVE EXAMINATION   *Special Questions to Ask*

Endocrine and metabolic disorders may produce subtle symptoms that progress so gradually the person may be unaware of the significance of such findings. This requires careful interviewing to screen for potential physical and psychologic changes associated with hormone imbalances or other endocrine or metabolic disorders.

As always, it is important to be aware of client medications (whether over-the-counter or prescribed), the intended purpose of these drugs, and any potential side effects.

- Have you noticed any decrease in your muscle strength recently? **(GH imbalance, FSH-LH deficiency, ACTH imbalance, Addison's disease, hyperthyroidism, hypothyroidism)**

- Have you had any muscle cramping or twitching? **(Metabolic alkalosis)**

- Do you take antacids on a daily basis?

  - If yes, how much and how often? **(Muscle fasciculation and cramping—metabolic alkalosis)**

- Do you frequently have unexplained fatigue? **(Hyperparathyroidism, hypothyroidism, GH deficiency, ACTH imbalance, Addison's disease)**

- What daily activities seem to be too difficult or tiring? **(Muscle weakness due to cortisol and aldosterone hypersecretion and adrenocortical insufficiency, hypothyroidism)**

- Do you notice general muscle and joint aches and pains that seem to persist despite rest? **(Hypothyroidism, Addison's disease)**

- Have you noticed tingling or spasms around the mouth, arms, or legs? **(Hypoparathyroidism, hypothyroidism)**

- Do you have frequent headaches? **(Tumor, primary aldosteronism, hypoglycemia, metabolic acidosis, Paget's disease)**

  - If yes, determine the location, frequency, intensity, duration, precipitating/relieving factors.

- Have you ever undergone head/neck radiation or cranial surgery? **(Thyroid cancer, pituitary dysfunction)**

- Have you recently had a head injury? **(Pituitary dysfunction)**

- Have you ever been told you are diabetic or that you have "sugar"?

- Have you noticed any disturbances in your vision such as blurred vision, double vision, loss of peripheral vision, or sensitivity to light? **(Thyrotoxicosis, hypoglycemia, DM)**

- Have you had an increase in your thirst or the number of times you need to urinate? **(Aldosteronism, DM, diabetes insipidus)**

- Have you noticed any change in the color of your urine? **(Dark urine: ochronosis)**

- Have you had an increase in your appetite? **(DM, hyperthyroidism)**

- Do you bruise easily? **(Cushing's syndrome, excessive secretion of cortisol causes capillary fragility; small bumps/injuries produce bruising)**

- When you injure yourself, do your wounds heal slowly? **(GH excess, ACTH excess, Cushing's syndrome)**

- Have you noticed any unusual intolerance to heat (sweat profusely) or cold? **(TSH imbalance)**

- Have you noticed any increase in your collar size (goiter growth), difficulty in breathing or swallowing? **(Goiter, Graves' disease, hyperthyroidism).**
  - ■ **To the physical therapist:** observe also for hoarseness.
- Have you noticed any changes in skin color? **(Addison's disease)** (e.g., overall skin color has become a darker shade of brown or bronze; occurrence of black freckles; darkening of palmar creases, tongue, mucous membranes)

For the Client Known to Be Taking Corticosteroids

- Have you ever been told that you have osteoporosis or brittle bones, fractures, or back problems? **(Wasting of bone matrix in Cushing's syndrome)**
- Have you ever been told that you have Cushing's syndrome?
- Do you have any difficulty in going up stairs or getting out of chairs? **(Muscle wasting secondary to large doses of cortisol)**

For the Client with Diagnosed DM

- What type of insulin do you take? (see Table 9-8)
- What is your schedule for taking your insulin?
  - ■ **To the physical therapist:** coordinate exercise programs according to the time of peak insulin action. Do not schedule exercise during peak times.
- Do you ever have episodes of hypoglycemia or insulin reaction?
  - ■ If yes, please describe the symptoms that you experience.
- Do you carry a source of sugar with you in case of an emergency?
  - ■ If yes, what is it and where do you keep it in case I need to retrieve it?
- Have you ever had diabetic ketoacidosis ("diabetic coma")?
  - ■ If yes, please describe any symptoms you may have had that I can recognize if this occurs during therapy.
- Do you use the fingerstick method for testing your own blood glucose levels?
  - ■ **To the physical therapist:** you may want to ask the person to bring the test kit for use before or during exercise.
- Do you have difficulty in maintaining your blood glucose levels within acceptable ranges (80 to 120 mg/dl)?
  - ■ If yes, **to the physical therapist:** you may want to take a baseline of blood glucose levels before initiating an exercise program.
- Do you ever have burning, numbness, or a loss of sensation in your hands or feet? **(Diabetic neuropathy)**

CASE STUDY

REFERRAL

Paul Martin, a 45-year-old diabetic client with IDDM, has been receiving whirlpool therapy for a foot ulcer during the last 2 weeks. Today, when he came to the clinic, he appeared slightly lethargic and confused. He indicated to you that he has had a "case of the flu" since early yesterday and that he had vomited once or twice the day before and once that morning before coming to the clinic. His wife, who had driven him to the clinic, said that he seemed to be "breathing fast" and urinating more frequently than usual. He has been thirsty, so he has been drinking "7-Up" and water, and those fluids "have stayed down okay."

PHYSICAL THERAPY INTERVIEW

When did you last take your insulin? (Client may have forgotten because of his illness, forgetfulness, confusion, or just being afraid to take it while feeling sick with the "flu")

What type of insulin did you take?

Do you have a source of sugar with you? If yes, where do you keep it? (This question should be asked during the initial physical therapy interview.)

Have you contacted your physician about your condition?

Have you done a recent blood glucose level (fingerstick)? If yes, when was the last time that this test was done?

What were the results?

To his wife: Your husband seems to be confused and is not himself; how long has he been like this? Have you observed any strong breath odor since this "flu" started? (Make your own observations regarding breath odor at this time.)

If possible, have the client perform a fingerstick blood glucose test on himself. This type of client should be sent immediately to his physician without physical therapy treatment. If he is hypoglycemic (unlikely under these circumstances), this condition should be treated immediately. It is more likely that this client is hyperglycemic and may have diabetic ketoacidosis. In either case, he should not be driving, and arrangements should be made for transport to the physician's office.

References

Aisenbrey, J.A.: Exercise in the prevention and management of osteoporosis. Physical Therapy 67(7): 1100–1104, 1987.

Aloia, J.F.: The osteoporosis: Pathogenesis and diagnosis. Clinical Rheumatology in Practice 4(3):100–113, 1986.

Alspach, J.: Core Curriculum for Critical Care Nursing. Philadelphia, W.B. Saunders, 1991.

Ashinsky, D.: Hemochromatosis. Postgraduate Medicine 91(4):127–145, 1992.

Atkins, C.J., MacIvor, A., and Smith, P.M.: Chondrocalcinosis and arthropathy. Quarterly Journal of Medicine 34:71–82, 1969.

Aurbach, G.D., Marx, S.J., and Spiegel, A.M.: Metabolic bone disease. In Wilson, J.B., and Foster, D.W. (eds.): Williams' Textbook of Endocrinology, 7th ed. Philadelphia, W.B. Saunders, 1985a, pp. 1218–1255.

Aurbach, G.D., Marx, S.J., and Spiegel, A.M.: Parathyroid hormone, calcitonin and the calciferols. *In* Wilson, J.B., and Foster, D.W. (eds.): Williams Textbook of Endocrinology, 7th ed. Philadelphia, W.B. Saunders, 1985b, pp. 1137–1217.

Axford, J.S., Bomford, A.B., Revell, P., Watt, I., and Hamilton, E.D.B.: Grand Rounds in Rheumatology: A case of hemochromatosis arthritis. Journal of Rheumatology *31*:547–553, 1992.

Beard, L., Kumar, A., and Estep, H.L.: Bilateral carpal tunnel syndrome caused by Graves' disease. Archives of Internal Medicine *145*:345–346, 1985.

Becker, K.L., Ferguson, R.H., and McConahey, W.M.: The connective tissue diseases and symptoms associated with Hashimoto's thyroiditis. New England Journal of Medicine *268*:277–280, 1963.

Benson, E.A., and Rosenthal, N.R.: Endocrinologic and related metabolic disorders. *In* Ramsey, P.G., and Larson, E.B. (eds.): Medical Therapeutics, 2nd ed. Philadelphia, W.B. Saunders, 1993, pp. 428–463.

Berkow, R., and Fletcher, A.J. (eds.): The Merck Manual of Diagnosis and Therapy, 16th ed. Rahway, New Jersey, Merck Sharp & Dohme Research Laboratory, 1992.

Birch, C.: Nursing care of clients with thyroid and parathyroid disorders. *In* Black, J.M., and Matassarin-Jacobs, E. (eds.): Luckmann and Sorensen's Medical-Surgical Nursing, 4th ed. Philadelphia, W.B. Saunders, 1993, pp. 1809–1836.

Bluestone, R., Bywaters, E.G.L., Hartog, M., et al.: Acromegalic arthropathy. Annals of Rheumatic Disease *30*:243–258, 1971.

Bridgman, J.F.: Periarthritis of the shoulder and diabetes mellitus. Annals of Rheumatic Disease *31*:69–71, 1972.

Butts-Krakoff, D.: Structure and function: Assessment of clients with metabolic disorders. *In* Black, J.M., and Matassarin-Jacobs, E. (eds.): Luckmann and Sorensen's Medical-Surgical Nursing, 4th ed. Philadelphia, W.B. Saunders, 1993, pp. 1757–1774.

Butts-Krakoff, D., and Black, J.M.: Nursing care of clients with endocrine disorders of the pancreas. *In* Black, J.M., and Matassarin-Jacobs, E. (eds.): Luckmann and Sorensen's Medical-Surgical Nursing, 4th ed. Philadelphia, W.B. Saunders, 1993, pp. 1775–1808.

Carette, S., and LeFrançois, L.: Fibrositis and primary hypothyroidism. Journal of Rheumatology *15*(9):1418–1421, 1988.

Cassmeyer, V.: Management of persons with diabetes mellitus and hypoglycemia. *In* Phipps, W., Long, B., Woods, N., and Cassmeyer, V. (eds.): Medical-Surgical Nursing: Concepts and Clinical Practice, 4th ed. St. Louis, Mosby–Year Book, 1991a, pp. 1091–1136.

Cassmeyer, V.: Management of persons with problems of the pituitary, thyroid, parathyroid and adrenal glands. *In* Phipps, W., Long, B., Woods, N., and Cassmeyer, V. (eds.): Medical-Surgical Nursing: Concepts and Clinical Practice, 4th ed. St. Louis, Mosby–Year Book, 1991b, pp. 1021–1086.

Chernecky, C.C., Krech, R., and Berger, B.: Laboratory Tests and Diagnostic Procedures. Philadelphia, W.B. Saunders, 1993.

Cirullo, J.A.: Osteoporosis. Clinical Management *9*(1):15–19, 1989.

Conrad, M.E.: Sickle cell disease and hemochromatosis. American Journal of Hematology *38*:150–152, 1991.

Degland, J., and Vallerand, A.: Davis Drug Guide for Nurses. Philadelphia, F.A. Davis, 1993.

Donahue, R., and Orchard, T.: Diabete mellitus and macrovascular complications: An epidemiological perspective. Diabetes Care *15*(9):1141–1155, 1992.

Dorfman, H., Solnica, J.H., Di Menza, C., and DeSeze, S.: Les arthropathic hemochromatoses: resultats d'une enquete prospective portant sur 54 malades. La semaine des hôpitaux (Paris) *45*:516–523, 1969.

Dorwart, B.B., and Schumacher, H.R.: Joint effusions, chondrocalcinosis and other rheumatologic manifestations in hypothyroidism. American Journal of Medicine *59*:780–790, 1975.

Dymock, I.W., Hamilton, E.B.D., Laws, J.W., and Williams, R.: Arthropathy of haemochromatosis. Clinical and radiological analysis of 63 patients with iron overload. Annals of Rheumatic Disease *29*:469–476, 1970.

Fairbanks, V.F., and Baldus, W.P.: Disorders of iron metabolism. *In* Williams, W.J., Beutler, E., Erslev, A.J. (eds.): Hematology, 4th ed. New York, McGraw-Hill, 1990, pp. 752–756.

Feibel, J.H., and Campa, J.F.: Thyrotoxic neuropathy. Journal of Neurology, Neurosurgery, and Psychiatry *39*:491, 1976.

Ferraccioli, G.: Neuroendocrinologic findings in fibromyalgia syndrome. Journal of Rheumatology *17*(7):869–873, 1990.

Fitzgerald, P.A.: Endocrine disorders. *In* Tierney, L.M., McPhee, S.J., and Papadakis, M.A. (eds.): Current Medical Diagnosis and Treatment. Norwalk, Connecticut, Appleton and Lange, 1994, pp. 912–1012.

Flexner, J.M.: Hemochromatosis: Diagnosis and treatment. Comprehensive Therapy *17*(11):7–9, 1991.

Forsham, P.H.: Disorder of the adrenal glands. *In* Smith, D.R. (ed.): General Urology, 11th ed. Los Altos, California, Lange Medical Publications, 1984, pp. 444–463.

Frohman, L.A., Felig, P., Broadus, A.E., and Baxter, J.D.: The clinical manifestations of endocrine disease. *In* Felig, P., Baxter, J.D., Broadus, A.E., and Frohman, L.A. (eds.): Endocrinology and Metabolism, 2nd ed. New York, McGraw-Hill, 1987, pp. 23–24.

Gallagher, J.C., Melton, L.J., and Riggs, B.L.: Examination of prevalence rates of possible risk factors in a population with a fracture of the proximal femur. Clinical Orthopedics (153):158–165, 1980.

Gilliland, B.C., and Gardner, G.C.: Rheumatic disorders. *In* Ramsey, P.G., and Larson, E.B. (eds.): Medical Therapeutics, 2nd ed. Philadelphia, W.B. Saunders, 1993, pp. 488–521.

Golding, D.N.: Hypothyroidism presenting with musculoskeletal symptoms. Annals of the Rheumatic Diseases *29*:10–14, 1970.

Gray, P., and Lugwig-Beymer, P.: Alterations of hormonal regulation. *In* McCance, K., and Huethen, S. (eds.): Pathophysiology: The Biologic Basis for Disease in Adults and Children. St. Louis, C.V. Mosby, 1990, pp. 594–645.

Grokoest, A.W., and Demartini, F.E.: Systemic disease and carpal tunnel syndrome. Journal of the American Medical Association *155*:635–637, 1954.

Grossman, L.A., Kaplan, H.J., Ownby, F.D., and Grossman, M.: Carpal tunnel syndrome—initial manifestation of systemic disease. Journal of the American Medical Association *176*:259–261, 1961.

Guyer, P.B.: Paget's disease of bone: The anatomical distribution. Metabolic Bone Disease and Related Research. *4*:239, 1981.

Guyton, A.: Human Physiology and Mechanisms of Disease, 5th ed. Philadelphia, W.B. Saunders, 1992.

Hahn, T.J.: Metabolic bone disease. *In* Kelley, W.N., Harris, E.D., Ruddy, S., et al. (eds.): Textbook of Rheumatology, 3rd ed. Philadelphia, W.B. Saunders, 1989, pp. 1714–1748.

Hall, A.: Joint and periarticular pain. *In* Blacklow, R.S. (ed.): MacBryde's Signs and Symptoms, 6th ed. Philadelphia, J.B. Lippincott, 1983, pp. 211–226.

Heaney, R.P., Recker, R.R., and Saville, P.D.: Menopausal changes in calcium balance performance. Journal of Laboratory and Clinical Medicine *92*:953–963, 1978.

Hellmann, D.B.: Arthritis and musculoskeletal disorders. *In* Tierney, L.M., McPhee, S.J., and Papadakis, M.A. (eds.): Current Medical Diagnosis and Treatment. Norwalk, Connecticut, Appleton and Lange, 1994, pp. 664–710.

Holland H.K., and Spivack, J.L.: Hemochromatosis. Medical Clinics of North America *73*(4):831–845, 1989.

Ingbar, S.H.: The thyroid gland. *In* Wilson, J.B., and Foster, D.W. (eds.): Williams' Textbook of Endocrinology, 7th ed. Philadelphia, W.B. Saunders, 1985, pp. 682–815.

Ingbar, S.H., and Woeber, K.A.: The thyroid gland. *In* Williams, R.H. (ed.): Williams' Textbook of Endocrinology, 6th ed. Philadelphia, W.B. Saunders, 1981, pp. 117–248.

Isley, W.: Thyroid disease. *In* Civetta, J., Taylor, R., and Kirby, R. (eds.): Critical Care. Philadelphia, J.B. Lippincott, 1988, pp. 1415–1424.

Kapoor, A., and Sibbitt, W.L.: Contractures in diabetes mellitus: The syndrome of limited joint mobility. Seminars in Arthritis and Rheumatism *18*:168–180, 1989.

Khaleeli, A.A., Levy, R.D., Edwards, R.H.T., et al.: The neuromuscular features of acromegaly: A clinical and pathological study. Journal of Neurology, Neurosurgery, and Psychiatry *47*:1009–1015, 1984.

Kruse, K., et al.: Hypocalcemic myopathy in idiopathic hypoparathyroidism. European Journal of Pediatrics *138*:280–282, 1982.

Layton, M.W., Fudman, E.J., Barkan, A., et al.: Acromegalic arthropathy: Characteristics and response to therapy. Arthritis and Rheumatism *31*:1022–1027, 1988.

Layzer, R.B.: CNS (Contemporary Neurology Series) Neuromuscular Manifestations of Systemic Disease. Philadelphia, F.A. Davis, 1985.

Lehman, M.K.: Acid-base imbalance. *In* Phipps, W., Long, B., Woods, N., and Cassmeyer, V. (eds.): Medical-Surgical Nursing: Concepts and Clinical Practice, 4th ed. St. Louis, Mosby–Year Book, 1991, pp. 569–575.

Lehman, M.K., Soltis, B., and Cassmeyer, V.: Fluid and electrolyte imbalance. *In* Phipps, W., Long, B., Woods, N., and Cassmeyer, V. (eds.): Medical-Surgical Nursing: Concepts and Clinical Practice, 4th ed. St. Louis, Mosby–Year Book, 1991, pp. 535–567.

Leon, A.: Diabetes. *In* Skinner, J. (ed.): Exercise Testing and Exercise Prescription for Special Cases; Theoretical Basis and Clinical Application, 2nd ed. Philadelphia, Lea and Febiger, 1993, pp. 153–183.

Locke, S., Lawrence, D.G., and Legg, M.A.: Diabetic amyotrophy. American Journal of Medicine *34*:775–785, 1963.

Loriaux, T.C.: Nursing care of clients with adrenal, pituitary, and gonadal disorders. *In* Black, J.M., and Matassarin-Jacobs, E. (eds.): Luckmann and Sorensen's Medical-Surgical Nursing, 4th ed. Philadelphia, W.B. Saunders, 1993, pp. 1837–1862.

Louthrenoo, W., and Schumacher, H.R.: Musculoskeletal clues to endocrine or metabolic disease. Journal of Musculoskeletal Medicine *7*(9):33–56, 1990.

Lumley, W.: Controlling hypoglycemia and hyperglycemia. Nursing 88 *18*:34, 1988.

MacKinnon, J.L.: Osteoporosis: A review. Physical Therapy *68*(10):1533–1540, 1988.

Mallette, L.E., Patten, B.M., and Engel, W.K.: Neuromuscular disease in secondary hyperparathyroidism. Annals of Internal Medicine *82*:474–483, 1975.

Mankin, H.J.: Rickets, osteomalacia, and renal osteodystrophy. Journal of Bone and Joint Surgery *56A*:101–128, 1974.

Marshall, B.: The Endocrine System. New York, Torstar Books, 1986.

McComas, A.J., Sica, R.E.P., and McNabb, A.R. (eds.): Evidence for reversible motor neuron dysfunction in thyrotoxicosis. Journal of Neurology, Neurosurgery, and Psychiatry *37*:548, 1974.

Moskowitz, R.W., et al.: Crystal-induced inflammation associated with chronic renal failure treated with periodic hemodialysis. American Journal of Medicine *47*:450–460, 1969.

National Osteoporosis Foundation: Osteoporosis and Women: A Major Public Health Problem. Washington, D.C., 1991a.

National Osteoporosis Foundation: The Older Person's Guide to Osteoporosis. Washington, D.C., 1991b.

National Osteoporosis Foundation: Stand UP to Osteoporosis: Your Guide to Staying Healthy and Independent Through Prevention and Treatment. Washington, D.C., 1992.

Nelson, D.H.: Diagnosis and treatment of Addison's disease. *In* DeGroot, L.J. (ed.): Endocrinology, 2nd ed. Vol. 2. New York, Grune and Stratton, 1989, pp. 1193–1201.

Niederau, C.: Survival and causes of death in cirrhotic and in non-cirrhotic patients with primary hemochromatosis. New England Journal of Medicine *313*:1246, 1985.

Norris, F.H., and Panner, B.J.: Hypothyroid myopathy: Clinical, electromyographical, and ultrastructural observations. Archives of Neurology *14*:574–589, 1966.

O'Toole, M. (ed.): Miller-Keane Encyclopedia and Dictionary of Medicine, Nursing and Allied Health, 5th ed. Philadelphia, W.B. Saunders, 1992.

Pastan, R.S., and Cohen, A.S.: The rheumatologic manifestations of diabetes mellitus. Medical Clinics of North America *62*:829–839, 1978.

Patten, B.M., Bilezikian, J.P., Mallette, L.E., et al.: Neuromuscular disease in primary hyperparathyroidism. Annals of Internal Medicine *80*:182–193, 1974.

Phalen, G.S.: The carpal tunnel syndrome: Seventeen years' experience in diagnosis and treatment of six hundred and fifty-four hands. Journal of Bone and Joint Surgery *48A*(2):211–228, 1966.

Pinnell, S.R., and Murad, S.: Disorders of collagen. *In* Scriver, C.R., et al.: The Metabolic Basis of Inherited Disease, 6th ed. New York, McGraw-Hill, 1987.

Preston, E.T.: Avulsion of both quadriceps tendons in hyperparathyroidism. Journal of the American Medical Association *221*:406–407, 1972.

Purtilo, D.T., and Purtilo, R.B.: A Survey of Human Diseases, 2nd ed. Boston, Little, Brown, 1989.

Ramsay, I.D.: Thyrotoxic myopathy—electromyography. Quarterly Journal of Medicine *34*:255, 1965.

Ramsay, I.D.: Muscle dysfunction in hyperthyroidism. Lancet *2*:931, 1966.

Ramsay, I.D.: Thyroid Disease and Muscle Dysfunction. Chicago, Year Book Medical Publishers, 1974.

Rauscher, N.A.: Nursing care of clients with musculoskeletal disorders. *In* Black, J.M., and Matassarin-Jacobs, E. (eds.): Luckmann and Sorensen's Medical-Surgical Nursing, 4th ed. Philadelphia, W.B. Saunders, 1993, pp. 1901–1914.

Richart, R.M., and Lindsay, R.: Osteoporosis and its relationship to estrogen. Contemporary Obstetrics/Gynecology *24*:201–224, 1984.

Rubin, L.A., Fam, A.G., Rubenstein, J., et al.: Erosive azotemic osteoarthropathy. Arthritis and Rheumatism *27*:1086–1094, 1984.

Salter, R.B.: Textbook of Disorders and Injuries of the Musculoskeletal System, 2nd ed. Baltimore, Williams & Wilkins, 1983.

Sartoris, D.J.: Radiologic manifestations of degenerative joint disease. Journal of Musculoskeletal Medicine *7*(2):29–43, 1990.

Schott, G.D., and Wills, M.R.: Muscle weakness in osteomalacia. Lancet *1*:626–629, 1976.

Schteingart, D.: Principles of endocrine and metabolic control mechanisms. *In* Price, S., and Wilson, L. (eds.): Pathophysiology Clinical Concepts of Disease Processes. St. Louis, Mosby–Year Book, 1992a, pp. 831–839.

Schteingart, D.: Pancreas: Glucose metabolism and diabetes mellitus. *In* Price, S., and Wilson, L. (eds.): Pathophysiology; Clinical Concepts of Disease Processes. St. Louis, Mosby–Year Book, 1992b, pp. 881–892.

Schteingart, D.: Disorders of the pituitary gland. *In* Price, S., and Wilson, L. (eds.): Pathophysiology;

Clinical Concepts of Disease Processes. St. Louis, Mosby–Year Book, 1992c, pp. 840–848.

Schteingart, D.: Adrenal cortex: Disorders of hyposecretion. *In* Price, S., and Wilson, L. (eds.): Pathophysiology; Clinical Concepts of Disease Processes. St. Louis, Mosby–Year Book, 1992d, pp. 877–880.

Schteingart, D.: Diseases of the thyroid gland. *In* Price, S., and Wilson, L. (eds.): Pathophysiology; Clinical Concepts of Disease Processes. St. Louis, Mosby–Year Book, 1992e, pp. 849–857.

Schteingart, D.: Disorders of calcium metabolism. *In* Price, S., and Wilson, L. (eds.): Pathophysiology; Clinical Concepts of Disease Processes. St. Louis, Mosby–Year Book, 1992f, pp. 858–862.

Schumacher, H.R., and Holdsworth, D.E.: Ochronotic arthropathy, I: Clinicopathologic studies. Seminars in Arthritis and Rheumatism *6*:207–246, 1977.

Shapira, D.: Alcohol Abuse and Osteoporosis. Seminars in Arthritis and Rheumatism, *19*(6):371–376, June, 1990.

Sinaki, M.: A new back support in rehabilitation of osteoporosis program-exercise: Posture training support. Presented at the Third International Symposium on Osteoporosis. Copenhagen, Denmark, Oct. 14–20, 1990.

Sinaki, M., Limburg, P.J., Rogers, J.W., Khosla, S., and Murtaugh, P.A.: Back muscle strength in osteoporotic compared with normal women. Presented at the Third International Symposium on Osteoporosis. Copenhagen, Denmark, Oct. 14–20, 1990.

Singer, F.R.: Metabolic bone disease. *In* Felig, P., Baxter, J.D., Broadus, A.E., and Frohman, L.A. (eds.): Endocrinology and Metabolism, 2nd ed. New York, McGraw-Hill, 1987, pp. 1454–1499.

Sinnett, P.: National Conference of the Australian Physiotherapy Association. Sydney, Australia, 1993.

Starkman, H.S., Gleason, R.E., Rand, L.I., et al.: Limited joint mobility (LJM) of the hand in patients with diabetes mellitus: Relation to chronic complications. Annals of Rheumatic Disease *45*:130–135, 1986.

Strowig, S., and Raskin, P.: Glycemic control and diabetic complications. Diabetes Care *15*(9):1126–1138, 1992.

Travell, J.G., and Simons, D.G.: Myofascial Pain and Dysfunction: The Trigger Point Manual. Vol. I. Baltimore, Williams & Wilkins, 1983.

Utiger, R.D.: Hypothyroidism. *In* DeGroot, L.J. (ed.): Endocrinology, 2nd ed. Vol. 2. New York, Grune & Stratton, 1988, pp. 471–488.

Wade, J.P., and Liang, M.H.: Avoiding common pitfalls in the diagnosis of gout. Journal of Musculoskeletal Medicine *5*(8):16–27, 1988.

Weinstein, J.D., Dick, H.M., and Granthan, S.A.: Pseudogout, hyperparathyroidism, and carpal-tunnel syndrome. Journal of Bone and Joint Surgery *50A*:1669–1674, 1968.

Whedon, G.D.: Osteoporosis. New England Journal of Medicine *6*:397–398, 1981.

Wilson, J.B., and Foster, D.W.: Williams' Textbook of Endocrinology, 7th ed. Philadelphia, W.B. Saunders, 1985.

Wohlgethan, J.R.: Frozen shoulder in hyperthyroidism. Arthritis and Rheumatism *30*:936–939, 1987.

Wyngaarden, J.B., and Kelley, W.N.: Gout. *In* Stanbury, J.B., Wyngaarden, J.B., and Fredrickson, D.S., et al.: The Metabolic Basis of Inherited Disease, 6th ed. New York, McGraw-Hill, 1989.

Bibliography

Becker, K.L., Ferguson, R.H., and McConahey, W.M.: The connective tissue diseases and symptoms associated with Hashimoto's thyroiditis. New England Journal of Medicine *268*:277–280, 1963.

Blacklow, R.S. (ed.): MacBryde's Signs and Symptoms, 6th ed. Philadelphia, J.B. Lippincott, 1983.

Bland, J.H., and Frymoyer, J.W.: Rheumatic syndromes of myxedema. New England Journal of Medicine *282*:1171–1174, 1970.

Braverman, L.E., and Utiger, R.D. (ed.): Werner and Ingbar's The Thyroid, 6th ed. Philadelphia, J.B. Lippincott, 1991.

DeGroot, L.J. (ed.): Endocrinology, 2nd ed. Vol. 2. New York, Grune & Stratton, 1989.

Elborn, J.S., Kelly, J., and Roberts, S.D.: Pseudogout, chondrocalcinosis and the early recognition of haemochromatosis. Ulster Medical Journal *61*(1):119–123, 1992.

Fessel, W.J.: Myopathy of hypothyroidism. Annals of Rheumatic Disease *27*:590–595, 1968.

Golding, D.N.: Hypothyroidism presenting with musculoskeletal symptoms. Annals of Rheumatic Disease *29*:10–14, 1970.

Greenspan, F.S., and Forsham, P.H.: Basic and Clinical Endocrinology, 3rd ed. Norwalk, Connecticut, Appleton & Lange, 1990.

Hochberg, M.C., Kopes, G.M., Edwards, C.Q., Barnes, H.V., and Arnett, F.C.: Hypothyroidism presenting as a polymyositis-like syndrome. Arthritis and Rheumatism *19*:1363–1366, 1976.

Lammers, J.E., Lyles, K.W., Shipp, K.M., and Pieper, C.F.: Impairments of mobility and function in patients with Paget's disease. American Geriatrics Society, 1992.

Lyles, K.W., Gold, D.T., Shipp, K.M.: Exercise for patient's with Paget's disease of bone. Newsletter of the Paget's Disease Foundation *12*(2):3, 1990.

Lyles, K.W., Gold, D.T., Shipp, K.M., et al.: Spinal osteoporosis: Association with impaired functional status. American Federation for Clinical Research, 1991.

Purnell, D.C., Daly, D.D., and Lipscomb, P.R.: Carpal-tunnel syndrome associated with myxedema. Archives of Internal Medicine *108*:751–756, 1961.

Richter, E., Ruderman, N., and Schneider, S.: Diabetes and exercise. American Journal of Medicine *70*:201, 1981.

Stanbury, J.B., Wyngaarden, J.B., Fredrickson, D.S., et al.: The Metabolic Basis of Inherited Disease, 6th ed. New York, McGraw-Hill, 1989.

Tourian, A., and Sidbury, J.B.: Phenylketonuria and hyperphenylalaninemia. *In* Stanbury, J.B., Wyngaarden, J.B., Fredrickson, D.S., et al.: The Metabolic Basis of Inherited Disease, 6th ed. New York, McGraw-Hill, 1989.

Wilke, W.S., Sheeler, L.R., and Makarowski, W.S.: Hypothyroidism with presenting symptoms of fibrositis. Journal of Rheumatology *8*:626–631, 1981.

Appendix

Osteoporosis Screening Evaluation

NAME _____   DATE _____

	YES	NO
1. Do you have a small, thin body?	☐	☐
2. Are you Caucasian or Asian?	☐	☐
3. Have any of your blood-related family members had osteoporosis?	☐	☐
4. Are you a postmenopausal woman?	☐	☐
5. Do you drink 2 or more ounces of alcohol each day? (1 beer, 1 glass of wine, or 1 cocktail = 1 ounce of alcohol)	☐	☐
6. Do you smoke more than 10 cigarettes each day?	☐	☐
7. Are you physically inactive? (walking or similar exercise at least three times per week is average)	☐	☐
8. Have you had both ovaries (with or without a hysterectomy) removed before age 40 years without treatment (estrogen or premarin)?	☐	☐
9. Have you been taking thyroid medication, antiinflammatories, or seizure medication for more than 6 months?	☐	☐
10. Have you ever broken your hip, spine, or wrist?	☐	☐
11. Do you drink four or more servings of caffeine (carbonated beverages, tea, coffee, chocolate) per day?	☐	☐
12. Is your diet low in dairy products and other sources of calcium? (three servings of dairy products or two doses of a calcium supplement per day are average)	☐	☐

If you answer "yes" to 3 or more of these questions, you may be at greater risk for developing osteoporosis, or "brittle bone disease," and you should contact your physician for further information.

10

Overview of Oncologic Signs and Symptoms

■ ■ ■ ■ ■ ■ ■ ■ ■ ■

Clinical Signs and Symptoms of:

Breast Cancer
Metastasized Breast Cancer
Acute and Chronic Leukemias
Multiple Myeloma
Hodgkin's Disease
Non-Hodgkin's Lymphoma
AIDS-NHL
Soft Tissue Sarcoma

Osteosarcoma
Ewing's Sarcoma
Chondrosarcoma
Paraneoplastic Syndromes
Brain Tumors
Increased Intracranial Pressure
Spinal Cord Tumors

A 56-year-old man has come to you for an evaluation without a referral. He has not seen any type of physician for at least 3 years. He is seeking an evaluation on the insistence of his wife, who has noticed that his collar size has increased two sizes in the last year and that his neck looks "puffy." He has no complaints of any kind (including pain or discomfort), and he denies any known trauma; however, his wife insists that he has limited ability in turning his head when backing the car out of the driveway. What questions would be appropriate for your first physical therapy interview with this client? What test procedures will you carry out during the first session? If you suggest to this man that he should see his physician, how would you make that recommendation? (See the Case Study at the end of the chapter.)

Cancer in its early stages is often asymptomatic, yet it is the second leading cause of death in the United States. Only heart disease claims more lives. There are over 1 million new cases of cancer in the United States each year and 510,000 deaths. One in four Americans develops at least one cancer in his or her lifetime. In the past, cancer was invariably fatal. Today, however, one in three people is cured with medical treatment (Matassarin-Jacobs and Petardi, 1993). An additional 600,000 new cases of nonmelanomatous skin cancer are diagnosed every year.

Figure 10–1 summarizes current United States figures for cancer incidence and deaths by site and sex. Although prostate and breast cancers are the most common malignancies in men and women, respectively, the cancer most commonly causing death is still lung cancer (Rugo, 1993).

CANCER

Definition

Cancer is the uncontrolled growth and reproduction of cells. Cancer cells differ from normal cells in their structure, size, function, and rate of growth. In the malignant cell, normal restraints on growth are ineffective, and rapid cellular proliferation results. The cause or causes of the genetic changes within a cell that result in malignancy are still poorly understood, but it is believed that the basic disturbance occurs in the regulatory functions of cellular deoxyribonucleic acid (DNA). This defect in growth regulation differentiates a malignant growth from one that is benign and from normal tissues. Benign tumors involve cellular proliferation of mature cells growing slowly in an encapsulated manner. A benign tumor, unlike a cancerous tumor, does not usually invade the normal tissue around it and does not have the capacity to spread to other parts of the body.

The spread of cancer cells from their primary site to secondary sites is called metastasis. Cancer cells can spread throughout the body through the bloodstream, through the lymphatic system, or by local invasion and infiltration into surrounding tissues. At secondary sites, the malignant cells continue to reproduce, and new tumors or lesions develop.

Cancer describes a group of more than 150 disease processes characterized by un-controlled growth and spread, eventually interfering with one or more vital functions of the host and possibly leading to death. Thus, cancer is not a singular, specific disease but is instead a variable group of tissue responses.

Survival (Matassarin-Jacobs and Petardi, 1993)

Generally, if there is no detectable recurrence of cancer 5 years after the initial diagnosis, the person is considered cured. Although the 5-year determination is arbitrary, the probability that the cancer will recur decreases with each passing year after treatment. As mentioned, although half a million Americans die from cancer each year, 7 million are alive with a cancer diagnosis, and at least 40 per cent of those people were diagnosed 5 or more years ago. Many people considered "cured," however, have physical limitations and movement dysfunctions that interfere with their daily lives. Even without complete remission, cancer often can be controlled to provide longer survival time and improved quality of life, but these factors are not reflected in survival rates.

There is a known lower survival rate in African-Americans for most cancer classifications. This difference may be due to a variety of factors, including limited access to health care, little or no medical insurance, no primary health care provider, homelessness, poverty, lack of knowledge regarding early diagnosis and treatment, and greater exposure to carcinogens.

Staging (Beahrs et al., 1992)

The practice of dividing cancer cases into groups according to *stages* arose from the fact that survival rates were higher for cases in which the disease was localized than for those in which the disease had extended beyond the organ or site of ori-

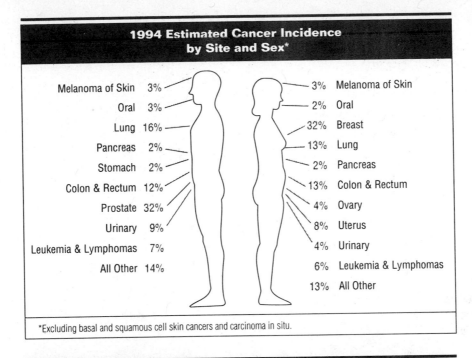

1994 Estimated Cancer Incidence by Site and Sex*

	Men	Women	
Melanoma of Skin	3%	3%	Melanoma of Skin
Oral	3%	2%	Oral
Lung	16%	32%	Breast
Pancreas	2%	13%	Lung
Stomach	2%	2%	Pancreas
Colon & Rectum	12%	13%	Colon & Rectum
Prostate	32%	4%	Ovary
Urinary	9%	8%	Uterus
Leukemia & Lymphomas	7%	4%	Urinary
All Other	14%	6%	Leukemia & Lymphomas
		13%	All Other

*Excluding basal and squamous cell skin cancers and carcinoma in situ.

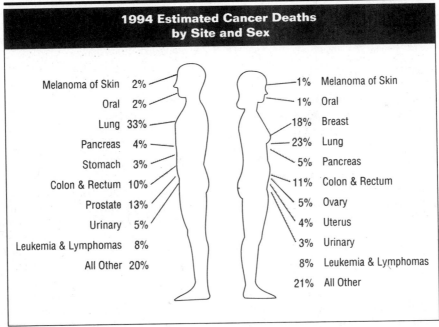

1994 Estimated Cancer Deaths by Site and Sex

	Men	Women	
Melanoma of Skin	2%	1%	Melanoma of Skin
Oral	2%	1%	Oral
Lung	33%	18%	Breast
Pancreas	4%	23%	Lung
Stomach	3%	5%	Pancreas
Colon & Rectum	10%	11%	Colon & Rectum
Prostate	13%	5%	Ovary
Urinary	5%	4%	Uterus
Leukemia & Lymphomas	8%	3%	Urinary
All Other	20%	8%	Leukemia & Lymphomas
		21%	All Other

Figure 10–1

Cancer incidence and deaths by site and sex—1994 estimates. (From Boring, C.S., Squires, T.S., Tong, T., and Montgomery, S.: Cancer Statistics. Atlanta, American Cancer Society, 1994.)

TNM CLINICAL CLASSIFICATION

PRIMARY TUMOR (T)

T_x	Primary tumor cannot be assessed
T_0	No evidence of primary tumor
T_{is}	Carcinoma in situ
$T_1 T_2 T_3 T_4$	Increasing size and/or local extent of the primary tumor

NODES (N)

N_x	Regional lymph nodes cannot be assessed
N_0	No regional lymph node metastasis
$N_1 N_2 N_3$	Increasing involvement of regional lymph nodes

METASTASIS (M)

M_x	Presence of distant metastasis cannot be assessed
M_0	No distant metastasis
M_1	Distant metastasis

From Beahrs, O.H., Henson, D.E., Hutter, R.V.P., and Kennedy, B.J. (eds.): American Joint Committee on Cancer: Manual, Staging of Cancer, 4th ed. Philadelphia, J.B. Lippincott, 1992, pp. 6–7.

---

gin. The stage of disease at the time of diagnosis may reflect not only the rate of growth and extension of the neoplasm but also the type of tumor and the tumor-host relationship.

One classification scheme proposed by the American Joint Committee on Cancer (AJCC) can be incorporated into a form for staging for universal application. This classification is identical with that of the Union Internationale Contre le Cancer (UICC) and is a combination of several other existing systems.

Tumors are staged according to three basic components (see TNM Clinical Classification): primary tumor (T), regional nodes (N), and metastases (M). Subscripts are used with each component to denote size and degree of involvement; for example, 0 indicates undetectable, and 1, 2, 3, and 4 indicate a progressive increase in size or involvement (O'Toole, 1992).

Tissue Changes

Normal tissue contains cells of uniform size, shape, maturity, and nuclear structure. The nucleus of each normal cell contains the proper chromosomal number and composition for the species; when mitosis, or cell division, takes place, the splitting of the chromosomal material occurs in an orderly, sequenced process. Normal cells also have the characteristic of cell *differentiation.*

Differentiation refers to the specialized structure and function of any given cell and to the extent to which each cell resembles its normal parent cell. In malignant cells, differentiation is altered and may be lost completely, so that the malignant cell may not be recognizable in relationship to its parent cell. In this case, it may become difficult or impossible to identify the malignant cell's tissue of origin.

Dysplasia

A variety of other tissue changes can occur in the body. Some of these changes are benign and others denote a malignant or premalignant state. Dysplasia is a general category that indicates a disorganization of cells in which an adult cell varies from its normal size, shape, or organization. This is often due to chronic irritation and is seen with changes in cervical (uterine) epithelium owing to long-standing irritation of the cervix. Dysplasia may reverse itself or may progress to cancer.

Metaplasia

Metaplasia is the first level of dysplasia (early dysplasia). It is a reversible, benign, but abnormal change in which one adult cell changes from one type to another. For example, the most common type of epithelial metaplasia is the change of columnar epithelium of the respiratory tract to squamous epithelium (Hogan, 1991). Although metaplasia usually gives rise to an orderly arrangement of cells, it may sometimes produce disorderly cellular patterns (i.e., cells varying in size, shape, and orientation to one another) (Groenwald, 1993a).

Loss of cellular differentiation is called *anaplasia.* Anaplasia is the most advanced form of metaplasia and is a characteristic of malignant cells only.

Hyperplasia

Hyperplasia refers to an increase in the number of cells in a tissue or part of a tissue, resulting in increased tissue mass. This type of change can be a normal consequence of certain physiologic alterations *(physiologic hyperplasia),* such as increased breast mass during pregnancy, wound healing, or bone callus formation. *Neoplastic hyperplasia,* however, is the increase in cell mass due to tumor formation and is an abnormal process.

Tumors

Tumors, or neoplasms, are "new growths" and may be benign or malignant. The mass of tissue comprising the new growth is a neoplasm that enlarges at the expense of its host. It acts as a parasite by competing for nutrients and threatening the survival of the host. An example of a benign neoplasm is the common wart that does not invade or metastasize. The classic example of a malignant neoplasm is a cancerous solid tumor (Groenwald, 1993a). A *primary* neoplasm of a given structure arises from cells that are normally "local inhabitants" of that structure, whereas a *secondary* neoplasm arises from cells that have metastasized from another part of the body. For example, a primary neoplasm *of* bone arises from within the bone structure itself, whereas a secondary neoplasm occurs *in* bone as a result of metastasized cancer cells from another (primary) site.

Malignant tumors do not respond to the rules that govern normal tissue growth. However, there can be considerable differences in the rate of growth of malignant tumors. Some tumors are very slow growing, even in a malignant state, and are easily removed. Other tumors may grow very rapidly initially and continue to grow rapidly; others may grow slowly at first, then undergo change and grow very fast later. A variety of factors affect the growth rate and pattern of tumors, including host immunocompetence, the rate of individual cell replication, the proportion of total cell population that is actively dividing, and the rate of cell loss from the tumor (Hogan, 1991).

Neoplasms are divided into three cate-

Table 10–1
CATEGORIES OF NEOPLASM

Benign Tumors	Invasive Tumors	Metastatic Tumors

Nonmetastatic
Noninvasive; benign
Structure typical of tissue
    of origin
	Nonmetastatic
	Malignant
	Consists of a large percentage
	    of dividing cells with many
	    abnormal chromosomes
		Metastatic
		Malignant
		Able to invade and transfer
		    disease from one organ to
		    another not directly connected
		    with the first organ

Well differentiated Slow growing	Undifferentiated cells	Undifferentiated cells

gories: benign, invasive, and metastatic (Table 10–1). Within the categories of invasive and metastatic tumors, four large subcategories of malignancy have been identified. These subcategories are classified according to the cell type of origin (Table 10–2).

Tumors can be classified according to cellular maturity and cellular differentiation. When a tumor has completely lost identity with the parent tissue, it is considered to be undifferentiated. In general, the less differentiated a tumor becomes, the worse the prognosis.

Neoplasms are also classified according to the extent of the tumor, as in staging, shown in TNM Clinical Classification.

CURRENT THEORIES OF ONCOGENESIS

Current cancer research has centered around the oncogene or "cancer gene," dysfunction of the immune system, and environmental features of oncogenesis.

Oncogene

The study of viruses as carcinogens is one of the most rapidly advancing areas in cancer research today and led to the discovery of oncogenes (Howley, 1993). The word "oncogene" is a generally accepted misnomer; it is used as a collective term

Table 10–2
SUBCATEGORIES OF MALIGNANCY BY CELL TYPE OF ORIGIN

Carcinomas	Sarcomas	Lymphomas	Leukemias

Arise from epithelial
    cells:
    breast
    colon
    pancreas
    skin
    large intestine
    lungs
    stomach
	Develop from connective
	    tissues:
	    fat
	    muscle
	    bone
	    cartilage
	    synovium
	    fibrous tissue
		Originate in lymphoid
		    tissues:
		    lymph nodes
		    spleen
		    intestinal lining
			Cancers of the hematologic
			    system:
			    bone marrow

Metastasize via lymphatics	Metastasize hematogenously Local invasion	Spread by infiltration	Invasion and infiltration

for a set of growth-regulatory genes that can contribute to the development of cancer after various types of pathologic activation (Klein, 1993). Oncogenes are small segments of genetic DNA that have the ability to transform normal cells into malignant cells, independently or incorporated with a virus (Matassarin-Jacobs and Petardi, 1993).

Even though animals have evolved a complex system to control cell growth, repair, and reproduction, cancer escapes this regulation because the mutations that lead to cancer are mutations of the same genes that regulate normal growth (Yarbro, 1993). Two types of oncogenes or growth-control genes have been identified. The first type, identified as oncogenes (also called proto-oncogenes), are dominant genes that code for proteins that stimulate growth. The second type, identified as anti-oncogenes, are recessive genes that code for proteins that suppress cell growth (Yarbro, 1993).

In addition, two types of cancer-causing mutations have been identified. One type is *somatic mutation,* a mutation that occurs in ordinary cells of body organs owing to carcinogenic exposure throughout a person's lifetime. A second type of mutation, *germ cell mutation,* is a mutation that is transmitted to the next generation at conception and is the cause of hereditary cancers. Most cancers are a combination of both types of mutations and involve alterations in both oncogenes and anti-oncogenes (Yarbro, 1993).

It is now known that oncogenes participate in many different types of tumors and can be involved at different stages of tumorigenesis and viral oncology. A growing number of oncogenes have been identified as being involved in the process of tumor growth, invasion, and metastasis (Liotta and Stetler-Stevenson, 1993). Because of the discovery of the oncogene and the relationship of oncogenes to viruses, gene therapy as a potential treatment for cancer has begun.

Human gene therapy involves the removal of a small piece of tumor from which immune cells called tumor-infiltrating lymphocytes are then extracted. These extracted lymphocytes are then genetically altered to make them more toxic to cancer cells and are reinjected into the person along with other tumor-killing activators such as interleukin-2. From this step, scientists are now testing a number of possible cancer vaccines and the possibility of using viruses as carriers of genetically altered material for use in gene therapy (Culver et al., 1993).

Dysfunction of the Immune System

Dysfunction of the immune system may predispose the body to the development of cancer. When the immune system response is altered, blocked, or overpowered by a large number of malignant cells, recognition and subsequent "attack" may be ineffective or incomplete and cancer growth begins to increase (Braun and Groenwald, 1993). People with genetic immune system defects are more likely to develop leukemia or lymphoma than are people who are immunocompetent. This theory is consistent with what happens when the immune system breaks down in people with acquired immunodeficiency syndrome (AIDS) and in clients who have been selectively immunosuppressed to prevent rejection of organ transplants.

Several other commonly occurring factors alter normal immune function, such as stress, malnutrition, advancing age, and chronic disease (Matassarin-Jacobs and Petardi, 1993). Cancer itself also appears to suppress the immune system both early and late in the disease.

Environmental Causes of Oncogenesis

There may be many probable causes of tumor growth, and more than one precipitating factor may be needed to produce

Table 10-3
DIFFERENTIATION OF COMMON MALIGNANT TUMORS BY AGE

Age 0–8 Yrs	Age 8–40 Yrs	Age 40–55 Yrs	Age 55–75 Yrs
Neuroblastoma	Osteogenic sarcoma	Secondary osteogenic sarcoma	Metastatic carcinoma of the breast
Ewing's sarcoma	Chondrosarcoma	Secondary chondrosarcoma	Metastatic carcinoma of the prostate
Lymphoma	Ewing's sarcoma	Multiple myeloma	Secondary osteogenic sarcoma
Osteogenic sarcoma	Lymphoma	Metastatic carcinoma of the breast	Secondary chondrosarcoma
	Secondary osteogenic sarcoma or chondrosarcoma	Primary osteogenic sarcoma	Multiple myeloma
	Metastatic carcinoma of the thyroid	Neurogenic sarcoma	Other metastatic tumors
	Metastatic carcinoma of the breast		

From D'Ambrosia, R.: Musculoskeletal Disorders: Regional Examination and Differential Diagnosis, 2nd ed. Philadelphia, J.B. Lippincott, 1986.

each individual tumor. There are probably at least 500 different cancer-causing agents. Researchers suspect that cancer results from multiple agents working together (Matassarin-Jacobs and Petardi, 1993).

Environmental and occupational factors, such as consumption of alcohol, smoking cigarettes, drinking contaminated water, diet (natural chemicals, food toxins, or additives), occupation (e.g., industrial carcinogens, asbestos, agricultural chemicals), and ultraviolet and ionizing radiation (background radiation), may contribute to the development of specific cancers (Shields and Harris, 1993). Some of the most common chemical carcinogens include tar, soot, asphalt, chemical dyes, hydrocarbons (e.g., benzene), crude paraffin oil, fuel oils, nickel, and arsenicals (Matassarin-Jacobs and Petardi, 1993).

One accepted premise is that cancer develops as a result of genetic alteration caused by one or more of these etiologic agents. These alterations result in uncontrolled cellular reproduction and growth. When a defective cell divides, the new cells contain the defective genetic code within the DNA. Over time, defective cells divide and multiply and the malignancy grows (Matassarin-Jacobs and Petardi, 1993).

Predisposing Factors (Matassarin-Jacobs and Petardi, 1993)

In addition to the environmental and occupational carcinogens, other predisposing factors such as age, sex, geographic location, stress, heredity, and hormonal status influence the host's vulnerability to various etiologic agents. The physical therapist must pay close attention to the client's age in correlation with a personal or family history of cancer (Table 10–3).

Many cancers, such as prostate, colon, ovarian, and some chronic leukemias, have increased incidence in older clients. This correlation between age and incidence of cancer is thought to be due to an accumulation of premalignant changes over a long period of time, making susceptibility more likely simply because of increased total exposure to carcinogens. The incidence of cancer doubles after 25 years of age and increases with every 5-year increase in age. In addition, as individuals age, the immune system becomes less able to respond to cancer cell invasion (immune response failure theory).

Other cancers occur within very narrow age ranges. Testicular cancer is found in men from about 20 to 40 years of age.

Breast cancer shows a sharp increase after 45 years of age. Ovarian cancer is more common in women over 55 years of age. A number of cancers occur mainly in childhood, such as Ewing's sarcoma, acute leukemia, Wilms' tumor, and retinoblastoma.

Women are more susceptible to certain types of cancer than men and vice versa. However, more men than women have died from all types of cancer, which apparently relates to higher incidence and mortality of lung cancer. More women are smoking, and lung cancer is now the leading cause of death from cancer in both sexes.

The roles of geographic location, diet, heredity, and stress as predisposing factors of cancer are under investigation. For example, it is hypothesized that chronic emotional and physical stress may cause hormonal or immunologic changes or both to the hypothalamus, the portion of the pituitary gland that regulates hormone and immune systems. These changes may enhance the growth and proliferation of cancer cells.

METASTASES (Liotta et al., 1993)

Approximately 30 per cent of clients with newly diagnosed cancers have clinically detectable metastases. At least 30 per cent to 40 per cent of the remaining clients clinically free of metastases harbor occult metastases. Only a third of newly diagnosed clients might potentially be cured by local therapeutic modalities alone, and that number may be optimistic.

Unfortunately, most clients suffer from multiple sites of metastatic disease, not all of which may present at any one time. The formation of metastatic colonies is a continuous process, commencing early in the growth of the primary tumor and increasing with time.

Metastases have the potential to metastasize; the presence of large, identifiable metastases in a given organ is frequently accompanied by a greater number of micrometastases that may have been disseminated more recently from the primary tumor or the metastasis.

The size and age variation in metastases, their dispersed anatomic locations, and their heterogeneous composition hinder complete surgical removal of disease and limit the effective concentration of anticancer drugs that can be delivered to tumor cells in metastatic colonies.

A metastatic colony is the end-result of a complicated series of tumor-host interactions called the *metastatic cascade*. Once a primary tumor is initiated and starts to move by local invasion, tumor angiogenesis occurs—i.e., blood vessels from surrounding tissue grow into the solid tumor. Tumor cells invade host blood vessels and are discharged into the venous drainage (Folkman, 1993). For rapidly growing tumors, millions of tumor cells can be shed into the circulation every day (Liotta et al., 1974; Liotta et al., 1993). Only a very small percentage of circulating tumor cells initiate metastatic colonies (Schirrmacher, 1985). Tumors generally lack a well-formed lymphatic network, so communication of tumor cells with lymphatic channels occurs only at the tumor periphery and not within the tumor mass. Lymphatic and hematogenous dissemination occur in parallel (Liotta and Stetler-Stevenson, 1993).

Although there is no clear explanation of the exact mechanism of metastasis, the metastatic sites of many tumors are fairly predictable. The predilection of certain tumors for particular sites may be due to the ability of the tumor to live within only certain tissues, or it may be due to some other unknown factors. The five most common sites of metastasis are the lymph nodes, liver, lung, bone, and brain (Black and Matassarin-Jacobs, 1993).

Mechanisms

Routes of spread include local invasion, lymphatic spread, and distant spread by

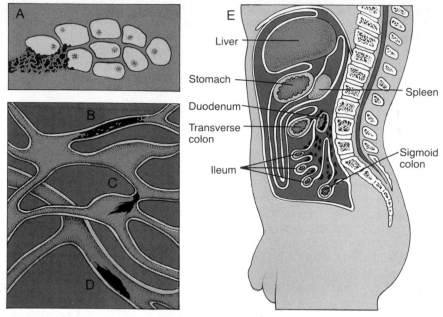

Figure 10–2

Some modes of dissemination of cancer. *A*, Direct extension into neighboring tissue. *B*, Permeation along lymphatic vessels. *C*, Embolism via lymphatic vessels to the lymph nodes. *D*, Embolism via blood vessels. *E*, Invasion of a body cavity by diffusion. (Based on Phipps, J.S., et al. [eds.]: Medical-Surgical Nursing: Concepts and Clinical Practice, 4th ed. St. Louis, C.V. Mosby, 1991.)

the bloodstream (Fig. 10–2). *Local invasion* refers to tumors that continue to grow at the original site of development. Tumors that remain localized are benign tumors and may not be troublesome unless they interfere mechanically with some body function. Some tumors invade nearby parts of the body, and this invasion may include spread into major organs, such as the bowel or bones. Tumors that grow rapidly and spread or destroy tissue are known as malignant tumors (American Medical Association, 1987).

The *lymph system* is a network of tiny vessels designed to remove excess fluid and unwanted substances, such as bacteria, from the body's tissues. If a tumor invades locally into these abundant lymph vessels, it may spread along them to lymph nodes nearby. Lymph nodes (or glands) filter out foreign material by producing lymphocytes (a type of immune cell in the

blood), which aid the lymph node in trapping cancer cells. Where lymph nodes drain into subclavian veins, cancer cells can enter the bloodstream (Groenwald, 1993b).

Hematogenous spread (i.e., via the bloodstream) occurs as cells of malignant neoplasms penetrate thin-walled capillaries. If the tumor invades a blood vessel, then cancer cells may break off into the bloodstream and may be carried to other parts of the body. As blood vessels become progressively smaller, these cells become trapped, and cancer may develop at that point. The pattern of spread depends on the direction of the blood flow from the original tumor (Groenwald, 1993b). Most cells released into the bloodstream are eliminated quickly, but the greater the number released by the primary tumor, the greater the probability that some cells will survive to form metastases. Larger tumors release greater numbers of cells, which increases the chances of survival and metastasis (Groenwald, 1993b).

The usual mode of spread and eventual location of metastases vary with the type of cancer and the tissue from which the cancer arises. For example, prostatic carcinomas typically spread via the lymphatics to the bones of the pelvis and vertebrae. Primary cancers of the bone, such as osteogenic sarcoma, metastastize initially to the lungs. For some cancers, such as malignant melanoma, no typical pattern exists, and metastases may occur anywhere (Baird, 1991).

Metastases usually reproduce the cellular structure of the primary growth well enough to enable a pathologist to determine the site of the primary tumor. For example, bone metastases from a carcinoma of the thyroid not only exhibit a microscopic structure similar to the original tumor but may also produce thyroid hormone (Baird, 1991).

Central Nervous System

Many primary tumors may lead to central nervous system (CNS) metastases. Lung carcinomas account for approximately half of all metastatic brain lesions. Breast carcinoma, the second leading type of primary tumor involved in brain metastases, accounts for approximately 15 per cent of clients with metastases to the CNS. Metastatic disease in the brain is both life-threatening and emotionally debilitating. Metastatic brain tumors can increase intracranial pressure, obstruct the normal flow of cerebrospinal fluid, change mentation, and reduce sensory and motor function (Wegman, 1993).

Primary tumors of the CNS rarely develop metastases outside the CNS despite the highly invasive capacity of these tumors. When it does take place, spread occurs via the cerebrospinal fluid or by direct extension. Spinal cord and nerve root compression cause either insidious or rapid loss of neurologic function. This compression phenomenon occurs in approximately 5 per cent of persons with systemic cancer caused by carcinomas of the lung, breast, prostate, and kidney. Lymphoma and multiple myeloma may also result in spinal cord and nerve root compression. The spinal cord is most often compressed anteriorly by direct growth of a tumor (Wegman, 1993).

Pulmonary System

Pulmonary metastases are the most common of all metastatic tumors because venous drainage of most areas of the body is through the superior and inferior venae cavae into the heart, making the lungs the first organ to filter malignant cells. Parenchymal metastases are asymptomatic until tumor cells have expanded and reached the parietal pleura, where pain fibers are stimulated. Pleural pain and dyspnea may be the first two symptoms experienced by the person (Belcher, 1992). Tumor cells from the lung embolizing via the pulmonary veins and carotid artery can result in metastases to the CNS. Lung cancer is the most common primary tumor to metastasize to the brain. In any individual, any neurologic sign may be the presentation of a silent lung tumor (Gudas, 1987).

Hepatic System

Liver metastases are among the most ominous signs of advanced cancer. The liver filters blood coming in from the gastrointestinal (GI) tract, making it a primary metastatic site for tumors of the stomach, colorectum, and pancreas. The client has abdominal pain and tenderness with general malaise and fatigue.

Skeletal System

Bone metastases represent the initial site of metastatic disease in a large proportion of cancer cases and are generally ominous in terms of prognosis (Belcher, 1992). The primary symptom associated with bone metastases is pain. Although lung, breast, and prostate are the three primary sites responsible for most metastatic bone disease, tumors of the thyroid and kidney, lymphoma (cancer of the lymphatic system, including Hodgkin's disease), and melanoma (skin cancer) can also metastasize to the skeletal system. Metastatic involvement of the vertebrae may result in epidural spinal cord compression with resultant quadriplegia or paraplegia and possibly death. The client who presents with spinal cord symptoms caused by metastatic epidural disease and resultant compression may have only transient symptoms with proper medical treatment (Gudas, 1987).

ONCOLOGIC PAIN (Hogan, 1991; Snyder, 1986)

Cancer pain is a common pain syndrome because one in four people in the United States develops cancer. Cancer pain is uncommon in some cancers such as leukemia. However, pain occurs in 60 per cent to 80 per cent of clients with solid tumors.

This pain syndrome has multiple causes. Some pain is caused by pressure on or displacement of nerves. Pain may also result from interference with blood supply or from blockage within hollow organs. A common cause of cancer pain is metastasis of cancer to the bone. This type of pain can occur as a result of pathologic fracture with resultant muscle spasms; if the spine is involved, nerves may be affected. Pain may also result from iatrogenic causes such as surgery, radiation therapy, and chemotherapy. Immobility and inflammation also can lead to pain.

Treatment of this pain syndrome is difficult because it has a variety of causes. Bone pain usually responds to a combination of radiation therapy with nonsteroidal antiinflammatory drugs (NSAIDs), whereas other pain may require narcotic analgesics.

Signs and Symptoms Associated with Levels of Pain

The severity of pain varies from one client to another, but certain signs and symptoms are characteristic of particular levels of pain. For example, in *mild-to-moderate superficial pain,* a sympathetic nervous system response is usually elicited with hypertension, tachycardia, and tachypnea (rapid, shallow breathing). In *severe or visceral pain,* a parasympathetic nervous system response is more characteristic, with hypotension, bradycardia, nausea, vomiting, tachypnea, weakness, or fainting (Snyder, 1986). Depression and anxiety may increase the client's perception of pain, requiring additional psychologic and emotional support.

Biologic Mechanisms

Five biologic mechanisms have been implicated in the development of chronic cancer pain. The characteristics of the pain depend on tissue structure as well as on the mechanisms involved.

Bone Destruction

Bone destruction secondary to infiltration by malignant cells or resulting from metastatic lesions is the first and most common of the biologic mechanisms causing chronic cancer pain. Bone metastases cause increased release of prostaglandins and subsequent bone breakdown and resorption. The client's pain threshold is reduced through sensitization of free nerve endings. Bone pain may be mild to intense. Maladaptive outcomes of bone destruction may include sharp continuous pain that increases on movement or ambulation. The rich supply of nerves and tension or pressure on the sensitive periosteum or endosteum may cause bone pain. Other factors contributing to the intense discomfort reported by clients include limited space for relief of pressure, altered local metabolism, weakening of the bone structure, and pathologic fractures ranging in size from microscopic to large (Bartzdorf and Catlin, 1990).

Obstruction

Obstruction of a hollow visceral organ and ducts such as the bowel, stomach, or ureters is a second physiologic factor in the development of chronic cancer pain. Viscus obstruction is most often due to the obstruction of an organ lumen by tumor growth. In the GI or genitourinary tracts, obstruction results in either a severe, colicky, crampy pain or true visceral pain that is dull, diffuse, boring, and poorly localized. If a vein, artery, or lymphatic channel is obstructed, venous engorgement, arterial ischemia, or edema, respectively, will result. In these cases, pain is described as being dull, diffuse, burning, and aching. Obstruction of the ducts leading from the gallbladder and pancreas is common in cancer of these organs, although jaundice is more frequently an earlier symptom than pain. Cancer of the throat or esophagus can obstruct these organs, leading to difficulties in eating or speaking (Hogan, 1991).

Infiltration or Compression

Infiltration or compression of peripheral nerves is the third physiologic factor that produces chronic cancer pain and discomfort. Pressure on nerves from adjacent tumor masses and microscopic infiltration of nerves by tumor cells result in continuous, sharp, stabbing pain generally following the pattern of nerve distribution. The invading cells affect the conduction of impulses by the nervous system and sometimes result in constant, dull, poorly localized pain and altered sensation.

Blockage of the blood in arteries and veins, again both by pressure from tumor masses nearby and by infiltration, can decrease oxygen and nutrient supply to tissues. This deficiency can be perceived as pain similar in origin and character to cardiac pain, or angina pectoris, which is chest pain from insufficient supply of oxygen to the heart (Foley, 1986). Hyperesthesia or paresthesia may result.

Infiltration or Distention

Infiltration or distention of integument (skin) or tissue is the fourth physiologic phenomenon resulting in chronic, severe cancer pain. This type of pain is secondary to the painful stretching of skin or tissue because of underlying tumor growth. This stretching produces severe, dull, aching, and localized pain, with the severity of the pain increasing concurrently with increase of tumor size. Pain associated with headaches secondary to brain tumors is thought to be due to traction on pain-sensitive intracranial structures (Hogan, 1991).

Inflammation, Infection, and Necrosis of Tissue

Inflammation, infection, and necrosis of tissue may be the fifth and final cause of cancer pain. Inflammation with its accompanying symptoms of redness, edema, pain, heat, and loss of function may progress to infection, necrosis, and sloughing of tissue. If the inflammatory process alone is present, the pain is characterized by a sensitive tenderness. If, however, necrosis and tissue sloughing have occurred, pain may be excruciating (Hogan, 1991).

LABORATORY AND DIAGNOSTIC STUDIES

Numerous procedures are used in the detection, diagnosis, and treatment of cancer. Assessment of the client with cancer involves careful, systematic evaluation and screening of a person's medical, social, cultural, and psychologic background, as well as thorough and systematic physical examination. The common procedures used in the detection, diagnosis, and evaluation of the cancer client include the following (Belcher, 1992):

- X-ray
- Mammography
- Lymphangiography
- Magnetic resonance imaging (MRI)
- Computed tomography (CT scan)
- Ultrasonography
- Contrast scanning (e.g., bone, liver)
- Lumbar puncture/spinal tap
- Pleural fluid tap
- Gastric washing
- Papanicolaou (Pap) smear
- Fiberoptic scope procedures (e.g., bronchoscopy, endoscopy, colonoscopy)
- Biopsy (surgical and/or needle)
- Hormone receptor assays (e.g., estrogen and progesterone)
- Chromosomal analyses

In addition to these studies, many blood studies are clinically useful and significant in the diagnosis and treatment of cancer. Blood studies include blood chemistries (electrolytes, enzymes, hormones, amino acids), hematology (red blood cells, white blood cells, platelets), tumor markers, and tumor antigen studies.

Tumor markers are substances produced and secreted by tumor cells and are found in the blood serum of clients with cancer. Increased levels of these markers in combination with other data are used to monitor the presence or progress of the disease. The level of the tumor marker seems to correlate with the extent of the disease process. For example, in clients with colorectal cancer, levels of carcinoembryonic antigen (CEA) usually relate directly to the extent of tumor growth and the response of the tumor to treatment (Belcher, 1992). Other examples of tumor markers are CA 125 (ovarian cancer), prostate-specific antigen (PSA) (prostate cancer), and alpha-fetoprotein (AFP) (testicular and liver cancers).

Tumor-associated antigens are identifiable in blood serum and are expressed by tumors and viruses, which then generate an immune response. Viral antigens are products expressed by virally transformed cells and are associated with certain types of lymphomas and nasopharyngeal cancers (Belcher, 1992).

CANCER TREATMENT (Hamburgh, 1992)

Modalities

For many years, three basic modalities of cancer treatment have been used, either alone or in combination: surgery, radiation therapy, and chemotherapy. In recent years, two newer treatment modalities have received increased attention. These include biologic response modifiers and bone marrow transplantation.

Surgery is probably the oldest type of cancer treatment and remains one of the most important treatments for solid tumors. Surgery can be curative in people with localized cancer, but because about 70 per cent of clients have evidence of micrometastases at the time of diagnosis, combining surgery with other modalities is usually necessary to achieve better response rates (Dietrick-Gallagher and Brasher, 1991).

Radiation therapy is also a major treatment modality. Approximately 60 per cent of all people with cancer will be treated with radiation therapy at some time during the course of their disease. Radiation can now be delivered to the client with maximal therapeutic effect and minimal toxicity and destruction of healthy tissue (Iwamoto, 1991).

Chemotherapy, or the use of chemical agents to destroy cancer cells, has a very large role in the treatment of cancer. A major advantage of chemotherapy is its applicability to the treatment of widespread or metastatic disease, because surgery and radiation are more useful for treatment of localized lesions. In the United States today, approximately 50 anticancer drugs and hormones are commercially available (Peterson, 1991).

Biologic response modifiers (BRMs) constitute the fourth cancer treatment modality. These agents change or modify the relationship between tumor and host by strengthening the host's biologic response to tumor cells. Recent technologic advances have prompted a renewed interest in BRMs, and they are now an important area in cancer research and treatment (Ersek, 1991).

Bone marrow transplantation is used for cancers that are responsive to high doses of chemotherapy or radiation therapy. These high doses kill cancer cells but are also toxic to bone marrow. Because bone marrow transplantation provides a method for "rescuing" clients from bone marrow destruction, higher doses of chemotherapy can be given, with better antitumor results. Many of the leukemias, lymphomas, multiple myelomas, and some other solid tumor cancers such as testicular cancer, small cell lung cancer, and breast cancer can be treated with bone marrow transplantation. Bone marrow for transplantation can be obtained from an identical twin, a sibling, or the person's own stored bone marrow. As with any organ transplant, the problem of organ or tissue rejection is a major consideration (Schilter and Rossman, 1991).

Side Effects (McGarvey, 1990; Watchie, 1992)

Cancer treatment has many side effects because the goal of treatment is to remove or to kill certain tissues. In any situation, healthy tissue also is usually sacrificed.

The pharmaceuticals used in chemotherapy are cytotoxic (destructive), designed to kill dividing cells selectively by blocking the ability of DNA and RNA to reproduce and by lysing cell membranes. All types of dividing cells, not just the cancer cells, are affected.

In addition, a combination of drugs (each causing cell death through different pharmacologic mechanisms) is traditionally used for greater efficacy in the systemic treatment of some cancers (e.g., breast cancer). Hence, an overlap of toxicities may result in greater side effects (Miller, 1992).

The effects of treatment for cancer can be debilitating physiologically, physically, and psychologically. Common physical side effects include severe mucositis, mouth sores, nausea and vomiting, fluid retention, pulmonary edema, cough, headache, malaise, fatigue, dyspnea, and loss of hair. Emotional and psychologic side effects are present but less evident.

Aggressive chemotherapeutic agents and chest irradiation can cause cardiopulmonary dysfunction, especially in the treatment of Hodgkin's disease and breast and lung cancers. High-dose radiation can result in pericardial fibrosis (scarring of the pericardium) and constrictive pericarditis (inflammation of the pericardium). These conditions are usually asymptomatic until the client starts to exercise, and then exertional dyspnea is the first symptom. Other causes of dyspnea include deconditioning, anemia, peripheral arterial disease, and increased physiologic demand for oxygen because of fever or infection.

Side effects associated with radiation treatment include edema, immunosuppression (bone marrow suppression), mucositis, hair loss, burns, and radiation sickness. Radiation sickness is characterized by headaches, diarrhea, nausea, vomiting, and fatigue. During radiation therapy, the client may be more tired than usual. Resting throughout exercise is important, as are adequate nutrition and hydration.

The skin in the irradiated area may become red or dry and should be exposed to the air but protected from the sun and from tight clothing. Gels, lotions, oils, or other topical agents should not be used over the irradiated skin without a physician's approval. Clients may have other side effects, depending on the areas treated. For example, radiation to the lower back may cause nausea, vomiting, or diarrhea because the lower digestive tract is exposed to the radiation (National Cancer Institute, 1991).

Radiation-related pulmonary toxicity may occur, presenting in one of two forms: *acute radiation pneumonitis* (lung inflammation) or *late radiation fibrosis* (connective tissue overgrowth). Symptoms of acute radiation pneumonitis occur 1 to 3 months after treatment and include dyspnea on exertion, nonproductive cough, and low-grade fever. Late radiation fibrosis develops 9 to 12 months after radiation therapy but can take up to 2 years to develop. This fibrosis is a form of restrictive pulmonary disease characterized by reduced pulmonary function, particularly decreased lung volumes.

▼ Side Effects of Cancer Treatment

- Severe mucositis
- Headache
- Dyspnea
- Mouth sores
- Diarrhea, nausea, and vomiting
- Fluid retention/edema
- Cough
- Fever
- Hair loss
- Malaise, fatigue
- Pulmonary edema
- Radiation sickness
- Bone marrow suppression (infection, anemia, bleeding)

Because bone marrow suppression is a common and serious side effect of many chemotherapeutic agents and can be a side effect of radiation therapy in some instances, it is extremely important to monitor the hematology values in clients receiving these treatment modalities. It is very important to review these values before any type of vigorous physical therapy is initiated. A guideline used by some physical therapy exercise programs is the Winningham Contraindications for Aerobic Exercise. According to these guidelines, aerobic exercise is contraindicated in chemotherapy clients when laboratory values are as follows (Winningham et al., 1986):

Platelet count	$<50,000/mm^3$
Hemoglobin	<10 g/dl
White blood cell count	$<3000/mm^3$
Absolute granulocytes	$<2500/mm^3$

EARLY WARNING SIGNS

For many years, the American Cancer Society has publicized seven warning signs of cancer, the appearance of which could indicate the presence of cancer and the need for a medical evaluation. The following mnemonic is often used as a helpful reminder of these warning signs:

Changes in bowel or bladder habits
A sore that does not heal in 6 weeks
Unusual bleeding or discharge
Thickening or lump in breast or elsewhere
Indigestion or difficulty in swallowing
Obvious change in a wart or mole
Nagging cough or hoarseness

Awareness of these signals is useful, but it is generally agreed that these symptoms do not always reflect early curable cancer, nor does this list include all the possible signs for the different types of cancer.

For the physical therapist, idiopathic proximal muscle weakness may be an early sign of cancer. This syndrome of proximal muscle weakness is referred to as *carcinomatous neuromyopathy*. It is accompanied by a diminution of two or more deep tendon reflexes (ankle jerk usually remains intact) (Croft and Wilkinson, 1965). Muscle weakness may occur secondary to hypercalcemia, which is typically found in people with multiple myeloma, a form of plasma cell cancer that affects bone marrow.

Pain is rarely an early warning sign of cancer, even in the presence of unexplained bleeding. Bleeding is an important sign of cancer, but a cancer is generally well established by the time bleeding occurs. Bleeding develops secondary to ulcerations in the central areas of the tumor or by pressure on or rupture of local blood vessels. As the tumor continues to grow, it may enlarge beyond its capacity to obtain necessary nutrients, resulting in devitalization of portions of the tumor. This process of invading and compressing local tissue, shutting off blood supply to normal cells, is called necrosis (Baird, 1991). Tissue necrosis leads ultimately to secondary infection, severe hemorrhage, and the development of pain when regional sensory nerves become involved. Other symptoms can include pathologic fractures, anemia, and thrombus formation.

SKIN AND BREAST CANCERS

Skin cancer and breast cancer are two of the more common cancers about which clients will ask physical therapists for advice. During the observation/inspection portion of any examination, the physical therapist may observe skin lesions that may need further medical investigation. For these reasons, this special section on skin and breast cancer is included.*

---

* Other specific types of cancer affecting organ systems are discussed individually in each related chapter.

Additionally, the woman presenting with chest, breast, axillary, or shoulder pain of unknown etiology must be questioned regarding breast self-examinations. Any recently discovered lumps or nodules must be examined by a physician. The client may need education regarding breast self-examination, and the physical therapist can provide this valuable information. Techniques of breast self-examination are commonly available in written form for the physical therapist or the client who is unfamiliar with these methods (Giuliano, 1993; Williams and Williams, 1986).

Skin Cancer

Skin cancer is the most common cancer diagnosed in the United States. It affects men and women equally but seldom occurs in children before puberty (Spitz, 1948).

The incidence of cutaneous melanoma (a tumor arising from the melanocytic system of the skin and other organs) increased 80 per cent from 1973 to 1980 and faster in white men than any other cancer from 1973 to 1988. This tumor accounts for 1 per cent of all cancers in the United States; its behavior is unpredictable, ranging from spontaneous regression to rapid progression to death. Death from malignant melanoma is increasing at a faster rate than death from any other malignant neoplastic disease except lung cancer (Goldstein and Odom, 1993; Press et al., 1993). Almost half of all melanoma deaths occur in men older than age 50 years, but melanoma frequently affects young people. The median age for people with melanoma is the early 40s (Sober, 1991).

The cause of skin cancer is well known. Prolonged or intermittent exposure to ultraviolet (UV) radiation from the sun, especially when it results in sunburn and blistering, plays a key role in the induction of skin cancer, especially malignant melanoma. The majority of all nonmelanoma skin cancers occur on parts of the body unprotected by clothing (face, neck, fore-

---

RISK FACTORS FOR THE DEVELOPMENT OF MALIGNANT MELANOMA

- Family history of malignant melanoma
- Blond or red hair
- Marked freckling on the upper back
- History of three or more blistering sunburns prior to age 20 years
- History of 3 or more years in an outdoor summer job during adolescence
- Presence of actinic keratosis (sharply outlined horny growth e.g., wart or callus)

From Friedman, R.J., Rigel, D.S., Silverman, M.K., Kopf, A.W., and Vossaert, K.A.: Malignant melanoma in the 1990s. CA—A Cancer Journal for Clinicians *41*(4):201–225, 1991.

---

arms, and backs of hands) and in people who have received considerable exposure to sunlight (Nicol, 1993).

All adults are at risk for skin cancer regardless of skin tone and hair color; however, some people are at much greater risk than others (see Risk Factors for the Development of Malignant Melanoma). In general, people with red, blond, or light-brown hair with light complexions and maybe freckles, many of Celtic or Scandinavian origin, are most susceptible; people of African or Asian origin are least susceptible. The most severely affected people usually have a history of long-term occupational or recreational sun exposure.

Types. The several different kinds of skin cancer are distinguished by the types of cells involved. Basal cell carcinoma, squamous cell carcinoma, and malignant melanoma are the three most common types of skin cancer. More than 90 per cent of all skin cancers fall into the first two classifications.

Basal Cell Carcinoma. Basal cell carcinoma involves the bottom layer of the epidermis of the face, neck, head, ears, or hands. Occasionally, basal cell carcinoma may appear on the trunk, especially the upper back and chest. The majority of cases are caused by chronic overexposure to UV radiation, and only a few cases can be linked to arsenic (e.g., occupational chemicals, insecticides, drinking water),

burns, radiation exposure (mainly in the form of therapeutic radiation used in the past to treat acne and other skin conditions), scars, or genetic predisposition.

Squamous Cell Carcinoma. Squamous cell carcinoma arises from the top of the epidermis and is the second most common skin cancer in whites. It is found on areas often exposed to the sun, typically the rim of the ear, the face, the lips and mouth, and the dorsa of the hands. These tumors are potentially dangerous because they may infiltrate surrounding structures, metastasize to lymph nodes, and become fatal (Nicol, 1993).

Malignant Melanoma. Malignant melanoma is the most serious form of skin cancer; it arises from pigmented cells in the skin called melanocytes. Whites have ten times the incidence that African-Americans do. UV radiation continues to be one of the most important causes of malignant melanoma; however, melanoma can appear anywhere on the body, not just on sun-exposed areas. The majority of malignant melanomas appear to be associated with the intensity rather than the duration of sunlight exposure, in contrast to basal and squamous cell carcinomas (Nicol, 1993).

Metastases. Basal cell carcinoma rarely metastasizes. Primary tumors that metastasize typically are located on the head and neck, are large and locally invasive, and are not cured with repeated surgery and radiation therapy. Once metastasis is recognized, the mean survival time is approximately 1 year. Dissemination of the neoplasm occurs via lymphatics and venous circulation. Most metastases are found in regional lymph nodes, but bone, lung, and liver are involved in up to 20 per cent of cases (Cannon and Schneidman, 1982; Patterson and Geronemus, 1989).

Squamous cell carcinoma metastasizes to regional lymph nodes and eventually to distant sites, including bone, brain, and lungs. The likelihood of metastasis depends on the anatomic site, previous inflammation, or injury at that site. Squamous cell carcinomas arising from normal skin may be rapidly invasive and metastasize frequently, but those developing in sun-damaged skin may have a lower incidence of metastasis. Lesions arising in sites of chronic cutaneous injury such as thermal burns and decubitus ulcers have a higher rate of metastasis (Patterson and Geronemus, 1989).

The most common sites of distant metastases associated with malignant melanoma are the skin and subcutaneous tissue. The second most common initial sites of metastasis are the lungs and surrounding visceral pleura. Any anatomic site may be involved, including skin, subcutaneous tissue, lungs, lymph nodes, GI tract, spleen, liver, CNS, and bone, and malignant melanoma is fatal within a year.

Clinical Signs and Symptoms. Basal cell carcinoma occurs mostly on sun-exposed skin. These lesions grow slowly, attaining a size of 1 to 2 cm in diameter, often after years of growth. Metastases almost never occur, but neglected lesions may ulcerate and produce great destruction, ultimately invading vital structures (Goldstein and Odom, 1994; Miller, 1991). There are a number of common forms of basal cell carcinoma (Harrist and Clark, 1994):

■ Pearly papule resembles a pearl 2 to 3 mm in diameter. It is covered by tightly stretched epidermis, which is laced with small delicate, branching vessels (telangiectasia)

■ Rodent ulcer is a small crater in the center of the pearl

■ Superficial basal carcinoma appears as a scaly, red, sharply demarcated plaque

■ Morphea-like basal cell carcinoma is an ill-defined pale, tough, scar-like tumor

■ Pigmented basal cell carcinoma grossly resembles malignant melanoma of the superficial spreading or nodular type

Squamous cell carcinoma lesions appear as small red, conical, hard nodules that occasionally ulcerate. The lesions characteristically arise on the backs of the hands or on the face but are also common on the lips and ears (Harrist and Clark, 1994). Premalignant lesions include sun-damaged skin or dysplasias (whitish discolored areas), scars, radiation-induced keratosis, and chronic ulcers. Invasive tumors are firm and increase in elevation and diameter. The surface may be granular and bleed easily (Huether and Kravitz, 1994).

The clinical characteristics of early malignant melanoma are similar regardless of anatomic site (Ackerman, 1981; Friedman et al., 1991). Unlike benign pigmented lesions, which are generally round and symmetric, the shape of an early malignant melanoma is often asymmetric. Although benign pigmented lesions tend to have regular margins, the borders of early malignant melanomas are often irregular. Compared with benign pigmented lesions, which are more uniform in color, macular malignant melanomas are usually variegated, ranging from various hues of tan and brown to black, sometimes intermingled with red and white. The diameters of malignant melanomas are often 6 mm or larger when first identified. During observation and inspection, the physical therapist should be alert to any potential signs of skin cancer. The major warning sign of melanoma is some change in a mole or "beauty mark." The Skin Cancer Foundation advocates the use of the ABCD method of early detection of melanoma and dysplastic (abnormal in size or shape) moles.

> **A: asymmetry:** (uneven edges, lop-sided in shape, one half unlike the other half)
> **B: border:** irregularity, irregular edges scalloped or poorly defined edges
> **C: color:** black, shades of brown, red, white, occasionally blue
> **D: diameter:** larger than a pencil eraser

Other signs that may be important include

- Irritation and itching
- Tenderness, soreness, or new moles developing around the mole in question
- A sore that keeps crusting and does not heal within 6 weeks

If any of these signs and symptoms are present in a client whose skin lesion(s) has not been examined by a physician, a medical referral is recommended. If the client is planning a follow-up visit with the physician within the next 2 to 4 weeks, then the client is advised to point out the mole or skin changes at that time. If no appointment is pending, then the client is encouraged to make a specific visit either to the family/personal physician or to a dermatologist.

Treatment. There are many treatment choices for cutaneous carcinoma, including primary surgery to excise the lesion, adjuvant chemotherapy, radiotherapy, or cryotherapy. Combination treatments have no proven effect on myeloma (Press et al., 1993; Steele et al., 1993). Immunotherapy and hormonal therapy are currently investigational and are not used to treat cutaneous carcinomas, but they may be an accepted standard in the future (Patterson and Geronemus, 1989).

Prognosis. Both basal cell carcinoma and squamous cell carcinoma are slow-growing tumors that have a cure rate of 95 per cent or greater with early treatment (Nicol, 1993). Survival figures for squamous cell carcinoma that has metastasized reflect the aggressive behavior of those neoplasms; in one study, only 25 per cent of clients with metastases were alive at 5 years, 13 per cent at 10 years, and 8 per cent at 15 years (Epstein et al., 1968).

The prognosis for malignant melanoma depends on multiple factors, including tumor thickness, the person's age, and the presence of metastases (number and location of sites). The depth of vertical invasion of a primary melanoma is the most important prognostic factor determining the risk of recurrence or dissemination (Balch et al., 1989; Goldstein and Odom, 1993; Press et al., 1993).

The disease-free interval before development of metastatic disease may be about 10 years (Press et al., 1993). In one study, median survival time for clients with a single distant metastatic site was 7 months; for clients with two sites, it was 4 months; and for those with three sites, it was 2 months (Patterson and Geronemus, 1989).

Breast Cancer

The breast is the most common site of cancer in women, and cancer of the breast is second only to lung cancer as a cause of death from cancer among women. A woman's probability of developing breast cancer increases throughout her life. The mean and median ages of women with breast cancer are 60 and 61 years, respectively. There will be about 182,000 new cases of breast cancer and about 46,000 deaths from this disease in women in the United States this year. At the present rate of incidence, 1 of every 9 American women will develop breast cancer during her lifetime (Carpenter, 1993; Giuliano, 1993). However, there are indicators that this increase in incidence is primarily caused by educational efforts toward early detection and that a decrease in breast cancer mortality should be the result of this effort in a few years (Garfinkel, 1993).

Table 10−4

FACTORS ASSOCIATED WITH BREAST CANCER

Gender	Women > men
Race	White
Age	Advancing age Peak incidence: 45−70 years Mean and median age: 60−61 (women) 60−66 (men)
Family History	North America or Northern European birthplace Breast cancer in any first-degree relative (mother, daughter, or sister), especially bilateral or premenopausal
Previous Medical History	Endometrial cancer; previous breast cancer Previous cancer of uterus, ovary, or colon Diabetes Obesity Mammary dysplasia (benign fibrocytic breast disease) Exposure to ionizing radiation
Menstrual History	Early menarche (under age 12 years) Late menopause (after age 50 years)
Pregnancy	Never pregnant Late first pregnancy (over 30 years)

Adapted from Giuliano, A.E.: Breast. *In* Schroeder, S.A., et al.: Current Medical Diagnosis and Treatment. Norwalk, Connecticut, Appleton & Lange, 1992.

While the frequency of breast cancer in men is strikingly less than that in women, the disease in both sexes is remarkably similar in epidemiology, natural history, and response to treatment. Men with breast cancer are 5 to 10 years older than women at the time of diagnosis, with mean or median ages between 60 and 66 years. This apparent difference may occur because symptoms in men are ignored for a longer period and the disease is diagnosed at a more advanced stage (Donegan, 1991).

Risk Factors (Table 10−4). The cause of breast cancer has not been definitely established. Genetic predisposition and hormonal factors may be involved (Carpenter, 1993). A predisposing gene for breast and ovarian cancer (BRCA-1) has been mapped to the long arm of chromosome 17. The disease is linked to this gene in almost all families having members with breast and ovarian cancer and in half of those families whose members have only breast cancer. All cases of bilateral breast cancer and ovarian cancer appear to be linked to this gene (Black and Solomon, 1993; Hall et al., 1992; Porter et al., 1993).

Heredity, race, hormonal influences, and diet are all being considered as scientific investigations continue to reveal potential risk factors. The presence of any of these factors may become evident during the interview with the client and alert the physical therapist to potential neuromusculoskeletal complaints of a systemic origin that would require a medical referral. At the same time, it should be remembered that many women diagnosed with breast cancer have no identified risk factors. More than 70 per cent of breast cancer cases are not explained by established risk factors (Garfinkel, 1993). There is no history of breast cancer among female relatives in over 90 per cent of breast cancer clients (Giuliano, 1993).

First-degree relatives (mother, daughters, or sisters) of women with breast cancer have two to three times the risk of developing breast cancer than the general female population; relatives of women with bilateral breast cancer have five times the normal risk. Women who have never been pregnant and women whose first full-term pregnancy was after age 30 years have a slightly higher incidence of breast cancer than multiparous women (Carpenter, 1993; Giuliano, 1993). Other factors, such as a history of mammary dysplasia (benign fibrocystic breast disease), can contribute to increased risk.

Breast cancer can occur in both premenopausal and postmenopausal women, with the peak incidence occurring between 45 and 70 years of age. Age itself represents a risk factor, because the incidence of breast cancer is highest in women over 50 years of age.

Early menarche (onset of menstrual function) or late menopause increases the risk of breast cancer. However, late menarche, an oophorectomy (removal of ovaries) before menopause, and artificial menopause are associated with a lower incidence of breast cancer (Giuliano, 1993).

White people have a slightly higher incidence of breast cancer than nonwhites, and the obese, diabetic person seems to be at higher risk. Exposure to ionizing radiation appears to be a risk factor. The risk increases with increasing doses of radiation, particularly with exposure before age 20 years (Donegan, 1991; Hall, 1993). For example, survivors of the atomic bombs dropped on Japan and women who received multiple fluoroscopies for tuberculosis or radiation treatment for mastitis during their adolescent or childbearing years are at increased risk. Irradiation was used

or a variety of other medical conditions, including gynecomastia, thymic enlargement, eczema of the chest, chest burns, pulmonary tuberculosis, mediastinal lymphoma, and other cancers (Donegan, 1991).

Risk factors under study as possible causes of increased incidence of breast cancer include

- Oral contraceptives
- Exogenous hormones (e.g., postmenopausal estrogen hormone replacement)
- Above average weight and height
- High-fat diet
- Alcohol consumption
- Ovarian-pituitary dysfunction
- Genetic factors

Metastases (Carpenter, 1993). Metastases have been known to occur up to 25 years after the initial diagnosis of breast cancer. On the other hand, breast cancer can be a rapidly progressing, terminal disease. All distant visceral sites are potential sites of metastases. Bone is the most frequent site of metastases from breast cancer in men and women. Other primary sites of involvement are lymph nodes, remaining breast tissue, lung, brain, CNS, and liver, but this widely metastasizing disease has been found in almost every remote site (Beahrs et al., 1992). Women with metastases to the liver or CNS have a poorer prognosis.

Knowledge of the usual metastatic patterns of breast cancer and the common complications can aid early recognition and effective treatment. Spinal cord compression, usually from extradural metastases, may present as back pain, leg weakness, and bowel/bladder symptoms.

Clinical Signs and Symptoms (Giuliano, 1993). Breast cancer usually consists of a nontender, firm, or hard lump with poorly delineated margins, caused by local infiltration. Breast cancer in women has a predilection for the outer upper quadrant of the breast. Slight skin or nipple retraction is an important sign. Watery, serous, or bloody discharge from the nipple is an occasional

▼ *Clinical Signs and Symptoms of*
Breast Cancer

- Nontender, firm or hard lump
- Skin or nipple retraction
- Discharge from nipple
- Erosion, retraction, enlargement, itching of the nipple
- Redness or skin rash
- Generalized hardness, enlargement, or shrinking of the breast
- Axillary mass
- Swelling of the arm
- Bone or back pain
- Weight loss
- Jaundice

▼ *Clinical Signs and Symptoms of*
Metastasized Breast Cancer

- Back pain
- Leg weakness
- Bowel/bladder symptoms

early sign but is more often associated with benign disease.

The presenting complaint in about 70 per cent of persons with breast cancer is a lump (usually painless) in the breast. About 90 per cent of breast masses are discovered by the individual. Less frequent symptoms are breast pain, nipple discharge, erosion/retraction/enlargement/itching of the nipple, redness, generalized hardness, or enlargement or shrinking of the breast. Rarely, an axillary mass, swelling of the arm, or bone pain from metastases may be the first symptom. Back or bone pain, jaundice, or weight loss may be the result of systemic metastases, but these symptoms are rarely seen on initial presentation.

A tumor of any size in male breast tissue presents with skin fixation and ulceration and deep pectoral fixation more often than a tumor of similar size in female breast tissue does because of the small size of male breasts. Lump masses that occur in the upper outer quadrant of the breast (usually women) involve the breast tissue overlying the pectoral muscle. During palpation, breast tissue lumps move easily over the pectoral muscle, compared with a lump within the muscle tissue itself. Later signs of malignancy include fixation of the tumor to the skin or underlying muscle fascia.

A suspicious finding should be checked by a physician, especially in the case of the woman with identified risk factors. For this reason, it is always important to ask the client about risk factors identified in the text and previous medical history and to correlate this information with objective findings.

Treatment. Pathologic Stage I (primary tumor less than 2 cm, negative nodes), Stage II (primary tumor less than 5 cm, positive nodes), and operable Stage III (primary tumor 5 cm or more with or without positive nodes, no local contraindication to resection) may be managed by a variety of approaches. Excisional biopsy, lumpectomy, mastectomy, irradiation, adjuvant chemotherapy, and hormonal therapy are commonly employed (Press et al., 1993). Autologous bone marrow transplantation with high-dose chemotherapy is currently under investigation as a treatment for women with metastatic disease (Affronti, 1990).

Prognosis (Giuliano, 1993). The stage of breast cancer is the single most reliable indicator of prognosis. Clients with disease localized to the breast and no evidence of regional spread after microscopic examination of the lymph nodes have by far the most favorable prognosis. Estrogen and progesterone receptors appear to be an important prognostic variable. Clients with hormone receptor–negative tumors and no evidence of metastases to the axillary lymph nodes have a much higher recurrence rate than do clients with hormone receptor–positive tumors and no regional metastases.

Cancer of the breast has been classified in Stages I to IV of disease progression (Miller, 1992):

Stage I	The tumor is usually less than 2 cm in diameter and has invaded extraductal breast tissue. There is no evidence of cancer in the lymph nodes and no evidence of metastasis.
Stage II	The tumor may be up to 5 cm in diameter and the lymph nodes may or may not be involved. There is no evidence of metastasis.
Stage III	The tumor may be larger than 5 cm in diameter with the presence of lymph node involvement. There is no evidence of metastasis.
Stage IV	There is evidence of metastasis to at least one body organ.

When cancer is localized to the breast with no evidence of regional spread after pathologic examination, the clinical cure rate with most accepted methods of medical therapy is 75 per cent to 90 per cent. When the axillary lymph nodes are involved with tumor, the survival rate drops to 40 per cent to 50 per cent at 5 years and less than 25 per cent at 10 years. Most people who develop breast cancer will ultimately die of that disease. The mortality rate of people with breast cancer exceeds that of age-matched normal controls for nearly 20 years. After 20 years, the mortality rates are equal, although deaths that occur among breast cancer clients are often directly the result of tumor.

The prognosis of breast cancer is poorer in men than in women. The crude 5- and 10-year survival rates for Stage I breast cancer in men are 58 per cent and 38 per cent, respectively.

Prevention. Women who are at greater than normal risk of developing breast cancer should be identified by their physicians, taught the techniques of breast self-examination, and followed carefully. Screening programs involving periodic physical examination and mammography of asymptomatic high-risk women increase the detection rate of breast cancer and improve the survival rate by as much as 30 per cent (Giuliano, 1993).

Both the American Cancer Society (ACS) and the National Cancer Institute (NCI) now recommend that women receive mammograms every year or two after age 40 years. However, the American College of Physicians recommends beginning routine mammograms at age 50 years. The research results in the area of mammographic accuracy and age remain controversial (AMA Council, 1989; Davies et al., 1993; Eddy et al., 1989; Feig and Ehrlich, 1990; McLelland, 1991, 1989; Stacey-Clear et al., 1993; Threatt, 1992; Whitman et al., 1993).

Case Example. A 67-year-old woman presented with loss of functional left shoulder motion (e.g., she could no longer reach the top shelf in her kitchen) as her only complaint. During the Past Medical History portion of the interview, she mentioned that she had had a stroke 10 years ago; her current physician was unaware of this information. Examination revealed mild loss of strength in the left upper extremity accompanied by mild sensory and proprioceptive losses. Palpation of the shoulder and pectoral muscles produced breast pain; the client had been aware of this pain, but she had attributed it to a separate medical problem. She was reluctant to report her breast pain to her physician. Objectively, there were positive trigger points of the left pectoral muscles and loss of accessory motions of the left shoulder.

Physical therapy treatment to eliminate trigger points and restore shoulder motion resolved the breast pain during the first week. Despite her positive response to physical therapy treatment, given the age of this client, her significant past medical history for cerebrovascular injury, and the residual paresis, medical referral was still indicated. At the first follow-up visit, a letter was sent with the client briefly summarizing the initial objective findings, her progress to date, and the current concerns. She returned for an additional week of physical therapy to complete the home program for her shoulder. A medical evaluation ruled out breast disease, but medical treatment (medication) was indicated related to her cardiovascular system.

GYNECOLOGIC CANCERS

Cancers of the female genital tract account for about 15 per cent of all new cancers diagnosed in women. Although gynecologic cancers are the fourth leading cause of deaths from cancer in women in the United States, most of these cancers are highly curable when detected early. The most common cancers of the female genital tract are uterine endometrial cancer, ovarian cancer, and cervical cancer (Tombes, 1991).

Endometrial Cancer

Cancer of the uterine endometrium or lining is the most common gynecologic cancer, usually occurring in women between the ages of 55 and 70 years. Factors associated with an increased risk of endometrial cancer include obesity, hypertension, diabetes, a history of infertility, failure to ovulate, and prolonged estrogen therapy (Tombes, 1991).

The American Cancer Society recommends that a uterine tissue sample be obtained from all high-risk women at menopause. A dilatation and curettage (D&C) is performed to confirm a diagnosis of this type of cancer. Seventy-five per cent of women with this disease are diagnosed in the early stages of the cancer.

Clinical Signs. Clinical manifestations (Tombes, 1991) include

■ Vaginal bleeding during or after menopause (extremely significant sign)

■ Persistent, irregular premenopausal bleeding, especially in obese women

Treatment. Treatment for this type of cancer includes a total abdominal hysterectomy and bilateral salpingo-oophorectomy (TAH-BSO) (removal of the uterus, fallopian tubes, and ovaries). The surgery may also involve removal of the surrounding lymph nodes.

In most cases, some form of radiation therapy is recommended for all but earliest-stage disease. In women with advanced or recurrent disease, a regimen of chemotherapy, hormonal agents, or both may be combined with other treatment modalities. Five-year survival rates range from about 90 per cent of clients with Stage I disease to less than 10 per cent of clients with Stage IV disease (metastasis to other organs) (Tombes, 1991).

Ovarian Cancer

Ovarian cancer is the second most common reproductive tract cancer in women and accounts for over half of all deaths from gynecologic cancers. The incidence of ovarian cancer peaks between the ages of 40 and 70 years. Risk increases with advancing age. Other factors that may influence the development of ovarian cancer (Tombes, 1991) include

■ Nulliparity (never pregnant)

■ History of breast, endometrial, or colorectal cancer

■ Family history of ovarian cancer

■ Infertility

■ Early menopause

■ Exposure to asbestos or talc

■ High-fat diet

Early lesions are difficult to detect even with the use of CT scans, ultrasonography, and MRI. Not all ovarian tumors are palpable. An exploratory laparotomy is usually performed for diagnostic and staging purposes. Staging involves intraoperative examination of peritoneal surfaces and pelvic and abdominal organs.

Because the early-stage symptoms are quite nonspecific, most women do not seek medical attention until the disease is advanced.

Clinical Signs and Symptoms. Clinical manifestations (Tombes, 1991) include

- Persistent vague gastrointestinal complaints
- Abdominal discomfort
- Indigestion
- Early satiety
- Mild anorexia in a woman 40 years of age or older
- Ascites, pain, and pelvic mass (advanced disease)

Treatment. Treatment includes surgery (total abdominal hysterectomy with BSO) and tumor debulking (removal of part or all of tumor to decrease tumor size). These are performed for all stages of ovarian cancer. Either chemotherapy or radiotherapy is used after surgery, depending on the extent of the disease. External beam radiation is given to early-stage clients with little or no residual tumor. Chemotherapy is commonly used in women with advanced disease.

Investigational approaches to the treatment of ovarian cancer include the instillation of chemotherapeutic, biologic, or radioactive agents through peritoneal catheters—a procedure similar to peritoneal dialysis. This treatment option is usually limited to women with small amounts of residual disease in the peritoneal cavity after surgery (Tombes, 1991). Many clients will also have a second-look operation when therapy is completed to evaluate the effectiveness of treatment and to plan future treatment options.

Cervical Cancer

Cancer of the cervix is the third most common gynecologic malignancy. Since the widespread introduction of the Pap smear as a standard screening tool, the diagnosis of cervical cancer at the invasive stage has decreased significantly, while the highly curable preinvasive carcinoma in situ (CIS) has increased. CIS is more common in women 30 to 40 years of age, whereas invasive carcinoma is more frequent in women over age 40 years (Tombes, 1991). Risk factors associated with the development of cervical cancer include

- Early age at first sexual intercourse
- Early age at first pregnancy
- Low socioeconomic status
- History of any sexually transmitted disease
- History of multiple sex partners
- Women whose mothers used the drug diethylstilbestrol (DES) during their pregnancy

Viral infection also may be involved in the development of this cancer, and this factor is currently under investigation.

Because early cervical cancer may be totally asymptomatic, the Pap smear is one of the most important screening tools available for this disease. Pap smears are highly accurate and permit early detection of precancerous changes in cervical cells. Eradication of such lesions can prevent the development of invasive or metastatic cancer (Tombes, 1991).

The American Cancer Society recommends that all women age 18 years and over and those under 18 years who are sexually active have an annual Pap smear and pelvic examination. After three negative annual examinations, the Pap smear may be performed less frequently at the advice of the physician. Women with risk factors for cervical cancer should be advised to have an annual Pap smear.

Women with abnormal Pap smears undergo a procedure that visualizes the cervical canal (colposcopy) and identifies abnormal areas to be biopsied. In some cases, conization, or removal of a cone-shaped section of cervical tissue, may be necessary to obtain adequate tissue for diagnosis (Tombes, 1991).

Clinical Signs and Symptoms. Early cervical cancer has no symptoms. Clinical symptoms related to advanced disease include painful intercourse; postcoital, coital, or intermenstrual bleeding; and a watery, foul-smelling vaginal discharge.

Treatment. Treatment is planned according to the stage of disease and grade of cervical dysplasia. For women with preinvasive cervical cancer (Stage 0) who want to retain their fertility, conization to remove the diseased tissue is the treatment of choice. Close follow-up is essential owing to risk of recurrent disease with such minimal intervention. Follow-up treatment is also necessary for women with early disease, using laser surgery, cryosurgery, or electrocautery (Tombes, 1991).

Later-stage disease is treated with hysterectomy or intracavitary radiation. As the disease stages advance, the radical nature of the surgery increases, and radical hysterectomy, pelvic lymphadenectomy, or full pelvic irradiation can be done. Radiation alone also can be used in women with mid-stage disease. Chemotherapy is sometimes used in clients with recurrent disease or nodal metastases, but its usefulness may be limited by lack of effective agents and because of the decreased blood supply to pelvic tumors and the subsequent lack of transport of chemotherapy to this region of the body.

CANCERS OF THE BLOOD AND LYMPH SYSTEM

Cancers arising from the bone marrow include acute leukemias, chronic leukemias, multiple myelomas, and some lymphomas. These cancers are characterized by the uncontrolled growth of blood cells. The major lymphoid organs of the body are the lymph nodes and the spleen (Fig. 10–3). Cancers arising from these organs are called malignant lymphomas and are categorized as either Hodgkin's disease or non-Hodgkin's lymphoma.

Like leukemia, lymphoma affects a body system that communicates with every other organ system. However, instead of arising in the blood system, this cancer arises in the lymphatic system, a network of nodes, vessels, and organs that provides a major defense against infection. The lymphatic vessels carry lymph, which is a clear, colorless fluid containing infection-fighting white blood cells (WBCs, or leukocytes) throughout the body. Along these vessels, small oval glands (lymph nodes) trap and help destroy foreign particles and agents that cause disease. Lymphoma usually originates in these nodes but arises occasionally in other lymphoid tissues, such as the spleen or the intestinal lining.

The causes of leukemia and lymphoma are not yet known. Among the predisposing factors of leukemia are ionizing radiation, occupational exposure to the chemical benzene, and exposure to drugs such as alkylating agents and nitrosoureas used in chemotherapy (Linker, 1993). The presence of primary immune deficiency and infection with the human leukocyte virus (HTLV-1) is another factor associated with leukemia. Other predisposing factors of lymphoma include infection and immunologic defects resulting from illness or from medical treatment such as kidney transplants. Diagnosis must be made by a biopsy.

Leukemia (Pavel et al., 1993)

Leukemia is a malignant disease of the blood-forming organs. It accounts for 8 per cent of all human cancers and is the most common malignancy in children and young adults. One half of all leukemias are classified as *acute,* with rapid onset and progression of disease resulting in 100 per cent mortality within days to months without appropriate therapy. Acute leukemias are most common in children from 2 to 4 years

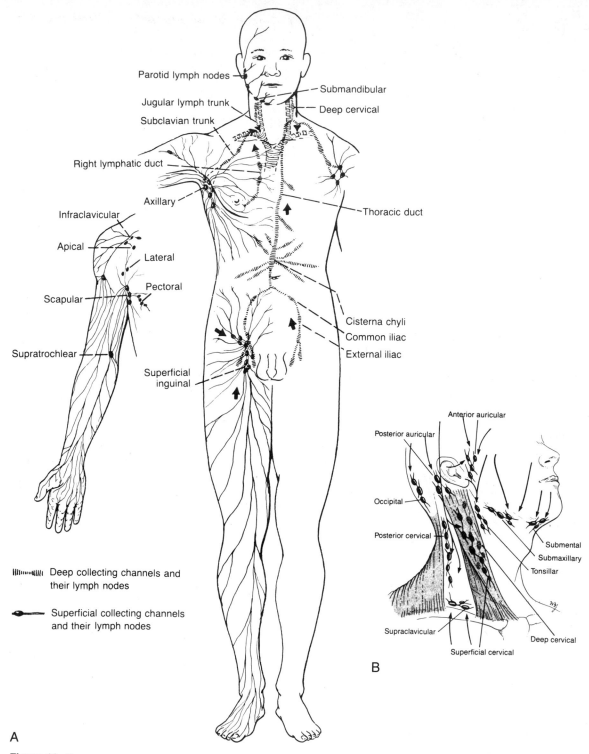

Figure 10-3

A, Major lymphoid organs of the body: lymph nodes and the spleen. (From Jacob, S.W., and Francone, C.A.: Elements of Anatomy and Physiology, 2nd ed. Philadelphia, W.B. Saunders, 1989.) *B*, Lymph nodes of the neck and their drainage. (From Swartz, M.: Textbook of Physical Diagnosis. Philadelphia, W.B. Saunders, 1989.)

of age, with a peak incidence again at age 65 years and older. The remaining leukemias are classified as *chronic,* which have a slower course and occur in people between the ages of 25 and 60 years.

Leukemia develops in the bone marrow and is characterized by abnormal multiplication and release of WBC precursors. The disease process originates during WBC development in the bone marrow or lymphoid tissue. In effect, leukemic cells become arrested in "infancy," with most of the clinical manifestations of the disease being related to the absence of functional "adult" cells, which are the product of normal differentiation (Schiffer, 1993).

With rapid proliferation of leukemic cells, the bone marrow becomes overcrowded with immature WBCs, which then spill over into the peripheral circulation. Crowding of the bone marrow by leukemic cells inhibits normal blood cell production. Decreased red blood cell (erythrocyte) production results in anemia and reduced tissue oxygenation. Decreased platelet production results in thrombocytopenia and risk of hemorrhage. Decreased production of normal WBCs results in increased vulnerability to infection, especially because leukemic cells are functionally unable to defend the body against pathogens. Leukemic cells may invade and infiltrate vital organs such as the liver, kidneys, lung, heart, or brain.

The two major forms of acute leukemia are *lymphocytic* leukemia, which involves the lymphocytes and lymphoid organs, and *nonlymphocytic* leukemia, which involves hematopoietic stem cells that differentiate into myeloid cells (monocytes, granulocytes, erythrocytes, and platelets).

From these two broad categories, leukemias are further classified according to the specific malignant cell line. Acute lymphoblastic leukemia (ALL) accounts for 80 per cent of all childhood leukemias and is caused by the malignant proliferation of precursor lymphocytes called lymphoblasts (Wujcik, 1993). ALL presents most often in children 2 to 10 years of age.

Acute nonlymphocytic leukemia (ANLL, formerly known as acute myelogenous leukemia or AML) is characterized by aberrations in the growth of megakaryocytes, monocytes, granulocytes, and erythrocytes. ANLL affects adults of all ages and is the most common leukemia in adults (Wujcik, 1993).

Chronic leukemia has two groups: chronic myelogenous leukemia (CML) and chronic lymphocytic leukemia (CLL). CML originates in the pluripotent stem cell. Initially, the marrow is hypercellular with a majority of normal cells. After a relatively slow course, the client with CML invariably enters a blast crisis that resembles acute leukemia. In 90 per cent of cases of CML, a chromosome abnormality (called the Philadelphia chromosome) can be identified during cell division.

CLL is a form of leukemia characterized by the proliferation of early B lymphocytes. It is an indolent form of leukemia most often seen in men over 50 years of age. It is the only leukemia with a possible genetic predisposition. Progression of the disease may take as long as 15 years.

Clinical Signs and Symptoms. Most of the clinical findings in acute leukemia are due to bone marrow failure (fatigue, bleeding, infection), which results from replacement of normal bone marrow elements by the malignant cells. The abnormal bleeding is caused by a lack of blood platelets required for clotting. Infections are due to a depletion of competent WBCs needed to fight infection.

For women, the abnormal bleeding may be prolonged menstruation leading to anemia. The Special Questions for Women (see Chapter 2) may elicit this kind of valuable information, which would then require medical referral. Less common manifestations include direct organ infiltration; clients may experience easy bruising of the skin or abnormal bleeding from the nose, urinary tract, or rectum (Linker, 1993).

Lymphoproliferative malignancies such as leukemia and lymphoma may also involve the synovium and may lead to symp-

▼ *Clinical Signs and Symptoms of*
Acute and Chronic Leukemias

- Abnormal bleeding
- Easy bruising of the skin
- Petechiae
- Epistaxis (nosebleeds) and/or bleeding gums
- Hematuria (blood in the urine)
- Rectal bleeding
- Infections, fever
- Weakness
- Easy fatigability
- Enlarged lymph nodes
- Bone and joint pain
- Weight loss
- Loss of appetite
- Pain or enlargement in the left upper abdomen (enlarged spleen)

toms suggestive of a rheumatic disease. The most common presentation is a child with ALL who has joint pain and swelling that mimics juvenile rheumatoid arthritis (JRA) (Gilkeson and Caldwell, 1990; Schaller, 1972).

The arthritic symptoms in such a child may be a consequence of leukemic synovial infiltration, hemorrhage into the joint, synovial reaction to an adjacent tumor mass, or crystal-induced synovitis (Gilkeson and Caldwell, 1990).

Asymmetric involvement of the large joints is most commonly observed. Pain that is disproportionate to the physical findings may occur, and joint symptoms are often fleeting. Less frequent rheumatic manifestations of leukemia in children are back pain secondary to infiltration of the meninges by leukemic cells and long bone pain (Gilkeson and Caldwell, 1990).

Treatment (Schiffer, 1993; Silver et al.,

1993). The treatment of leukemia is targeted at destroying neoplastic cells and maintaining a sustained remission. The treatment plan is determined by the disease classification, the presence or absence of prognostic factors, and disease progression. Radiation therapy may be administered as an adjunct to chemotherapy if leukemic cells infiltrate the nervous system, skin, rectum, and testes. Transfusions of red blood cells and platelets are required until the marrow can produce mature ones.

The most important advances in the treatment of CML have been the use of recombinant interferons and bone marrow transplantation. Bone marrow transplantation is currently the best treatment option for ANLL for those under 40 years of age who have a suitable matched donor.

Prognosis. Advances in therapy during the last several decades have significantly improved the chances for remission and even a cure. However, the prognosis for clients with ALL is less favorable if any of the following factors exist:

- Presentation in younger or older age groups
- Male sex
- High leukocyte count (over 100,000) at time of diagnosis
- CNS involvement
- Chromosomal abnormalities

The prognostic factors are less clearly defined in ANLL, and the long-term prognosis is usually poor. Blast crisis results in the death of more than 70 per cent of clients with CML. Death usually occurs within 6 months of onset.

Multiple Myeloma (Pavel et al., 1993)

Multiple myeloma, also known as plasma cell myeloma, is a primary malignant bone tumor associated with widespread osteolytic lesions (decreased areas of bone density), appearing radiographically as punched-out defects of bone (O'Toole,

1992). Excessive growth of plasma cells originating in the bone marrow destroys bone tissue.

This disease can develop at any age from young adulthood to advanced age but peaks among people between the ages of 50 and 70 years. Incidence is 3 to 4 cases per 100,000 (Press et al., 1993). It is more common in men and African-Americans. No etiologic or risk factors have been identified (Pavel et al., 1993).

Clinical Signs and Symptoms. The onset of multiple myeloma is usually gradual and insidious. Most clients pass through a long presymptomatic period that lasts 5 to 20 years. Early symptoms involve the skeletal system, particularly the pelvis, spine, and ribs. Some clients have backache or bone pain that worsens with movement (Pavel et al., 1993). The presence of an abnormal immunoglobulin in the urine (Bence Jones protein) is also diagnostic of multiple myeloma.

Bone pain is the most common symptom of myeloma; it is caused by infiltration of the plasma cells into the marrow with subsequent destruction of bone. Initially, the skeletal pain may be mild and intermittent, or it may develop suddenly as a severe pain in the back, rib, leg, or arm, often the result of an abrupt movement or effort that has caused a spontaneous (pathologic) bone fracture (Linker, 1993). The pain is often radicular and lancinating to one or both sides and is aggravated by movement (Salmon and Cassady, 1993).

As the disease progresses, more and more areas of bone destruction develop. Symptoms associated with bone pain usually subside within days to weeks after initiation of systemic chemotherapy. If left untreated, this disease will result in skeletal deformities, particularly of the ribs, sternum, and spine. Diffuse osteoporosis develops, accompanied by a negative calcium balance. Orthopedic back braces are generally poorly tolerated; however, the newer lightweight supports with Velcro fasteners are useful (Salmon and Cassady, 1993).

Drainage of calcium and phosphorus from damaged bones eventually leads to the development of renal stones, particularly in immobilized clients (Pavel et al., 1993). Renal insufficiency is the second most common cause of death, after infection, in clients with multiple myeloma (Fang, 1993).

To rid the body of the excess calcium (hypercalcemia), the kidneys increase the output of urine, which can lead to serious dehydration if there is an inadequate intake of fluids. This dehydration may be compounded by vomiting. Clients who have symptoms of hypercalcemia (confusion, increased urination, loss of appetite, abdominal pain, constipation, and vomiting) should seek immediate medical care, because this condition can be life-threatening.

In addition to bone destruction, multiple myeloma is characterized by disruption of red blood cell, leukocyte, and platelet production, which results from plasma cells crowding the bone marrow. Impaired production of these cell forms causes anemia, increased vulnerability to infection, and bleeding tendencies.

Approximately 10 per cent of people with myeloma have amyloidosis, deposits of insoluble fragments of a monoclonal protein resembling starch. These deposits cause tissues to become waxy and immobile and may affect nerves, muscles, and ligaments, especially the carpal tunnel area of the hand. Carpal tunnel syndrome with pain, numbness, or tingling of the hands and fingers may develop.

More serious neurologic complications may occur in 10 per cent to 15 per cent of clients with multiple myeloma. Spinal cord compression is usually observed early or in the late relapse phase of disease. Back pain is usually present as the initial symptom, with radicular pain that is aggravated by coughing or sneezing. Motor or sensory loss and bowel/bladder dysfunction are signs of more extensive compression. Paraplegia is a late, irreversible event (Salmon and Cassady, 1993).

Renal insufficiency may be the result of

> ### Clinical Signs and Symptoms of
> ### Multiple Myeloma
>
> - Skeletal/bone pain (especially pelvis, spine, and ribs)
> - Spontaneous fracture
> - Osteoporosis
> - Spinal cord compression
> - Recurrent bacterial infections (especially pneumococcal pneumonias)
> - Anemia with weakness and fatigue
> - Carpal tunnel syndrome
> - Hypercalcemia: confusion, increased urination, loss of appetite, abdominal pain, constipation, and vomiting

amyloidosis, with resultant hypertension and the nephrotic syndrome. Renal amyloidosis complicated by hypercalcemia contributes to the development of progressive renal insufficiency (Fang, 1993).

Treatment and Prognosis. All clients diagnosed with multiple myeloma should be monitored, but not all people with multiple myeloma require treatment (Press et al., 1993). Symptoms, physical findings, and laboratory data are taken into consideration. Adequate hydration and mobility help minimize the development of hypercalcemia.

Treatment varies and includes no medical therapy with regular follow-up for serum analysis, no treatment until symptoms develop or progression occurs, and drug therapy, chemotherapy, or radiation for symptomatic, progressive myeloma. Chemotherapy is the preferred initial treatment.

There is a 70 per cent to 75 per cent response rate to chemotherapy, but relapse almost always occurs when chemotherapy is discontinued. Interferon appears to be beneficial in prolonging the duration of remission. Radiation therapy and large doses of steroids and possibly a laminectomy may be performed when spinal cord compression occurs (Pavel et al., 1993).

Bone marrow transplantation is being investigated for use in myeloma therapy (Barlogie et al., 1987). Prognosis is affected by the presence of renal failure, hypercalcemia, or extensive bony disease, but median survival of clients with myelomas is 3 years (Linker, 1993).

Hodgkin's Disease (Pavel et al., 1993)

Hodgkin's disease is a chronic, progressive, neoplastic disorder of lymphatic tissue characterized by the painless enlargement of lymph nodes with progression to extralymphatic sites such as the spleen and liver. Hodgkin's disease can occur at any age, but the most common age of incidence (3 cases per 100,000) in the United States is 20 to 40 years with a second peak of frequency between 50 and 60 years of age. Men are affected more often than women, and boys are affected five times more often than girls.

The cause of lymphoma is unknown. However, clients who develop long-term immunosuppression owing to illness, therapeutic treatment, or drug abuse have an increased incidence of this disease. There appears to be a higher risk of Hodgkin's disease in clients with high titers of Epstein-Barr virus or a history of mononucleosis.

Metastases. The exact mechanism of growth and spread of Hodgkin's disease remains unknown. The disease may progress by extension to adjacent structures or via the lymphatics, because lymphoreticular cells inhabit all tissues of the body except the CNS. Hematologic spread may also occur, possibly by means of direct infiltration of blood vessels.

Clinical Signs and Symptoms. Hodgkin's disease usually presents as a painless, enlarged lymph node, often in the neck, underarm, or groin. The physical therapist may palpate these nodes during a cervical spine, shoulder, or hip examination (see Fig. 10–3). Lymph nodes are evaluated on the basis of size, consistency, mobility, and tenderness. Lymph nodes up to 1 cm in diameter of soft to firm consistency that move freely and easily without tenderness are considered within normal limits. Lymph nodes greater than 1 cm in diameter that are firm and rubbery in consistency or tender are considered suspicious. Enlarged lymph nodes associated with infection are more likely to be tender than slow-growing nodes associated with cancer.

Because lymph nodes enlarge in response to infections throughout the body, referral to a physician is not necessary upon finding enlarged lymph nodes unless these nodes persist for more than 4 weeks or involve more than one area. However, the physician should be notified of these findings, and the client should be advised to have the lymph nodes checked at the next follow-up visit with the physician. As always, *changes* in size, shape, tenderness, and consistency raise a red flag. Supraclavicular nodes are common metastatic sites for occult lung and breast cancers, whereas inguinal nodes implicate tumors arising in the legs, perineum, prostate, or gonads (Press et al., 1993).

Other early symptoms may include unexplained fevers, night sweats, weight loss, and pruritus (itching). The itching occurs more intensely at night and may result in severe scratches because the client is unaware of scratching during the sleep state. The fever typically peaks in the late afternoon, and night sweats occur when the fever breaks during sleep. Fatigue, malaise, and anorexia may accompany progressive anemia. Some clients with Hodgkin's disease experience pain over the involved nodes after ingesting alcohol.

Symptoms may arise when enlarged lymph nodes obstruct or compress adjacent structures, causing edema of the face, neck, or right arm secondary to superior vena cava compression, or causing renal failure secondary to urethral obstruction. Obstruction of bile ducts as a result of liver

▼ **Clinical Signs and Symptoms of**

Hodgkin's Disease

- Painless, progressive enlargement of unilateral lymph nodes, often in the neck
- Pruritus (itching) over entire body
- Unexplained fevers, night sweats
- Anorexia and weight loss
- Anemia, fatigue, malaise
- Jaundice
- Edema
- Nonproductive cough, dyspnea, chest pain, cyanosis
- Nerve root pain
- Paraplegia

damage causes bilirubin to accumulate in the blood and discolor the skin. Mediastinal lymph node enlargement with involvement of lung parenchyma and invasion of the pulmonary pleura progressing to the parietal pleura may result in pulmonary symptoms, including nonproductive cough, dyspnea, chest pain, and cyanosis.

Dissemination of disease from lymph nodes to bones may cause compression of the spinal cord, leading to paraplegia. Compression of nerve roots of the brachial, lumbar, or sacral plexus can cause nerve root pain.

Treatment. Treatment varies according to the stage at diagnosis. Stage I and Stage II disease are treated with radiation therapy and supplemental chemotherapy. Clients with Stage III disease may receive radiation coupled with an aggressive multiagent chemotherapy regimen. Stage IV disease is treated with a multiagent drug regimen.

Prognosis. The complete remission rate for clients with Hodgkin's disease is 75 per cent to 90 per cent. The recurrence rate varies with the stage of disease and is 10 per cent to 20 per cent. When untreated, clients with Hodgkin's disease have a life

---

MODIFIED ANN ARBOR STAGING CLASSIFICATION FOR HODGKIN'S DISEASE

Stage I   Single lymph node region or extralymphatic site (I_E)

Stage II   Two or more node sites on one side of the diaphragm

Stage III   Involved sites on both sides of the diaphragm

Stage IV   Disseminated (multifocal) involvement of an extralymphatic site, with or without associated lymph node involvement

---

From Glick, J.H.: Hodgkin's disease. *In* Wyngaarden, J.B., et al. (eds.): Cecil Textbook of Medicine, 19th ed. Philadelphia, W.B. Saunders, 1992.

---

expectancy of 5 years. Hodgkin's is divided into categories or stages according to the microscopic appearance of the involved lymph nodes, the extent and severity of the disorder, and the prognosis. The classic TNM system is replaced by Stage I to IV groupings (see Modified Ann Arbor Staging Classification for Hodgkin's Disease), because it is usually not possible to determine the primary tumor site (Beahrs et al., 1992). Stages are subdivided by the absence (A) or presence (B) of fever (more than 38° C, or 102° F), night sweats, or weight loss (more than 10 per cent of body weight in the last 6 months) (Press et al., 1993).

Non-Hodgkin's Lymphoma
(Pavel et al., 1993)

Non-Hodgkin's lymphoma (NHL) is a group of lymphomas affecting lymphoid tissue and occurring in people of all ages (9 per 100,000). It is more common in adults in their middle and older years (40 to 60 years); it is more common in men than in women in a ratio of 5:3. Non-Hodgkin's lymphomas present a clinical picture broadly similar to that of Hodgkin's disease, except that the disease is usually initially more widespread. The disease starts in the lymph node, although involvement of extranodal sites is more commonly seen in the non-Hodgkin's lymphomas than in Hodgkin's disease (Beahrs et al., 1992).

The histologic classification of non-Hodgkin's lymphoma has been an area of considerable controversy. The staging system used for Hodgkin's disease has been extended to the non-Hodgkin's lymphomas. Non-Hodgkin's lymphomas can be classified on the basis of pattern of node involvement (follicular or diffuse) and bulk of disease at individual sites, which is often more useful than other classification systems (Beahrs et al., 1992).

Clinical Signs and Symptoms. The most common manifestation is painless enlargement of one or more peripheral lymph nodes (O'Toole, 1992). Systemic symptoms are not as commonly associated with the non-Hodgkin's lymphomas as with Hodgkin's disease. Clients with non-Hodg-

▼ *Clinical Signs and Symptoms of*
Non-Hodgkin's Lymphoma

- Enlarged lymph nodes
- Fever
- Night sweats
- Weight loss
- Bleeding
- Infection
- Red skin and generalized itching of unknown etiology

kin's lymphomas often have remarkably few symptoms, even though many node areas or extranodal sites are involved. When systemic symptoms are seen, they are subdivided into A and B categories, as with Hodgkin's disease.

As with all cancers of the lymph system, a surgical biopsy is required to confirm the diagnosis and stage the disease. Other follow-up tests, such as x-ray studies, blood and bone marrow studies, and CT scans, may be used.

Treatment and Prognosis. Treatment protocols vary greatly. Treatment may include chemotherapy, radiotherapy, and bone marrow transplantation. With appropriate medical treatment, approximately 50 per cent of people with disseminated large cell lymphomas may be cured (Linker, 1993).

Prognosis overall is poorer than that for Hodgkin's disease. Without effective treatment, non-Hodgkin's lymphomas are very quickly fatal. Stage I is rarely observed, because non-Hodgkin's lymphoma is not usually diagnosed at this stage. If the disease is detected during this early stage, remissions have been achieved by use of involved field radiotherapy alone. Aggressive lymphomas are usually less widespread on diagnosis but grow rapidly and involve the CNS. The cure rate for aggressive tumors with treatment is significantly better than for the slower-growing, low-grade types, presumably because rapidly growing cells are more susceptible to chemotherapy and radiation therapy.

investigation; profound cellular immmunodeficiency plays a central role in lymphomagenesis. Although the HIV genome appears to be absent in AIDS-NHL tumor cells, this cancer is associated with other viruses that are likely to at least have a role in tumorigenesis. For example, Epstein-Barr virus (EBV) often accompanies non-Hodgkin's lymphoma, with genomic sequences detectable in about 50 per cent of AIDS-related lymphomas (Cremer et al., 1990; Neri et al., 1991; Shibata et al., 1991). It is generally accepted that EBV acts in the pathogenesis of lymphoma owing to the alteration in balance between host and the latent EBV infection in immunodeficiency states, with an increased activity of the virus.

Other predisposing factors include age and sex. The median age at diagnosis of HIV-related non-Hodgkin's lymphoma is 38 years, compared with 56 years for HIV-negative clients with non-Hodgkin's lymphoma. Women are at relatively less risk of developing lymphoma than are men. The percentage of AIDS cases with non-Hodgkin's lymphoma is shown not to vary between risk groups (homosexuals versus intravenous drug abusers) (Beral et al., 1991). Non-Hodgkin's lymphoma is more likely to develop among clients who have Kaposi's sarcoma, a history of herpes simplex infection, and a lower neutrophil count (Chachoua et al., 1989).

Clinical Signs and Symptoms. The most common presentations of HIV-related non-Hodgkin's lymphoma are systemic B symptoms (which may suggest an infectious

Acquired Immunodeficiency Syndrome–Non-Hodgkin's Lymphoma (AIDS-NHL)

(Broder and Karp, 1992; Safai et al., 1992)

Only recently has AIDS-NHL emerged as a major sequela of HIV infection. It now occurs frequently in clients who survive other consequences of AIDS (Gail et al., 1991; Pluda et al., 1990).

The etiology of AIDS-NHL is still under

Clinical Signs and Symptoms of

AIDS-NHL

- Painless, enlarged mass
- Fever
- Night sweats
- Weight loss

process), a rapidly enlarging mass lesion, or both. At the time of diagnosis, approximately 75 per cent of clients will have advanced (Stage III/IV) disease. Extranodal disease frequently involves any part of the body, with the most common locations being the CNS, bone marrow, gastrointestinal tract, and liver.

Treatment. The treatment of non-Hodgkin's lymphoma in the setting of HIV infection has been much less effective than in clients without immunodeficiency. Treatment with cytotoxic agents in this population exacerbates the already existing immune impairment and leaves clients with prolonged neutropenia and at further risk for opportunistic infections.

Effective treatment requires use of multiple modalities to target the various interactive factors underlying tumor pathogenesis in the immunosuppressed, HIV-infected host. Combined cytotoxic antitumor agents are directed against both RNA and DNA viral cofactors and aim toward inhibiting growth factors that specifically drive tumor cell proliferation. Investigations involving suppression of the malignant clone while sparing normal host tissue by targeting and modifying the activity of specific overexpressed or aberrant genes continue.

Prognosis. In one study, the median survival among 254 clients with AIDS-NHL was only 5 months. Death was most often due to opportunistic infections and to progressive lymphoma (Safai et al., 1992).

SARCOMA

By definition, sarcoma is a fleshy growth and refers to a large variety of tumors arising in the connective tissues that are grouped together because of similarities in pathologic appearance and clinical presentation. Tissues affected include

- Connective tissue such as bone and cartilage (discussed subsequently under Bone Tumors)
- Muscle
- Fibrous tissue

- Fat
- Synovium

The different types of sarcomas are named for the specific tissues affected (e.g., fibrosarcomas are tumors of the fibrous connective tissue; osteosarcomas are tumors of the bone; and chondrosarcomas are tumors arising in cartilage [Table 10–5]).

As a general category, sarcoma differs from carcinoma in the origin of cells comprising the tumor. As mentioned, sarcomas arise in connective tissue (embryologic mesoderm), whereas carcinomas arise in epithelial tissue (embryologic ectoderm) (i.e., cellular structures covering or lining surfaces of body cavities, small vessels, or visceral organs). Carcinomas affect structures such as the skin, large intestine, stomach, breast, and lungs. Generally, carcinomas tend to metastasize via the lymphatics, whereas sarcomas are more likely to metastasize hematogenously (Gudas, 1987).

Malignant neoplasms or new growths that develop as *primary* lesions in the musculoskeletal tissues are relatively rare, representing less than 1 per cent of malignant disease of all age groups and 6.5 per cent of all cancers in children under the age of 15 years (American Cancer Society, 1993). *Secondary* neoplasms that develop in bone as metastases from a primary neoplasm elsewhere (especially metastatic carcinoma) are common.

Soft Tissue Tumors

Little is known about important epidemiologic or etiologic factors in clients with soft tissue sarcomas. There is no proven genetic predisposition to the development of soft tissue sarcomas. There are two peaks of incidence in human sarcoma development: early adolescence and the middle decades (Hellman, 1993). Although soft tissue sarcomas can arise anywhere in the body, approximately 60 per cent of sarcomas occur in the extremities, and three times more frequently in the lower extrem-

Table 10–5
CLASSIFICATION OF SOFT TISSUE AND BONE TUMORS

Tissue of Origin	Benign Tumor	Malignant Tumor
Connective Tissue		
Fibrous	Fibroma	Fibrosarcoma
Cartilage	Chondroma: Enchondroma, Chondroblastoma	Chondrosarcoma
Bone	Osteoma	Osteosarcoma
Bone marrow		Leukemia
		Multiple myeloma
		Ewing's sarcoma
Adipose (fat)	Lipoma	Liposarcoma
Synovial	Ganglion, giant cell of tendon sheath	Synovial sarcoma
Muscle		
Smooth muscle	Leiomyoma	Leiomyosarcoma
Striated muscle	Rhabdomyoma	Rhabdomyosarcoma
Endothelium (Vascular/Lymphatic)		
Lymph vessels	Lymphangioma	Lymphangiosarcoma
		Kaposi's sarcoma
Lymphoid tissue		Lymphosarcoma (lymphoma)
		Lymphatic leukemia
Blood vessels	Hemangioma	Hemangiosarcoma
Neural Tissue		
Nerve fibers and sheaths	Neurofibroma	Neurofibrosarcoma
	Neuroma	Neurogenic sarcoma
	Neurinoma (neurilemmoma)	
Glial tissue	Gliosis	Glioma
Epithelium		
Skin and mucous membrane	Papilloma	Squamous cell carcinoma
	Polyp	Basal cell carcinoma
Glandular epithelium	Adenoma	Adenocarcinoma

Data from Purtilo, D.T., and Purtilo, R.B.: A Survey of Human Disease, 2nd ed. Boston, Little, Brown, 1989; and Phipps, W., et al.: Medical: Surgical Nursing: Concepts and Clinical Practice, 4th ed. St. Louis, C.V. Mosby, 1990.

ity than in the upper extermity. A full 75 per cent of lower-extremity sarcomas occur at or above the knee.

Metastases. Soft tissue sarcomas rarely spread to regional lymph nodes. The poor prognosis of most people with soft tissue sarcomas is due to the tendency of these lesions to invade aggressively into surrounding tissues and for early hematogenous dissemination, usually to the lungs. Soft tissue sarcomas invade locally along anatomic planes, such as nerve fibers, muscle bundles, fascial planes, and blood vessels. Most clients with soft tissue sarcomas present without obvious clinical metastases. Approximately 80 per cent of all lesions that recur after surgery do so within 2 years (Cantin et al., 1968).

Clinical Signs and Symptoms. Soft tissue sarcomas most often present as asymptomatic soft tissue masses. Because these lesions arise in compressible tissues and are often far from vital organs, symptoms are few until the lesions are large compared with the anatomic part.

Often, the neoplasm goes unnoticed until

▼ *Clinical Signs and Symptoms of*
Soft Tissue Sarcoma

- Persistent swelling or lump in a muscle (most common finding)
- Pain
- Pathologic fracture
- Local swelling
- Warmth of overlying skin

the client has some trauma or injury that requires medical attention (e.g., x-ray study to rule out fracture). Pain is the most significant symptom of rapidly growing neoplasms. Initially mild and intermittent, the pain from a neoplasm becomes progressively more severe and more constant.

There are no reliable physical signs to distinguish between benign and malignant soft tissue lesions; consequently, all soft tissue lumps that persist or grow should be reported immediately to the physician.

Treatment and Prognosis. Surgery alone, surgery combined with radiation, surgery combined with radiation and intraarterial chemotherapy, and radiation alone have been used for the treatment of soft tissue sarcomas. Amputation may be required, but limb salvation to preserve limbs of clients with sarcomas of soft tissues of the extremities is becoming an important part of medical treatment (Davis and Mellette, 1991).

Prognostic factors of importance in clients with soft tissue sarcomas include histologic grade, site, size (more than 5 cm in diameter implies a worse prognosis than smaller size), and lymph node involvement. The site of a sarcoma often influences resectability and thus local control and cure. Lesions in the trunk, especially those in the retroperitoneum, mediastinum, and head and neck, often involve vital structures before they become clinically apparent. They are usually large, and local control by any approach is less likely for them than for tumors on the extremities or torso. In the extremities, the exact site of the lesion is also of prognostic importance. Distal lesions are generally more curable than proximal lesions. Size is a major factor in achieving local control by surgery and radiation.

Bone Tumors (Malawer et al., 1993)

Benign and malignant (primary) bone tumors are relatively rare, accounting for less than 1 per cent of total deaths from cancer. Excluding multiple myeloma, the ratio of benign to malignant bone tumors is approximately 7:1. Primary bone cancer affects children and young adults most commonly, whereas secondary bone tumors or metastatic neoplasms occur in adults with primary cancer (e.g., cancer of the prostate, breast, lungs, kidneys, thyroid). The two most common childhood sarcomas of the bone are osteosarcoma (osteogenic sarcoma) and Ewing's sarcoma; both have a poor prognosis. This text is limited to the most common forms of bone tumors. The reader is referred to a more comprehensive text for a detailed discussion of all the soft tissue and bone tumors (DeVita et al., 1993; Holland et al., 1993).

A history of sudden onset of severe pain usually indicates the complication of a pathologic fracture (a break in an already weakened bone). Local swelling can be detected when the lesion protrudes beyond the normal confines of the bone. The swelling of a benign lesion is usually firm and nontender. In the presence of a rapidly growing malignant neoplasm, however, the swelling is more diffuse and frequently tender (Fig. 10–4). The overlying skin may be warm owing to the highly vascularized nature of neoplasms. If the lesion is close to a joint, function in that joint may be disturbed, with painful and restricted range of motion (Salter, 1983).

Bone pain (especially pain on weight bearing) that persists for more than 1 week and grows worse at night, often awakening the person, is usually the most common

Figure 10–4

A, Benign bone tumors have a characteristic sclerotic rim around the periphery of the lesion. The lesion is usually well defined, and there is no evidence of the erosion of the cortex or soft tissue mass. *B,* Malignant bone tumors can have lytic or sclerotic components. It is frequently difficult to know the extent of the lesion within the bone, because there is no well-defined sclerotic rim around the tumor. The destructive process is diffuse within the medullary cavity of the bone, and the tumor may break through the cortex of the bone, thus producing a Codman triangle. Frequently, there is an associated soft tissue mass. Differential diagnosis of this lesion is between an osteogenic sarcoma and a chondrosarcoma. (Adapted from DeVita, V.T., Jr., and Hellman, S. [eds.]: Cancer; Principles and Practice of Oncology. Philadelphia, J.B. Lippincott, 1982.)

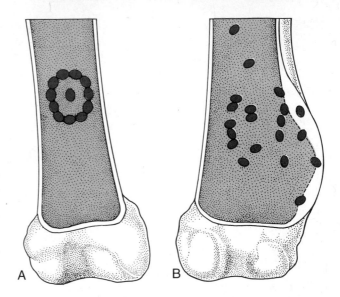

A   B

symptom of bone cancer. The pain is often associated with trauma during a game or exercise and may be dismissed in children as "growing pains."

Occasionally, a growing bone mass is the first sign of disease. Diagnosis is made by x-ray study and surgical biopsy, requiring immediate attention to suspicious symptoms by referral to the client's physician.

Osteosarcoma

Osteosarcoma (also known as osteogenic sarcoma) is the most common type of bone cancer, occurring between the ages of 10 and 25 years; it is more common in boys. Although it can involve any bones in the body, because it arises from osteoblasts the usual site is the epiphyses of the long bones, where active growth takes place (e.g., lower end of the femur, upper end of the tibia or fibula, and upper end of the humerus). In general, 80 per cent to 90 per cent of osteosarcomas occur in the long bones; the axial skeleton is rarely affected. The growth spurt of adolescence is a peak time for the development of osteosarcoma. Half of all osteosarcomas are located in the upper leg above the knee, where the most active epiphyseal growth occurs.

Metastases. Bone tumors, unlike carcinomas, disseminate almost exclusively through the blood; bones lack a lymphatic system. Metastases to the lungs, pleurae, lymph nodes, kidneys, and brain and to other bones are common and occur early in the disease process (Snyder, 1986; Williams and Williams, 1986). Hematogenous spread is to the lungs first and to other bones second.

With the use of adjuvant chemotherapy, the skeletal system has become a more common site of initial relapse (Giuliano et al., 1984; Jaffe et al., 1983). Local recurrence of either a benign or a malignant lesion is due to inadequate removal of the primary tumor. Most local recurrences develop within 24 months of attempted removal.

Clinical Signs and Symptoms. Osteosarcoma usually presents with pain in a lesional area, usually around the knee in clients with femur or tibia involvement (Rosen, 1993). The pain is initially mild and intermittent but becomes progressive, more severe, and constant over time.

Most lesions produce pain as the tumor starts to expand the bony cortex and stretch the perineum. A tender lump may develop, and a bone weakened by erosion

▼ *Clinical Signs and Symptoms of*
Osteosarcoma

- Pain and swelling of the involved body part
- Loss of motion and functional movement of adjacent joints
- Tender lump
- Pathologic fracture
- Occasional weight loss
- Malaise
- Fatigue

▼ *Clinical Signs and Symptoms of*
Ewing's Sarcoma

- Increasing and persistent pain
- Increasing and persistent swelling over a bone (localized over the area of tumor)
- Decrease in movement if a limb bone is involved
- Fever
- Fatigue
- Weight loss

of the metaphyseal cortex may break with little or no stress. This pathologic fracture often brings the person into the medical system, at which time a diagnosis is established by x-ray study and surgical biopsy. This neoplasm is highly vascularized, so that the overlying skin is usually warm.

Treatment and Prognosis. Local recurrence, especially in clients who have undergone therapy, may be associated with a poor prognosis. It is interesting that the majority of clients who are long-term survivors of sustained metastatic bone disease are those with breast and prostate cancer as the primary disease (Gudas, 1992).

Although amputation has been the standard treatment of most bony sarcomas, limb-sparing surgery has been developed for both malignant and aggressive benign tumors. Today, more than 90 per cent of clients with extremity sarcomas (bone or soft tissue) are treated with limb-sparing techniques (Davis and Mellette, 1991). Preoperative and adjuvant chemotherapy has dramatically increased overall survival. The survival rate has risen from 15 per cent to 20 per cent in the 1960s to 55 per cent to 80 per cent in the 1990s.

Ewing's Sarcoma (Pizzo et al., 1993)

Ewing's sarcoma is a relatively rare but malignant tumor of bones that is most common between the ages of 5 and 16 years, with a slightly greater incidence in boys than in girls. Ewing's sarcoma rarely occurs in people of African origin (Arthur, 1986). Almost any bone can be involved, but typically the pelvis, femur, tibia, ulna, and metatarsal are the most frequent sites for Ewing's sarcoma.

Metastases. Metastasis is predominantly hematogenous (to lungs and bone), although lymph node involvement may occur. Metastasis usually occurs late in the disease process and is associated with poor survival rates (Snyder, 1986; Williams and Williams, 1986).

Clinical Signs and Symptoms. Ewing's sarcoma is a rapidly growing tumor that often outgrows its blood supply and quickly erodes the bone cortex, producing a soft, tender, palpable mass. Systemic symptoms such as fatigue, weight loss, and intermittent fever may be present, especially in clients with metastatic disease. Fever may occur when products of bone degeneration enter the bloodstream. In addition, the blood supply to local areas of bone may be compromised, with resultant avascular necrosis of bone (Salter, 1983).

Less common presentations of Ewing's sarcoma include primary rib tumor associated with a pleural effusion and respiratory symptoms, mandibular lesions presenting with chin and lip paresthesias, primary vertebral tumor with symptoms of nerve root or spinal cord compression, and primary sacral tumor with neurogenic bladder. Neurologic symptoms may occur secondary to nerve entrapment by the tumor.

Treatment and Prognosis. Prognosis depends greatly on whether metastasis is present at the time of diagnosis. Multimodality therapy (surgery, radiation therapy, chemotherapy) has increased the proportion of long-term disease-free survivors from less than 15 per cent to more than 50 per cent over the past two to three decades. Even so, Ewing's sarcoma has a 50 percent mortality rate (Hellman, 1993).

Case Example. A 17-year-old male high school athlete noted low back pain 6 weeks ago. He was unable to identify a specific traumatic event or injury but noted that he had been "training pretty hard" the last 2 weeks. Spinal motions were all within normal limits with no apparent step suggestive of spondylolisthesis. There were no obvious postural changes such as a scoliotic shift or unusual kyphosis/lordosis of the spinal curves. The only positive evaluation findings included a mild left foot drop and an absent left ankle jerk. Pain was intensified on weight bearing and on movement of any kind. Pain was not relieved by rest or aspirin. There was no fever or recent history of sore throat, upper respiratory or ear infection, and so on. After 1 week in physical therapy, the pain began radiating into the posterior aspect of the left thigh. He had also noted for the first time paresthesias along the lateral side of the left leg. The pain had increased rather markedly over the past 2 weeks.

The therapist might assume that the physical therapy treatment aggravated this client's condition, causing increased symptoms. However, given the unknown etiology of pain, symptoms inconsistent with musculoskeletal conditions (e.g., unrelieved by rest), combined with the recent change in symptoms and the presence of positive neurologic symptoms, this client was returned to the physician before continuing further therapy.

A blood test performed at that time indicated the white blood count was 10,000 mm³ (normal range = 4300 to 10,800 mm³). Further testing, including a radiograph, resulted in a diagnosis of Ewing's sarcoma.

Chondrosarcoma

Chondrosarcoma, the most common malignant cartilage tumor, occurs most often in adults over 40 years of age. However, when it does occur in the younger age group, it tends to be a higher grade of malignancy and capable of metastases (Rosen, 1993).

It occurs most commonly in some part of the pelvic or shoulder girdles or long bones, such as the femurs. Chondrosarcomas are the most common malignant tumors of the sternum and scapula.

Chondrosarcoma is usually a relatively slow-growing malignant neoplasm that arises either spontaneously in previously normal bone or as a result of malignant change in a preexisting benign bone tumor (osteochondromas and enchondromas or chondromas) (Baird, 1991; Salter, 1983; Williams and Williams, 1986).

Metastases. Chondrosarcomas are graded I, II, and III. The majority of chondrosarcomas are either Grade I or II. The metastatic rate of moderate-grade lesions is 15 per cent to 40 per cent; in high-grade lesions, it is 75 per cent. Grade III lesions have the same metastatic potential as osteosarcomas (Malawer et al., 1993).

Clinical Signs and Symptoms. Clinical presentation of chondrosarcoma varies. *Peripheral chondrosarcomas* (arising from bone surface) grow slowly and may be un-

---

▼ *Clinical Signs and Symptoms of*
Chondrosarcoma

- Back or thigh pain
- Sciatica
- Bladder symptoms
- Unilateral edema

detected and quite large. Local symptoms develop only because of mechanical irritation; otherwise, pain is not a prominent symptom. Pelvic chondrosarcomas are often large and present with pain referred to the back or thigh, sciatica caused by sacral plexus irritation, urinary symptoms from bladder neck involvement, or unilateral edema due to iliac vein obstruction.

Conversely, *central chondrosarcomas* (arising within bone) present with dull pain, and a mass is rare. Pain, which indicates active growth, is an ominous sign of a central cartilage lesion. Metastases develop late, so that the prognosis of chondrosarcoma is considerably better than that of osteosarcoma (Salter, 1983).

Treatment and Prognosis. The treatment of chondrosarcoma is surgical removal with limb-sparing. Adjuvant chemotherapy has not proved effective. The overall survival rate for chondrosarcoma is 52 per cent. Adequate surgical removal is the main determinant of recurrence. In general, chondrosarcomas occurring during childhood have worse prognoses than those occurring during adulthood (Aprin et al., 1982).

NEUROLOGIC MANIFESTATIONS OF MALIGNANCY (Bunn and Ridgway, 1993; Rugo 1993)

Neurologic problems occur frequently in people with cancer. The most frequent neurologic complications are caused directly by three phenomena: tumor metastases to the brain; endocrine, fluid, and electrolyte abnormalities; and paraneoplastic syndromes, or "remote effects" of tumors on the CNS.

When tumors produce signs and symptoms at a distance from the tumor or its metastasized sites, these "remote effects" of malignancy are collectively referred to as *paraneoplastic syndromes*. For example, when tumors secrete hormones, such as adrenocorticotropin (ACTH), which are distributed by the circulation and act on target organs at a site other than the location of the tumor, a paraneoplastic syndrome may occur (Croft and Wilkinson, 1965).

The etiologies of these syndromes are not well understood. In contrast to the hormone syndromes in which the cancer directly produces a substance that circulates in blood to produce symptoms, the neurologic syndromes are generally produced by cancer stimulation of antibody production (Odell, 1993).

Several of the disorders are suspected to have an autoimmune basis. The strongest evidence for an autoimmune disorder is the Lambert-Eaton myasthenic syndrome (LEMS). In this syndrome, autoantibodies directed against the presynaptic calcium channels at the neuromuscular junction cause impaired release of acetylcholine from presynaptic nerve terminals, resulting in muscle weakness (Dropcho et al., 1989; Henson and Posner, 1993; Nagel et al., 1988; Odell, 1993).

The most common cancer associated with paraneoplastic syndromes is small cell cancer of the lung. This association is thought to be due to its neuroectodermal origin. The paraneoplastic syndromes are often considered to be from aberrant hormonal or metabolic effects not associated with a cancer's normal tissue equivalent. Clinical findings may resemble those of primary endocrine, metabolic, hematologic, or neuromuscular disorders.

The mechanisms for such remote effects can be classified into three groups:

- Effects initiated by a tumor product (e.g., carcinoid syndrome)

- Effects due to the destruction of normal tissues by tumor (e.g., hypercalcemia from osteolytic skeletal metastases)

- Effects due to unknown mechanisms, such as unidentified tumor products or circulating immune complexes stimulated by the tumor (e.g., osteoarthropathy due to bronchogenic carcinoma)

The paraneoplastic syndromes are of considerable clinical importance because they may accompany relatively limited neoplastic growth and provide an early clue to

Table 10–6

PARANEOPLASTIC SYNDROMES HAVING MUSCULOSKELETAL MANIFESTATIONS

Malignancy	Rheumatic Disease	Clinical Features
Lymphoproliferative disease (leukemia)	Vasculitis	Necrotizing vasculitis
Plasma cell dyscrasia	Cryoglobulinemia	Vasculitis; Raynaud's phenomenon; arthralgia; neurologic symptoms
Hodgkin's disease	Immune complex disease	Nephrotic syndrome
Ovarian cancer	Reflex sympathetic dystrophy	Palmar fasciitis and polyarthritis
Carcinoid syndrome	Scleroderma	Scleroderma-like changes: anterior tibia
Colon cancer	Pyogenic arthritis	Enteric bacteria cultured from joint
Mesenchymal tumors	Osteogenic osteomalacia	Bone pain, stress fractures
Renal cell cancer (and other tumors)	Severe Raynaud's phenomenon	Digital necrosis
Pancreatic cancer	Panniculitis	Subcutaneous nodules, especially in males

Adapted from Gilkeson, G.S., and Caldwell, D.S.: Rheumatologic associations with malignancy. Journal of Musculoskeletal Medicine 7(1):72, 1990.

the presence of certain types of cancer. The course of the paraneoplastic syndrome usually parallels the course of the tumor. Therefore, effective medical treatment (rather than physical therapy) should result in resolution of the syndrome. Likewise, recurrence of the cancer may be first recognized by the return of systemic symptoms. The metabolic or toxic effects of the syndrome may constitute a more urgent hazard to life than the underlying cancer (e.g., hypercalcemia, hyponatremia).

These syndromes occur in 10 to 20 per cent of all cancer clients (Croft and Wilkinson, 1965). Paraneoplastic syndromes may be the first sign of a malignancy that may be cured if detected early. Paraneoplastic syndromes with musculoskeletal manifestations are listed in Table 10–6.

Even such nonspecific symptoms as anorexia, malaise, weight loss, and fever are truly paraneoplastic and probably due to the production of specific factors by the tumor itself. For example, anorexia is a common symptom in clients with cancer, especially people with lung carcinoma, hypernephroma, and carcinoma of the pan-

creas. This has been attributed to tumor production of the protein tumor necrosis factor (TNF), also called cachectin. Fever may be seen in clients with cancer in the absence of infection. Fever could be produced either by tumor induction of pyrogen formation by host white cells or by

Clinical Signs and Symptoms of
Paraneoplastic Syndromes

- Fever
- Skin rash
- Clubbing of the fingers
- Pigmentation disorders
- Arthralgias
- Paresthesias
- Thrombophlebitis
- Proximal muscle weakness
- Anorexia, malaise, weight loss

direct tumor production of a pyrogen (Bernheim et al., 1979; Odell, 1993).

Gradual, progressive muscle weakness during a period of weeks to months (especially of the pelvic girdle muscles) may occur. Proximal muscles are most likely to be involved. The weakness does stabilize. Reflexes of the involved extremities are present but are diminished.

Paraneoplastic syndromes may be related to rheumatologic complaints. For example, the important clinical features of carcinoma polyarthritis are

- Asymmetric joint involvement
- Involvement of primarily the lower extremities
- Concurrent arthritis and malignancy
- Explosive onset
- Late age of onset

This condition can be differentiated from rheumatoid arthritis by these features (Gilkeson and Caldwell, 1990).

Other rheumatologic conditions associated with paraneoplastic syndromes include myopathies such as dermatomyositis (DM) and polymyositis (PM); arthropathies such as hypertrophic osteoarthropathy, amyloidosis, and carcinoma polyarthritis; and various conditions like necrotizing vasculitis, scleroderma, and a lupus-like syndrome that resembles systemic lupus erythematosus (SLE) (Gilkeson and Caldwell, 1990).

Table 10–7
MUSCULAR DISORDERS ASSOCIATED WITH MALIGNANCY

Dermatomyositis and polymyositis
Type II muscle atrophy
Myasthenia gravis
Lambert-Eaton myasthenic syndrome (LEMS)
Metabolic myopathies
Primary neuropathic diseases
   Amyotrophic lateral sclerosis
   Amyloidosis

From Gilkeson, G.S., and Caldwell, D.S.: Rheumatologic associations with malignancy. Journal of Musculoskeletal Medicine 7(1):70, 1990.

In clients who do have malignancy and DM/PM, the myositis may precede, follow, or arise concurrently with the malignancy. No particular type of cancer has been found to predominate in people with DM/PM, but these clients are generally older and respond poorly to medical treatment for the myositis.

A list of muscular disorders associated with malignancy is provided in Table 10–7.

Primary Central Nervous System Tumors (Aminoff, 1993)

Primary tumors of the CNS arise within the CNS and include tumors that lie within the spinal cord (intramedullary), within the dura mater (extramedullary), or outside the dura mater (extradurally). About 80 per cent of CNS tumors occur intracranially, and 20 per cent affect the spinal cord and peripheral nerves. Of the intracranial lesions, about 60 per cent are primary, and the remaining 40 per cent are metastatic lesions, often multiple and most commonly from the lung, breast, kidney, and gastrointestinal (GI) tract.

CNS tumors are associated with a high mortality, despite advances in treatment with surgery and radiation. Brain tumors occur in people of all ages, with peak incidences at 5 to 10 years of age and 50 to 55 years of age. They are second only to leukemia as a cause of death in children. The incidence is also increasing in people over 75 years of age, which adds gerontology as an additional component in client care.

In 1993, an estimated 17,500 new cases of CNS tumors were identified, with a slightly higher ratio of men to women in all age groups. This figure compares with 12,000 cases in 1987. The increased incidence over the last 5 years is unaccounted for. Heredity is not a significant risk factor in brain tumors, except for tumors of neurofibromatosis and tuberous sclerosis (Schnell, 1993a). Risk factors under investigation include brain trauma, history of infection/inflammation, and living under high-voltage power lines (Fuller, 1993).

Virtually every cell type within the CNS can give rise to a neoplasm. However, tumors commonly develop from the neurons themselves. Intraaxial tumors originate from glial (support) cells within the cerebrum, cerebellum, or brain stem. These tumors infiltrate and invade brain tissue. Extraaxial tumors have their origin in the skull, meninges, cranial nerves, or pituitary gland. These tumors have a compressive effect on the brain (Schnell, 1993a).

Gliomas comprise 40 per cent to 50 per cent of primary brain tumors. Less frequently they occur within the spinal canal, where the condition is predominantly benign.

Any CNS tumor, even if well-differentiated and histologically benign, is potentially dangerous owing to the lethal effects of increased intracranial pressure and tumor location near critical structures. For example, a small, well-differentiated lesion in the pons or medulla may be more rapidly fatal than a massive liver cancer.

Primary CNS tumors rarely metastasize outside the CNS; there is no lymphatic drainage available, and hematogenous spread is also unlikely. In most cases, CNS spread is contained in the cerebrospinal axis, involving local invasion or CNS seeding through the subarachnoid space and the ventricles.

Brain Tumors

Metastases. Melanoma frequently metastasizes to the neuraxis (CNS), causing transient paralysis or paresis of motor and sensory function. In brain tumors as well as metastasized melanoma, clients may present with a wide variety of neurologic symptoms and syndromes, mimicking presentation of a cardiovascular accident (CVA), with early return of function (Gudas, 1987).

At the University of California, San Francisco, which has a large primary CNS tumor program, almost 10 per cent of spinal tumors originate as metastases from an intracranial primary CNS tumor. Neoplasms disseminate by local invasion or through the cerebrospinal fluid pathways (Levin et al. 1993).

Clinical Signs and Symptoms. Headaches occur in 30 per cent to 50 per cent of persons with brain tumors and are usually bioccipital or bifrontal. They are usually intermittent and of increasing duration, and may be intensified by a change in posture or by straining. The headache is characteristically worse on awakening owing to differences in CNS drainage in the supine and prone positions and usually disappears soon after the person arises. It may be intensified or precipitated by any activity that increases intracranial pressure, such as straining during a bowel movement, stooping, lifting heavy objects, or coughing.

Often, the pain can be relieved by aspirin, acetaminophen, or other moderate painkillers. Vomiting with or without nausea (unrelated to food) occurs in about 25 per cent to 30 per cent of people with brain tumors and often accompanies headaches. If the tumor invades the meninges, the headaches will be more severe (Shapiro, 1986).

Focal manifestations of a space-occupying brain lesion are caused by the local compression or destruction of the brain tissue as well as by compression secondary to edema (Snyder, 1986). Papilledema (edema and hyperemia of the optic disc) may be the first sign of intracranial tumors. Visual changes do not occur until prolonged papilledema causes optic atrophy (Schnell, 1993a).

Specific symptoms depend on where the tumor is located. For example, if a tumor is growing in the motor cortex, the client may develop isolated extremity weakness. If the tumor is developing in the cerebellum, coordination may be affected. Seizures occur in approximately one third of persons with metastatic brain tumors (Glucksberg and Singer, 1982).

Treatment and Prognosis (Schnell, 1993a). Intervention depends on the type and location of an intracranial tumor and the client's condition. Chemotherapy, radiation therapy, and surgical management are the primary treatment options.

▼ *Clinical Signs and Symptoms of*
Brain Tumors

- Altered mentation
- Increased sleeping
- Difficulty in concentration
- Memory loss
- Increased irritability
- Poor judgment in decision making
- Headaches
- Papilledema

Both benign and malignant intracranial tumors are potentially fatal. The outcome depends on the tumor location, size, and type. Benign tumors (e.g., neurinomas, meningiomas) may be cured with early diagnosis and surgery. However, gliomas and metastatic intracranial tumors are often fatal. These tumors are the subject of extensive ongoing research.

Intracranial tumors cause death by infiltration and compression of brain tissue. Not only are the tumors space-occupying lesions, but also they often produce con-

▼ *Other Clinical Signs and Symptoms of*
Brain Tumors (Schnell, 1993a)

- Seizures (without previous history)
- Sensory changes
- Muscle weakness
- Bladder dysfunction
- Positive Babinski reflex
- Increased lower extremity (LE) reflexes compared with upper extremity reflexes
- Decreased coordination
- Ataxia
- Paralysis
- Clonus (ankle or wrist)

▼ *Possible Late Signs of*
Increased Intracranial Pressure
(Schnell, 1993a)

- Pupillary change
- Changes in vital signs
- Elevated systolic blood pressure
- Bradycardia
- Slow, irregular respirations

siderable cerebral edema. Brain tumors progressively cause intracranial pressure (ICP), which causes brain stem herniation and death.

Spinal Cord Tumors

Spinal tumors are similar in nature and origin to intracranial tumors but occur much less often. They are most common in young and middle-aged adults, and they occur most often in the thoracic spine because of its length, proximity to the mediastinum, and proximity to direct metastatic extension from lymph nodes involved with lymphoma, breast cancer, or lung cancer.

Metastases. Most metastasis is disseminated by local invasion. Spinal cord tumors account for less than 15 per cent of brain tumors. As mentioned, 10 per cent of spinal tumors are themselves metastasized neoplasms from the brain.

One other means of dissemination is through the intervertebral foramina. The extradural space communicates through the intervertebral foramina with adjacent extraspinal compartments, such as the mediastinum and retroperitoneal space. In most cases, extradural tumors are metastatic, reaching the extradural space and then adjacent extraspinal spaces through this foraminal connection (Levin et al., 1993). Tumors within the spinal cord (intramedullary) or outside the spinal cord (extramedullary) may metastasize to the dural tube to become intradural tumors.

Clinical Signs and Symptoms. Back pain at the level of the spinal cord lesion occurs in over 80 per cent of cases and may be aggravated by lying down, weight bearing, sneezing, or coughing (Rugo, 1993b). Discomfort may be thoracolumbar back pain in a beltlike distribution; the pain may extend to the groin or to the legs (Snyder, 1986). The pain may be constant or intermittent, a dull ache or a sharp, knifelike sensation. Pain occurs most often at rest; pain occurring at night can awaken an individual from sleep; the person reports that it is impossible to go back to sleep.

Clinical manifestations of spinal tumors vary according to their location. Spinal cord compression is the most common pathologic feature of all tumors within the spinal column; symptoms occur in the body below the level of the tumor. Early characteristics of spinal cord compression include pain, sensory loss, muscle weakness, and muscle atrophy. Less commonly, chest or abdominal pain may occur, caused by nerve root compression from epidural

---

Clinical Signs and Symptoms of

Spinal Cord Tumors

- Pain
- Decreased sensation
- Spastic muscle weakness
- Progressive muscle weakness
- Muscle atrophy
- Paraplegia or quadriplegia
- Thoracolumbar pain
- Unilateral groin or leg pain
- Pain at rest and/or night pain
- Bowel/bladder dysfunction (late finding)

---

tumor(s). Bowel and bladder dysfunction are late findings (Rugo, 1993b).

Pain associated with *extramedullary tumors* can be located primarily at the site of the lesion or may refer down the ipsilateral extremity, with radicular involvement from nerve root compression, irritation, or occlusion of blood vessels supplying the cord. Progressive cord compression is manifested by spastic weakness below the level of the lesion, decreased sensation, and increased weakness (Schnell, 1993b).

Intramedullary tumors produce more variable signs and symptoms. High cervical cord involvement causes spastic quadriplegia and sensory changes. Tumors in descending areas of the spinal cord produce motor and sensory changes appropriate to functions of that level (Schnell, 1993b).

Treatment. Intervention for spinal tumors is usually surgery, radiation therapy, or both. Immediate surgery is indicated if compression of the cord or nerve roots is evident. Complete surgical removal of an intramedullary tumor is rare, but partial resection followed by radiation may improve the client's condition clinically. Treatment of early lesions may avoid significant compromise completely. Although clients who present with paralysis may not recover function, physical therapy treatment is indicated to relieve pain and to limit the extent of further progression (Rugo, 1993b).

Prognosis. Primary spinal cord tumors usually produce a slow onset of symptoms, whereas metastatic tumors are characterized by rapid development of symptoms. Severe cord compression destroys the cord and produces paraplegia or quadriplegia. Marked improvement and even complete restoration of function can occur with treatment if the tumor is encapsulated (e.g., meningioma or lipoma). Prognosis is poor in the presence of cord necrosis from compression or interrupted blood flow.

Overview   CANCER PRESENCE AND PAIN

SKIN (Melanoma only)

Location:	Women: arms, legs, back, face
	Men: head, trunk
	African-Americans: palms, soles, under the nails
Referral:	None
Description:	Usually painless
	Sore that does not heal
	Irritation and itching
	Cluster mole formation
	Tenderness and soreness around a mole
Intensity:	Mild
Duration:	Constant
Associated Signs and Symptoms:	None

■ ■ ■ ■ ■ ■ ■ ■ ■ ■ ■

BREAST (Fig. 10-5)

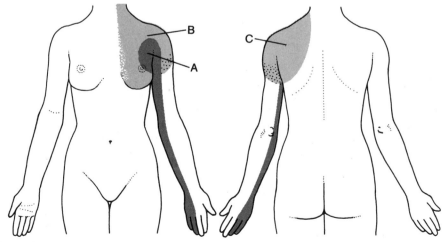

Figure 10-5

Pain arising from the breast. *A*, Mammary pain referred into the axilla along the medial aspect of the arm. *B*, Referral pain to the supraclavicular level and into the neck. *C*, Diffusion around the thorax through the intercostal nerves. Pain may be referred to the back and to the posterior shoulder.

Location:	Changes or pain occur anywhere on the breast or nipple
Referral:	May be painless
	Around the chest into the axilla, to the back at the level of the breast, occasionally into the neck and posterior aspect of the shoulder girdle
	Along the medial aspect of the ipsilateral arm to the 4th and 5th digits
Description:	Usually painless
	Involvement of breast tissue may result in sharp cutting or sharp aching
Intensity:	Mild to severe
Duration:	Intermittent to constant
Associated Signs and Symptoms:	May have no other symptoms
	May report discharge or bleeding from the breasts or nipples
	Distorted shape of the breast or nipple
	Enlarged tender lymph nodes
	Dimpling of the skin surface over the breast
	Unusual rash on the breast or nipple
	Unusual prominence of the veins over the breast

■ ■ ■ ■ ■ ■ ■ ■ ■ ■ ■ ■

LEUKEMIA

Location:	Usually painless, may have pain in the left abdomen
Referral:	None
Description:	Dull pain in the abdomen and may occur only on palpation
Intensity:	Mild to moderate
Duration:	Intermittent (with applied pressure)
Associated Signs and Symptoms:	Unusual bleeding from the nose or rectum, or blood in urine
	Prolonged menstruation
	Easy bruising of the skin
	Fatigue
	Dyspnea
	Weight loss, loss of appetite
	Fevers and sweats

■ ■ ■ ■ ■ ■ ■ ■ ■ ■ ■ ■

MULTIPLE MYELOMA

Location:	Skeletal pain, especially in the spine, sternum, rib, leg, or arm
Referral:	According to the location of the tumor

Description: Sharp, knifelike
Intensity: Moderate to severe
Duration: Intermittent, progressing to constant
Associated Signs
and Symptoms: Hypercalcemia: dehydration (vomiting), polyuria
                Spontaneous bone fracture
                Carpal tunnel syndrome

■ ■ ■ ■ ■ ■ ■ ■ ■ ■ ■

HODGKIN'S DISEASE

Location: Lymph glands, usually unilateral neck or groin
Referral: According to the location of the metastases
Description: Usually painless, progressive enlargement of lymph nodes
Intensity: Not applicable
Duration: Not applicable
Associated Signs
and Symptoms: Fever peaks in the late afternoon, night sweats
                Anorexia and weight loss
                Severe itching over the entire body
                Anemia, fatigue, malaise
                Jaundice
                Edema
                Nonproductive cough, dyspnea, chest pain, cyanosis

■ ■ ■ ■ ■ ■ ■ ■ ■ ■ ■

NON-HODGKIN'S LYMPHOMA

Location: Peripheral lymph nodes
Referral: Not applicable
Description: Usually painless enlargement
Intensity: Not applicable
Duration: Not applicable
Associated Signs
and Symptoms: Fever, night sweats
                Weight loss
                Bleeding
                Generalized itching and reddened skin

SOFT TISSUE TUMORS

Location:	Any connective tissue (e.g., tendon muscle, cartilage, fat, synovium, fibrous tissue)
Referral:	According to the tissue involved
Description:	Persistent swelling or lump, especially in the muscle
Intensity:	Mild, increases progressively to severe
Duration:	Intermittent, increases progressively to constant
Associated Signs and Symptoms:	Local swelling with tenderness and skin warmth
	Pathologic fracture

■ ■ ■ ■ ■ ■ ■ ■ ■ ■ ■

BONE TUMORS

Location:	Can affect any bone in the body, depending on the specific type of bone cancer
Referral:	According to pattern and location of metastases
Description:	Sharp, knifelike, aching bone pain
	Occurs on movement and weight bearing, with pathologic fractures
	Pain at night preventing sleep
Intensity:	Initially mild, progressing to severe
Duration:	Usually intermittent, progressing to constant
Associated Signs and Symptoms:	Fatigue and malaise
	Weight loss
	Swelling over localized areas of tumor
	Soft, tender palpable mass over bone
	Loss of range or motion and joint function if limb bone is involved
	Fever
	Sciatica
	Unilateral edema

■ ■ ■ ■ ■ ■ ■ ■ ■ ■ ■

PARANEOPLASTIC SYNDROMES

Location:	Remote sites from primary neoplasm
Referral:	Organ dependent
Description:	Asymmetric joint involvement

Lower extremities primarily
Concurrent arthritis and malignancy
Explosive onset at late age
See Tables 10–6 and 10–7

Intensity: Symptom dependent
Duration: Symptom dependent
Associated Signs
and Symptoms: Fever

Skin rash

Clubbing of the fingers

Pigmentation disorders

Arthralgias

Paresthesias

Thrombophlebitis

Proximal muscle weakness

Anorexia, malaise, weight loss

Rheumatologic complaints

■ ■ ■ ■ ■ ■ ■ ■ ■ ■ ■

PRIMARY CENTRAL NERVOUS SYSTEM: BRAIN TUMORS

Location: Intracranial
Referral: Specific symptoms depend on tumor location
Headaches
Description: Bioccipital or bifrontal headache
Intensity: Mild to severe
Duration: Worse in morning upon awakening
Diminishes or disappears soon after rising

Aggravating
Factors: Activity that increases intracranial pressure (e.g., straining during bowel movements, stooping, lifting heavy objects, coughing, bending over)
Prone/supine position at night during sleep

Relieving
Factors: Pain medications, including aspirin, acetaminophen
Associated Signs
and Symptoms: Papilledema
Altered mentation:
Increased sleeping
Difficulty in concentrating

Memory loss
Increased irritability
Poor judgment
Vomiting unrelated to food accompanies headaches
Seizures
Neurologic findings:
Positive Babinski reflex
Clonus (ankle or wrist)
Sensory changes
Decreased coordination
Ataxia
Muscle weakness
Increased LE deep tendon reflexes
Transient paralysis

■ ■ ■ ■ ■ ■ ■ ■ ■ ■ ■

PRIMARY CENTRAL NERVOUS SYSTEM: SPINAL CORD TUMORS

Location:	Intramedullary (within the spinal cord)
	Extramedullary (within the dura mater)
	Extradural (outside the dura mater)
Referral:	Back pain at the level of the spinal cord lesion
	Pain may extend to the groin or legs
Description:	Dull ache; sharp, knifelike sensation
Intensity:	Mild to severe, progressive; night pain
Duration:	Intermittent, progressing to constant, or constant
Aggravating Factors:	(Back pain) Lying down/rest
	Weight bearing
	Sneezing or coughing
Associated Signs and Symptoms:	Muscle weakness
	Muscle atrophy
	Sensory loss
	Paraplegia/quadriplegia
	Chest or abdominal pain
	Bowel/bladder dysfunction (late findings)

PHYSICIAN REFERRAL

Early detection of cancer can save a person's life. Any suspicious sign or symptom discussed in this chapter should be investigated immediately by a physician. This is true especially in the presence of a positive family history of cancer, a previous personal history of cancer, the presence of environmental risk factors, and/or in the absence of medical or dental (oral) evaluation during the previous year.

Any recently discovered lumps or nodules must be examined by a physician. Any suspicious finding by report, on observation, or by palpation should be checked by a physician. Finding enlarged, tender lymph nodes does not require a referral to a physician unless these lymph nodes persist and involve more than one area, because lymph nodes enlarge in response to infections throughout the body.

However, the physician should be notified of your findings, and the client should be advised to have the lymph nodes checked at the next follow-up visit with the physician. If the nodes remain enlarged over a long period (4 weeks or more), then the client should be encouraged to contact the physician to discuss the need for follow-up. The exception is with people who have enlarged, *painless* lymph nodes. These people should notify their physician of these findings and make an appointment for follow-up at the physician's discretion.

If any signs of skin lesions are described by the client or if they are observed by the physical therapist, and the client has not been examined by a physician, a medical referral is recommended. If the client is planning a follow-up visit with the physician within the next 2 to 4 weeks, then that client is advised to indicate the mole or skin changes at that time. If no appointment is pending, then the client is encouraged to make a specific visit either to the family/personal physician or to a dermatologist.

Systemic Signs and Symptoms Requiring Physician Referral

The physical therapist is advised to ask the client further questions whenever any of the following signs and symptoms are reported or observed, because they may indicate cancer or some other systemic disease. The client should therefore be referred to a physician for further evaluation.

Arthralgias	Itching/scratching
Bleeding mole	Jaundice
Bone pain	Loss of appetite
Change in bowel habits	Lump or thickening
Change in urinary habits	Pain at night disturbing sleep
Change in voice	Pain on weight bearing
Chronic cough	Persistent nausea, vomiting, and neurologic findings
Clubbing of the fingers	
Drowsiness/confusion	Prolonged menstruation
Dysphagia	(Proximal) muscle weakness
Dyspnea	Restlessness
Epistaxis	Sore that does not heal
Fatigue, general malaise	Unusual bleeding
Fevers and sweats	Unusual discharge
Headache	Unusual skin lesions or rash
Hemoptysis (spitting blood)	Wheezing
Hoarseness	

Key Points to Remember

- Spinal cord compression from metastases may present as back pain, leg weakness, and bowel/bladder symptoms.
- Back pain may precede the development of neurologic signs and symptoms in any person with cancer.
- Signs of nerve root compression may be the first indication of cancer, in particular lymphoma, multiple myeloma, or cancer in the lung, breast, prostate, or kidney.
- The five most common sites of metastasis are the lymph nodes, liver, lung, bone, and brain.
- The presence of jaundice in association of any atypical presentation of back pain may indicate liver metastasis.
- Lung, breast, prostate, thyroid, and the lymphatics are the primary sites responsible for most metastatic bone disease.
- Monitoring physiologic responses (vital signs) to exercise is important in the immunosuppressed population. Watch closely for early signs (dyspnea, pallor, sweating, and fatigue) of cardiopulmonary complications of cancer treatment.

- To determine appropriate exercise levels for clients who are immunosuppressed, review blood test results (WBCs, RBCs, hematocrit, platelets).
- Besides the seven early warning signs of cancer, the physical therapist should watch for idiopathic muscle weakness accompanied by decreased deep tendon reflexes.
- Any woman presenting with chest, breast, axillary, or shoulder pain of unknown etiology must be screened for breast cancer.
- Changes in size, shape, tenderness, and consistency of lymph nodes raise a red flag. Supraclavicular nodes and inguinal nodes are common metastatic sites for cancer.
- No reliable physical signs distinguish between benign and malignant soft tissue lesions; all soft tissue lumps that persist or grow should be reported immediately to the physician.

SUBJECTIVE EXAMINATION | *Special Questions to Ask*

Special questions to ask will vary with each client and the clinical signs and symptoms presented at the time of the evaluation. The physical therapist should refer to the specific chapter representing the client's current complaints. The case study provided here is one example of how to follow up with necessary questions to rule out a systemic origin of musculoskeletal findings.

A previous history of drug therapy and current drug use may be important information to obtain because prolonged use of drugs such as phenytoin (Dilantin) or immunosuppressive drugs such as azathioprine (Imuran) and cyclosporine may lead to cancer. Postmenopausal use of estrogens has been linked with endometrial cancer.

A previous personal/family history of cancer may be significant, especially any history of breast, colorectal, or lung cancers that demonstrates genetic susceptibility.

Using the seven early warning signs of cancer as a basis for follow-up, one or all of these questions may be appropriate:

- Have you noticed any changes in your bowel movement or in the flow of urination?

  - If yes, ask pertinent follow-up questions as suggested in Chapter 7.

  - If the client answers "No," it may be necessary to provide prompts or examples of what changes you are referring to (e.g., difficulty in starting or continuing the flow of urine, numbness or tingling in the groin or pelvis).

- Have you noticed any sores that have not healed properly?

  - If yes, where are they located? How long has the sore been present? Has your physician examined this area?

- Have you noticed any unusual bleeding (for women: including prolonged menstruation, or *any* bleeding for the postmenopausal woman) or prolonged discharge from any part of your body?

  - If yes, where? How long has this been present? Has your physician examined this area?

- Have you noticed any thickening or lump of any muscle, tendon, bone, breast, or anywhere else?

  - If yes, where? How long has this been present? Has your physician examined this area?*

  - If no (for women): do you examine your own breasts? How often do you examine them, and when was the last time you did a breast self-examination?

- Do you have any pain, swelling, or unusual tenderness in the breasts? **(Pain can be a symptom of cancer; cyclic pain is common with normal breasts, use of oral contraceptives, and fibrocystic disease)**

  - If yes, is this pain brought on by strenuous activity? **(Spontaneous/systemic or related to specific cause/musculoskeletal**—e.g., use of one arm, part of under-wire bra, exercise)

- Have you noticed any rash on the breast or discharge from the nipple? **(Medications such as oral contraceptives, phenothiazines, diuretics, digitalis, tricyclic tranquilizers, reserpine, methyldopa, and steroids can cause clear discharge from the nipple; blood-tinged discharge is always significant)**

- Have you noticed any difficulty in eating or swallowing? Have you had a chronic cough, recurrent laryngitis, hoarseness, or any difficulty with speaking?

  - If yes, how long has this been happening? Have you discussed this with your physician?

---

* An asymptomatic mass that has been present for years and causes only cosmetic concern is usually benign, whereas a painful mass of short duration that has caused a decrease in function may be malignant (Wilkins and Sim, 1986).

- Have you had any change in digestive patterns? Have you had increasing indigestion or unusual constipation?
  - If yes, how long has this been happening? Have you discussed this with your physician?
- Have you had a recent, sudden weight loss, such as 10 to 15 pounds in 2 weeks without dieting?
- Have you noticed any obvious change in color, shape, or size of a wart or mole?
  - If yes, what have you noticed? How long has this wart or mole been present? Have you discussed this problem with your physician?
- Have you had any unusual headaches or changes in your vision?
  - If yes, please describe. **(Brain tumors: bioccipital or bifrontal)**
  - Can you attribute these to anything in particular?
  - Do you vomit (unrelated to food) when your headaches occur? **(Brain tumors)**
- Have you been more tired than usual or experienced persistent fatigue during the last month?
- Can you think of any time during the past week when you may have bumped yourself, fallen, or injured yourself in any way? (Ask when in the presence of local swelling and tenderness.) **(Bone tumors)**
- Have you noticed any bone pain or problems with any of your bones? Is the pain affected by movement? **(Fractures cause sharp pain that increases with movement. Bone pain from systemic causes usually feels dull and deep and is unrelated to movement)**
- Have you ever been exposed to chemical agents or irritants, such as asbestos, asphalt, aniline dyes, benzene, herbicides, fertilizers, wood dust, or others? **(Environmental causes of cancer)**

CASE STUDY

REFERRAL

A 56-year-old man has come to you for an evaluation without referral. He has not been examined by a physician of any kind for at least 3 years. He is seeking an evaluation on the insistence of his wife, who has noticed that his collar size has increased two sizes in the last year and that his neck looks "puffy." He has no complaints of any kind (including pain or discomfort), and he denies any known trauma, but his wife insists that he has limited ability in turning his head when backing the car out of the driveway.

PHYSICAL THERAPY INTERVIEW

First read the client's Family/Personal History form with particular interest in his personal or family history of cancer, the presence of allergies or asthma, the use of medications or over-the-counter drugs, previous surgeries, available x-ray studies of the neck or spine, and/or history of cigarette smoking (or other tobacco use). An appropriate lead-in to the following series of questions may be, "Because you have not seen a physician before your appointment with me, I will ask you a series of questions to find out if your symptoms require examination by a physician rather than treatment in this office."

Current Symptoms

What have you noticed different about your neck that brings you here today?

When did you first notice that your neck was changing (in size or shape)?

Can you remember having any accidents, falls, twists, or any other kind of potential trauma at that time?

Do you ever notice any pain, stiffness, soreness, or discomfort in your neck or shoulders?

> If yes, please describe (as per the outline in the Core Interview, Chapter 2).

Does this or any other pain ever awaken you at night or keep you awake? **(Night pain associated with cancer)**

> If yes, follow up with appropriate questions. (See the Physical Therapy Interview.)

Associated Symptoms

Have you noticed any numbness or tingling in your arms or hands?

Have you noticed any swollen glands, lumps, or thickened areas of skin or muscle in your neck, armpits, or groin? **(Cancer screen)**

Do you have any difficulty in swallowing? Do you have recurrent hoarseness, influenza-like symptoms, or a persistent cough or cold that never seems to go away? **(Cancer screen)**

Have you noticed any low-grade fevers or night sweats? **(Systemic disease)**

Have you had any recent unexplained weight gain or loss? (You may need to explain that you mean a gain or loss of 10 to 15 pounds in as many days without dieting.) Have you had a loss of appetite? **(Cancer screen or other systemic disease)**

Do you ever have any difficulty with breathing or find yourself short of breath at rest or after minimal exercise? **(Dyspnea)**

Do you have frequent headaches or do you experience any dizziness, nausea, or vomiting? **(Systemic disease, carotid artery affected)**

FUNCTIONAL CAPACITY

What kind of work do you do?

Do you have any limitations caused by this condition that affect you in any way at work or at home? **(Occupational disease, limitations of activities of daily living (ADL) skills)**

Do you have difficulty when driving or turning your head?

Final Questions

How would you describe your general health?

Have you ever been diagnosed with cancer of any kind?

Is there anything that you would like to tell me that you think is important about your neck or your health in general?

TEST PROCEDURES DURING THE FIRST SESSION TO ASSESS THE MUSCULOSKELETAL SYSTEM

Observation/Inspection

Observe for presence of swelling anywhere, tender or swollen lymph nodes (cervical, supraclavicular, and axillary), changes in skin temperature, unusual moles or warts. Perform a brief posture screen (general postural observations may be made while you are interviewing the client). Palpate for carotid and upper extremity pulses. Check vital signs and **TAKE THE CLIENT'S ORAL TEMPERATURE!**

Cervical AROM/PROM

Assess for muscle tightness, loss of joint motion (including accessory movements if indicated by a loss of passive motion). Assess for compromise of the vertebral artery, and, if negative, clear the cervical spine by using a quadrant test with overpressure (e.g., Spurling's test) and assess accessory movements of the cervical spine. Perform tests for thoracic outlet syndrome. Palpate the anterior cervical spine for pathologic protrusion while the client swallows.

Temporomandibular Joint (TMJ) Screen

Clear the joint above (i.e., TMJ) using AROM, observation, and palpation specific to the TMJ.

Shoulder Screen

Clear the joint below (i.e., shoulder) by using a screening examination (e.g., AROM/PROM and quadrant testing).

Neurologic Screen

Deep tendon reflexes, sensory screen (e.g., gross sensory testing for light touch), manual muscle test (MMT) screening using break testing of the upper quadrant, grip strength. If test(s) is abnormal, consider further neurologic testing (e.g., balance, coordination, stereognosia, in-depth sensory examination, dysmetria).

It is always recommended that the physical therapist give the client ongoing verbal feedback during the examination regarding evaluation results, such as, "I notice you can't turn your head to the right as much as you can to the left—from checking your muscles and joints, it looks like muscle tightness, not any loss of joint movement." . . . or . . . "I notice your reflexes on each side aren't the same (your right arm reacts more strongly than the left)—let's see if we can find out why."

RECOMMENDATION FOR PHYSICIAN VISIT

I noticed on your intake form that you haven't listed the name of a personal or family physician. Do you have a physician?

If yes, when was the last time you saw your physician? Have you seen your physician for this current problem?

Give the client a brief summary of your findings while making your recommendations; for example, "Mr. X., I notice today that although you don't have any ongoing neck pain, the lymph nodes in your neck and armpit are enlarged but not particularly tender. Otherwise, all of my findings are negative. Your loss of motion on turning your head is not unusual for a person your age and certainly would not cause your neck to increase in size or shape.

"Given the fact that you have not seen a physician for almost 3 years, I strongly recommend that you see a physician of your choice, or I can give you the names of several to choose from. In either case, I think some medical tests are necessary to rule out any underlying medical problem. For instance, a neck x-ray would be recommended before physical therapy treatment is started."

If the client has indicated a positive family history of cancer, it might be appropriate to suggest, "Given your positive family history of previous medical illnesses, the 3 years since you have seen a physician, and the lack of musculoskeletal findings, I strongly recommend . . . etc." It is important to provide the client with all the information available to you, but without causing undue alarm and emotional stress that could actually prevent the client from seeking further testing.

If the client does give the name of a physician, you may ask for written permission (disclosure release) to send a copy of your results to the physician. If the client does not have a physician and requests recommendations from you, then you may offer to send a copy of your results to the physician with whom the client makes an appointment. If you think that a problem may be potentially serious and you want this person to receive adequate follow-up without causing alarm, you may offer to let him make the appointment from your office, suggest that your secretary or receptionist make the appointment for him, or even offer to make the initial telephone contact yourself.

RESULT

This client did comply with the physical therapist's suggestion to see a physician and was diagnosed as having Hodgkin's disease (a cancer of the lymph system) without constitutional symptoms (i.e., without evidence of weight loss, fever, or night sweats). Medical treatment was initiated, and physical therapy treatment was not warranted.

References

Ackerman, A.B.: Clinical diagnosis of malignant melanoma in situ. *In* Ackerman, A.B. (ed.): Pathology of Malignant Melanoma. New York, Masson Publishing USA, 1981, pp. 57–58.

Affronti, M.L., et al.: Autologous bone marrow transplant for the treatment of advanced breast cancer. Innovations in Oncology Nursing 6(4):2–6, 19–21, 1990.

AMA Council on Scientific Affairs: Mammographic screening in asymptomatic women aged 40 years and older. Journal of the American Medical Association 261:2535, 1989.

American Cancer Society: 1993 Cancer Facts and Figures. Atlanta, 1993.

American Medical Association: Cancer: Facts You Should Know. Chicago, AMA Patient Information Service, 1987.

Aminoff, M.J.: Nervous system: Primary and metastatic spinal tumors. *In* Holland, J.F., Frei, E., Bast, R.C., Kufe, D.W., Morton, D.L., and Weichselbaum, R.R. (eds.): Cancer Medicine, 3rd ed. Vols. 1 and 2. Philadelphia, Lea & Febiger, 1993, pp. 729–785.

Aprin, H., Riserborough, E.J., and Hall, J.E.: Chondrosarcoma in children and adolescents. Clinical Orthopedics 166:226–232, 1982.

Arthur, D.C.: Genetics and cytogenetics of pediatric cancers. Cancer 58:534, 1986.

Baird, S.B. (ed.): A Cancer Source Book for Nurses, 6th ed. Atlanta, American Cancer Society Professional Education Publication, 1991.

Balch, C.M., Houghton, A., and Peters, L.: Cutaneous melanoma. *In* DeVita, V.T., Hellman, S., and Rosenberg, S.A. (eds.): Cancer: Principles and Practice of Oncology, 4th ed. Philadelphia, J.B. Lippincott, 1993, pp. 1612–1661.

Barlogie, B., Aleninian, R., Dicke, K.A., Zagars, G., Spitzer, G., Jagannath, S., and Horwitz, L.: High-dose chemoradiotherapy and autologous bone marrow transplantation for resistant multiple myeloma. Blood 70(3): 869–872, 1987.

Bartzdorf, U., and Catlin, D.: Pain syndromes. *In* Haskell, C. (ed.): Cancer Treatment, 3rd ed. Philadelphia, W.B. Saunders, 1990, pp. 874–883.

Beahrs, O.H., Henson, D.E., Hutter, R.V.P., and Kennedy, B.J. (eds.): American Joint Committee on Cancer Manual, Staging of Cancer, 4th ed. Philadelphia, J.B. Lippincott, 1992.

Belcher, A.: Cancer nursing. *In* Mosby's Clinical Nursing Series. St. Louis, Mosby–Year Book, 1992.

Beral, V., Peterman, T., Berkelman, R., and Jaffe, H.: AIDS-associated non-Hodgkin lymphoma. Lancet 1: 805–809, 1991.

Bernheim, H.A., Block, L.H., and Atkins, E.: Fever: Pathogenesis, pathophysiology and purpose. Annals of Internal Medicine 91:261, 1979.

Black, D.M., and Solomon, E.: The search for the familial breast/ovarian cancer gene. Trends in Genetics 9(1):22–26, 1993.

Black, J.M., and Matassarin-Jacobs, E. (eds.): Luck-

mann and Sorensen's Medical-Surgical Nursing, 4th ed. Philadelphia, W.B. Saunders, 1993.

Braun, D., and Groenwald, S.: Relation of the immune system to cancer. *In* Groenwald, S., Frogge, M., Goodman, B., and Yarbro, C. (eds.): Cancer Nursing; Principles and practice, 3rd ed. Boston, Jones and Bartlett Publishers, 1993, pp. 70–83.

Broder, S., and Karp, J.E.: The challenge of HIV-associated malignancies. CA—A Cancer Journal for Clinicians 42(2):69–73, 1992.

Bunn, P.A., and Ridgway, E.C.: Paraneoplastic syndromes. *In* DeVita, V.T., Hellman, S., and Rosenberg, S.A. (eds.): Cancer: Principles and Practice of Oncology, 4th ed. Philadelphia, J.B. Lippincott, 1993, pp. 2026–2071.

Cannon, J.R., and Schneidman, D.W.: Recent developments in adnexal pathology. *In* Moschella, S.L. (ed.): Dermatology Update. New York, Elsevier, 1982, p. 217.

Cantin, J., McNeer, G.P., Chu, F.C., et al.: The problem of local recurrence after treatment of soft tissue sarcoma. Annals of Surgery 168:47–53, 1968.

Carpenter, L.: Nursing care of the client with breast disorders. *In* Black, J.M., and Matassarin-Jacobs, E. (eds.): Luckmann and Sorensen's Medical-Surgical Nursing, 4th ed. Philadelphia, W.B. Saunders, 1993, pp. 2173–2196.

Chachoua, A., Krigel, R., Lafleur, F., et al.: Prognostic factors and staging classification of patients with epidemic Kaposi's sarcoma. Journal of Clinical Oncology 7:774–780, 1989.

Cremer, K.J., Spring, S.B., and Gruber, J.: Role of human immunodeficiency virus type 1 and other viruses in malignancies associated with acquired immunodeficiency disease syndrome. Journal of the National Cancer Institute 82:1016–1024, 1990.

Croft, P.B., and Wilkinson, M.W.: The incidence of carcinomatous neuropathy in patients with various types of carcinoma. Brain 88:427, 1965.

Croft, P.B., and Wilkinson, M.W.: The incidence of carcinomatous neuropathy with special reference to carcinoma of the lung and breast. *In* Brain, W.R., and Norris, F.H., Jr. (eds.): The Remote Effects of Cancer on the Nervous System. New York, Grune & Stratton, 1965, pp. 44–54.

Culver, K.W., Walbridge, S., Blaese, R.M., and Oldfield, E.H.: In situ retroviral-mediated gene transfer for the treatment of brain tumors in rats. Cancer Research 531(1):83–88, 1993.

Davies, R.J., A'Hern, R.P., Parsons, C.A., and Moskovic, E.C.: Mammographic accuracy and patient age: A study of 297 patients undergoing breast biopsy. Clinical Radiology 47(1):23–25, 1993.

Davis, T.E., and Mellette, S.: Cancer rehabilitation: A special report. Report of the Task Force on Medical Rehabilitation Research—NIH. Rehabilitation in Oncology 3:5–14, 1991.

DeVita, V.T., Hellman, S., and Rosenberg, S.A. (eds.): Cancer; Principles and Practice of Oncology, 4th ed. Philadelphia, J.B. Lippincott, 1993.

Dietrick-Gallagher, M., and Brasher, E.: Surgical oncology. *In* Baird, S. (ed.): A Cancer Source Book for

Nurses, 6th ed. Atlanta, American Cancer Society Publication, 1991, pp. 56–62.

Donegan, W.L.: Cancer of the breast in men. CA—A Cancer Journal for Clinicians 41(6):339–354, 1991.

Dropcho, E.J., Stanton, C., and Oh, S.J.: Neuronal anti-nuclear antibodies in a patient with Lambert-Eaton myasthenic syndrome and small-cell lung carcinoma. Neurology 39:249, 1989.

Eddy, D.M., et al.: The value of mammography screening in women under age 50 years. Journal of the American Medical Association 259:1512, 1989.

Epstein, E., Epstein, N.E., Bragg, K., et al.: Metastases from squamous cell carcinomas of the skin. Archives of Dermatology 97:245, 1968.

Ersek, M.: Biological response modifiers. In Baird, S. (ed.): A Cancer Source Book for Nurses, 6th ed. Atlanta, American Cancer Society Publication, 1991, pp. 83–90.

Fang, L.S.: Renal diseases. In Ramsey, P.G., and Larson, E.B. (eds.): Medical Therapeutics, 2nd ed. Philadelphia, W.B. Saunders, 1993, pp. 192–237.

Feig, S.A., and Ehrlich, S.M.: Estimation of radiation risks from screening mammography: Recent trends and comparison with expected benefits. Radiology 174:638, 1990.

Foley, K.M., Cancer and pain. In Holleb, A.I. (ed.): The American Cancer Society Cancer Book. New York, Doubleday and Company, 1986, pp. 225–237.

Folkman, J.: Tumor angiogenesis. In Holland, J.F., et al. (eds.): Cancer Medicine, 3rd ed. Vols. 1 and 2. Philadelphia, Lea & Febiger, 1993, pp. 153–170.

Friedman, R.J., Rigel, D.S., Silverman, M.K., Kopf, A.W., and Vossaert, K.A.: Malignant melanoma in the 1990s. CA—A Cancer Journal for Clinicians 41(4): 201–225, 1991.

Fuller, K.: Neurologic deficits with cancer. Combined Sections Meeting, American Physical Therapy Association, San Antonio, Texas, February 4, 1993.

Gail, M.H., Pluda, J.M., Rabkin, C.S., et al.: Projections of the incidence of non-Hodgkin's lymphoma related to acquired immunodeficiency syndrome. Journal of the National Cancer Institute 83:695–701, 1991.

Garfinkel, L.: Current trends in breast cancer. CA—A Cancer Journal for Clinicians 43(1):5–6, 1993.

Gilkeson, G.S., and Caldwell, D.S.: Rheumatic associations with malignancy. Journal of Musculoskeletal Medicine 7(1):64–79, 1990.

Giuliano, A.E.: Breast. In Tierney, L.M., McPhee, S.J., Papadakis, M.A., and Schroeder, S.A. (eds.): Current Medical Diagnosis and Treatment. Norwalk, Connecticut, Appleton & Lange, 1993, pp. 538–560.

Giuliano, A.E., Feig, S., and Eilber, F.: Changing metastatic patterns of osteosarcoma. Cancer 54:2160–2164, 1984.

Glick, J.H.: Hodgkin's disease. In Wyngaarden, J.B., et al. (eds.): Cecil Textbook of Medicine, 19th ed. Philadelphia, W.B. Saunders, 1992, pp. 955–963.

Glucksberg, H., and Singer, J.W.: Cancer Care. New York, Chas. Scribner's Sons, 1982.

Goldstein, S.M., and Odom, R.B.: Skin and appendages. In Tierney, L.M., McPhee, S.J., Papadakis, M.A., and Schroeder, S.A. (eds.): Current Medical Diagnosis and Treatment. Norwalk, Connecticut, Appleton & Lange, 1993, pp. 64–124.

Goldstein, S.M., and Odom, R.B.: Skin and appendages. In Tierney, L.M., McPhee, S.J., and Papadakis, M.A. (eds.): Current Medical Diagnosis and Treatment. Norwalk, Connecticut, Appleton & Lange, 1994, pp. 89–149.

Groenwald, S.: Differences between normal and cancer cells. In Groenwald, S., Frogge, M., Goodman, M., and Yarbro, C. (eds.): Cancer Nursing; Principles and Practice, 3rd ed. Boston, Jones and Bartlett, 1993a, pp. 47–57.

Groenwald, S.: Invasion and metastasis. In Groenwald, S., Frogge, M., Goodman, M., and Yarbro, C. (eds.): Cancer Nursing; Principles and Practice, 3rd ed. Boston, Jones and Bartlett, 1993b, pp. 58–69.

Gudas, S.: The physical therapy challenge in disseminated cancer. Oncology Section Newsletter of the APTA 5:3, 1987.

Gudas, S.: Directives in cancer rehabilitation. Clinical Management 12(4):32–36, 1992.

Hall, E.J.: Principles of carcinogenesis: Physical. In DeVita, V.T., Hellman, S., and Rosenberg, S.A. (eds.): Cancer; Principles and Practice of Oncology, 4th ed. Philadelphia, J.B. Lippincott, 1993, pp. 213–227.

Hall, J.M., Friedman, L., Guenther, C., Lee, M.K., Weber, J.L., Black, D.M., and King, M.C.: Closing in on a breast cancer gene on chromosome 17q. American Journal of Human Genetics 50(6):1235–1242, 1992.

Hamburgh, R.R.: Principles of cancer treatment. Clinical Management 12(4):37–41, 1992.

Harrist, T.J., and Clark, W.H.: The skin. In Rubin, E., and Farber, J.L. (eds.): Pathology, 2nd ed. Philadelphia, J.P. Lippincott, 1994, pp. 1176–1237.

Hellman, D.B.: Arthritis and musculoskeletal disorders. In Tierney, L.M., McPhee, S.J., Papadakis, M.A., and Schroeder, S.A.: Current Medical Diagnosis and Treatment. Norwalk, Connecticut, Appleton & Lange, 1993, pp. 637–682.

Henson, J.W., and Posner, J.B.: Neurological complications. In Holland, J.F., et al. (eds.): Cancer Medicine, 3rd ed. Vols. 1 and 2. Philadelphia, Lea & Febiger, 1993, pp. 2268–2286.

Hogan, R.: Cancer. In Phipps, W., Long, B., Woods, N., Cassmeyer, V. (eds.). Medical-Surgical Nursing; Concepts and Clinical Practice, 4th ed. St. Louis, Mosby–Year Book, 1991, pp. 327–404.

Holland, J.F., et al. (eds.): Cancer Medicine, 3rd ed. Vols. 1 and 2. Philadelphia, Lea & Febiger, 1993.

Holleb, A.I. (ed.): The American Cancer Society Cancer Book. New York, Doubleday & Company, 1986.

Howley, P.M.: Principles of carcinogenesis: Viral. In DeVita, V.T., Hellman, S., and Rosenberg, S.A. (eds.): Cancer; Principles and Practice of Oncology, 4th ed. Philadelphia, J.B. Lippincott, 1993, pp. 182–199.

Huether, S.E., and Kravitz, M.: Structure, Function, and Disorders of the Integument. In McCance, K.L., and Huether, S.E. (eds.): Pathophysiology: The Biologic Basis for Disease in Adults and Children, 2nd ed., 1994, pp. 1512–1560.

Iwamoto, R.: Radiation therapy. *In* Baird, S. (ed.): A Cancer Source Book for Nurses, 6th ed. Atlanta, American Cancer Society Publication, 1991, pp. 63–72.

Jaffe, N., Smith, E., Abelson, H., et al.: Osteogenic sarcoma. Alterations in the pattern of pulmonary metastases with adjuvant chemotherapy. Journal of Clinical Oncology *1*:251–254, 1983.

Klein, G.: Oncogenes. *In* Holland, J.F., et al. (eds.): Cancer Medicine, 3rd ed. Vols. 1 and 2. Philadelphia, Lea & Febiger, 1993, pp. 65–77.

Levin, V.A., Gutin, P.H., and Leibel, S.: Neoplasms of the central nervous system. *In* DeVita, V.T., Hellman, S., and Rosenberg, S.A. (eds.): Cancer; Principles and Practice of Oncology, 4th ed. Philadelphia, J.B. Lippincott, 1993, pp. 1679–1737.

Linker, C.A.: Blood. *In* Tierney, L.M., McPhee, S.J., Papadakis, M.A., and Schroeder, S.A. (eds.): Current Medical Diagnosis and Treatment. Norwalk, Connecticut, Appleton & Lange, 1993, pp. 387–439.

Liotta, L.A., Kleinerman, J., and Saidel, G.M.: Quantitative relationships of intravascular tumor cells, tumor vessels, and pulmonary metastases following tumor implantation. Cancer Research *34*:997, 1974.

Liotta, L.A., and Stetler-Stevenson, W.G.: Principles of molecular cell biology of cancer: Cancer metastasis. *In* DeVita, V.T., Hellman, S., and Rosenberg, S.A. (eds.): Cancer; Principles and Practice of Oncology, 4th ed. Philadelphia, J.B. Lippincott, 1993, pp. 134–149.

Liotta, L.A., Stetler-Stevenson, W.G., and Steeg, P.S.: Invasion and metastasis. *In* Holland, J.F., et al. (eds.): Cancer Medicine, 3rd ed. Vols. 1 and 2. Philadelphia, Lea & Febiger, 1993, pp. 138–153.

Malawer, M.M., Link, M.P., and Donaldson, S.S.: Sarcomas of bone. *In* DeVita, V.T., Hellman, S., and Rosenberg, S.A. (eds.): Cancer; Principles and Practice of Oncology, 4th ed. Philadelphia, J.B. Lippincott, 1993, pp. 1509–1566.

Matassarin-Jacobs, E., and Petardi, L.: Basic concepts of neoplastic disorders. *In* Black, J.M., and Matassarin-Jacobs, E. (eds.): Luckmann and Sorensen's Medical-Surgical Nursing, 4th ed. Philadelphia, W.B. Saunders, 1993, pp. 473–500.

McGarvey, C. (ed.): Physical Therapy for the Cancer Patient. New York, Churchill Livingstone, 1990.

McLelland, R.: Challenges and progress with mammography. Cancer *64*(12 Suppl):2664, 1989.

McLelland, R.: Screening mammography. Cancer *67* (4 Suppl):1129, 1991.

Miller, L.T.: Post-surgery breast cancer outpatient program. Clinical Management *12*(4):50–56, 1992.

Miller, S.J.: Biology of Basal Cell Carcinoma. Journal American Academy of Dermatology *24*(1):161, 1991.

Nagel, A., Engel, A.G., Lang, B., Newsom-Davis, J., and Fukuoka, T.: Lambert-Eaton myasthenia syndrome IgG depletes presynaptic membrane active zone particles by antigenic modulation. Annals of Neurology *24*:552, 1988.

National Cancer Institute (NCI): Multiple Myeloma. Bethesda, U.S. Department of Health and Human Services, December 1991.

Neri, A., Barriga, F., Inghirami, G., et al.: Epstein-Barr virus infection precedes clonal expansion in Burkitt's and acquired immunodeficiency syndrome-associated lymphoma. Blood *77*:1092–1095, 1991.

Nicol, N.: Nursing care of clients with integumentary disorders. *In* Black, J.M., and Matassarin-Jacobs, E. (eds.): Luckmann and Sorensen's Medical-Surgical Nursing, 4th ed. Philadelphia, W.B. Saunders, 1993, pp. 1955–1984.

Odell, W.D.: Ectopic hormones and humoral syndromes of cancer. *In* Holland, J.F., et al. (eds.): Cancer Medicine, 3rd ed. Vols. 1 and 2. Philadelphia, Lea & Febiger, 1993, pp. 896–904.

O'Toole, M. (ed.): Miller-Keane Encyclopedia and Dictionary of Medicine, Nursing and Allied Health, 5th ed. Philadelphia, W.B. Saunders, 1992.

Patterson, J.A.K., and Geronemus, R.G.: Cancers of the skin. *In* DeVita, V.T., Hellman, S., and Rosenberg, S.A. (eds.): Cancer; Principles and Practice of Oncology, 3rd ed. Vols. 1 and 2. Philadelphia, J.B. Lippincott, 1989, pp. 1469–1498.

Pavel, J., Plunkett, A., and Sink, B.: Nursing care of clients with hematologic disorders. *In* Black, J.M., and Matassarin-Jacobs, E. (eds.): Luckmann and Sorensen's Medical-Surgical Nursing, 4th ed. Philadelphia, W.B. Saunders, 1993, pp. 1335–1404.

Peterson, J.: Chemotherapy. *In* Baird, S. (ed.): A Cancer Source Book for Nurses, 6th ed. Atlanta, American Cancer Society Publication, 1991, pp. 73–82.

Pizzo, P.A., Horowitz, M.E., Poplack, D.G., Hays, D.M., and Kun, L.E.: Solid tumors in childhood. *In* DeVita, V.T., Hellman, S., and Rosenberg, S.A. (eds.): Cancer; Principles and Practice of Oncology, 4th ed. Philadelphia, J.B. Lippincott, 1993, pp. 1738–1791.

Pluda, J.M., Yarchoan, R., Jaffe, E.S., et al.: Development of non-Hodgkin's lymphoma in a cohort of patients with severe human immunodeficiency virus (HIV) infection on long-term antiretroviral therapy. Annals of Internal Medicine *113*:276–282, 1990.

Porter, D.E., Cohen, B.B., Wallace, M.R., Carothers, A., and Steel, C.M.: Linkage mapping in familial breast cancer: Improved localisation of a susceptibility locus on chromosome 17q12-21. International Journal of Cancer *53*(2):188–198, 1993.

Press, O.W., Collins, C., Mortimer, J., and Livingston, R.: Oncologic therapeutics. *In* Ramsey, P.G., and Larson, E.B. (eds.): Medical Therapeutics, 2nd ed. Philadelphia, W.B. Saunders, 1993, pp. 374–427.

Rosen, G.: Neoplasms of the bone and soft tissue. *In* Holland, J.F., et al. (eds.): Cancer Medicine, 3rd ed. Vols. 1 and 2. Philadelphia, Lea & Febiger, 1993, pp. 1825–1858.

Rugo, H.S.: Cancer: The paraneoplastic syndromes. *In* Tierney, L.M., McPhee, S.J., Papadakis, M.A., and Schroeder, S.A.: Current Medical Diagnosis and Treatment. Norwalk, Connecticut, Appleton & Lange, 1993, pp. 40–63.

Safai, B., Diaz, B., and Schwartz, J.: Malignant neoplasms associated with human immunodeficiency virus infection. CA—A Cancer Journal for Clinicians 42(2):74–95, 1992.

Salmon, S.E., and Cassady, J.R.: Plasma cell neoplasms. In DeVita, V.T., Hellman, S., and Rosenberg, S.A. (eds.): Cancer; Principles and Practice of Oncology, 4th ed. Philadelphia, J.B. Lippincott, 1993, pp. 1984–2025.

Salter, R.B.: Textbook of Disorders and Injuries of the Musculoskeletal System, 2nd ed. Baltimore, Williams & Wilkins, 1983.

Schaller, J.: Arthritis as a presenting manifestation of malignancy in children. Journal of Pediatrics 81:793–796, 1972.

Schiffer, C.A.: Acute myeloid leukemia in adults. In Holland, J.F., et al. (eds.): Cancer Medicine, 3rd ed. Vols. 1 and 2. Philadelphia, Lea & Febiger, 1993, pp. 1907–1933.

Schilter, L., and Rossman, E.: Bone marrow transplantation. In Baird, S. (ed.): A Cancer Source Book for Nurses, 6th ed. Atlanta, American Cancer Society Publication, 1991, pp. 91–99.

Schirrmacher, V.: Cancer metastasis: Experimental approaches, theoretical concepts and impacts for treatment strategies. Advances in Cancer Research 43:1, 1985.

Schnell, S.: Nursing care of clients with cerebral disorders. In Black, J.M., and Matassarin-Jacobs, E. (eds.): Luckmann and Sorensen's Medical-Surgical Nursing, 4th ed. Philadelphia, W.B. Saunders, 1993a, pp. 705–772.

Schnell, S.: Nursing care of clients with disorders of the spinal cord, peripheral nerves and cranial nerves. In Black, J.M., and Matassarin-Jacobs, E. (eds.): Luckmann and Sorensen's Medical-Surgical Nursing, 4th ed. Philadelphia, W.B. Saunders, 1993b, pp. 793–826.

Shapiro, W.R.: Tumors of the brain. In Holleb, A.I. (ed.): The American Cancer Society Cancer Book. New York, Doubleday & Company, 1986, pp. 277–296.

Shibata, D., Weiss, L.M., Nathwani, B.N., et al.: Epstein-Barr virus in benign lymph node biopsies from individuals infected with the human immunodeficiency virus is associated with concurrent or subsequent development of non-Hodgkin's lymphoma. Blood 77:1527–1533, 1991.

Shields, P.G., and Harris, C.C.: Principles of carcinogenesis: Chemical. In DeVita, V.T., Hellman, S., and Rosenberg, S.A. (eds.): Cancer; Principles and Practice of Oncology, 4th ed. Philadelphia, J.B. Lippincott, 1993, pp. 200–213.

Silver, R.T., Morton, D.L., Antman, K.H., and Toepper, J.: Soft tissue sarcoma. In Holland, J.F., et al. (eds.): Cancer Medicine, 3rd ed. Vols. 1 and 2. Philadelphia, Lea & Febiger, 1993, pp. 1858–1887.

Snyder, C.C.: Oncology Nursing. Boston, Little, Brown, 1986.

Sober, A.: Cutaneous melanoma: Opportunity for cure. CA—A Cancer Journal for Clinicians 41(4):197–198, 1991.

Spitz, S.: Melanomas of childhood. Americal Journal of Pathology 24:591–609, 1948.

Stacey-Clear, A., McCarthey, K.A., Hall, D.A., Pile-Spellman, E., White, G., Hulka, C.A., Whitman, G.J., Halpern, E.F., and Kopans, D.B.: Mammographically detected breast cancer: Location in women under 50 years old. Radiology 186(3):677–680, 1993.

Steele, G.D., Winchester, D.P., Mench, H.R., and Murphy, G.P.: Clinical highlights from the National Cancer Data Base. CA—A Cancer Journal for Clinicians 43(2):71–82, 1993.

Threatt, B.: Early detection of breast cancer. Journal of the American Medical Women's Association 47(5):152–154, 1992.

Tombes, M.B.: Gynecologic malignancies. In Baird, S. (ed.): A Cancer Source Book for Nurses, 6th ed. Atlanta, American Cancer Society, 1991, pp. 228–241.

Watchie, J.: Cardiopulmonary complication of cancer treatment. Clinical Management 12(4):92–95, 1992.

Wegman, J.: Central nervous system cancers. In Groenwald, S., Frogge, M., Goodman, B., and Yarbro, C. (eds.): Cancer Nursing; Principles and Practice, 3rd ed. Boston, Jones and Bartlett, 1993, pp. 959–983.

Wilkins, R.M., and Sim, F.H.: Evaluation of bone and soft tissue tumors. In D'Ambrosia, R.D. (ed.): Musculoskeletal Disorders: Regional Examination and Differential Diagnosis, 2nd ed. Philadelphia, J.B. Lippincott, 1986.

Williams, C., and Williams, S.: Cancer: A Guide for Patients and Their Families. New York, John Wiley & Sons, 1986.

Winningham, M.L., McVicar, M., and Burke, C.: Exercise for cancer patients: Guidelines and precautions. The Physician and Sportsmedicine 14:121–134, 1986.

Wujcik, D.: Leukemia. In Groenwald, S., Frogge, M., Goodman, B., and Yarbro, C. (eds.): Cancer Nursing; Principles and Practice, 3rd ed. Boston, Jones and Bartlett, 1993, pp. 1149–1173.

Yarbro, J.: Milestones in our understanding of the causes of cancer. In Groenwald, S., Frogge, M., Goodman, B., and Yarbro, C. (eds.): Cancer Nursing; Principles and Practice, 3rd ed. Boston, Jones and Bartlett, 1993, pp. 28–46.

Bibliography

Bland, K.I., and Copeland, E.M.: The Breast: Comprehensive Management of Benign and Malignant Diseases. Philadelphia, W.B. Saunders, 1991.

Boring, C.C., Squires, T.S., and Tong, T.: Cancer statistics: 1993. Cancer Journal for Clinicians 43(2):7–26, 1993.

Brooks, P.M.: Rheumatic manifestations of neoplasia. Current Opinions in Rheumatology 4:90, 1992.

Caldwell, D.S.: Musculoskeletal syndromes associated with malignancy. In Kelley, W.N., et al. (eds.): Textbook of Rheumatology, 3rd ed. Philadelphia, W.B. Saunders, 1989.

DeVita, V.T., Hellman, S., and Rosenberg, S.A. (eds.): Cancer; Principles and Practice of Oncology, 4th ed. Philadelphia, J.B. Lippincott, 1993.

Edelhart, M., and Lindenmann, J.: Interferon: The New Hope for Cancer. New York, Ballantine (Division of Random House), 1982.

Hall, T.C.: The paraneoplastic syndromes. *In* Rubin, P. (ed.): Clinical Oncology for Physicians and Students: A Multidisciplinary Approach, 7th ed. Philadelphia, W.B. Saunders, 1993.

Layzer, R.B.: Neuromuscular Manifestations of Systemic Disease. Philadelphia, F.A. Davis, 1985.

McWhorter, W.P., and Eyre, H.J.: Impact of mammographic screening on breast cancer diagnosis. Journal of the National Cancer Institute 82:153, 1990.

Moossa, A.R., Schimpff, S.C., and Robson, M.C.: Comprehensive Textbook of Oncology, 2nd ed. Boston, Williams and Wilkins, 1991.

Panem, S.: The Interferon Crusade. Washington, D.C., The Brookings Institution, 1984.

Posner, J.B.: Paraneoplastic syndromes. Neurologic Clinics 9:919, 1991.

Richardson, G.E., and Johnson, B.E.: Paraneoplastic syndromes in thoracic malignancies. Current Opinions in Oncology 3:320, 1991.

Robertson, C.L.: A private breast imaging practice: Medical audit of 25,788 screening and 1,077 diagnostic examinations. Radiology 187(1):75–79, 1993.

Sayre, R.S., and Marcoux, B.C.: Exercise and autologous bone marrow transplants. Clinical Management 12(4):78–82, 1992.

Weinberger, M., Saunders, A.F., Bearon, L.B., Gold, D.T., Brown, J.T., Samsa, G.P., and Loehrer, P.J.: Physician-related barriers to breast cancer screening in older women. Journal of Gerontology 47(Spec No):111–117, 1992.

White, E.: Projected changes in breast cancer due to trend in delayed childbearing. American Journal of Public Health 77:495–497, 1987.

White, E.W., Lee, C.Y., and Kristal, A.R.: Evaluation of the increase in breast cancer incidence in relation to mammography use. Journal of the National Cancer Institute 82:1546–1552, 1990.

Overview of Immunologic Signs and Symptoms

■ ■ ■ ■ ■   ■ ■ ■ ■ ■   ■

Clinical Signs and Symptoms of:

Early Symptomatic HIV Infection
Advanced Symptomatic HIV Infection
HIV Neurologic Disease
Myasthenia Gravis
Guillain-Barré Syndrome (Acute Idiopathic Polyneuritis)
Multiple Sclerosis
Rheumatoid Arthritis
Sjögren's Syndrome
Systemic Lupus Erythematosus
Limited Cutaneous Systemic Sclerosis

Diffuse Cutaneous Systemic Sclerosis
Scleroderma
Polymyositis/Dermatomyositis
Mixed Connective Tissue Disease
Ankylosing Spondylitis
Reiter's Syndrome
Psoriatic Arthritis
Lyme Disease
Bacterial Arthritis
Fibromyalgia Syndrome

Immunology, one of the few disciplines with a full range of involvement in all aspects of health and disease, is one of the most rapidly expanding fields in medicine today. Keeping current is difficult at best considering the volume of new immunologic information generated by clinical researchers each year. The information presented here is a simplistic representation of the immune system and should be supplemented by the reader with any of the texts referenced.

Immunity denotes protection against infectious organisms. The immune system is a complex network of specialized organs and cells that has evolved to defend the body against attacks by "foreign" invaders. Immunity is provided by lymphoid cells residing in the immune system. This system consists of central and peripheral lymphoid organs (Fig. 11–1).

By circulating its component cells and substances, the immune system maintains an early warning system against both exogenous microorganisms (infections produced by bacteria, viruses, parasites, and fungi) and endogenous cells that have become neoplastic.

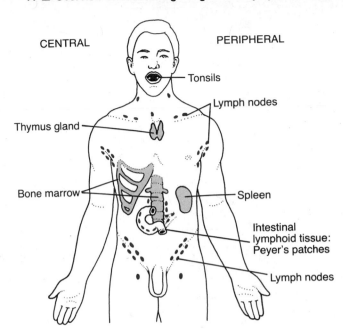

Figure 11–1
Organs of the immune system.

Understanding the interactions of antigens and antibodies is basic to understanding how the immune system functions. These interactions are discussed later in this chapter.

Immunologic responses in humans can be divided into two broad categories: humoral immunity, which takes place in the body fluids (humors) and is concerned with antibody and complement activities; and cell-mediated or cellular immunity, which involves a variety of activities designed to destroy or at least contain cells that are recognized by the body as being alien and harmful. Both types of responses are initiated by lymphocytes and are discussed in the context of lymphocytic function (O'Toole, 1992).

IMMUNE SYSTEM PHYSIOLOGY

Organs of the Immune System

The lymphoid system includes organs and tissues in which lymphocytes predomi-

nate, as well as cells that circulate in peripheral blood. Central and primary organs include (Lydyard and Grossi, 1993)

- Bone marrow
- Thymus (see Fig. 11–1)

  Peripheral or secondary organs include:

- Lymph nodes and lymph vessels of the lymphatic system (see Fig. 10–3)
- Spleen
- Tonsils
- Intestinal lymphoid tissue: Peyer's patches and appendix

Central Lymphoid Organs

The *bone marrow* and the *thymus gland* play a role in developing the principal cells of the immune system. All the cells involved in the immune response are derived from undifferentiated stem cells of the bone marrow. The stem cell has the potential for developing into any of the body's blood cells (Fig. 11–2). Various signals and

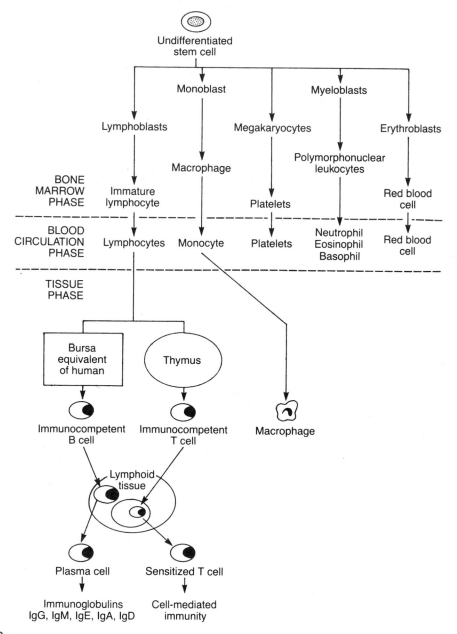

Figure 11−2

Development of cells of the immune system. (From Phipps, W., Long, B., and Woods, N.: Medical-Surgical Nursing: Concepts and Clinical Practice, 4th ed. St. Louis, C.V. Mosby, 1991, p. 165.)

influences within the body's replicative mechanism control this process.

The primary cells of the immune system develop from the lymphocytic cell popula-

tion. One population of lymphocytic cells undergoes change and differentiation in the thymus gland (thymus-dependent). These cells are called *T cells* and become respon-

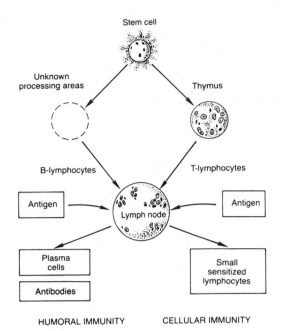

Figure 11-3

Origin of B lymphocytes and T lymphocytes responsible for cellular and humoral immunity. In response to antigens, B lymphocytes and T lymphocytes are sensitized by lymphoid tissue. (From O'Toole, M. (ed): Miller-Keane: Encyclopedia and Dictionary of Medicine, Nursing, and Allied Health, 5th ed. Philadelphia, W.B. Saunders, 1992, p. 870.)

sible for initiating the cell-mediated immune responses. Another population of lymphocytes undergoes maturation in sites other than the thymus gland (thymus-independent) and are called *B cells.* The B cells are responsible for the production of the immunoglobulins (antibodies) and mediate the body's humoral response (Lydyard and Grossi, 1993) (Fig. 11-3).

Peripheral Lymphoid Organs

Both B cells and T cells are distributed throughout the tissue of the peripheral lymphoid organs. *Lymph nodes,* small oval organs, are located throughout the body, most abundantly in the head and neck, axillae, abdomen, and groin (see Fig. 10-3). They contain lymphocytes (B cells, T cells)

and macrophages and comprise webbed areas that filter and enmesh antigens (foreign substances). The nodes are linked by a network of lymphatic vessels similar in physical properties to blood vessels.

The lymph vessels carry lymph, a clear fluid derived from interstitial fluid that contains lymphocytes and flows from connective tissue spaces throughout the body via lymphatic capillaries (Lydyard and Grossi, 1993). As the lymph passes through lymph nodes, antigens are filtered out and more lymphocytes are picked up. These lymphocytes are then carried to the bloodstream, which delivers them to tissues throughout the body and returns them eventually to the lymphatic system, where they are used again.

The *spleen* is the chief site of the immune system's filtering response to antigens. It is rich in lymphocytes and cells of the monocyte-macrophage lineage and represents the single largest collection of lymphoid tissue in the body (Lydyard and Grossi, 1993). In addition to its role of erythrocyte production in the fetus, the spleen acts as a reservoir for cellular elements of the peripheral blood (platelets, lymphocytes, and monocytes) and also acts to keep the blood free of unwanted substances, including wastes and infecting organisms. The blood is delivered to the spleen by the splenic artery and passes through smaller branch arteries into a network of channels lined with leukocytes known as phagocytes. These phagocytes clear the blood of old erythrocytes, damaged cells, parasites, and other toxic or foreign substances (O'Toole, 1992). Because of the remarkable phagocytic capacity of the spleen and its active participation in the host immune response to foreign antigen, the spleen is often responsible for many of the clinical and laboratory manifestations of a variety of infectious, malignant, autoimmune, and hereditary disorders (Lydyard and Grossi, 1993).

The remaining peripheral lymphoid organs (tonsils, Peyer's patches, appendix) are masses of lymphoid tissue containing lymphocytes and thymus-dependent areas.

Tonsils are small, round masses of lymphoid tissue located on each side of the back of the throat. These tissues filter the circulating lymph of any bacteria or foreign material that may enter the body, especially through the mouth and nose (O'Toole, 1992). *Peyer's patches* consist of aggregates of lymphoid nodules located in the submucosa of the intestinal wall. A Peyer's patch contains a varying number of B cells and T cells as well as a collection of lymphocytes that do not demonstrate either B-cell or T-cell markers. The (vermiform) appendix, an appendage near the juncture of the small intestine and the large intestine, is lined with large lymphatic nodules that atrophy in adult life and apparently become nonfunctional.

Functions of the Lymphoid System

The lymphoid system has four main functions (Wright and Long, 1991):

- To bring B cells and T cells to maturity
- To concentrate antigens from throughout the body into a few lymphoid organs
- To circulate lymphocytes through these organs so that any antigen is quickly exposed to antigen-specific lymphocytes
- To carry antigen-specific lymphocytes and antibodies to the blood and tissues

An *antigen* is any substance (exogenous or endogenous) capable of eliciting an immune response because the body recognizes it as being "foreign." Antigens are sometimes referred to as "nonself" molecules. The body recognizes molecules as being "self" or "nonself" by identifying epitopes (markers) that protrude from the molecule surface. An antigen is usually a protein, polysaccharide, or lipid that can be contained within microorganisms, such as fungi, parasites, bacteria, and viruses.

When an antigen enters the body, lymphoid cells function together to eliminate it. Within the lymph nodes, macrophages prepare or process antigens so that lymphocytes can mount a response to invasion. Synthesis of antibody by B lymphocytes is one type of response to antigenic stimulation.

Antibodies are serum proteins produced by plasma cells (cells derived from B lymphocytes). Antibodies bind to specific antigens and begin processes that induce lysis (destruction) or phagocytosis (engulfing) of an offending antigen. Another possible response to antigenic invasion is the growth of new T lymphocytes that have receptors on their surfaces for the antigen. T lymphocytes that have received an antigenic stimulus are called sensitized T-cell lymphocytes. In this situation, no circulating antibody is produced, but sensitized T cells are released into the circulation. These cells then migrate to the site of the antigen's entrance and begin a direct attack on the invading antigen. Most antigens, however, do not cause purely one or the other of these reactions but usually induce a combination of both. The type of antigen introduced will determine which of these immune responses will occur.

Cells of the Immune System: White Blood Cells (Table 11-1)

The immune system stockpiles a tremendous arsenal of immunocompetent cells. By storing just a few cells specific for each potential invader, it has room for the entire array. When an antigen appears, the few specifically matched cells of the immune system are stimulated to multiply (Purtilo and Purtilo, 1989).

Lymphocytes

Lymphocytes are the white blood cells that bear the major responsibility for carrying out both cell-mediated and humoral immunity. The two major classes of lymphocytes are the *T cells* (which are processed in the thymus) and the *B cells* (which grow to maturity in the bone marrow independent of the thymus). Both

Table 11–1
CATEGORIES OF WHITE BLOOD CELLS AND THEIR FUNCTIONS

Leukocyte Type	% in Normal Leukocytes	Function
Lymphocytes	34	
B lymphocytes		Humoral immunity; production of specific antibodies against viruses, bacteria, and other proteins
T lymphocytes		Cell-mediated immunity, including delayed hypersensitivity and graft rejection; regulation of immune response
Monocytes	4	Phagocytosis of microorganisms and cell debris; cooperation in immune response
Granulocytes		
Neutrophils	59	Phagocytosis and killing of bacteria; release of pyrogen that produces fever
Eosinophils	2.7	Phagocytosis of antigen-antibody complexes; killing of parasites
Basophils	0.3	Release of chemical mediators of immediate hypersensitivity

B cells and T cells include a number of different subsets, all of which have different functions (Table 11–2).

B cells are the precursors of antibody-producing plasma cells; T-cell subclasses either promote or suppress the immune response, kill antigens directly, or participate in other immune responses, such as delayed hypersensitivity (Wright and Long, 1991). These reactions, which are often referred to as cell-mediated immune responses, are introduced by antigen-specific T cells and are slow to develop, beginning 18 to 24 hours after antigen exposure. They reach maximum response by 48 hours and subside by 3 to 7 days.

Approximately two thirds of the lymphocytes circulating in the peripheral blood are T lymphocytes, 15 per cent are B lymphocytes, and the remaining lymphocytes are made up of uncommitted lymphocytes (lymphocytes without surface antigens) called *null cells.* Such cells are seen in ac-

Table 11–2
COMPARATIVE FUNCTIONS OF THE T LYMPHOCYTES AND B LYMPHOCYTES

B Lymphocytes *Short-Lived*	T Lymphocytes *Long-Lived*
Humoral immunity	Cell-mediated immunity
Specific antigen recognition	Specific antigen recognition
Synthesis of antibody; most effective in pyrogenic infections and toxic reactions	Macrophage stimulation, complement activation, destruction of intracellular pathogens; graft rejection; immunologic surveillance; stimulation of B-cell antibody production by helper cells
Immediate hypersensitivity reaction (allergy)	Delayed hypersensitivity reactions (skin test to antigens)
Transferable by plasma	Transfer uncommon, occurs only via cells
Mostly in blood	Mostly in lymph tissue

From Gurevich, I.: The competent internal immune system. Nursing Clinics of North America *20*:156, 1985.

tive systemic lupus erythematosus and other disease states discussed later in this chapter. All lymphocytes recirculate from the blood to the lymph nodes via the lymphatic vessels (O'Toole, 1992).

B Cells. B cells are responsible for humoral-mediated immunity and derive from hematopoietic stem cells that mature in the bone marrow (or in lymphoid organs other than the thymus). B cells secrete soluble substances called antibodies. Every B cell is programmed to make only one specific antibody that coats foreign cells or agents, making them susceptible to lymphocytotoxicity or neutrophil and macrophage ingestion. A given antibody exactly matches a specific invading antigen. Stimulation of B cells to produce antibody is a complex process that usually requires interactions among macrophages, T cells, and B cells (Wright and Long, 1991). The exact mechanism of this process is not clearly understood.

When the B cell encounters its triggering antigen, the B cell gives rise to many cells called plasma cells. Every plasma cell is essentially a factory for producing millions of identical antibodies. Scientists have identified five classes of antibodies or antigen-specific immunoglobulins: IgG, IgM, IgA, IgE, and IgD. Special functions are served by each class of immunoglobulin.*

T Cells. T cells are responsible for cell-mediated immunity and are derived from hematopoietic stem cells at T-cell precursors that mature into T cells within the thymus. T-cell subgroups include the regulatory helper and suppressor T cells, which respectively enhance or suppress the development of immune responses, particularly antibody production. Helper T cells stimulate B-cell proliferation and differentiation into antibody-secreting plasma cells. These helper cells also aid in B-cell activation by producing soluble, nonspecific mediators called lymphokines. Suppressor T cells reduce the immune response by limiting the amount of T-cell help available to activate B cells, thus protecting the body from the excesses of its own defense (Guyton, 1992). T lymphocytes are capable of the following (Purtilo and Purtilo, 1989):

■ Killing intracellular viruses, bacteria, and fungi

■ Rejecting transplanted organs*

■ Defending against neoplastic cells by providing immunologic surveillance that eliminates these cancer cells

Lymphokines. Lymphokines are soluble mediators that are produced by activated lymphocytes (through complex interactions among macrophages and subsets of T cells). They facilitate intracellular communication between macrophages, B cells, T cells, and lymphoid cells (Guyton, 1992). The reader may appreciate the complexity of the immune system by noting the following identified lymphokines:

■ Chemotactic factor (CF)

■ Macrophage-activating factor (MAF)

■ Migration-inhibiting factor (MIF)

■ Transfer factor (TF)

■ Blastogenic factor (BF)

■ Lymphotoxin, B-cell growth factor (BCGF)

■ T-cell replacement factor (TRF)

■ Interleukin-1 (IL-1); also known as lymphocyte-activating factor

■ Interleukin-2 (IL-2); also known as T-cell growth factor

■ Interferon

The nomenclature of these lymphokines generally describes their predominant biologic activity. For example, chemotactic and migratory inhibitory factors affect cell motility; activation factors enhance such

---

* The reader is referred to an immunology text for specific details concerning the known actions of these immunoglobulins.

* Tissues or cells from another individual, unless an identical twin, can also act as antigens; because a transplanted organ is seen as "foreign" or "nonself," the body's natural response is to reject it.

cellular processes as phagocytosis and induce further mediator release. Mitogenic factors stimulate cell proliferation, whereas cytotoxic factors target cell lysis and death. Interferons are a heterogeneous group of glycoproteins secreted by a variety of human cell types in response to viral infection and a variety of other stimuli. Although described initially as antiviral factors, these glycoproteins have other biologic effects, particularly in immuno-regulation. Once released, interferons interact with surrounding cells to induce the synthesis and secretion of other soluble factors that are actually responsible for the various activities ascribed to the interferons (Guyton, 1992).

Monocytes and Macrophages

Monocytes and macrophages are large cells that act as scavengers (or phago-cytes), engulfing and digesting microorganisms and other antigenic particles, such as bacteria, fungi, dead tissue, antigen-antibody complexes, and tumor cells. Originating in the stem cell, monocytes circulate in the blood for 24 hours before migrating to the tissues where they develop into macrophages. Macrophages line the lungs and intestines and are often referred to by different names depending on their location. For example, dendritic macrophages are found in lymph nodes; Kupffer's cells are found in the liver; and tissue histiocytes are found in connective tissue surrounding skin and muscle (Guyton, 1992).

Macrophages are the chief cells of the mononuclear phagocyte system. Macrophages not only phagocytize foreign matter, but also play a crucial role in initiating the immune response by "presenting" antigens to T cells in a special way that allows the T cell to recognize them. In addition, macrophages and monocytes secrete powerful chemical substances called *monokines* that help direct and regulate the immune response.

Granulocytes and Mast Cells

Granulocytes, like macrophages and monocytes, are phagocytes and are thus capable of enveloping and destroying invaders. They contain granules filled with potent chemicals that enable them to digest microorganisms. These chemicals also contribute to inflammatory reactions and are responsible for the symptoms of allergy. Neutrophils, eosinophils, basophils, and mast cells are examples of granulocytes (Guyton, 1992).

Along with the major immune cells (B cells and T cells and macrophages), granulocytes and mast cells participate in immunologic reactions. As discussed in Chapter 5, *granulocytes* (neutrophils, eosinophils, and basophils) are participants in phagocytosis, allergic reactions, and specific antibody (IgE) response important in anaphylactic reactions, respectively. *Mast cells* are thought to be derived from circulating basophils and are most abundant in organs or tissues that are exposed to the environment (e.g., skin and mucosa of the gastrointestinal and respiratory tracts). These cells serve an important role in the immediate hypersensitivity reaction to foreign antigen by releasing chemicals (e.g., histamine, heparin, hyaluronic acid) that produce the redness, warmth, and swelling of the inflammatory allergic response (Guyton, 1992).

Immune Response

When an antigen enters the body, a wide spectrum of response mechanisms can be activated. The specific response pattern depends on (Wright and Long, 1991)

■ Amount of antigen introduced

■ Site of introduction

■ Type of antigen introduced

Each immune response is a unique sequence of events determined by the nature of the antigen. Chemical toxins and a large number of inert environmental substances, such as asbestos and smoke particles, are normally attacked only by phagocytes and are handled efficiently at a local site. Organic antigens such as viruses, single-cell bacteria, protozoa, and fungi elicit the full range of immunologic responses. An excessively large, sustained antigen dose can overwhelm defenses at the local site and can exhaust the entire defense system (Wright and Long, 1991).

Microorganisms entering the body must find a route past the body's first line of defense: the outer protection of skin and mucous membranes; ciliated epithelium of the respiratory tract; and antimicrobial factors in tears, saliva, and breast milk. The second line of the body's defense includes the macrophages and neutrophils that do not react to specific antigens but can recognize antigenic material and attempt to destroy it (Wright and Long, 1991).

Once an antigen has overcome the first-line and second-line barriers, the immune response begins to function to destroy the antigen. Two types of immunity can be summoned for use: immunity occurring in the blood and tissue fluid outside the cells, provided by B-lymphocyte cells that produce antibodies (humoral immunity), and immunity taking place inside or on the surface of cells, provided by T-lymphocyte cells (cell-mediated immunity). These two distinct mechanisms usually work together to provide a defense against immunologic threats.

When an antigenic substance is introduced into the body, it is taken directly to a regional lymphoid tissue where it is processed and then presented to reactive B cells or T cells in the regional lymph node. During this interaction, the specific B cell or T cell is stimulated to begin proliferation and differentiation. Lymphokines, released from cells involved in the presenting process, further signal the lymphocyte to divide and differentiate (Wright and Long, 1991).

If the antigen is the type that activates a *humoral response* the first time the body is exposed to the antigen, the B-cell system responds by synthesizing circulating antibody from plasma cells. The first exposure of the body to an antigen is followed by a latent phase, during which no antibody levels are detected. This latent phase is then followed by a *primary response,* when serum antibodies increase rapidly, plateau, and finally decline (Wright and Long, 1991).

Because the reaction and production of antibody are not immediate, the antigen has time to spread during the body's first exposure. However, an immunologic memory develops so that when subsequent contact occurs with the same antigen, the antibodies are produced faster and at higher concentrations. This rapid response to a second contact is called the *secondary response* and is the basis for immunization.

The reaction between antibody and antigen activates serum proteins called complement. Complement usually circulates in the bloodstream as a series of inactive proteins produced by mononuclear phagocytes. Once the antigen is "captured" by the antibody, complement proteins receive a signal to activate. When activated, complement breaks down into enzymes that are then capable of destroying antigens. Complement enzymes actually poke holes in the cell membranes of the antigen (many bacteria and some viruses), causing intracellular fluid to leak out and resulting in cell destruction (Wright and Long, 1991). With rare exceptions, complement proteins bind only to cells already "labeled" with antibodies, so that healthy tissues are protected from the effects of these powerful enzymes.

If the antigens are such that they are physically or structurally inaccessible to attack from antibodies (e.g., viruses, some fungi, bacteria harbored inside cells, and cancer cells), then cell-mediated immunity is the main line of defense in combating these antigens. A cell-mediated reaction begins when an antigen binds with an antigen receptor on the surface of a T lymphocyte. The antigen is then presented to the lymph node T cells, and there is proliferation and differentiation of T cells. Instead of circulatory antibodies, sensitized T lymphocytes are then released into the circulation and are differentiated into five subsets:

- Helper T cells (T_h): stimulate production of killer T cells and, in combined response, stimulate B-cell production and differentiation
- Killer T cells (T_k): activated by helper T cells, directly attack and kill the antigen or cells labeled with the antigen (including cancer cells)
- Lymphokine-producing T cells: produce mediators such as lymphokines, which further stimulate T-cell production and, in a combined response, stimulate antibody production from B cells
- Suppressor T cells (T_s): slow down or stop the activities of both T cells and B cells so that the attack can be stopped when the antigen is conquered
- Memory T cells (T_m): generated during an initial exposure to the antigen, can mount a quick response after reexposure to the same antigen

Once these differentiated T lymphocytes are released into the circulation, the activated T cells seek out the antigen at the site of injection and destroy it. Between 24 and 48 hours are required for the development of inflammation at the site of local invasion.

Chemical examples of cellular immune reactions include

- Delayed hypersensitivity
- Allograft rejection
- Contact allergies
- Immunity to tumors and intracellular parasites

Most antigens do not cause a purely humoral or purely cell-mediated response but activate both types of protective mechanisms. The remarkable power of the immune system is best appreciated by the pathologic results that accompany its failure, whether that occurs with the common overreaction of the system known as allergies or the devastating immunodeficient effects of the human immunodeficiency virus (HIV), which causes acquired immunodeficiency syndrome (AIDS).

IMMUNE SYSTEM PATHOPHYSIOLOGY

Immune disorders involve dysfunction of the immune response mechanism, causing overresponsiveness or blocked, misdirected, or limited responsiveness to antigens. These disorders may result from a developmental defect, infection, malignancy, trauma, metabolic disorder, or drug use. Immunologic disorders may be classified as (Long and Wright, 1991)

- Immunodeficiency
- Hypersensitivity
- Autoimmunity
- Immunoproliferative disorders

When the immune system is underactive or *hypoactive,* it is referred to as being immunodeficient. When the immune system becomes overactive or *hyperactive,* a state of hypersensitivity exists, leading to immunologic diseases such as allergies.

T cells act as modulators of immune reactions, so that along with clearance of antigen by macrophages, death of antibody-producing plasma cells, and certain humoral factors, the immune response ultimately ceases. Abnormalities in this control system lead to immunodeficiency, autoimmunity, and possibly hematologic diseases, such as aplastic anemia (Long and Wright, 1991).

Autoimmune disorders occur when the immune system fails to distinguish self from nonself and misdirects the immune response against the body's own tissues. The resultant abnormal tissue reaction and tissue damage may cause systemic manifestations varying from minimal localized symptoms to systemic multiorgan involvement with severe impairment of function and life-threatening organ failure (Long and Wright, 1991).

Immunoproliferative disorders occur when abnormal reproduction or multiplication of the cells of the lymphoid system results in leukemia, lymphoma, and other related disorders. These have been covered in other parts of this text and are not discussed in this chapter.

Immunodeficiency Disorders

Acquired Immunodeficiency Syndrome (Mann et al., 1992)

HIV is a cytopathogenic virus that causes AIDS. In the past 10 years, HIV has been identified as the causative agent, its genes have been mapped and analyzed, drugs that act against it have been found and tested, and vaccines against the HIV infection have been under development.

Acquired refers to the fact that the disease is not inherited or genetic but develops as a result of a virus, as described later. *Immuno* refers to the body's immunologic system, and *deficiency* indicates that the immune system is underfunctioning, resulting in a group of signs or symptoms that occur together called a *syndrome*. People who are HIV-infected are vulnerable to serious illnesses called "opportunistic" infections or diseases, so named because they use the opportunity of lowered resistance to infect and destroy. These infections and diseases would not be a threat to most people whose immune systems functioned normally. *Pneumocystis carinii* pneumonia (PCP) continues to be a major cause of morbidity and mortality in the AIDS population (Liles and Ramsey, 1993).

Two types of viruses have been identified: HIV-1, found worldwide, and HIV-2, found mainly in West Africa. The routes of transmission are the same for both types of virus. HIV is a lentivirus, consisting of an RNA genome wrapped in viral protein and cellular membrane. Cells most affected are primarily the subset of immune system cells that "help" others in their tasks (T-helper cells or T4 lymphocytes), but a wide range of other cell types from the immune system to the gut and the brain may be included. Opportunistic infections most commonly occur when the T4 cell count drops below 200 (normal range is between 700 and 1300 T4 cells/mm^3) (Bova and Matassarin-Jacobs, 1993).

Once inside the cell, the virus transcribes its genes from RNA to DNA, which can then be inserted into the cell's own genes. At some point, it will make copies of its genes, direct the cell to make the protein it needs, and start to reproduce itself. Some form of activation must occur for viral replication to begin; the exact mechanism is still being investigated.

Incidence. As of January, 1992, an estimated 11.8 million adults and 1.1 million children—a total of 12.9 million people worldwide (1 million in the United States alone)—had been infected with HIV. Of the 11.8 million HIV-infected adults, 4.7 million are women, representing 40 per cent of the global total. AIDS strikes during the prime of life; it affects clients mostly between the ages of 20 and 49 years.

In the United States, at least 40,000 to 80,000 new HIV infections are estimated to have occurred during 1992, and 1993 estimates are at least as high. By 1995, an additional 6.9 million people worldwide will become infected with HIV (5.7 million adults and 1.2 million children). HIV/AIDS is *pandemic*, affecting all inhabited continents. Although the virus itself is old, its significant worldwide spread appears to have started only in the mid-1970s. Everywhere in the world, HIV spreads through the same basic and narrowly circumscribed routes —sex, blood, and mother-to-fetus or infant.

Population groups at greatest risk include commercial sex workers (prostitutes) and their clients, homosexual men, injection drug users (IDUs), blood recipients, hemophiliacs, dialysis recipients, organ transplant recipients, fetuses of HIV-infected mothers, and people with sexually transmitted diseases (STDs). The latter group is estimated to have several times higher the risk for HIV infection compared with those having no STDs (Wasserheit, 1992).

Transmission (Curran, 1992; Mann et al., 1992). Transmission of HIV occurs through horizontal transmission (from either sexual contact or parenteral exposure to blood and blood products) or through vertical transmission (from HIV-infected mother to infant). HIV is not transmitted through casual contact such as the shared use of food, towels, cups, razors, or toothbrushes, or even by kissing (Koop, 1986). Transmission always involves exposure to some body fluid from an infected client. The greatest concentrations of virus have been found in blood, semen, cerebrospinal fluid, and cervical/vaginal secretions. HIV has been found in low concentrations in tears, saliva, and urine, but no cases have been transmitted by these routes. Several cases of HIV transmission through breast milk have been reported (Bova and Matassarin-Jacobs, 1993).

Sexual Transmission. Sexual activity remains the number one route of transmission in the United States. Sexual activity between men and between men and women can result in transmission of HIV. At the time of this writing, sexual activity between women has resulted in only two reported cases of HIV infection (Bova and Matassarin-Jacobs, 1993).

Transmission of infectious agents in genital secretions tends to be more efficient from men to women. Presumably, this discrepancy is largely a function of anatomy, as the vagina and cervix provide a large surface area for infection and a natural reservoir for microorganisms. Women not only are more vulnerable to acquiring STDs but also are less likely to seek treatment and more likely to be misdiagnosed when they seek medical attention. Signs, symptoms, and laboratory test results may be less reliable in women (Erhardt and Wasserheit, 1991). For these and other reasons, women and infants sustain a disproportionate share of major STD complications, including pelvic inflammatory disease (PID), infertility, ectopic pregnancy, fetal wastage, neonatal blindness, and genital malignancy.

Injection Drug Use. Although there are significant variations among countries, the main drug injected worldwide is heroin, followed by cocaine and amphetamines. Any injectable drug, legal or illegal, can be associated with HIV transmission. It is not injection drug use that spreads HIV, but the sharing of HIV-infected IV drug needles among individuals.

Despite the perception that only intravenous injection is dangerous, HIV can be transmitted through subcutaneous and intramuscular injection as well. Public health organizations have changed their terminology in order to reflect this, substituting the acronym IDU (injection drug user) for the earlier term IVDU (intravenous drug user).

Injection drug users who sterilize their drug paraphernalia with a 1:10 solution of bleach to water before passing the needles are less likely to spread HIV.*

Blood and Blood Products. Parenteral transmission occurs when there is direct blood-to-blood contact with a client infected with HIV. This can occur through sharing of contaminated needles and drug paraphernalia ("works"), through transfusion of blood or blood products, by accidental needlestick injury to a health care worker, or from blood exposure to nonintact skin or mucous membranes. Health care workers who have contact with clients with AIDS and who follow routine instructions for self-protection are a very low risk group (see the Appendix in Chapter 8 detailing universal precautions). The rate of transmission to a health care worker from a needlestick involving a known HIV-positive client is 0.47 per cent (Bova and Matassarin-Jacobs, 1993).

There are two major types of blood products. The first group is obtained from whole blood itself and includes both cells

---

* For further information regarding this or other AIDS-related questions, contact the National AIDS Hotline (1-800-342-2437).

AIDS AT A GLANCE

- **What it is:** AIDS, acquired immune deficiency syndrome, is a contagious disease that destroys the T cells, a key component of the body's immune system.

- **What causes it:** AIDS is caused by the human immunodeficiency virus (HIV), spread through sexual contact, needles or syringes shared by injection drug users (IDUs), transfusion of infected blood or blood products, or perinatal transmission (from infected birthing mother to her baby).

- **Who gets it:** Primary persons infected with HIV have been homosexual men and IDUs. The Centers for Disease Control and Prevention (CDC) estimates that heterosexual contact is responsible for 3 per cent of male cases and 34 per cent of female cases. One million Americans are infected.

- **Diagnosis:** Screening for AIDs is conducted by testing blood for the presence of antibodies to the AIDs virus or detection of pieces of proteins or genetic material from the virus. The test indicates only if a person has been exposed to the virus. There is a typical 6-month window of latency when those infected test negative.

- **Prognosis:** According to the CDC, a person with a positive test has a 20 to 30 per cent chance of developing AIDS over a 5-year period. At present, there is no cure, and death occurs as a result of "opportunistic" infections or cancers that the immunosuppressed body cannot resist.

- **Treatment:** Numerous types of drugs for AIDS are under investigation, including an effective AIDS vaccine. At present, two antiviral drugs that attack HIV have been approved: AZT (azidothymidine), now called zidovudine (ZDU), and ddl (dideoxyinosine or didanosine).

---

in the blood (red blood cells, platelets, and buffy coat elements) and plasma. The second group is derived by separating the plasma into different components (fractionation), such as albumin, immune serum globulin, and factor VIII (antihemophilia factor).

HIV infection through blood transfusions or receipt of blood or blood products for people with *hemophilia* or other coagulation disorders has accounted for approximately 5 per cent of the global burden of HIV infection. This burden would have been multiplied many times if factors VII and IX, used for people with hemophilia, had been HIV contaminated. This potential catastrophe has been averted because the method of preparation involves physical and chemical processes that completely inactivate HIV.

However, heat-treated factor VIII concentrates were not available in the United States until 1984. This means that almost all hemophiliacs born before 1985 have been infected with HIV. Approximately 70 to 90 per cent of all persons with hereditary clotting disorders in the United States have been infected with HIV. In the developed world, AIDS is now the leading cause of death in people with hemophilia.

Additionally, HIV is being transmitted heterosexually from infected men with hemophilia to spouses or sexual partners in what is termed *the second wave* of infection, and on to children born to infected couples.

Mother to Fetus/Infant. Although the mechanism is not completely clear, it is believed that perinatal transmission of HIV can occur at various stages of gestation. Fifty to eighty per cent of babies born to infected mothers will not be infected with HIV. The incidence of AIDS in infants directly correlates with the geographic distribution of injection drug use in the United States.

Breast Milk. Initial concern about postnatal transmission (transmission from HIV-infected mother to infant after childbirth) was raised when HIV was found in colostrum and breast milk (Bucens et al., 1988; Ruff et al., 1991; Thiry et al., 1985; Vonesch, 1991).

However, finding the virus in breast milk did not mean that breast feeding would become a significant transmission route. Several reasons were proposed for this, including the inability of HIV to survive in the inhospitable environment of the digestive tract and the presence of anti-HIV antibodies in breast milk (Belec et al., 1990; Van de Perre et al., 1988). This remains a controversial area, and the extent and precise circumstances of transmission remain unknown.

Clinical Signs and Symptoms (Hollander and Katz, 1993). Many individuals with HIV infection remain asymptomatic for years, with a mean time of approximately 10 years between exposure and development of AIDS. Systemic complaints such as weight loss, fevers, and night sweats are common. Cough or shortness of breath may occur with HIV-related pulmonary disease. GI complaints include changes in bowel function, especially diarrhea.

Cutaneous complaints are common and

▼ *Clinical Signs and Symptoms of*
Early Symptomatic HIV Infection

- Fever
- Night sweats
- Chronic diarrhea
- Fatigue
- Minor oral infections
- Headache
- (Women): vaginal candidiasis
- Cough
- Shortness of breath
- Cutaneous changes (rash, nail bed changes, dry skin)

▼ *Clinical Signs and Symptoms of*
Advanced Symptomatic HIV Infection

- Kaposi's sarcoma
  - Multiple, purple blotches and bumps on skin
- Opportunistic diseases (e.g., tuberculosis, *Pneumocystis carinii*, pneumonia, lymphoma, thrush; herpes I and II; toxoplasmosis)
  - Persistent dry cough
  - Fever, night sweats
  - Easy bruising
  - Thrush (thick, white coating on the tongue or throat, accompanied by a sore throat)

---

include dry skin, new rashes, and nail bed changes. Because virtually all these findings may be seen with other diseases, a combination of complaints is more suggestive of HIV infection than any one symptom.

Any woman at risk for AIDS should be aware of the possibility that recurrent or stubborn cases of vaginal candidiasis may be an early sign of infection with HIV. Pregnancy, diabetes, contraceptive pills, and antibiotics are also commonly linked to these fungal infections.

Diagnosis. The national Centers for Disease Control and Prevention's new definition of AIDS, which took effect January 1, 1993, includes anyone with laboratory evidence of HIV infection and a T-cell count of less than 200, tuberculosis, recurrent pneumonia, or cervical cancer. These are added to an existing list of 23 diseases that denote a diagnosis of full-blown AIDS.

Prognosis and Treatment. AIDS has an extremely high mortality rate; over 90 per cent of clients who develop the most severe form of the disease will die within 4 years of an AIDS diagnosis (Bova and Matassarin-Jacobs, 1993). The challenge is not what drug will "cure" AIDS, but rather what combination of drug therapy will most effectively fight off opportunistic infections and slow the progression of HIV.

Treatment of HIV infection can be divided into four categories: therapy for opportunistic infections and malignancies, antiviral treatment, hematopoiesis-stimulating factors, and prophylaxis of opportunistic infections, particularly PCP (Hollander and Katz, 1993). Many clients choose to add supplemental therapy such as nutrition and exercise to the already-existing drug therapy.

Zidovudine (also known as Retrovir and ZDV, and formerly as AZT) is an antiretroviral agent that has been shown to prolong survival and reduce mortality in clients with HIV infection. Antiretroviral chemotherapy controls the replication of the virus and thereby delays further destruction of the immune system (Liles and Ramsey, 1993). Side effects from the medication include

- Nausea
- Headaches
- Muscle pain
- Weakness
- Fatigue

Vaccines both to prevent HIV transmission and to treat those persons already infected are being developed, but these may be as much as 5 to 10 years from general distribution (Bova and Matassarin-Jacobs, 1993). Prevention is still the most effective means of eliminating HIV/AIDS.

HIV and Other Diseases (Greenberg, 1992)

AIDS is a unique disease—no other known infectious disease causes its damage through a direct attack on the human immune system. Because the immune system is the final mediator of human host–infectious agent interactions, it was anticipated early that HIV infection would com-plicate the course of other serious human diseases.

This has proved to be the case, particularly for tuberculosis and certain sexually transmitted infections like syphilis and the genital herpes virus. Cancer has been linked with AIDS since 1981; this link was discovered with the increased appearance of a highly unusual malignancy, Kaposi's sarcoma. Since then, HIV infection has been associated with a second malignancy, non-Hodgkin's lymphoma (NHL).

KAPOSI'S SARCOMA

This disease was first recognized as a malignant tumor of the inner walls of the heart, veins, and arteries in 1873 in Vienna, Austria. Prior to the AIDS epidemic, Kaposi's sarcoma (KS) was a rare tumor that primarily affected older people of Mediterranean and Jewish origin. How the HIV infection or HIV-related immunodeficiency contributes to the onset of KS is unknown.

Clinically, KS in HIV-infected, immunodeficient persons occurs more often as purplish-red lesions of the trunk and head. The lesion is not painful; it can be flat or indurated and over time frequently progresses to a nodule (Bova and Matassarin-Jacobs, 1993). The mouth and many internal organs (especially those of the gastrointestinal and respiratory tracts) may be involved either symptomatically or subclinically.

Prognosis depends on the status of the individual's immune system. People who die of AIDS usually succumb to opportunistic infections rather than to KS.

NON-HODGKIN'S LYMPHOMA

Approximately 3 per cent of AIDS diagnoses in all risk groups and in all areas originate through discovery of non-Hodgkin's lymphoma (Casabona et al., 1991). In the United States, 3000 to 4000 AIDS-related NHL cases were expected to occur in 1993, constituting about 10 per cent of all cases of NHL (Gail et al., 1991; Rabkin et al., 1991).

HIV generally infects T cells, but NHL tumors are almost always of B-cell origin. Analyses of genetic material from these tumors confirm that HIV is not present in the genome, suggesting that immunodeficiency is the major causative factor (Biggar, 1990). The incidence of NHL increases with age and as the immune system weakens.

Treatment and Prognosis. These malignancies are difficult to treat because clients often cannot tolerate the further immunosuppression that treatment causes. As with KS, prognosis depends largely on the initial level of immunity. Clients with adequate immune reserves may tolerate therapy and respond reasonably well. However, in people with severe immunodeficiency, survival is only 4 to 7 months on average. Clients diagnosed with HIV-related brain lymphomas have a very poor prognosis, often surviving only 1 to 2 months (Krown, 1993).

TUBERCULOSIS

Just a few years ago, tuberculosis (TB) was considered a stable, endemic health problem. Now, in association with the HIV/AIDS pandemic, tuberculosis is resurgent. The recent emergence of multiple drug–resistant TB, which has reached epidemic proportions in New York City, has created a serious and growing threat to the capacity of TB control programs.

In urban areas of the United States, the present upsurge in TB cases is occurring among young (aged 25 to 44 years) injection drug users, ethnic minorities, prisoners and prison staff due to poorly ventilated and overcrowded prison systems, homeless people, and immigrants from countries with a high prevalence of TB.

TB can be either subclinical (infection) or clinical (disease). Clinical TB develops through three different pathways: progressive primary infection, reactivation of latent infection, or exogenous reinfection, sometimes with multiple drug–resistant organisms in a host with a defective immune response.

The first major interaction between HIV and TB occurs as a result of the weakening of the immune system in association with progressive HIV infection. The great majority of people exposed to TB are infected but not clinically ill. Their subclinical TB infection is kept in check by an active, healthy immune system. However, when a TB-infected person becomes infected with HIV, the immune system begins to decline, and at a certain level of immune damage from HIV, the tuberculosis bacteria become active, causing clinical pulmonary TB.

TB is the only opportunistic infection associated with AIDS/HIV that is directly transmissible to household and other contacts. Therefore, each individual case of active TB is a threat to community health.

Clinical Signs and Symptoms (Sattler, 1992). Pulmonary TB is the most common manifestation of TB disease in HIV-positive clients. When TB precedes the diagnosis of AIDS, disease is usually confined to the lung, whereas when TB is diagnosed after the onset of AIDS, the majority of clients also have extrapulmonary TB, most commonly involving the bone marrow or lymph nodes. Fever, night sweats, wasting, cough, and dyspnea occur in the majority of clients (see also Chapter 4).

Diagnosis and Treatment. The standard tuberculin test is not reliable in people with HIV infection or AIDS because the weakened immune system may simply be unable to respond to the test (Centers for Disease Control, 1989). As a result, clinicians have to interpret the test differently for an HIV-infected person. The specific treatment of TB consists of different combinations of drugs. Preventing and controlling the spread of TB are the most cost-effective components of treatment.

HIV NEUROLOGIC DISEASE (Bova and Matassarin-Jacobs, 1993; Hollander and Katz, 1993)

HIV neurologic disease may be the presenting symptom of HIV infection and can involve the central and peripheral nervous systems. Signs and symptoms range from mild sensory polyneuropathy to seizures, hemiparesis, paraplegia, and dementia.

Central Nervous System Disease. CNS disease in HIV-infected clients can be divided into intracerebral space-occupying lesions, encephalopathy, meningitis, and spinal cord processes. Toxoplasmosis is the most common space-occupying lesion in HIV-infected clients. Presenting symptoms may include headache, focal neurologic deficits, seizures, or altered mental status.

AIDS dementia complex (HIV encephalopathy) is the most common neurologic complication and the most common cause of mental status changes in HIV-infected clients. It is characterized by cognitive, motor, and behavioral dysfunction. This disorder is similar to Alzheimer's dementia but has less impact on memory loss and a greater effect on time-related skills (i.e., psychomotor skills learned over time, such as learning to read or playing piano).

Early symptoms of AIDS dementia involve difficulty with concentration and memory, personality changes, irritability, and apathy. Depression and withdrawal occur as the dementia progresses. Motor dysfunction may accompany cognitive changes and may result in poor balance, poor coordination, and frequent falls.

In addition to the brain, neurologic disorders related to AIDS and HIV may affect the spinal cord, presenting as myelopathies. A vacuolar myelopathy often presents in the thoracic spine and causes gradual weakness, painless gait disturbance characterized by spasticity, and ataxia in the lower extremities progressing to include weakness of the upper extremities.

Peripheral Nervous System. Peripheral

▼ *Clinical Signs and Symptoms of*
HIV Neurologic Disease

- Difficulty with concentration and memory
- Personality changes (depression, withdrawal, apathy)
- Headaches
- Seizures
- Paralysis (hemiparesis, paraplegia)
- Motor dysfunction (balance and coordination)
- Gradual weakness of extremities
- Numbness and tingling (peripheral neuropathy)
- Radiculopathy

---

nervous system syndromes include inflammatory polyneuropathies, sensory neuropathies, and mononeuropathies. An inflammatory demyelinating polyneuropathy similar to Guillain-Barré syndrome occurs in HIV-infected clients.

Peripheral nerve disease is a common complication of the HIV infection. Cytomegalovirus (CMV), a highly host-specific herpes virus that infects the nerve roots, may result in an ascending polyradiculopathy characterized by lower extremity weakness progressing to flaccid paralysis. Progressive multifocal leukoencephalopathy (PML), localized lesions within the brain, causes demyelination in the brain and leads to death within a few months. The most common neuropathy develops into painful sensory neuropathy with numbness and burning or tingling in the feet, legs, or hands.

Prognosis and Treatment. Overall survival of people with AIDS is increasing, and the frequency of HIV dementia, therefore, can be expected to rise as individuals with AIDS live longer. The course of HIV dementia is variable, and progression cannot be predicted. Overall prognosis is poor, and end-stage dementia leaves the client lying in bed with a vacant stare, unable to ambulate and often incontinent. Symptomatic therapy is aimed at treating the depression or mania; ensuring safety is essential. Amitriptyline has been reported to have some benefit in treating the neuropathies.

Hypersensitivity Disorders (Bova and Matassarin-Jacobs, 1993)

Although the immune system protects the body from harmful invaders, an overactive or overzealous response is detrimental. Overreaction to a substance, or hypersensitivity, is often referred to as an allergic response. Although the word "allergy" is widely used, the term "hypersensitivity" is more appropriate. Hypersensitivity designates an increased immune response to the presence of an antigen (referred to as an allergen) that results in tissue destruction.

The two general categories of hypersensitivity reaction are immediate and delayed. These designations are based on the rapidity of the immune response. In addition to these two categories, hypersensitivity reactions are divided into four main types (I to IV).

Type I Anaphylactic Hypersensitivity ("Allergies")

ALLERGY AND ATOPY

Allergy refers to the abnormal hypersensitivity that takes place when a foreign substance (allergen) is introduced into the body of a person likely to have allergies. The body fights these invaders by producing the special antibody immunoglobulin E (IgE). This antibody (now a vital diagnostic sign of many allergies), when released into the blood, breaks down mast cells, which contain chemical mediators such as histamine that cause dilation of blood vessels and the characteristic symptoms of allergy.

Atopy differs from allergy because it refers to a genetic predisposition to produce large quantities of IgE, causing this state of clinical hypersensitivity. The reaction between the allergen and the susceptible person (i.e., allergy-prone host) results in the development of a number of typical signs and symptoms usually involving the gastrointestinal tract, respiratory tract, or skin.

Clinical Signs and Symptoms. Clinical signs and symptoms vary from one client to another according to the allergies present. Using the Family/Personal History form, each client should be asked what known allergies are present and what the specific reaction to the allergen would be for that particular person. The physical therapist can then be alert to any of these warning signs during treatment and can take necessary measures, whether that means grading exercise to the client's tolerance, controlling the room temperature, or appropriately using medications prescribed.

Treatment. Treatment may include avoidance of known allergens, environmental control (elimination of airborne allergens), medications, and immunotherapy, sometimes called desensitization. Desensitization, the regular injection of small quantities of allergen, helps immunize the person against the offending allergies. Steady exposure builds up high quantities of IgG antibodies in the bloodstream and creates competition between two classes of antibodies for the same antigen. Allergens that bind to IgG antibodies do not reach the IgE antibodies coating mast cells. Without the interaction of IgE antibodies, allergens, and mast cells, smaller amounts of histamine enter the body, making the allergic response less severe.

ANAPHYLAXIS

Anaphylaxis, the most dramatic and devastating form of type I hypersensitivity, is the systemic manifestation of immediate hypersensitivity. The implicated antigen is often introduced parenterally, such as by injection of penicillin or a bee sting. The activation and breakdown of mast cells

Table 11–3

CLINICAL ASPECTS OF ANAPHYLAXIS BY SYSTEM

System	Signs and Symptoms
General	Malaise, weakness
	Sense of illness
Dermal	Hives, erythema
Mucosal	Periorbital edema
	Nasal congestion and pruritus
	Flushing or pallor, cyanosis
Respiratory	Sneezing
	Rhinorrhea
	Dyspnea
Upper airway	Hoarseness, stridor
	Tongue and pharyngeal edema
Lower airway	Dyspnea
	Acute emphysema
	Air trapping: asthma, bronchospasm
	Chest tightness; wheezing
Gastrointestinal	Increased peristalsis
	Vomiting
	Dysphagia
	Nausea
	Abdominal cramps
	Diarrhea (occasionally with blood)
Cardiovascular	Tachycardia
	Palpitations
	Hypotension
	Cardiac arrest
Central nervous system	Anxiety, seizures

Adapted from Lawlor, G.J., and Rosenblatt, H.M.: Anaphylaxis. *In* Lawlor, G.J., and Fischer, T.J. (eds.): Manual of Allergy and Immunology: Diagnosis and Therapy, 2nd ed. Boston, Little, Brown, 1988, p. 228.

systematically causes vasodilation and increased capillary permeability, which promotes fluid loss into the interstitial space, resulting in the clinical picture of bronchospasms, urticaria (wheals or hives), and anaphylactic shock (Bova and Matassarin-Jacobs, 1993).

Initial manifestations of anaphylaxis may include local itching, edema, and sneezing. These seemingly innocuous problems are followed in minutes by wheezing, dyspnea, cyanosis, and circulatory shock. Clinical signs and symptoms of anaphylaxis are listed by system in Table 11–3.

Clients with previous anaphylactic reactions (and the specific signs and symptoms of that individual's reaction) should be identified by using the Family/Personal History form. Identification information should be worn at all times by people who have had previous anaphylactic reactions.

For identified and unidentified clients, immediate action is required when the person has a severe reaction. In such situations, the physical therapist is advised to call for emergency assistance.

Type II Hypersensitivity (Cytolytic or Cytotoxic)

These reactions are complement-dependent and thus involve IgG or IgM antibodies. The antigen-antibody complex and complement attach to a cell, usually a circulating blood cell, with resultant cell lysis. During blood transfusion, blood group incompatibility causes cell lysis, which results in a transfusion reaction. The antigen responsible for initiating the reaction is a part of the donor red blood cell membrane.

Clinical Signs and Symptoms. Manifestations of a transfusion reaction result from intravascular hemolysis of red blood cells and include

- Headache
- Back (flank) pain
- Chest pain similar to angina
- Nausea and vomiting
- Tachycardia and hypotension
- Hematuria
- Urticaria (skin reaction)

Treatment. Treatment is to stop the transfusion immediately and notify the physician.

Type III Hypersensitivity (Immune Complex)

Immune complex disease results from formation or deposition of antigen-antibody complexes in tissues. Immune complex–mediated inflammation is produced by IgG or IgM antibodies, antigen, and complement.

Larger complexes are rapidly cleared by phagocytic cells. Smaller complexes formed in response to antigen excess persist longer in the circulation because they are not so easily captured by phagocytic cells in the spleen and liver. Inflammation results and leads to acute or chronic disease of the organ system in which the immune complexes were deposited.

For example, the antigen-antibody complexes may form in the joint space, with resultant synovitis, as in rheumatoid arthritis. Antigen-antibody complexes are formed in the bloodstream and get trapped in capillaries or are deposited in vessel walls, causing urticaria, arthritis, arteritis, or glomerulonephritis.

Serum sickness is another type III hypersensitivity response that develops 6 to 14 days after injection with foreign serum (e.g., penicillin, sulfonamides, streptomycin, thiouracils, hydantoin compounds). Deposition of complexes on vessel walls causes complement activation with resultant edema, fever, inflammation of blood vessels and joints, and urticaria.

Clinical Signs and Symptoms. Clinical signs and symptoms are

- Fever
- Arthralgias
- Lymphadenopathy
- Urticaria

Treatment. Treatment is directed toward control of fever and pain with aspirin and antihistamines. A severe reaction may require steroids for control of the problem.

Type IV Hypersensitivity (Cell-Mediated or Delayed)

In cell-mediated hypersensitivity, sensitized T cells respond to antigens by releasing lymphokines, which direct phagocytic cell activity. This reaction occurs 24 to 72 hours after exposure to an allergen.

For example, type IV reactions occur after the intradermal injections of tuberculosis antigen. Graft-versus-host disease (GVHD) and transplant rejection are also type IV reactions. In GVHD, immunocompetent donor bone marrow cells (the graft) react against various antigens in the bone marrow recipient (the host), which results in a variety of clinical manifestations, including skin, gastrointestinal, and hepatic lesions.

Contact dermatitis is another type IV reaction that occurs after sensitization to an allergen, commonly a cosmetic, adhesive, topical medication, drug additive (such as lanolin added to lotions, ultrasound gels, or other preparations used in massage or soft tissue mobilization), or plant toxin (e.g., poison ivy).

With the first exposure, no reaction occurs; however, antigens are formed. On subsequent exposures, hypersensitivity reactions are triggered, which leads to itching, erythema, and vesicular lesions. Anyone with known hypersensitivity (identified through the Family/Personal History form) should have a small area of skin tested before use of large amounts of topical agents in the physical therapy clinic. Careful observation throughout treatment is required.

Organ Transplantation (Bova and Matassarin-Jacobs, 1993)

Histocompatibility

With recent advances in technology and immunology, organ and tissue transplantations are becoming commonplace. There are several types of transplants. *Syngeneic* transplants are between genetically identical members of the same species (identical twins); they are also called *isografts*. *Allogeneic* transplants are between individuals of the same species (e.g., human to human). *Autologous* transplants are grafts within the same organism (e.g., skin graft from leg to hand, on the same person). *Xenogeneic* transplants are between individuals of different species.

In all cases of graft rejection, the cause is incompatibility of cell-surface antigens. As expected, there is a better chance of graft acceptance with autologous or syngeneic transplants, because the cell-surface antigens are identical.

In the immunocompetent recipient, the client's immune system recognizes the transplanted tissue or organ as "foreign" and produces antibodies and sensitized lymphocytes against it. The cell-mediated delayed hypersensitivity response causes damage or destruction to the donated tissue. Graft rejection is the term describing the immune responses leading to graft destruction by the recipient's immune system.

Graft Rejection

Rejection is actually the body's normal immune response to the invasion of foreign tissue (the transplanted tissue or organ). Although this response is normal, it is not the desired response after a transplant.

The physiologic mechanisms in rejection (the normal immune response) involve B lymphocytes formation of antibodies and T lymphocytes production of cell-mediated immunity. Acute rejection is caused by the T-lymphocyte activity and chronic rejection by activity of B lymphocytes.

There are three basic kinds of rejection: hyperacute, acute, and chronic. Allografts transplanted into presensitized recipients may be rejected very quickly (within 48 hours) after the transplant. The symptoms of hyperacute rejection include general malaise and high fever. It is not treatable, and removal of the tissue is required.

Acute rejection usually occurs within 3 months but may occur as late as 2 years after the transplant. Treatment with immunosuppressant medications may still be followed by repeated episodes of acute rejection, leading to permanent organ damage.

Months or even years after the transplant, function of the transplanted tissue or organ may deteriorate gradually. Clients with chronic rejection may be asymptomatic. Others will demonstrate symptoms directly related to failure of the transplanted organ.

In renal transplants, there is a gradual increase in serum creatinine and blood urea nitrogen, electrolyte imbalance, weight gain, hypertension, decreasing urine output, and peripheral edema. In cardiac transplants, there is myocardial fibrosis and increasing blockage of the coronary arteries, which leads to myocardial ischemia and infarction. In liver transplants, there is a progressive thickening of the hepatic arteries and narrowing of the bile ducts, which leads to progressive liver failure. In pancreatic rejections, there is thickening of the vessels, which leads to fibrosis and a decrease in insulin secretion and hyperglycemia.

Treatment. Treatment is not usually successful for chronic rejection. It is a gradual, progressive deterioration. Antirejection medications may slow the process, so it is years before the organ fails completely and retransplantation is required.

Graft-Versus-Host Disease (GVHD)

A different type of rejection occurs when the transplanted material is an allogeneic bone marrow transplant. GVHD is a variation of the traditional graft rejection but involves the same immunologic principles.

GVHD occurs with bone marrow transplantation in which immunocompetent donor cells are infused into the immunosuppressed recipient. If rejection occurs, it is the immunocompetent T lymphocytes from the graft (i.e., the donated marrow) rather than the host cells that cause the problem.

GVHD can be acute or chronic. Acute GVHD manifests itself 1 to 100 days after transplant; chronic GVHD usually occurs or persists later than 100 days. The major organs affected by GVHD are the skin, liver, and gastrointestinal tract. Skin involvement often begins with an erythematous rash, which may progress to a severe, sloughing stage.

Liver disease may present clinically as right upper quadrant (including right shoulder) pain and signs of hepatitis. Gastrointestinal manifestations of GVHD include nausea, vomiting, and mild to severe diarrhea.

Treatment. Graft rejection can be decreased by the use of agents that interfere with the body's immune response. The major drugs used in immunosuppressive therapy are cyclosporine (Sandimmune; cyclosporine A); azathioprine (Imuran); and glucocorticoids (Long and Wright, 1991). Clients receiving these drugs will be at risk for developing opportunistic infections and side effects common to glucocorticoid therapy, such as osteoporosis and other musculoskeletal abnormalities. It is important for the physical therapist to be aware of the potential dangers of infections in these clients and to monitor clients for any musculoskeletal problems related to the use of glucocorticoids.

Neurologic Disorders

Some neurologic disorders encountered by the physical therapist display features that suggest an immunologic basis for the disorder. Such diseases include myasthenia gravis, Guillain-Barré syndrome, and multiple sclerosis. Other dysfunctions, such as amyotrophic lateral sclerosis (ALS) and acute disseminated encephalomyelitis, also associated with immunologic dysfunction but seen less often by the physical therapist, are not discussed.

Myasthenia Gravis (Ozuna, 1993; Andreoli, 1993)

Myasthenia gravis (MG) is a disease of unknown cause in which there is motor weakness due to a disorder of neuromuscular transmission. The largest proportion of the group of disorders known as MG has an immunologic basis, with autoimmune mechanisms causing a block or destruction of the acetylcholine receptor lying within the postsynaptic muscle membrane.

In MG, an autoaggressive antibody response directed against acetylcholine receptor protein at the myoneural junction is directly involved in disease pathogenesis. This deactivation of acetylcholine (necessary for normal impulse transmission to muscles) receptor sites occurs when antibodies to acetylcholine receptors block and remove the receptor sites from the postsynaptic membrane. Without acetylcholine, the nerve impulses fail to pass across the neuromuscular junction and stimulate contraction of the muscles.

These antibodies may also activate the complement system, leading to further damage at the myoneural junction. In MG, often other autoantibodies and other associated diseases are present, such as thyroiditis, systemic lupus erythematosus, and rheumatoid arthritis. In most cases, an association with a pathologic thymus gland (either thymic hyperplasia or a thymoma) occurs, necessitating the removal of the thymus gland.

Myasthenia gravis may begin at any time in life, including in the newborn infant, but there are two major peaks of onset. In early-onset MG, at age 20 to 30 years, women are more often affected than men. In late-onset MG, after age 50 years, men are more often affected.

Clinical Signs and Symptoms. Clinically, the disease is characterized by weakness and fatigability; symptoms show fluctuations in intensity and are more severe late in the day or after prolonged activity.

Skeletal muscle weakness is often the first symptom noted, especially affecting the extraocular muscles and producing ptosis and diplopia. The weakness is due primarily to postactivation exhaustion and lasts for 10 to 30 minutes. This weakness fluctuates with superimposed illness, menses, and air temperature (worsening with warming).

Proximal muscles are affected more than distal muscles, and difficulty in climbing stairs, rising from chairs, combing the hair, or even holding up the head occurs. Cra-

▼ *Clinical Signs and Symptoms of*
Myasthenia Gravis

- Muscle fatigability and proximal muscle weakness, aggravated by exertion
- Respiratory failure from progressive involvement of respiratory muscles
- Ptosis (extraocular muscle weakness resulting in drooping of the upper eyelid)
- Diplopia (double vision)
- Dysarthria (speech disturbance)
- Severe quadriparesis
- Bulbar involvement
  - Alteration in voice quality
  - Dysphagia (speech impairment)
  - Nasal regurgitation
  - Choking, difficulty in chewing

nial muscles, neck muscles, respiratory muscles, and muscles of the proximal limbs are the primary areas of muscular involvement. Neurologic findings are normal except for muscle weakness.

The muscular weakness is believed to be caused by the presence of circulating antibodies that are directed against the postsynaptic acetylcholine receptors at the neuromuscular junction. It is not clear what events initiate the formation of these antibodies. There is no muscular atrophy or loss of sensation. Muscular weakness ranges from mild to life-threatening (when involving respiratory muscles) (O'Toole, 1992).

Diagnosis. Diagnosis is difficult because laboratory tests for immune-related neurologic disorders rarely prove to be conclusive. Physicians must rely on the client's history and clinical findings in association with supportive information from electrodiagnostic tests involving the injection of anticholinesterase drugs. Injection of these drugs elicits a sudden, brief improvement in muscle function (which is measured by improvement in the loss of amplitude of

the evoked motor potential) of the person with MG; the same injection worsens the symptoms of a cholinergic person.

Prognosis and Treatment. Prognosis has improved with improved medical treatment. Improvement and remission within 5 years occurs in up to 90 per cent of clients undergoing medial treatment. Serious exacerbations of the illness (myasthenic crisis), including respiratory involvement (especially in the elderly population suffering from other complicating diseases), account for most deaths from MG.

Medical treatment is aimed at increasing the effectiveness of acetylcholine released at the myoneural junction by preventing its breakdown. Treatment may include the use of anticholinesterase, immunosuppressive and corticosteroid drugs, thymectomy (removal of the thymus to suppress production of the antibody), and plasmapheresis (plasma exchange to remove the circulating autoantibodies, used for the severely ill client who has not responded to other treatments). Physical therapy may be indicated as supportive care in MG to assist the client in recovering motor skills.

Guillain-Barré Syndrome (Acute Idiopathic Polyneuritis)

Guillain-Barré syndrome is a demyelinative disease that affects the peripheral nervous system (especially spinal nerves) and is characterized by an abrupt onset of paralysis. The disease affects all age groups, and incidence is not related to race or sex. The exact cause of the disease is unknown, but it frequently occurs after an infectious illness. Upper respiratory infections, vaccinations, or viral infections such as measles, hepatitis, or mononucleosis commonly precede acute idiopathic polyneuritis by 1 to 3 weeks.

Like MG, acute idiopathic polyneuritis may be an autoimmune disease that occurs after surgery, a viral infection, or immunization as a result of a viral antigen's triggering an autoimmune reaction to myelin. Evidence of a cell-mediated immune response includes serum specimens containing antinerve and antimyelin antibodies, the presence of lymphocytes infiltrating the peripheral nerve sheaths, and low levels of immune complexes and complement components (Long and Wright, 1991).

Clinical Signs and Symptoms. The onset of acute idiopathic polyneuritis is generally characterized by a rapidly progressive weakness for a period of 3 to 7 days. It is usually symmetric, involving first the lower extremities, then the upper extremities, and then the respiratory musculature. Weakness and paralysis are frequently preceded by paresthesias and numbness of the limbs, but actual objective sensory loss is usually mild and transient.

Although muscular weakness is usually described as bilateral, progressing from the legs upward toward the arms, this syndrome may be missed when the client presents with unilateral symptoms that do not progress proximally. Muscular weakness of the chest may present early in this disease process as respiratory compromise. Respiratory involvement as such may be unnoticed until the person develops more severe symptoms associated with the Guillain-Barré syndrome.

Cranial nerves, most commonly the facial nerve, can be involved. The tendon reflexes are decreased or lost early in the course of the illness.

Diagnosis. Medical diagnosis is usually based on the history and presenting clinical signs and symptoms associated with this syndrome. Laboratory studies may be used to support the diagnosis but are not usually required in typical cases.

Prognosis and Treatment. The progression of paralysis varies from one client to another, often with full recovery from the paralysis. Usually symptoms develop over a period of 1 to 3 weeks, and the progression of paralysis may stop at any point. Once the weakness reaches a maximum (usually during the second week), the client's condition plateaus for days or even

▼ *Clinical Signs and Symptoms of*

Guillain-Barré Syndrome (Acute Idiopathic Polyneuritis)

- Muscular weakness (bilateral, progressing from the legs to the arms to the chest and neck)
- Diminished deep tendon reflexes
- Paresthesias (without loss of sensation)
- Fever, malaise
- Nausea

weeks before spontaneous improvement and eventual recovery begin, extending over a period of 6 to 9 months. The prognosis is favorable, with decreased mortality owing to improved medical technology that provides advanced respiratory care for clients with compromised pulmonary status. The incidence of residual neurologic deficits is higher than was previously recognized, and deficits may occur in as many as 50 per cent of all cases.

There is no immediate cure for this disease, but medical support is vital during the progression of symptoms, particularly in the acute phase when respiratory function may be compromised. Physical therapy is initiated at an early stage to maintain joint range of motion within the client's pain tolerance and to monitor muscle strength until active exercises can be initiated. The usual precautions for clients immobilized in bed are required to prevent complications during the acute phase. A major precaution is to provide active exercise at a level consistent with the client's muscle strength. Overstretching and overuse of painful muscles may result in a prolonged recovery period or a lack of recovery.

Multiple Sclerosis

Multiple sclerosis (MS) is the most common demyelinating disease of the CNS.

Symptoms appear usually between 20 and 40 years of age, with a peak onset at age 30 years. Onset is rare in children and in adults over the age of 50 years. Men and women are affected equally, but the disorder is uncommon in Asians, Africans, and African-Americans. Environmental factors may affect onset; MS is more common in the temperate (colder) climates of North America and Europe than in tropical areas.

Pathogenesis. The exact etiology of MS is still unknown. Proposed theories include

- Immune-mediated pathogenesis

- Infectious origin (slow or latent virus)

- Disorder of immune regulation characterized by a deficiency in suppressor T cells

The disease is characterized by inflammatory demyelinating (destructive removal or loss) lesions that later form scars known as plaques, which are scattered throughout the CNS white matter, especially the optic nerves, cerebrum, and cervical spinal cord. When edema and inflammation subside, some remyelination occurs, but it is often incomplete.

Marked infiltration of mononuclear cells, consisting mainly of T cells and macrophages, has been found in the plaques, supporting an immunologically mediated pathogenesis. Epidemiologic studies and the identification of increased immunoglobulin G (IgG) in the cerebrospinal fluid (CSF) support an infectious origin. Suppressor T-cell levels are known to decline just before an MS attack. This change, or perhaps an MS antigen present on suppressor T cells, allows a latent autoimmune reaction to occur. Multiple agents may be implicated as research continues. A genetic predisposition and a familial tendency have also been identified. Susceptibility to MS appears to depend on the genetically linked antigen system.

Evidence of active immune responses in immunoglobulin production in the CNS serum and in CSF is abundant. Activated T cells have been found in the blood and CSF of persons with MS in both clinically active and inactive stages of the disease. The exact role of these immune-control mechanisms is unclear. They have been suggested to be the direct cause of the demyelination or the result of the disease process itself. Perhaps a viral infection is the initial causative factor in triggering an autoimmune response that produces de-

---

▼ *Clinical Signs and Symptoms of*
Multiple Sclerosis

(Listed in declining order of frequency [Andreoli et al., 1993])

Symptoms

- Unilateral visual impairment
- Paresthesias
- Ataxia or unsteadiness
- Vertigo (sensation of rotation of self or surroundings)
- Fatigue
- Muscle weakness
- Bowel/bladder dysfunctions:
  - Frequency
  - Urgency
  - Incontinence
  - Retention
  - Hesitancy
- Speech impairment (slow, slurred speech)

Signs

- Optic neuritis
- Nystagmus
- Spasticity or hyperreflexia
- Babinski's sign
- Absent abdominal reflexes
- Dysmetria or intention tremor
- Labile or changed mood
- Lhermitte's sign

myelination. Inflammatory reactions and the production of antibodies then occur as the body reacts to the primary infection (Schenk, 1991).

Clinical Signs and Symptoms. Clinically, MS is characterized by multiple signs and symptoms and by fluctuating periods of remissions and exacerbations. The symptoms vary greatly, and the course of the disease is unpredictable. It is known that more than 60 per cent of the people diagnosed with MS are sensitive to the slightest changes in body temperature. Elevated temperatures worsen symptoms, whereas a decrease improves them. Heating the nerve shortens the duration of the nerve impulse, whereas cooling the nerve prolongs it. Cooling actually restores conduction in blocked nerves (Lab Tech Bulletin, 1990).

Symptoms may vary considerably in character, intensity, and duration. Symptoms can develop rapidly over a course of minutes or hours; less frequently, the onset may be insidious, occurring during a period of weeks or months. Symptoms depend on the location of the lesions, and early symptoms demonstrate involvement of the sensory, pyramidal, cerebellar, and visual pathways or disruption of cranial nerves and their linkage to the brain stem. Lhermitte's sign (electric shock–like sensation radiating to the extremities, initiated by neck flexion) is very suggestive of MS.

In early stages, a relatively complete remission of initial symptoms may occur. However, as the disease progresses, the remissions become less complete and neurologic dysfunction increases.

Diagnosis. The diagnosis of MS is difficult because of the wide variety of possible clinical manifestations and the resemblance that they bear to other neurologic disorders, hysteria, and alcohol intoxication. There is no definitive diagnostic test for MS; rather, the physician relies on objectively measured CNS abnormalities, a history of episodic exacerbations, and early remission of symptoms with progressive worsening of symptoms over time (O'Toole, 1992).

Prognosis and Treatment. The prognosis is difficult to predict and depends on several factors, including the person's age and the intensity of onset, the neurologic status at 5 years after the onset, and the course of exacerbations-remissions. The survival rate after the onset of symptoms is at least 25 years, and death typically results from either respiratory or urinary infection.

Medical treatment is directed at the overall disease process and the specific symptoms as these emerge. Some experiments are being conducted with pharmaceutical agents that slow the potassium ion flow and mimic, even magnify, the cooling effect on nerve conduction. The effect of such drugs has been to restore conduction in blocked demyelinated nerves, thereby alleviating MS symptoms (Lab Tech Bulletin, 1990).

There is no known cure or prevention for MS. Physical therapy is one of many disciplines used in the ongoing management of MS.

Autoimmune Disorders

Autoimmunity results from an inability to distinguish self from nonself, causing the immune system to direct immune responses against normal ("self") tissue. The body begins to manufacture antibodies directed against the body's own cellular components or specific organs. These antibodies are known as autoantibodies, and the diseases that they produce are called autoimmune diseases (Matassarin-Jacobs, 1993).

Autoimmune disorders involve disruption of the immunoregulatory mechanism, causing normal cell-mediated and humoral immune responses to turn self-destructive, which results in tissue damage. Autoimmune disorders may be related to disorders of T-cell subsets or defective recognition of antigens.

The exact cause of autoimmune diseases is not understood, but factors implicated in the development of autoimmune immunologic abnormalities may include

- Genetics (familial tendency)
- Sex hormones (women are affected more often than men by autoimmune diseases)
- Viruses
- Stress
- Cross-reactive antibodies
- Altered antigens
- Environment (e.g., exposure to sunlight, drugs that may destroy suppressor T-cells)

Recently, there have been case reports of various autoimmune diseases in women who have had silicone gel breast implants. These diseases include scleroderma (the most commonly reported disease), systemic lupus erythematosus (SLE), rheumatoid arthritis (RA), mixed connective tissue disease (MCTD), and Sjögren's syndrome. Organ-specific (breast) autoimmune disease is discussed briefly because of the associated musculoskeletal problems.

As yet, silicone breast implants have not been proved as a cause of musculoskeletal conditions, but concern about the safety of these implants led the Food and Drug Administration (FDA) to announce its policy to limit the use of these implants (Robertson, 1993). These limitations restrict use of implants except for breast reconstruction following surgery for cancer, burns, or traumatic injuries.

Another musculoskeletal syndrome described in women who have undergone augmentation mammoplasty has been termed *human adjuvant disease*. This condition includes symptoms of joint pain and/or swelling, fevers, weakness, fatigue, weight loss, swollen lymph nodes, or rash (Robertson, 1993). It has not been proved that removal of the implants will result in elimination of symptoms. Ongoing studies by the FDA are investigating the possible causal relationship between silicone breast implants and connective tissue disease.

Autoimmune disorders may be classified as organ-specific diseases or generalized (systemic) diseases. Organ-specific diseases involve autoimmune reactions limited to one organ.

Organ-specific autoimmune diseases include thyroiditis, Addison's disease, Graves' disease, chronic active hepatitis, pernicious anemia, ulcerative colitis, and insulin-dependent diabetes. These diseases have been discussed in the text appropriate to the organ involved and are not covered further in this chapter.

Generalized autoimmune diseases involve reactions in various body organs and tissues (e.g., SLE). Systemic autoimmune diseases lead to a sequence of abnormal tissue reaction and damage to tissue that may result in diffuse systemic manifestations. These diseases fall into two categories:

- Diffuse connective tissue diseases (previously known as collagen-vascular diseases)
- Spondyloarthropathies (arthritis associated with spondylitis)

Diffuse connective tissue diseases are more common in women and have a strong potential for multiorgan involvement in addition to arthritis and skin manifestations. Disorders that follow this pattern include

- Rheumatoid arthritis
- Systemic lupus erythematosus
- Scleroderma (progressive systemic sclerosis)
- Polymyositis/dermatomyositis
- Mixed connective tissue disease

Spondyloarthropathies represent a group of noninfectious, inflammatory, erosive, rheumatic diseases that target the sacroiliac joints, the bony insertions of the annuli fibrosi of the intervertebral discs, and the facet or apophyseal joints (Hadler, 1987). Spondyloarthropathies are more common in men who by gender have a familial tendency toward the development of a spondyloarthropathy disease. Clinical features described here are associated with the genetic marker human leukocyte anti-

> ▼ *History Associated With*
> **Spondyloarthropathies**
>
> ■ Insidious onset of each episode of backache
> ■ First episode of backache occurs before 30 years of age
> ■ Each episode lasts for months
> ■ Pain intensifies after rest
> ■ Pain lessens with movement
> ■ Family history of a spondyloarthropathy

gen (HLA-B27). The exact role of HLA in these disorders is still unknown. This group includes

■ Ankylosing spondylitis
■ Reiter's syndrome
■ Psoriatic arthritis
■ Arthritis associated with chronic inflammatory bowel disease (see the discussion in Chapter 6)

For most affected individuals, backache is the principal symptom of illness with a corresponding history similar to the following (Hadler, 1987):

Radiographic evidence of sacroiliitis is confirmatory, but years can pass before it is apparent (Hadler, 1987).

Rheumatoid Arthritis

RA is a chronic, systemic, inflammatory disorder of unknown etiology that can affect various organs but predominantly involves the synovial tissues of the diarthrodial joints (Andreoli et al., 1993). There are more than 100 rheumatic diseases affecting joints, muscles, and extraarticular systems of the body.

Incidence. Women are affected with RA two to three times more often than men; however, women who are taking or have taken oral contraceptives are less likely to develop RA. Although it may occur at any age, RA is most common in people between the ages of 20 and 40 years. The incidence of RA is about 1 to 3 per 100 (Matassarin-Jacobs, 1993).

Etiology. The etiologic factor or trigger for this process is as yet unknown. A multifactorial etiology is proposed, including bacterial or viral agents as possible triggering agents. The genetic factor of susceptibility to RA has been substantiated, as demonstrated by the presence of HLA-DR4 antibody, which has been shown to be present in more than 70 per cent of people with RA.

Extraarticular features, such as rheumatoid nodules, arteritis, neuropathy, scleritis, pericarditis, lymphadenopathy, and splenomegaly, occur with considerable frequency (Table 11-4). Once thought to be complications of RA, they are now recognized as being integral parts of the disease and serve to emphasize its systemic nature (Zvaifler, 1988).

The potential for renal, pulmonary, vascular, and cardiac involvement also contributes to RA's being included as a systemic disease. Although RA is a major subclassification within the category of diffuse connective tissue diseases, in this text rheumatic disease is discussed from an immunogenetic basis as an autoimmune disease.

Pathogenesis. (Matassarin-Jacobs, 1993). Not all of the immunologic mechanisms of RA are fully understood, but it is known that rheumatoid factor (antibody to IgG or IgM or both) is present in 60 per cent to 80 per cent of adults and approximately 20 per cent of children with RA. This factor is thought to participate in the pathogenesis of RA by forming an immune complex with human gamma globulin. These complexes lodge in the synovium and other connective tissues. The result is local and systemic inflammation.

The pathologic processes involved in RA are type III (immune complex) and type IV (cell-mediated) reactions. If unarrested, pathologic changes in RA cause membrane

Table 11–4

EXTRAARTICULAR MANIFESTATIONS OF RHEUMATOID ARTHRITIS

Organ System	Extraarticular Manifestations
Skin	Cutaneous vasculitis
	Rheumatoid nodules
Eye	Episcleritis
	Scleritis
	Scleromalacia perforans
	Corneal ulcers/perforation
	Uveitis
	Retinitis
	Glaucoma
	Cataract
Lung	Pleuritis
	Diffuse interstitial fibrosis
	Vasculitis
	Rheumatoid nodules
	Caplan's syndrome
	Pulmonary hypertension
Heart and	Pericarditis
Blood Vessels	Myocarditis
	Coronary arteritis
	Valvular insufficiency
	Conduction defects
	Vasculitis
	Felty's syndrome
Nervous System	Mononeuritis multiplex
	Distal sensory neuropathy

From Andreoli, T.E., et al.: Cecil Essentials of Medicine, 3rd ed. Philadelphia, W.B. Saunders, 1993, p. 566.

proliferation and ultimate erosion of articular cartilage and subchondral bone by passing through four stages: (1) synovitis, (2) pannus formation, (3) fibrous ankylosis, and (4) bony ankylosis.

In stage 1, synovitis, the involved joint or joints become inflamed with a proliferative type of inflammation, initially localized in the joint capsule, primarily in the synovial membrane (synovitis). Tissue thickens with edema and congestion.

In stage 2, pannus, a layer of inflammatory granulation derived from synovial membrane and extending over the articular surface into the joint interior gradually develops. It appears reddish and rough and adheres tightly to underlying cartilage by invasion and lysis, interfering with cartilage

nutrition. Additional destruction may occur as pannus granulation develops on contiguous areas and in subchondral bone, progressively damaging the joint capsule and subchondral bone.

In stage 3, fibrous ankylosis with subluxation and distortion of the affected joint occurs as granulation tissue becomes invaded with tough fibrous tissue and is converted to scar tissue that inhibits or prevents joint movement.

In stage 4, bony ankylosis, firm, bony union may then develop as the fibrous tissue calcifies and changes into osseous tissue.

Clinical Signs and Symptoms (Andreoli et al., 1993). In most people, the symptoms begin gradually during a period of weeks or months. Frequently malaise and fatigue prevail during this period, sometimes accompanied by diffuse musculoskeletal pain. Subsequently, specific joints exhibit pain, tenderness, swelling, and redness.

Inactivity, such as sleep or prolonged sitting, is commonly followed by stiffness. Morning stiffness lasting more than 30 minutes may occur when the person arises in the morning or after prolonged inactivity. The duration of morning stiffness is an accepted measure of the severity of the condition. Pain and stiffness increase gradually as RA progresses and may limit a person's ability to walk, climb stairs, open doors, or perform other activities of daily living (ADLs). Weight loss, depression, and low-grade fever can accompany this process (Bennett, 1988).

As indicated, the inflammatory process may be under way for some time before swelling, tissue reaction, and joint destruction are seen. When symptoms do occur, a symmetric pattern is characteristic, commonly involving the joints of the hands, wrists, elbows, and shoulders, usually sparing the distal interphalangeal (DIP) joints (Bennett, 1988).

Chronic synovitis of the elbows, shoulders, hips, knees, and/or ankles creates special secondary disorders. Destruction of the elbow articulations can lead to flexion contracture, loss of supination and pronation, and subluxation. When the shoulder is involved, limitation of shoulder mobility, dislocation, and spontaneous tears of the rotator cuff result in chronic pain.

The joints of the wrist are frequently affected in RA, with variable tenosynovitis of the dorsa of the wrists and, ultimately, interosseous muscle atrophy and diminished movement owing to articular destruction or bony ankylosis. Volar synovitis can lead to carpal tunnel syndrome.

In the feet, subluxation of the heads of the metatarsophalangeal joints and foreshortening of the extensor tendons give rise to "hammer toe" or "cock up" deformities. A similar process in the hands results in volar subluxation of the metacarpophalangeal joints and ulnar deviation of the fingers. An exaggerated inflammatory response of an extensor tendon can result in a spontaneous, often asymptomatic, rupture. Hyperextension of a proximal interphalangeal (PIP) joint and flexion of the DIP joint produce a swan neck deformity. The boutonniere deformity is a fixed flexion contracture of a PIP joint and extension of a DIP joint.

Involvement of the cervical spine by RA tends to occur late in more advanced disease. Inflammation of the supporting ligaments of C1-C2 eventually produces laxity, sometimes giving rise to atlantoaxial subluxation. Spinal cord compression can result from anterior dislocation of C1 or from vertical subluxation of the odontoid process of C2 into the foramen magnum.

Subcutaneous nodules, present in approximately 25 per cent to 35 per cent of clients with RA, occur most commonly in the subcutaneous or deeper connective tissues in areas subjected to repeated mechanical pressure, such as the olecranon bursae, the extensor surfaces of the forearms, the elbows, and the Achilles tendons (Guccione, 1988).

Diagnosis. The clinical diagnosis of RA is based on careful consideration of three factors: the clinical presentation of the client, which is elucidated through history taking and physical examination; the corroborating evidence gathered through laboratory tests and radiography; and the exclusion of other possible diagnoses (Guccione, 1988).

The physical presence of rheumatoid nodules and the presence of rheumatoid factor measured by laboratory studies are two indicators of RA, although some people with actual rheumatoid factors are missed by commonly available methods. This may account for the 20 per cent of the people with RA who are seronegative (Gall, 1988).

Classification of RA (Table 11–5) is difficult in the early course of the disease, when articular symptoms are accompanied only by constitutional symptoms such as fatigue and loss of appetite, which are common to a number of chronic diseases. A full array of clinical signs and symptoms may not be manifest for 1 to 2 years.

A diagnosis of RA is established on the presentation of four of the seven listed criteria with a duration of joint signs and symptoms for at least 6 weeks.

Additional laboratory tests of significance in the diagnosis and management of rheumatoid arthritis include the following:

■ White blood cell count

■ Erythrocyte sedimentation rate

Clinical Signs and Symptoms of
Rheumatoid Arthritis

- ■ Swelling in one or more joints
- ■ Early morning stiffness
- ■ Recurring pain or tenderness in any joint
- ■ Inability to move a joint normally
- ■ Obvious redness and warmth in a joint
- ■ Unexplained weight loss, fever, or weakness combined with joint pain
- ■ Symptoms such as these that last for more than 2 weeks

Table 11–5

AMERICAN RHEUMATISM ASSOCIATION CRITERIA FOR CLASSIFICATION OF RHEUMATOID ARTHRITIS*

Criteria	Definition
Morning stiffness	Morning stiffness in and around the joints lasting at least 1 hour
Arthritis of three or more joint areas	Simultaneous soft tissue swelling or fluid (not bony overgrowth alone) observed by a physician. The 14 possible joint areas are (right or left) PIP, MCP, wrist, elbow, knee, ankle, and MTP joints
Arthritis of hand joints	At least one joint area swollen as above in wrist, MCP, or PIP joint
Symmetric arthritis	Simultaneous bilateral involvement of the same joint areas as above (PIP, MCP, or MTP joints without absolute symmetry is acceptable)
Rheumatoid nodules	Subcutaneous nodules, over bony prominences or extensor surfaces
Serum rheumatoid factor	Abnormal amounts of serum rheumatoid factor
Radiographic changes	Radiographic changes typical of RA on posteroanterior hand and wrist radiographs, which must include erosions or bony decalcification localized to involved joints (osteoarthritis changes alone do not qualify)

* For classification purposes, a client is said to have RA if she or he has satisfied at least four of the above seven criteria. Criteria 1 through 4 must be present for at least 6 weeks. Clients with two clinical diagnoses are not excluded. Designation as classic, definite, or probable rheumatoid arthritis is no longer made.

Adapted from Harris, E.D., Jr.: Clinical features of rheumatoid arthritis. In Kelley, W.N., et al.: Textbook of Rheumatology, 4th ed. Philadelphia, W.B. Saunders, 1993, p. 874.

- Hemoglobin and hematocrit
- Urinalysis
- Rheumatoid factor assay

The number of white blood cells will increase in the presence of joint inflammation, as will the erythrocyte sedimentation rate. Anemia may be present, and the rheumatoid factor will be elevated in clients with active RA. If the client's urinalysis reveals any protein, blood cells, or casts, SLE should be suspected. This type of abnormal urinalysis would necessitate further diagnostic evaluation and immediate physician referral (Baum, 1993).

Prognosis and Treatment. Although RA is a systemic disease involving the connective tissues of other than the musculoskeletal system (e.g., lungs, heart, blood vessels, pleurae), RA itself is not usually the cause of death. More likely, this disease creates a progressive functional disability that can lead to a loss of income and work

capacity. Medical management with medication is geared toward the control of inflammation augmented by rest, minimizing emotional stress, preventing or correcting deformities, maintaining muscle performance, and maintaining cardiovascular endurance to provide the client with as independent a level of function as possible. Physical therapy in conjunction with occupational therapy assists in meeting this goal through various treatment techniques.

Sjögren's Syndrome (Moutsopoulos and Youinou, 1991; Talal et al., 1991)

In 1933, a Swedish physician, Henrik Sjögren (show-gren), wrote about a group of women whose chronic arthritis was accompanied by dry eyes and dry mouth. Since that time, clients with this combination of symptoms have been described as having Sjögren's syndrome (SS).

SS is a chronic inflammatory disorder of probable autoimmune nature in which the body destroys the exocrine (mucus-secreting) glands, particularly the salivary and lacrimal glands, as though they were foreign bodies. The glands are attacked by lymphocytes, impairing or destroying gland function and resulting in decreased or absent production of tears and saliva. The actual cause of this phenomenon is unknown, but both hereditary factors and viruses are being investigated as possible causes.

SS may occur alone (primary) or be associated with a connective tissue disease (secondary). These different forms of the illness are associated with different signs and symptoms, although the features of the Sjögren's component are basically the same in the two groups.

Clinical Signs and Symptoms. A triad of symptoms marks SS, including keratoconjunctivitis sicca (dry eyes), xerostomia (dry mouth), and a connective tissue disease that is most commonly RA but sometimes may be SLE, scleroderma, or polymyositis.

Primary SS (called sicca), or SS1, refers to dry eyes and dry mouth without any other connective tissue disease. Bulky enlargement of the glands around the face, jaw, and neck is somewhat more frequent in clients with primary SS. An underrecognized component of SS is thyroid dysfunction, usually seen as hypo- or underactive thyroid. Symptoms include recent onset of sluggishness, feeling cold, constipation, and deepening of the voice.

Seventy-five per cent of clients with SS1 have some type of pulmonary involvement. About one third have chronic obstructive pulmonary disease, in which the smaller or larger airways may be involved. The lung tissue itself (parenchyma) may be "clogged up" with lymphocytes, presenting as pseudolymphoma. The tissue of the lungs can develop scarring, which is referred to as interstitial lung disease. This condition is more often seen in clients with SS2 or when there is other organ involvement.

In *secondary SS*, or SS2, symptoms of dry eyes, dry mouth, and swollen salivary glands are accompanied by a disease affecting the body's connective tissue. Approximately 50 per cent of clients with SS have the secondary form.

The most common connective tissue disease found with SS is RA, but it may also involve SLE, scleroderma, polymyositis, or dermatomyositis. It is important to note that all people, including clients with SS, experience arthralgias and myalgias, and that these do not necessarily confirm a diagnosis of arthritis. For example, pain in the spine is rarely, if ever, associated with secondary SS or RA.

Clients with primary SS may be apprehensive about developing a connective tissue disease in the future. While this may happen, it is more common for the person with long-standing connective tissue disease to develop SS.

Xerophthalmia (dry, thick conjunctivae and corneas) and xerostomia, two characteristic symptoms of SS, have been reported with increasing frequency in people

---

Clinical Signs and Symptoms of
Sjögren's Syndrome

- Joint pain, primarily in the fingers, wrists, and knees, lasting a significant portion of the day
- Joint swelling in more than one joint
- Joint stiffness, especially in the morning, lasting 1 hour or more
- Extreme coldness associated with pain and color change in the fingertips and toes, especially in low temperatures
- Distinct rash on the face, involving the cheeks, especially worsened by sun exposure and accompanied by hair loss
- Dry eyes and dry mouth (difficulty in swallowing)
- Swollen salivary glands

with AIDS. Features that closely resemble idiopathic SS, including sicca symptoms, a positive Schirmer's test (measure of tear formation), abnormal salivary gland emptying, and abnormal salivary gland biopsies, have been reported in HIV-infected clients. As a result, it has been suggested that AIDS be an exclusionary disease for the diagnosis of idiopathic SS (Saag, 1992).

Diagnosis and Treatment. A number of tests are available for the diagnosis of SS, including measurement of saliva production, examination of the salivary glands, examination of cells from the lip to determine whether lymphocytes are present in the minor lip salivary glands, and blood tests, including ANA (antinuclear antibody) and Ig levels.

New laboratory tests have helped differentiate primary from secondary SS. The so-called Sjögren's antibodies (SS-A and SS-B) are positive more frequently in clients with primary SS (60 per cent to 80 per cent versus 5 per cent to 10 per cent). Antibodies against the salivary ducts are present in 20 per cent of clients with primary SS but in 70 per cent of clients with secondary SS.

Because there is no known cure for SS, the main goal of treatment is supportive, to reduce client discomfort and to avoid further damage by keeping the affected organs moist.

Specific treatment depends on symptoms and severity. No treatment has yet been found to restore glandular secretions. Artificial tears help lubricate dry eyes, and artificial salivas may provide temporary relief for the dry mouth. Antiinflammatory drugs may reduce the swelling and pain of the enlarged, inflamed glands. Immunosuppressive drugs may be necessary in clients with severe, life-threatening complications.

Systemic Lupus Erythematosus

SLE belongs to the family of rheumatic diseases. It is known to be a chronic, systemic, inflammatory disease characterized by injury to the skin, joints, kidneys, heart and blood-forming organs, nervous system, and mucous membranes.

Lupus comes from the Latin word for wolf, referring to the belief in the 1800s that the rash of this disease was caused by a wolf bite. The characteristic rash of lupus is red, leading to the term erythematosus (Matassarin-Jacobs, 1993).

There are three forms of lupus: discoid, systemic, and drug-induced. *Discoid lupus* is a limited form of the disease confined to the skin. Discoid lupus rarely develops into systemic lupus. Individuals who develop the systemic form probably had systemic lupus at the outset, with the discoid rash as the main symptom. Treatment of discoid lupus will not prevent its progression to the systemic form.

Systemic lupus is usually more severe than discoid lupus and can affect almost any organ or system of the body. For some people, only the skin and joints will be involved. In others, the joints, lungs, kidneys, blood or other organs, or tissues may be affected.

Drug-induced lupus occurs after the use of certain prescribed drugs. The symptoms of drug-induced lupus are similar to those of systemic lupus. The drugs most commonly connected with drug-induced lupus are hydralazine (used to treat high blood pressure or hypertension) and procainamide (used to treat irregular heart rhythms). About 4 per cent of the people who take these drugs will develop antibodies suggestive of lupus. Of those 4 per cent, only an extremely small number will develop overt drug-induced lupus. The symptoms usually fade when the medications are discontinued.

Etiology and Incidence. The exact cause of SLE is unknown, although it appears to result from an immunoregulatory disturbance brought about by the interplay of genetic, hormonal, and environmental factors. Some of the environmental factors that may trigger the disease are infections, antibiotics (especially those in the sulfa and penicillin groups), exposure to ultraviolet (sun) light, and extreme physical and emotional stress, including pregnancy (Lahita, 1992; Matassarin-Jacobs, 1993).

Although lupus is known to occur within families, no known gene is associated with SLE. Lupus can occur at any age, but it is most common in persons between the ages of 15 and 40 years. It occurs 10 to 15 times more often among adult women than among adult men. The symptoms are the same in men and women. People of African, American Indian, or Asian origin develop the disease more often than whites (Andreoli et al., 1993).

Hormonal factors may explain why lupus occurs more frequently in women than in men. The increase of disease symptoms before menstrual periods or during pregnancy supports the belief that hormones, particularly estrogen, may be involved. The incidence of SLE declines after menopause, but the exact hormonal reason for the greater prevalence of lupus in women and the cyclic increase in symptoms is unknown (McDuffie, 1990).

Pathogenesis. As with other autoimmune diseases, antibodies exist without any invading organisms and attack the body's own healthy tissues. Antinuclear antibody (ANA) is an unusual type of antibody that is found in the blood of almost all people with lupus. ANA often includes anti-DNA antibodies during the active phase of the disease. Antigen-antibody complexes accumulate throughout the body, causing inflammation, injury to tissues, and pain, as well as interfering with normal organ functions. As a result there can be damage to the joints, lymph nodes, spleen, liver, lungs, and gastrointestinal tract and internal bleeding of the kidneys and heart (Lahita, 1992).

What triggers the chain of events that leads to this abnormal autoimmune reaction in lupus is unknown. It is known that B cells capable of making autoantibodies are hyperactive, whereas suppressor cells are underactive, although it is unclear which defect comes first (McDuffie, 1990).

Clinical Signs and Symptoms. These follow no single characteristic pattern. Clients

▼ *Clinical Signs and Symptoms of*

Systemic Lupus Erythematosus (Lahita, 1992)

Although lupus can affect any part of the body, most people experience symptoms in only a few organs. This list of the most common symptoms associated with lupus is in order of prevalence.

Sign/Symptom	%
■ Achy joints (arthralgia)	95
■ Fever over 38° C (100° F)	90
■ Arthritis (swollen joints)	90
■ Skin rashes	74
■ Anemia	71
■ Kidney involvement	50
■ Pain in the chest on deep breathing (pleurisy)	45
■ Butterfly-shaped rash across the cheeks and nose	42
■ Sun or light sensitivity (photosensitivity)	30
■ Hair loss	27
■ Raynaud's phenomenon (fingers turning white or blue in the cold)	17
■ Seizures	15
■ Mouth or nose ulcers	12

may differ dramatically in the relative severity and pattern of organ involvement; two people with this diagnosis may have no symptoms in common.

The onset can be acute or insidious. The course of lupus is one of alternating exacerbations and remissions. Skin rash is one of the main symptoms of lupus. Exposure to ultraviolet light exacerbates this rash and causes flare-up of this and other symptoms.

Just how the sun causes skin rash flare-ups is largely unknown. One theory is that the DNA of people with lupus, when exposed to sunlight, becomes more antigenic. This increased antigenicity causes accelerated antigen-antibody reactions and thus more deposition of complexes in the skin. The photosensitivity is most commonly associated with SLE and not other rheumatologic diseases.

Every organ system may become involved (Table 11–6). Although these symptoms may not be present at disease onset, most people soon develop manifestations of multisystem disease. Either glomerulonephritis (usually mild) or cardiovascular manifestations are found in about half the people with SLE (O'Toole, 1992).

Distal sensory polyneuropathy has been reported in 5 per cent to 7 per cent of persons with SLE. This may evolve subacutely or may pursue an insidious, progressive course, starting in the lower extremities and spreading to the distal upper extremities. Numbness on the tip of the tongue and inside the mouth is a frequent complaint. Touch, vibration, and position sense are most prominently affected, and the distal limb reflexes are depressed (Layzer, 1985).

Diagnosis. Tests for autoantibodies, ANA, and DNA binding are the major diagnostic tests in SLE, but no one clinical abnormality or one single test definitively establishes the diagnosis.

The American College of Rheumatology has proposed that clients meeting 4 of the 11 criteria present in Table 11–7 be considered to have SLE. Although these criteria may be helpful diagnostically, they are not foolproof. It is possible for a client to fail to fulfill the criteria and still have SLE. It is also possible for a client to fulfill these criteria but not have SLE (Andreoli et al., 1993).

Prognosis and Treatment. SLE may run a very mild course confined to one or a few organs, or it may be a fatal disease. Although the prognosis has improved greatly in the last three decades, a significant mortality remains (Hollister, 1988).

Renal failure and CNS involvement were the leading causes of death until corticosteroids and cytotoxic agents came into widespread use. Since then, the complica-

Table 11–6
CLINICAL FEATURES OF SYSTEMIC LUPUS ERYTHEMATOSUS

- Skin
    - Rash of areas of the body exposed to ultraviolet light
    - Vasculitis (inflammation of cutaneous blood vessels)
    - Alopecia (loss of hair; baldness)
    - Raynaud's phenomenon
    - Subcutaneous nodules and thickening of the skin
- Joints and Muscles
    - Symmetric polyarthralgia or arthritis
    - Avascular necrosis of bone
    - Myalgias
- Polyserositis (inflammation of serous membranes with effusion)
    - Pleurisy
    - Pleuritic chest pain
    - Shortness of breath
    - Peritonitis with abdominal pain, anorexia, nausea, and vomiting
- Lungs
    - Pulmonary hypertension
    - Pneumothorax
    - Alveolar hemorrhage
    - Vasculitis
- Cardiovascular
    - Coronary artery disease
    - Myocarditis, usually without clinical signs
    - Pericarditis
    - Endocarditis
    - Stocking-glove peripheral neuropathy due to small vessel vasculitis
    - Vasculitis
        - Distal leg ulcers
        - Involution and scarring of the fingertips and nail beds
        - Gangrene of the fingertips
        - Alopecia (baldness or loss of hair)
- Kidney
    - Nephritis
    - Glomerulonephritis
    - Renal failure
    - Systemic hypertension contributing to renal dysfunction
- Central Nervous System
    - Disturbances of mentation (psychosis, depression)
    - Diplopia (double vision)
    - Convulsions
    - Cranial nerve palsies
    - Migraine headaches
    - Peripheral neuritis
    - Cerebrovascular accidents

Adapted from Fye, K.H., and Sack, K.E.: Rheumatic diseases. *In* Stites, D.P., Stobo, J.D., and Wells, J.Y.: Basic and Clinical Immunology, 8th ed. Norwalk, Connecticut, Appleton & Lange, 1994.

Table 11–7

CRITERIA USED FOR DIAGNOSIS OF SLE

Criterion	Definition
Malar rash	Rash over the cheeks
Discoid rash	Red, raised patches
Photosensitivity	Reaction to sunlight, resulting in the development of or increase in skin rash
Oral ulcers	Ulcers in the nose or mouth, usually painless
Arthritis	Nonerosive arthritis (bones around the joints do not become destroyed) involving two or more peripheral joints
Serositis	Pleuritis or pericarditis
Renal disorder	Excessive protein (greater than 0.5 gm/day or 3+ on test sticks) or cellular casts in urine (abnormal elements in the urine derived from red or white blood cells or kidney tubule cells)
Neurologic disorder	Seizures or psychosis in the absence of drugs or metabolic disturbances that are known to cause such effects
Hematologic disorder	Hemolytic anemia or leukopenia (WBC below 4000 cells per mm^3) Lymphopenia (less than 1500 lymphocytes per mm^3) Thrombocytopenia (less than 100,000 platelets per mm^3); not drug-induced
Immunologic disorder	Positive LE prep test, positive anti-DNA test, positive anti-Sm test, or false-positive syphilis test (VDRL)
Antinuclear antibody	Positive test for antinuclear antibodies (ANA); not drug-induced

From Lahita, R.G.: What Is Lupus? Rockville, Maryland, Lupus Foundation of America, 1992; adapted from Tan, E.M., et al.: Revised Criteria for the Classification of SLE. Arthritis and Rheumatism *25*:1271–1277, 1982.

tions of therapy, including atherosclerosis, infection, and cancer, have become common causes of death. The 10-year survival rate with SLE has improved greatly during the past decade and now approaches 80 per cent to 90 per cent (Andreoli et al., 1993).

Medical treatment is supportive for the underlying pathologies of SLE, because there is no specific treatment for SLE itself. Supportive measures are aimed at preventing or minimizing acute relapses and exacerbations of symptoms. Active disease is treated with topical steroids, salicylates for fever and joint pain, corticosteroids, and immunosuppressive agents (O'Toole, 1992). Physical therapy for muscle weakness and prevention of orthopedic deformities is often indicated.

Case Example. A 33-year-old woman with a known diagnosis of systemic lupus erythematosus came to the physical therapy clinic with the following report: "Three weeks ago, I was carrying a heavy briefcase with a strap around my shoulder. I put weight on my right leg and felt my hip joint slip in the back with immediate pain and I was unable to put any weight on that leg. I moved my hip around in the socket and was able to get immediate relief from the pain, but it felt like it could catch at any time." The client also reported that "it feels like my left hip is 2 inches higher than my right."

The client reported prolonged (over 7-year) use of prednisone, and a past medical history of proteinuria and compromised kidney function. Muscle weakness 2 years ago resulted in a muscle biopsy and a diagnosis of "abnormal" muscle tissue of unknown etiology. The client developed a staph infection from the biopsy, which resolved very slowly.

Other past medical history included a motor vehicle accident 2 years ago, at which time her knees went through the dashboard, which left both knees "numb" for a year after the accident.

Aggravating and relieving factors from this visit fit a musculoskeletal pattern of symptoms, and objective examination was consistent with lumbar/sacroiliac mechanical dysfunction with a multitude of other compounding factors, including bilateral posterior cruciate ligament laxity, poor posture, obesity, and emotional lability.

Physical therapy treatment was initiated but, a week later, when the client woke up at night to go to the bathroom, she swung her legs over the edge of her bed and experienced immediate hip and diffuse low back pain and lower extremity weakness. She went to the Emergency Department by ambulance and later was admitted to the hospital. She was evaluated by a neurologist (results unknown), recovered from her symptoms within 24 hours, and was released after a 3-day hospitalization. She was directed by her primary care physician to continue outpatient physical therapy services.

This case example is included to point out the complexity of treating a musculoskeletal condition in a client with a long-term chronic inflammatory disease process requiring years of steroidal antiinflammatory medications. Before including any resistive exercises, muscle energy techniques, or joint or self-mobilization techniques, the therapist must be aware of any clinically significant changes in bone density and the presence of developing osteoporosis.

After consulting with this client's physician, conservative symptomatic treatment was planned. Within 2 weeks, she experienced another middle-of-the-night acute exacerbation of symptoms. A subsequent magnetic resonance image resulted in a diagnosis of disc extrusion (annulus fibrosus perforated with discal material in the epidural space) at two levels (L4-L5, and L5-S1).

Scleroderma (Progressive Systemic Sclerosis) (PSS)

Scleroderma, one of the lesser known chronic disorders in the family of rheumatic diseases, affects joints, muscles, and connective tissue of the body. The word "scleroderma" means hard skin, with chronic hardening of the connective tissue found in many parts of the body, including the skin, blood vessels, synovium, skeletal muscle, and certain internal organs like the kidneys, lungs, heart, and gastrointestinal tract (O'Toole, 1992).

The exact cause of scleroderma is as yet unknown. Current theories suggest three possibilities: an immunologic reaction in which the skin attracts lymph cells that stimulate the production of collagen, hereditary factors related to abnormal serum proteins and antinuclear factors, and occupational exposure to silica dust (O'Toole, 1992).

It is known that the connective tissue cells of people who have scleroderma produce too much of the protein called collagen. This excess collagen is deposited in the skin and body organs, causing thickening and hardening of the skin (induration).

Incidence. The milder forms of scleroderma are most often seen in persons in the 30- to 50-year age group and affect women more than twice as often as men; however, the most severe forms usually affect men, African-Americans, and older persons.

Types. The three forms of PSS most often seen in a physical therapy practice are

- Localized scleroderma

- Limited scleroderma (lSSc)

- Diffuse systemic (generalized) scleroderma (dSSc)

Localized Scleroderma. Localized scleroderma primarily affects children and young (usually female) adults. This group of conditions does not have the typical visceral and serologic manifestations seen with systemic sclerosis (SSc).

This type of scleroderma may also be referred to as *morphea,* a condition in which there is connective tissue replacement of the skin and sometimes of the subcutaneous tissue, marked by the formation of ivory-white or pink patches, bands, or lines that are sometimes bordered by a purple areola. The lesions are firm but not hard and are usually depressed (O'Toole, 1992).

Limited Systemic Sclerosis. This is a form of systemic sclerosis that usually occurs in the third to fourth decade. The client may have a history of Raynaud's phenomenon for several years and subsequently presents with skin edema or tightening of hands, face, and feet. Clients with this form of PSS have a much lower frequency of serious internal organ involvement, although pulmonary hypertension and esophageal disease are not uncommon in lSSc (Andreoli et al., 1993).

lSSc is also called the CREST syndrome from its manifestations described by the following mnemonic:

- **C**alcinosis (abnormal deposition of calcium salts in the tissues; usually on the fingertips and over bony prominences)

- **R**aynaud's phenomenon

- **E**sophageal dysmotility

- **S**clerodactyly (chronic hardening and shrinking of the fingers and toes)

- **T**elangiectasia (spider-like hemangiomas formed by dilation of a group of small blood vessels; occurs most commonly on the fingers, face, lips, and tongue)

Diffuse Systemic Sclerosis. Although dSSc is less common than lSSc, it affects roughly one third of all clients with SSc, and it is by far the more debilitating because of the more frequent renal and pulmonary involvement. Truncal skin involvement is the hallmark of dSSc, and the disease is rapidly progressive. Clients with dSSc may face death from major organ failure within just a few years. An abrupt onset of swollen hands, face, and feet associated with Raynaud's phenomenon may occur. These changes may evolve over several weeks or months to include more proximal areas of the extremities as well as the thorax and abdomen (Istfan and LeRoy, 1990).

Pathogenesis. There are three stages in the clinical evolution of scleroderma:

- Edematous stage
- Sclerotic stage
- Atrophic stage

In the *edematous stage,* bilateral nonpitting edema is present in the fingers and hands and, rarely, in the feet. The edema can progress to the forearms, arms, upper anterior chest, abdomen, back, and face. After a few weeks to several months, edema is replaced by thick, hard skin.

The replacement of edema takes place in the *sclerotic stage,* when the skin becomes tight, smooth, and waxy and seems bound down to underlying structures. Accompanying changes include a loss of normal skin folds and skin hyperpigmentation and hypopigmentation. The face appears to be stretched and masklike, with thin lips and a "pinched" nose.

The skin changes may stabilize for prolonged periods (years) and may then either progress to the third *(atrophic) stage* or soften and return to normal. Actual atrophy of skin may occur, particularly over joints at sites of flexion contractures, such as the PIP joints and the elbows. Such thinning of the skin contributes to the development of ulcerations at these sites. Improvement of the skin (softening and return to normal) may occur to some extent in most people. Improvement typically begins centrally, so that the last areas to become clinically involved are the first to show regression (Medsger, 1988).

Not all people pass through all the stages. Subcutaneous calcification (calcinosis) is a late-developing complication that is considerably more frequent in lSSc. Sites of trauma are often affected, such as the fingers, forearms, elbows, and knees. These calcifications vary in size from tiny deposits to large masses (Fye and Sack, 1991; Medsger, 1988).

Clinical Signs and Symptoms (Andreoli et al., 1993). Raynaud's phenomenon and tight skin are the hallmarks of SSc. Virtually all clients with SSc have Raynaud's phenomenon, which is defined as episodic pallor of the digits following exposure to cold or stress associated with cyanosis, followed by erythema, tingling, and pain. Raynaud's phenomenon affects primarily the hands and feet and less commonly the ears, nose, and tongue.

The appearance of the skin is the most distinctive feature of SSc. By definition, clients with diffuse SSc have taut skin in the more proximal parts of extremities, in addition to the thorax and abdomen. However, the skin tightening of SSc begins on the fingers and hands in nearly all cases; therefore, the distinction between limited and diffuse SSc may be difficult to make early in the illness.

Articular complaints are very common in PSS and may begin at any time during the course of the disease. The arthralgias, stiffness, and frank arthritis seen may be difficult to distinguish from those of RA, particularly in the early stages of the disease. Involved joints include the metacarpophalangeals, PIPs, wrists, elbows, knees, ankles, and small joints of the feet. Flexion contractures, due to changes in the skin or joints, are common.

Muscle involvement is usually mild with weakness, tenderness, and pain of proximal muscles of the upper and lower extremities.

Involvement of the GI tract is the third most common manifestation of SSc, following only skin changes and Raynaud's phenomenon. Esophageal hypomotility occurs in more than 90 per cent of clients with either diffuse or limited SSc. Similar changes occur in the small intestine, resulting in reduced motility and causing intermittent diarrhea, bloating, cramping, malabsorption, and weight loss.

Although more than 90 per cent of clients with diffuse SSc have some form of cardiac involvement, and cardiac abnormalities are a significant cause of mortality

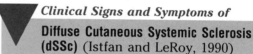

Clinical Signs and Symptoms of

Limited Cutaneous Systemic Sclerosis (lSSc) (Istfan and LeRoy, 1990)

- CREST syndrome
  - Raynaud's phenomenon persisting for years
  - Skin changes absent or limited to hands, face, feet, and forearms
- Significant late incidence of
  - Pulmonary hypertension
  - Trigeminal neuralgia
  - Skin calcifications
  - Telangiectasia (spider angiomas)

Clinical Signs and Symptoms of

Diffuse Cutaneous Systemic Sclerosis (dSSc) (Istfan and LeRoy, 1990)

- Raynaud's phenomenon
- Both trunk and extremity skin changes (swelling, thickening, hardening)
- Ulcerations of the fingers secondary to constriction of small blood vessels
- Polyarthralgia (joint pain affecting large and small joints with inflammation, stiffness, swelling, warmth, tenderness)
- Flexion contractures of large and small joints
- Muscle weakness
- Early and significant incidence of
  - Interstitial lung disease
  - Renal failure
  - GI disease
  - Myocardial involvement

in this group (Anvari et al., 1992), clinical evidence of myocardial involvement is uncommon (less than 10 per cent). Cardiac involvement can be manifested as cardiomyopathy, pericarditis, pericardial effusion, or arrhythymias.

Diagnosis. There is no specific test to

▼ *Clinical Signs and Symptoms of*
Scleroderma

Esophageal Involvement

- Muscle weakness of esophagus
- Dysphagia (difficulty in swallowing liquids or solids)
- Heartburn

Gastrointestinal Involvement

- Bloating
- Cramps
- Diarrhea or constipation

Lung Involvement

- Dyspnea on exertion (usually the first symptom)
- Chronic cough
- Pleurisy

confirm the diagnosis of scleroderma. Various medical tests including x-rays, skin biopsies, tests for antinuclear antibodies, gamma globulin, and others may be used to diagnose scleroderma. The symptoms of scleroderma often mimic those of other diseases, such as bursitis, osteoarthritis, RA, and other connective tissue diseases, which makes medical diagnosis difficult (O'Toole, 1992).

Prognosis and Treatment. The prognosis for systemic scleroderma (more serious form) depends on the extent of visceral involvement. Overall prognosis is poor if cardiac, pulmonary, or renal systems are affected at the time of diagnosis.

"Scleroderma renal crisis," the abrupt onset of accelerated hypertension, oliguria, and microangiopathic hemolysis, once accounted for the majority of deaths in SSc. At present, however, with the early diagnosis and treatment of hypertension, renal failure in SSc is less common. Clinically,

scleroderma renal crisis is usually observed in an individual with diffuse SSc whose disease is at a relatively early stage and who has rapid progression of skin involvement.

The leading cause of mortality in SSc is pulmonary disease. Interstitial lung disease with fibrosis, pulmonary hypertension, pleurisy, and pleural effusions are the pulmonary complications with SSc. The 10-year survival rate after first diagnosis for SSc is approximately 65 per cent (Medsger, 1988).

Medical treatment involves the use of agents that inhibit excessive collagen production, in addition to supportive and symptomatic measures. Drugs such as penicillamine, immunosuppressives, and antiinflammatories may be administered.

Physical therapy is essential in assisting clients with skin, joint, and muscle involvement to maintain range of motion, to prevent contractures, to increase the nutritional blood supply to the tissues, and to protect the joints through positioning, splinting, and modified ADLs.

Evaluation of the effectiveness of intervention in systemic sclerosis is difficult because of its slowly progressive nature, the frequent tendency toward spontaneous improvement, limitations in objective criteria for determining improvement or deterioration, and the influence of psychologic factors on many symptoms (Medsger, 1988).

Polymyositis/Dermatomyositis

Polymyositis (PM) and dermatomyositis (DM) are related illnesses belonging to the family of rheumatic diseases that result in damage to connective tissue, primarily muscles and skin. The major result of these diseases is weakness. There are actually five categories of inflammatory muscle disease that are distinguished under myositis (Oddis and Medsger, 1991):

- Polymyositis
- Dermatomyositis

■ Myositis with malignancy

■ Childhood polymyositis or dermatomyositis

■ Polymyositis associated with other inflammatory diseases (Sjögren's syndrome, mixed connective tissue disease, RA)

Polymyositis literally means "many muscles inflamed." It is a subacute or chronic generalized disorder of striated muscle and skin characterized clinically by progressive, symmetric muscular weakness and pathologically by scattered muscle fiber necrosis and inflammation, without a known infectious cause. As with other connective tissue diseases, these disorders are characterized by periods of remission and exacerbation and are chronically progressive (Matassarin-Jacobs, 1993).

When a rash is associated with PM, it is referred to as *dermatomyositis*. The rash occurs typically on the upper eyelids and generally with edema. An erythematous rash may also recur on other body surfaces, including the knees, the elbows, the V-region of the neck and upper chest, and across the back and shoulders. DM in children is notable for its more frequent extramuscular manifestations, generally owing to a systemic vasculitis that can involve almost any organ system (Andreoli et al., 1993).

Incidence. PM and DM are uncommon but not rare, with an annual incidence of 1 per 100,000. There is a female predominance (2:1), and African-American women are most frequently affected. Myositis can occur at any age, but its distribution is bimodal, with a small peak in children aged 5 to 14 years and a larger peak in adults aged 45 to 64 years. In children under age 16 years, DM is more common than PM. Myositis, especially dermatomyositis, with malignancy is found more often in persons over age 50 years and in a more equal sex ratio (Oddis and Medsger, 1991).

Clinical Signs and Symptoms. The onset of this connective tissue disorder is almost always gradual. The clinical hallmark of inflammatory myopathy is *proximal muscle weakness*. This symmetric muscle weakness increases during a period of weeks or months before diagnosis and is noticed first in the proximal limb muscles (usually the lower extremities first) and trunk. Facial muscles and distal muscles are not completely spared, but involvement is rare. Clients may have difficulty in lifting body parts, such as the head from a pillow or arms overhead, and similar difficulty is encountered when trying to rise from a chair or climb stairs.

Myalgias (muscle aches or tenderness) occur in about half of the clients. Initially, the muscles may be slightly swollen, but as the disease progresses, muscular atrophy and induration (hardening) become more noticeable, reflecting the deposition of fibrous tissue.

Musculotendinous contractures are a common complication and may begin to appear within the first 2 or 3 weeks. Muscle stretch reflexes are often depressed in the affected muscles.

Arthralgias/arthritis (inflammatory joint symptoms) are commonly present in PM/DM. These symptoms accompany or precede the onset of muscle weakness but usually occur early in the disease course. Symptoms are often mild, resolving quickly when corticosteroid therapy is initiated for the myositis (Oddis and Medsger, 1991).

Pulmonary complications of PM or DM may precede the appearance of muscle or skin manifestations. Dyspnea and a nonproductive cough are the most common of the pulmonary symptoms. Respiratory muscles are usually preserved until very late in the disease, but eventually weakness occurs and, together with pharyngeal weakness, disposes the client to interstitial pneumonia and pulmonary fibrosis. Nasal regurgitation of liquids and difficulty in swallowing from the pharyngeal weakness result in a tendency to aspirate liquids, causing aspiration pneumonia.

A small minority of people with PM/DM

(less than 10 per cent) have a concomitant *malignant tumor*. This tumor is more likely to occur in people over 40 or 50 years of age. Tumors are more likely to occur in people with DM than in those with PM.

The most common places for such tumors are in the lungs, ovaries, breasts, endometrium, prostate, colon, and stomach, but they may occur in or spread to other areas of the body (Andreoli et al., 1993). Other features of this disorder may include a mild transitory arthritis and Raynaud's phenomenon.

Diagnosis. In conjunction with the pres-

Clinical Signs and Symptoms of
Polymyositis/Dermatomyositis

- Symmetric proximal muscle weakness (shoulder and pelvic girdles)
- Symmetric distal muscle weakness (less common than proximal weakness)
- Respiratory muscle weakness
- Polyarthralgias
- Polyarthritis
- Myalgias
- Dysphagia (secondary to muscle weakness)
- Low-grade fever
- Weight loss
- Raynaud's phenomenon (rare)

Additional clinical signs and symptoms of **dermatomyositis:**

- Red, scaly thickening of the skin over bony prominences of extensor surfaces (e.g., elbows, knees, knuckles)
- Patchy, red skin rash on the face and around the eyes
- Periorbital edema (puffy eyelids)

ence of a characteristic skin rash and proximal muscle weakness, various tests may be used by the physician to determine the diagnosis. These tests may include muscle biopsy, serum enzyme levels (elevated muscle enzymes), and electromyogram (EMG) studies (Oddis and Medsger, 1991).

Prognosis and Treatment. The clinical course in these diseases is generally prolonged, with remissions and exacerbations. The prognosis depends on accompanying complications, such as malignant tumors or cardiac or pulmonary involvement, in which PM tends to be more severe.

Long remissions and even recovery in children have been observed, but death in adults can occur after severe and progressive muscle weakness and dysphagia with aspiration and subsequent aspiration pneumonia. As with other autoimmune disorders, medical treatment is supportive. The specific treatment for myositis varies from one person to another but usually includes medication (corticosteroids, immunosuppressants), exercise, and rest.

Physical therapy to improve muscle strength should not be initiated until the drug treatment takes effect. In the early stages of treating myositis, the muscle fibers are fragile and could be damaged further by exercises and other forms of physical therapy. The physical therapist treating a client with myositis should keep in close contact with the physician, who will be using physical examination and laboratory tests to determine the most opportune time for an exercise program.

Mixed Connective Tissue Disease
(Andreoli et al., 1993)

As many as 25 per cent of all clients with features suggestive of a connective tissue disease do not fit into a definitive diagnostic category such as SLE, RA, scleroderma, or myositis (PM/DM). Mixed connective tissue disease (MCTD) is a rheumatic disease syndrome that combines the clinical features of these other connective tissue diseases.

There is much confusion about the appropriate way to classify these diseases. Three terms used to describe such clients have been *early undifferentiated connective tissue disease* (EUCTD), *mixed connective tissue disease*, and *overlap syndrome*.

The terms MCTD and overlap syndrome are often used interchangeably; however, the designation of overlap syndrome is appropriate when a client exhibits features of more than one established diagnosis. For example, a client with RA who subsequently develops symptoms suggestive of SLE would be labeled as having an overlap syndrome.

The diagnosis of MCTD is generally reserved for clients with evidence of an overlap syndrome who also have very high titers of antibodies to a ribonucleoprotein (RNP). The presenting features of MCTD do not differentiate it from other diffuse connective tissue diseases. Antibodies to RNP constitute the only constant feature in clients with MCTD.

Incidence. The prevalence of MCTD is unknown, but it appears to be more common than PM and less frequent than SLE. Eighty per cent of the clients are female, and persons in any age group can be affected.

Clinical Signs and Symptoms. Raynaud's phenomenon, present in approximately 85 per cent of clients, may precede other disease manifestations by months or years. Skin changes, such as lupus-like rashes, erythematous patches over the knuckles, alopecia, and telangiectasia over the hands and face, may occur. Esophageal abnormalities and lung and cardiac involvement are not uncommon.

Renal disease is unusual, although death has occurred secondary to progressive renal failure in some people. Other findings in clients diagnosed with MCTD may in-

---

Clinical Signs and Symptoms of

Mixed Connective Tissue Disease
(in decreasing order of incidence)

- Polyarthritis or polyarthralgias
- Swollen hands (sausage-like appearance of fingers)
- Raynaud's phenomenon
- Abnormal esophageal motility
- Myositis (inflammation of a voluntary muscle)
- Proximal muscle weakness (with or without tenderness)
- Lymphadenopathy (disease of the lymph nodes)
- Sensory polyneuropathy (occurs in about 10 per cent of all cases) (Layzer, 1985)

---

clude fever, lymphadenopathy, splenomegaly, hepatomegaly, persistent hoarseness, and intestinal involvement similar to that seen in scleroderma.

Diagnosis. The medical diagnosis is easier to determine in clients in whom classic skin changes and Raynaud's phenomenon are associated with characteristic visceral complaints than in clients presenting with visceral or arthritic complaints without skin changes. In many cases, only the presence or absence of certain antinuclear antibodies makes it possible to differentiate scleroderma from MCTD (O'Toole, 1992).

Treatment and Prognosis. The pattern of organ system involvement is used by physicians to guide medical treatment with the client who has MCTD or overlap syndrome. Treatment varies with the presenting symptoms, combining the measures appropriate for each component disease.

Although the prognosis of clients with MCTD is favorable, serious and sometimes fatal complications such as pulmonary hypertension do occur. Clients with MCTD who have high titers of anti-RNP experience a relatively favorable prognosis and a low frequency of renal disease.

Spondyloarthropathies (Andreoli et al., 1993; Matassarin-Jacobs, 1993)

The spondyloarthropathies are a group of interrelated disorders that share certain epidemiologic, pathogenetic, clinical, and pathologic features. They are not seropositive for rheumatoid factor and characteristically have involvement of the sacroiliac joints, including peripheral inflammatory arthritis.

This group of diseases includes ankylosing spondylitis (AS) (also known as Marie-Strümpell disease or rheumatoid spondylitis), Reiter's syndrome, and psoriatic arthritis. The first two disorders are more common in men, and the latter disorder is more common in women.

The major characteristics of these disorders are progressive joint fibrosis (especially of the vertebral column in AS), synovitis, and inflammation of the skin, mucous membranes, and the site of ligament insertion into the bone.

All the disorders are treated with steroid therapy and aggressive physical therapy. Nonsteroidal antiinflammatory drugs (NSAIDs) may be used to treat joint pain.

Ankylosing Spondylitis

AS, or "crooked vertebrae," is a chronic, progressive inflammatory disorder of undetermined etiology. AS is actually more an inflammation of fibrous tissue affecting the entheses, or insertions of ligaments and capsules into bone, than of synovium, as is common in other rheumatic disorders. The sacroiliac joints, spine, and large peripheral joints are primarily affected.

Incidence. The prevalence of AS is about 0.2 per cent of the general population—approximately 2 million persons in the United States. Misdiagnosis is common, especially in women, and initial treatment is misdirected at mechanical low back pain or seronegative RA (Ramanujam and Schumacher, 1992).

Studies now suggest that the disease has a more uniform sex distribution, but it may be milder in women because they are less likely than men to have progressive spinal disease. Women tend to have more peripheral joint manifestations, thus leading to an inappropriate diagnosis (Calin, 1988). AS in women tends to evolve slowly both clinically and radiographically (Kidd et al., 1988).

AS has an uneven racial distribution and is more common among whites than African-Americans. It is rare among Africans and Japanese but common among persons of Chinese parentage (Ball, 1989).

Pathogenesis (Ramanujam and Schumacher, 1992). The pathogenesis of AS is unknown. Clients are seronegative for rheumatoid factor, and antinuclear antibodies are not seen. There may be a genetic predisposition, as 90 per cent of clients have the specific cell surface antigen labeled HLA-B27. The gene that determines this specific antigen may be linked to other genes that determine pathologic autoimmune phenomena or that lead to an increased susceptibility to infectious or environmental agents. As yet, there are no other data to confirm an autoimmune pathogenetic mechanism.

Epidemiologic studies suggest that environmental factors also may play a role. For example, sibling pairs with AS have similar dates of onset but not similar ages of onset (Will, 1990).

The most striking features of AS are the high degree of fibrosis, bony ankylosis, and inflammation that focus on bone, cartilage, and tendon-bone junctions (Calin, 1989). The disease typically involves ligamentous insertions, fibrocartilage, and the intervertebral discs.

Inflammation is nongranulomatous and causes disruption of the ligament fibers. Reactive bone is formed as part of a reparative process, causing ligaments to ossify. When this occurs in the sacrotuberous or sacrospinous ligaments or along the rami of the ischia, pubis, greater trochanter, and heels, the typical "whiskering" picture is produced radiographically.

This reparative process also forms linear bone ossification along the outer fibers of the annulus fibrosus of the disc, called syndesmophyte formation (Fig. 11–4). This bridging of the vertebrae is most prominent along the anterior longitudinal ligament and occurs earliest in the thoracolumbar area. Destructive changes of the upper and lower corners of the vertebrae at the site of insertion of the annulus fibrosus of the disc are responsible for the vertebral squaring. Late in the disease, the vertebral column takes on an appearance that is referred to as "bamboo" spine.

Clinical Signs and Symptoms. The classic presentation of AS is insidious onset of mid and low back pain and stiffness for more than 3 months in a person under age 40 years. It is usually worse in the morning, lasting more than 1 hour, and is characterized as either achy or sharp ("jolting"), typically localized to the pelvis, buttocks, and hips.

Paravertebral muscle spasm, aching, and stiffness are common, but some clients may have slow progressive limitation of motion with no pain at all. Most clients present with sacroiliitis as the earliest feature seen on x-ray films before clinical involvement extends to the lumbar spine.

On physical examination, decreased mobility in the anteroposterior and lateral planes will be symmetric. The Wright-Schöber test is used to confirm reduction in spinal motion associated with AS (Magee, 1992). The sacroiliac joint is rarely tender by direct palpation. As the disease progresses, loss of lumbar lordosis is easily observed.

Peripheral joint involvement usually (but not always) occurs after involvement of the spine. Typical extraspinal sites include the manubriosternal joint, symphysis pubis, shoulder, and hip joints.

Diminished chest expansion (less than 2 cm) occurs as a result of decreased rib movement secondary to vertebral and costovertebral fusion caused by syndesmo-

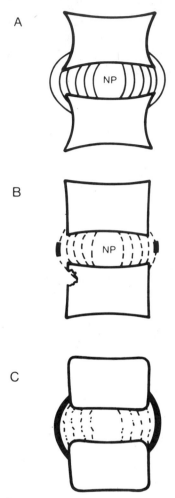

Figure 11–4

The pathogenesis of the syndesmophyte. The syndesmophyte, along with destruction of the sacroiliac joint, is the hallmark of the inflammatory spondyloarthropathies, such as ankylosing spondylitis. It should be distinguished from the osteophyte, which is characteristic of degenerative spondylosis. *A*, The normal intervertebral disk. The inner fibers of the annulus fibrosus are next to the nucleus pulposus (NP). The outer fibers insert into the periosteum of the vertebral body at least one third the distance toward the next end-plate. *B*, With early inflammation, the corners of the bodies are reabsorbed and appear to be square or even eroded. Fine deposits of amorphous apatite (calcium phosphate, a mineral constituent of bone) appear on radiographs at first as thin, delicate calcification on the outer fibers of the mid-annulus. *C*, The process progresses to bridging calcification, the syndesmophyte, extending from one midbody to the next; thus the spine takes on its "bamboo" appearance on radiographs. (From Hadler, N.M.: Medical Management of the Regional Musculoskeletal Diseases. Orlando, Florida, Grune & Stratton, 1984, p. 5.)

▼ *Clinical Signs and Symptoms of*
Ankylosing Spondylitis

Early Stages

- Intermittent, low-grade fever
- Fatigue
- Anorexia, weight loss
- Anemia
- Sacroiliitis (inflammation, pain, and tenderness in the sacroiliac joints)
- Spasm of the paravertebral muscles
- Intermittent low back pain (nontraumatic, insidious onset)

Advanced Stages

- Constant low back pain
- Ankylosis (immobility and consolidation or fusion) of the sacroiliac joints and spine
- Muscle wasting in shoulder and pelvic girdles
- Loss of lumbar lordosis
- Marked dorsocervical kyphosis
- Decreased chest expansion
- Arthritis involving the peripheral joints (hips and knees)
- Iritis or iridocyclitis (inflammation of the iris; occurs in 25 per cent of all cases)
- Carditis (10 per cent occurrence)
- Pericarditis and pulmonary fibrosis (rare)
- Fatigue and weight loss
- Low-grade fever

ease. Ocular symptoms may precede spinal symptoms by several weeks or even years. Pulmonary changes (chronic infiltrative or fibrotic bullous changes of the upper lobes) occur in 1 per cent to 3 per cent of persons with AS and may be confused with tuberculosis (Hakala et al., 1990).

Cardiomegaly, conduction defects, and pericarditis are well-recognized cardiovascular complications of AS. Occasionally, renal manifestations precede other symptoms of AS.

Complications (Ramanujam and Schumacher, 1992). The very stiff osteoporotic spine of clients with AS is prone to *fracture* from even minor trauma. The most common site of fracture is the lower cervical spine. Risk of neurologic damage may be compounded by the development of epidural hematoma from lacerated vessels.

Severe neck or occipital pain possibly referring to the retroorbital or frontal area is the presenting symptom of *atlantoaxial subluxation*. This underappreciated entity may be either an early or a late manifestation, but it is frequently seen in clients with persistent peripheral arthritis (Hunter, 1989; Suarez-Almazor and Russell, 1988).

Movement aggravates pain, and progressive myelopathy develops from cord compression, leading to motor/sensory disturbance in bladder and bowel control. The diagnosis of atlantoaxial subluxation is usually made from lateral x-ray views of the cervical spine in flexion and extension.

Spondylodiscitis (erosive and destructive lesions of vertebral bodies) is seen in clients with long-standing disease. Intervertebral disc lesions occur at multiple levels, especially in the thoracolumbar region.

Cauda equina syndrome is a late manifestation of the disease with an average interval of 24 years between onset of AS and the syndrome (Tullous et al., 1990). The initial deficit is loss of sensation of the lower extremities, along with urinary and rectal sphincter disturbances and/or perineal pain and weakness. Neurologic abnormalities in AS are usually related to nerve impingement or spinal cord trauma.

Spinal stenosis occurs as a result of bony

phytes. Chest wall stiffness seldom leads to respiratory disability as long as diaphragmatic movement is intact.

Extraarticular Features. Uveitis, conjunctivitis, or iritis occurs in nearly 25 per cent of clients and follows a course that is unrelated to the severity of the joint dis-

overgrowth of the spinal ligaments and facet joints. Symptoms are pain and numbness of the lower extremities brought on by walking and relieved by rest.

Pregnancy usually does not change symptoms in a woman already diagnosed with AS. Occasionally, severe sacroiliac joint fusion or hip involvement necessitates a cesarean section. The client must avoid using NSAIDs during pregnancy or breast-feeding.

Diagnosis. After 3 months of low back pain and stiffness of insidious onset, that is unrelieved by rest, the disease is usually diagnosed by demonstration of the appropriate features on physical examination and x-ray studies. X-ray films of the sacroiliac joints reveal osteoporosis and erosions early in the disease and sclerosis with fusion in advanced disease. Calcification of the anterior longitudinal ligament of the spine and squaring of the vertebrae are seen on lateral x-ray views of the spine. Ossification of the outer margins of the intervertebral disc (syndesmophyte formation) may lead to fusion of the spine (see Fig. 11–4).

Prognosis and Treatment. Although AS has serious consequences for some clients, most maintain a functional and productive life style. Of all the rheumatic diseases, AS is the most responsive to rehabilitation if it is recognized early and if treatment is initiated before the disease fuses the vertebrae and involves other organs.

Treatment is directed toward maintaining function and strength and includes the use of medications to decrease inflammation and relieve pain, making exercise possible. Client education toward preserving body posture and mechanics, and work modification as indicated, may be augmented by breathing exercises. Smoking is strongly discouraged because of the risk of associated restrictive lung disease.

Reiter's Syndrome

Reiter's syndrome is characterized by a triad of arthritis, conjunctivitis, and non-specific urethritis, although some clients develop only two of these three problems. Reiter's syndrome occurs mainly in young adult men between the ages of 20 and 40 years, although women and children can be affected.

Two forms have been identified: (1) cases associated with dysentery, and (2) a sexually transmitted form most often implicated with venereal infection. Characteristically, Reiter's syndrome develops 1 to 4 weeks following venereal exposure or diarrhea. The onset of Reiter's syndrome can be abrupt, occurring over several days or more gradually over several weeks.

HLA-B27 is found by serotyping in 80 per cent of white and 35 per cent of African-American clients. When it occurs in a woman, HLA-B27 is found in almost 100 per cent of the cases, which supports a genetic predisposition for the development of this syndrome after a person is exposed to certain bacterial infections or after sexual contact. Having HLA-B27 does not necessarily mean that the person will develop this syndrome but indicates that the person will have a greater chance of developing Reiter's syndrome than do people without this marker.

Reiter's syndrome can be differentiated from AS by the presence of urethritis and conjunctivitis, the prominent involvement of distal joints, and the presence of asymmetric radiologic changes in the sacroiliac joints and spine (Fye and Sack, 1991).

Clinical Signs and Symptoms. (Andreoli, 1993). *Arthritis* associated with Reiter's syndrome often presents precipitously and frequently affects the knees and ankles, lasting weeks to months. The distribution of the arthritis is asymmetric, and typically arthritis begins in the weight-bearing joints, especially of the lower extremities.

It may vary in severity from absence to extreme joint destruction. Involvement of the feet and spine is most common and is associated with HLA-B27 positivity. Affected joints are usually warm and edematous. Although the joints usually begin to improve after 2 or 3 weeks, many people continue to have pain, especially in the heels and back.

One third of the people with Reiter's syndrome have sacroiliac x-ray changes that may be asymmetric and are similar to those in AS. Small joint involvement, especially in the feet, is more common in Reiter's syndrome than in AS and is often asymmetric.

Inflammation at tendinous insertions into bone is common in Reiter's syndrome and causes plantar fasciitis, digital periostitis, or Achilles tendinitis.

The *conjunctivitis* of Reiter's syndrome is mild and characterized by irritation with redness, tearing, and burning usually lasting a few days, or less commonly as long as several weeks. The process is ordinarily self-limiting.

Urethritis manifested by burning and uri-nary frequency is often the earliest symptom. A profuse and watery diarrhea can precede the onset of urethritis in Reiter's syndrome.

Diagnosis. Diagnosis is based on the overall pattern of symptoms and on results of a physical examination. Diagnosis of Reiter's syndrome requires peripheral arthritis occurring in association with urethritis and lasting more than 3 or 4 weeks. Although no blood or urine tests will confirm Reiter's syndrome, these tests can be used to rule out similar diseases and to indicate evidence of infection. Testing for the HLA-B27 genetic marker also may assist in confirming the diagnosis but is not an absolute indicator of Reiter's syndrome.

Prognosis and Treatment. This syndrome demonstrates a self-limited (for 3 to 4 months) but relapsing course (sometimes recurring for 2 to 3 years). Joint deformity, ankylosis, and inflammation of the sacroiliac joint may occur with chronic or recurrent Reiter's syndrome. Heel pain is a particularly ominous predictor of eventual disability. Medical treatment is primarily with medication. Physical therapy during the recovery phase can offer the client symptomatic relief and can provide preventive and self-care measures to reduce joint trauma.

▼ *Clinical Signs and Symptoms of*
Reiter's Syndrome

- Low-grade fever
- Urethritis (when present, precedes other symptoms by 1 to 2 weeks)
- Conjunctivitis and iritis, bilaterally
- Polyarthritis (occurs several days or weeks after symptoms of infection appear)
- Sacroiliac joint changes
- Low back pain
- Small joint involvement, especially the feet: heel pain
- Plantar fasciitis
- Skin involvement: inflammatory hyperkeratotic lesions of the toes, nails, and soles resembling psoriasis
- May be preceded by bowel infection: diarrhea, nausea, vomiting
- Anorexia and weight loss

Psoriatic Arthritis (Mader and Gladman, 1993)

Psoriatic arthritis (PsA) is a chronic, recurrent, erosive, inflammatory arthritis associated with the skin disease psoriasis. It is not just a variant of RA but is a distinct disease. Psoriasis is quite common, affecting 1 per cent to 3 per cent of the general population. This arthritis occurs in one third of clients with psoriasis.

Incidence. In contrast to RA, there is no gender predilection in PsA; both sexes are affected equally. It can occur at any age although it usually occurs between the ages of 20 and 30 years. The onset of the arthritis may be acute or insidious and is usually preceded by the skin disease.

Pathogenesis. The cause of psoriasis and PsA is unknown. Genetic factors appear to play a role in the development of this disease, because psoriasis and rheumatic diseases are found in other family members. Both antinuclear antibodies and rheumatoid factor may be present in up to 10 per cent of PsA clients or in clients with psoriasis uncomplicated by arthritis. The presence of the histocompatibility complex marker HLA-B27 and other HLA antigens is not uncommon, and they occur in clients with peripheral arthritis and spondylitis.

The presence of these genetic markers may be associated with an increased susceptibility to unknown infectious or environmental agents or to primary abnormal autoimmune phenomena. As yet, no known immunologic pathogenetic mechanism has been demonstrated.

Clinical Signs and Symptoms. *Skin lesions* that characterize psoriasis are readily recognized as piles of well-defined, dry, erythematous, often overlapping silver-scaled papules and plaques. These may appear in small, easily overlooked patches or run together and cover wide areas. The scalp, extensor surfaces of the elbows and knees, back, and buttocks are common sites. The lesions, which do not usually itch, come and go.

Nail lesions, including pitting, transverse grooves, stippling, general discoloration, and destruction of the nail, are the only clinical feature that may identify clients with psoriasis in whom arthritis is likely to develop. The nail changes may be mistaken for those produced by a fungal infection.

Arthritis presents as an early and severe distal distribution (DIP joints of fingers and toes before involvement of MCP/MTP joints) in half of all clients with PsA, which distinguishes it from RA. Severe erosive disease may lead to marked deformity of the hands and feet, called arthritis mutilans.

Clients report pain and stiffness in the inflamed joints, with morning stiffness that lasts more than 30 minutes. Other evidence of inflammation includes pain on stressing the joint, tenderness at the joint line, and the presence of effusion. Painful symptoms are aggravated by prolonged immobility and reduced by physical activity.

Marked vertebral involvement can result in *ankylosis of the spine*. This differs from AS in a number of respects, most notably in the tendency for many of the syndesmophytes to arise not at the margins of the vertebral bodies but from the lateral and anterior surfaces of the bodies (McEwan, 1971). *Sacroiliac changes*, including erosions, sclerosis, and ankylosis similar to that in Reiter's syndrome, occur in 10 per cent to 30 per cent of clients with PsA.

Soft-tissue involvement occurs often in PsA. Enthesitis, or inflammation at the site of tendon insertion or muscle attachment to bone, is frequently observed at the Achilles tendon, plantar fascia, and pelvic bones. Also common are tenosynovitis of the flexor tendons of the hands, extensor carpi ulnaris, and other sites.

Dactylitis, which occurs in more than one third of PsA clients, is marked by diffuse swelling of the whole finger. Inflammation in this typical "sausage finger" extends to the tendon sheaths and adjacent joints.

Extraarticular features similar to those seen in clients with other seronegative spondyloarthropathies are frequently seen. These extraarticular lesions include iritis, mouth ulcers, urethritis, and less commonly, colitis and aortic valve disease.

▼ *Clinical Signs and Symptoms of*
Psoriatic Arthritis

- Fever
- Fatigue
- Nail bed changes
- Polyarthritis
- Psoriasis
- Sore fingers (sometimes sausage-like swelling)

Diagnosis. Seronegativity for rheumatoid factor used to be required for a diagnosis of PsA. However, because rheumatoid factor is present in the serum of more than 10 per cent of clients with uncomplicated psoriasis and in up to 15 per cent of healthy persons, PsA may be more accurately described as usually seronegative.

Presently, the diagnosis of PsA is based on both clinical and x-ray observations. Diagnosis is difficult in the absence of skin involvement, although not all people with psoriasis and arthritis have PsA. The skin disease may simply coexist with RA, osteoarthritis, arthritis associated with inflammatory bowel disease, or gout.

There are no specific laboratory tests for psoriasis or the arthritis associated with it. The pattern of joint involvement and tenderness, along with extraarticular features, is often helpful to the physician in distinguishing PsA from other disorders.

Prognosis and Treatment. In the past, PsA was believed to follow a relatively benign course, but it is now recognized that as many as 20 per cent of clients may sustain early and severe joint damage, with accompanying deformity and disability (Gladman et al., 1987).

Early treatment aimed at controlling inflammation is essential because inflammation is the major pathogenetic factor in PsA. Client education about the disease, the need for joint protection, and ergonomics is an important part of physical therapy.

Systemic treatment with NSAIDs is initiated; exacerbation of psoriasis necessitates a change in medications. If the arthritis does not respond to treatment with NSAIDs, other agents such as intramuscular gold compounds, sulfasalazine, methotrexate, and antimalarials may be introduced (Gladman, 1992; Gladman et al., 1992).

Infectious Arthritis (Williams, 1993)

Infectious agents are the known or suspected cause of a number of rheumatologic disorders, including *disseminated gonoccocal infection* causing multiple painful swollen joints, *Lyme disease,* in which a spirochetal infection may lead to an acute and then chronic systemic disease, and *acute rheumatic fever* associated with a β-hemolytic streptococcal organism. Other examples of arthritis associated with infection include polyarthritis associated with hepatitis B and parvovirus infection.

Acute rheumatic fever is discussed in Chapter 3 and will not be repeated in this chapter. General principles regarding arthritis as a direct result of infection, disseminated gonoccocal infection, and Lyme disease are included in this section.

In other forms of arthritis such as Reiter's syndrome, AS, SLE, MCTD, and PM/DM, the connection between arthritis and a presumed infection-induced triggering event is more tenuous. For this reason, these forms of arthritic conditions are covered earlier in this chapter under a different category.

General Principles

Arithritis as a direct result of infection is one of the most common musculoskeletal system disorders encountered in general medicine. The client presents with high fever, chills, an elevated white blood cell count, and general sepsis. There is usually a single painful, swollen joint, most often a knee, ankle, elbow, or shoulder. Aspirated synovial fluid is cloudy yellow or sometimes green or slightly bloody, and blood or synovial fluid culture is positive for staphylococci or pneumonococci.

Septic arthritis is seen frequently in elderly or debilitated clients and in clients who have diabetes or another disorder associated with immune suppression, such as RA or chronic renal failure, or following renal transplantation.

Disseminated Gonococcal Infection

Clients with acute disseminated gonococcal infection may present with high fever, sepsis, characteristic skin lesions near the anatomic region of joint involvement, oligoarthritis, and, frequently, localized manifestations of tenosynovitis.

Lyme Disease (Schoen and Rahn, 1991; U.S. Department of Health and Human Services, 1992)

In the early 1970s, a mysterious clustering of juvenile arthritis occurred among children in Lyme, Connecticut, and in surrounding towns. Medical researchers soon recognized the illness as a distinct disease, which they called Lyme disease. They were able to identify the deer tick infected with a spiral bacterium or spirochete (later named *Borrelia burgdorferi*) as the key to its spread.

Incidence. The number of reported cases of Lyme disease, as well as the number of geographic areas in which it is found, has been increasing. More than 40,000 Americans have now been diagnosed with Lyme disease. Lyme disease has been reported in nearly all of the United States, although most cases are concentrated in the coastal northeast, the mid-Atlantic states, Wisconsin, Minnesota, Oregon, and northern California. Children may be more susceptible simply because they spend more time outdoors and are more likely to be exposed to ticks.

The risk of Lyme disease exposure is seasonally limited by the tick's life cycle, the tick being more active during the spring and summer. The adult female, which also can transmit the disease, is active in the fall and on warm winter days. Migratory birds can spread Lyme disease by carrying infected ticks to areas where the disease was not previously endemic (Anderson, 1988).

Clinical Signs and Symptoms. In most people, the first symptom of Lyme disease is a red rash known as *erythema migrans* that starts as a small red spot that expands over a period of days or weeks, forming a circular, triangular, or oval rash. Sometimes the rash resembles a bull's eye because it appears as a red ring surrounding a central clear area. The rash can range in size from that of a dime to the entire width of a person's back, appearing within a few weeks of a tick bite and usually at the site of the bite, which is often the axilla or groin. As infection spreads, several rashes can appear at different sites on the body.

Erythema migrans is often accompanied by flu-like symptoms such as fever, headache, stiff neck, body aches, and fatigue. Although these symptoms resemble those of common viral infections, Lyme disease symptoms tend to persist or may occur intermittently over a period of several weeks to months.

Arthritis appears after several months after infection with *B. burgdorferi*. Slightly more than half of the people who are not treated with antibiotics develop recurrent attacks of painful and swollen joints that last a few days to a few months. About 10 per cent to 20 per cent of untreated clients will go on to develop chronic arthritis.

In most clients, Lyme arthritis is monoarticular or oligoarticular (few joints), most commonly affecting the knee, but the arthritis can shift from one joint to another. Other large joints, such as the shoulder and elbow, are also commonly affected. Involvement of the hands and feet is uncommon, and it is these features that help differentiate Lyme arthritis from RA.

Neurologic symptoms can appear because Lyme disease can affect the nervous system. Symptoms include stiff neck, severe headache associated with meningitis, Bell's palsy, numbness, pain or weakness in the limbs, or poor motor coordination. Memory loss, difficulty in concentrating, mood changes, and sleep disturbances have also been associated with Lyme disease.

Nervous system involvement can develop several weeks, months, or even years following an untreated infection. These symptoms last for weeks or months and may recur.

Cardiac involvement occurs in less than 1 per cent of the people affected by Lyme disease. Symptoms of irregular heartbeat, dizziness, and dyspnea occur several weeks

▼ *Clinical Signs and Symptoms of*
Lyme Disease

Early infection (one or more may be present at different times during infection)

■ Red rash

■ Flu-like symptoms (fever, headache, stiff neck, myalgias, fatigue)

■ Neurologic symptoms:
  ■ Severe headache (meningitis)
  ■ Bell's palsy
  ■ Numbness, pain, weakness of extremities
  ■ Poor motor coordination
  ■ Cognitive dysfunction: memory loss, difficulty in concentrating, mood changes, sleep disturbances

Less Common Symptoms

■ Eye problems such as conjunctivitis

■ Heart abnormalities and myocarditis

Late Infection

■ Arthritis, intermittent or chronic

---

after the infection and rarely last more than a few days or weeks. Recovery is usually complete (Steere et al., 1980).

Finally, although Lyme disease can be divided into early and later stages, each with a different set of complications, they may vary in duration, may overlap, or may even be absent. Clinical manifestations may first appear from 3 to 30 days after the tick bite but usually occur within 1 week (Steere et al., 1983).

Diagnosis. Lyme disease is still mistaken for other ailments, including Guillain-Barré, syndrome, multiple sclerosis, and fibromyalgia syndrome, and can be difficult to diagnose. The only distinctive hallmark unique to Lyme disease, the erythema migrans rash, is absent in at least one fourth of the people who become infected. Many people are unaware that they have been bitten by a tick.

Because some tests cannot distinguish Lyme disease antibodies from antibodies to similar organisms, clients may test positive for Lyme disease when their symptoms actually stem from other bacterial infections.

Unfortunately, the Lyme disease microbe itself is difficult to isolate or culture from body tissues or fluids. Most physicians look for evidence of antibodies against *B. burgdorferi* in the blood. In the first few weeks following infection, antibody tests are not reliable because a person's immune system has not produced enough antibodies to be detected. Antibiotics given early during infection also may prevent antibodies from reaching detectable levels. New methods to detect infection using highly sensitive genetic engineering techniques eventually may result in more accurate diagnosis.

Prognosis and Treatment. Nearly all people with Lyme disease can be effectively treated with an appropriate course of antibiotic therapy. In general, the sooner treatment is initiated, the quicker and more complete the recovery with less chance for the development of subsequent symptoms of arthritis and neurologic problems. Lyme disease can be difficult to treat in its later phases, and its prevention through the development of an effective vaccine is hampered by the elusive nature of the bacterium.

Lyme arthritis may be treated with oral antibiotics. In the case of severe arthritis, intravenous medications may be prescribed. To ease these clients' discomfort and further their healing, the physician may also give antiinflammatory drugs, draw fluid from affected joints, or surgically perform synovectomy (removal of the inflamed lining of the joints).

Following treatment for Lyme disease, some people still have persistent fatigue and achiness, which can take months to subside. Unfortunately, a bout with Lyme disease is no guarantee that the illness will be prevented in the future. The disease can strike more than once in the same individual if she or he is reinfected with the Lyme disease bacterium.

Avoiding deer ticks by avoiding areas of high grass and thick underbrush, minimizing skin exposure by wearing long, tucked-in, light-colored clothing, using repellents that contain a chemical called DEET (*N,N*-diethyl-M-toluamide), careful washing of clothes and body, and checking for ticks on all people and pets before going inside are the keys to prevention.

Case Example. A 54-year-old business executive developed searing neck and back pain and was diagnosed as having a cervical disc protrusion. He was sent to physical therapy but had a very busy travel schedule and was unable to make even half of his scheduled appointments.

He chose to discontinue physical therapy, until his symptoms worsened and the pain became so intense that he was unable to go to work some mornings. He also started experiencing numbness in his right arm along the ulnar nerve distribution. After a lengthy trial of physical therapy, there was no discernible improvement subjectively by client report or objectively as measured by functional improvement.

Anterior cervical discectomy was performed to remove the fifth cervical disc but with no change in symptoms postoperatively. There was significant right extremity paresis, with maximal functional loss of the right hand and continued neck and back pain.

This client was eventually discharged from further physical therapy services and underwent a second surgical procedure with no improvement in his condition. A year later, he telephoned the therapist to report that he had been diagnosed with Lyme disease. This man spent his vacations in the woods of Connecticut and Long Island, but this important piece of information was never gleaned from his past medical history.

Despite the lengthy time before diagnosis, the client was almost entirely recovered and ready to return to work after completing a course of antibiotics.

Bacterial Arthritis (Phillips and Goldberger, 1990)

Bacterial arthritis can be caused by a wide variety of organisms, including gonococci, staphylococci, streptococci, enterobacteria, *Pseudomonas* species, and *Haemophilus influenzae.* In most clients, bacterial arthritis begins with infection, such as sinusitis, bedsores, pneumonia, or septicemia, or an abdominal or genitourinary tract infection. The bacteria travel through the bloodstream and eventually invade and infect the synovium. Occasionally, bacterial arthritis results from a penetrating injury (including arthrocentesis) or from an infection in the periarticular tissues.

Many clients with bacterial arthritis have been immunocompromised by severe illness, particularly neoplasm, or by treatment with immunosuppressive drugs such as corticosteroids or cytotoxic agents.

Chronic arthritis in any form, especially RA, predisposes the joint to bacterial arthritis. Other predisposing factors include previous joint surgery, especially if a plastic or metal prosthesis has been implanted, and injection drug abuse.

Clinical Signs and Symptoms. Bacterial arthritis is typically monoarticular, begins abruptly, and is characterized by inflammatory symptoms of pain and swelling. Symptoms progressively worsen in 12 to 48 hours. In later stages, the infected joint is usually tender, warm, swollen, and red. Both active and passive motions are painful and almost always limited.

▼ *Clinical Signs and Symptoms of*
Bacterial Arthritis

- Constitutional symptoms, especially fever
- Monoarticular (single joint) involvement
- Inflammatory symptoms: redness, warmth, pain, swelling

Large joints, particularly the knee but also the shoulder, elbow, wrist, ankle, and hip, are affected more often than the small joints of the hands and feet. Infection can occur in the spine, with poorly localized back pain as the initial symptom. The sternoclavicular and sacroiliac joints often become infected in injection drug users.

Diagnosis. Symptoms are easily confused with those of other rheumatic diseases, making diagnosis difficult for the physician. Physical examination and synovial fluid analysis are the keys to diagnosis. X-ray films, arthrocentesis, and cultures of blood and other substances are the three most helpful diagnostic tools.

Prognosis and Treatment. Left untreated, bacterial arthritis causes cartilage and bone damage that can proceed rapidly to total joint destruction within a few weeks. Immediate hospitalization and parenteral antibiotic therapy are appropriate for most clients; treatment also includes joint aspiration, analgesics, and physical therapy, beginning in the acute phase to help control pain. As soon as the inflammation begins to resolve and the joint can be moved with relatively little pain, passive range of motion exercise is started, progressing to active range of motion exercise. With proper care, the prognosis for recovery with no residual joint damage is good.

Nonspecific Rheumatic Disorders

Fibromyalgia (Fibrositis*) Syndrome
(Fibromyalgia Network, 1992)

Fibromyalgia syndrome (FMS) is a condition presenting with generalized musculoskeletal pain in conjunction with tenderness to touch in a large number of specific areas of the body and an array of asso-

---

* The term *fibrositis* has now been officially replaced by the term *fibromyalgia*, which was introduced in 1981 (Wolfe et al., 1990; Yunus et al., 1981).

ciated symptoms, including sleep disturbance and fatigue (Harvey et al., 1993).

There is still much controversy over the exact nature of FMS and even debate over whether fibromyalgia is an organic disease with abnormal biochemical or immunologic pathology (Hunder et al., 1993). There is no doubt that FMS exists as a clinical musculoskeletal pain syndrome. Current theories suggest it may be genetically transferred as an autosomal dominant trait, characterized by neurohormonal imbalances that may be triggered by viral infection, traumatic event, or stress (Goldenberg, 1990). Because the field of FMS research is constantly changing, FMS is included here as a nonspecific category until a definitive answer is derived scientifically.

Fibromyalgia has been differentiated from myofascial pain in that FMS is considered a systemic problem with multiple tender points as one of the key symptoms. Myofascial pain is a localized condition specific to a muscle and may involve as few as one or several areas (Yunus et al., 1988).

The hallmark of myofascial pain syndrome is a trigger point, as opposed to tender points in FMS. Both disorders cause myalgia with aching pain and tenderness and exhibit similar local histologic changes in the muscle. Painful symptoms in both conditions are increased with activity, although fibromyalgia is more generalized aching whereas myofascial pain is more direct and localized (Wolfe, 1988).

Incidence. The prevalence of fibromyalgia is not well documented, in part because of a lack of consensus as to what constitutes the condition (Harvey et al., 1993). Up to 5 per cent of the general population may have FMS (Nies, 1992); Goldenberg (1989a) estimates that 6 million Americans have this condition. Clinical data indicate that it is a common diagnosis in rheumatologic practice (Goldenberg, 1988).

The condition is much more common in women than in men, reportedly occurring in women in from 73 per cent to 87 per cent of cases (Campbell et al., 1983; Goldenberg, 1989a). The age range of clients is 14 to 68 years, although it is rare in the elderly (Forseth and Gran, 1992; Harvey et al., 1993).

Pathogenesis. There are numerous theories, but no conclusive cause, for the development of FMS. The common hypotheses are presented here. For example, abnormal production of growth hormone in FMS may provide the link between the commonly described sleep disturbance in this client group and the widespread muscular pain. Eighty per cent of the body's growth hormone is secreted by the pituitary gland (under hypothalamic control) during deep level sleep, and it is crucial for normal muscle metabolism and tissue repair (Bennett et al., 1992).

Two separate reports have demonstrated that many FMS clients have a blunted response to thyrotropin-releasing hormone (Ferraccioli, 1990; Neeck and Riedel, 1992). Thyrotropin-releasing hormone is released by the hypothalamus to signal the pituitary gland to secrete thyroid-stimulating hormone, which regulates the thyroid's metabolic functions (e.g., body temperature, body weight). Standard laboratory tests of baseline thyroid-stimulating hormone, T3, and T4 tend to come out low-to-normal in FMS clients, but the function of the hypothalamic-pituitary-thyroid-axis seems impaired. Hypothyroidism is common in clients with FMS.

Other conditions or syndromes have been found to occur in association with FMS, including mitral valve prolapse, temporomandibular joint dysfunction syndrome, and chronic fatigue syndrome (CFS). It is possible that FMS and CFS are two names for the same syndrome. At present, CFS is thought to differ by the greater degree of fatigue, whereas clients with FMS tend to demonstrate more pain. Abnormal serotonin metabolism has been implicated in many of these syndromes (Pellegrino et al., 1989; Yunus et al., 1989).

The role of neurotransmitters such as serotonin, substance P, epinephrine, and norepinephrine has been studied in relation to FMS. Serotonin, a biogenic amine or central nervous system neurotransmitter that is made from tryptophan (an essential amino acid obtained from our diet), is necessary for restorative sleep and is also known to play a role in pain control, immune system function, vascular constriction/dilation, and even emotions that may contribute to such feelings as depression or anxiety. Several studies have found the concentration of serotonin end-products (metabolites) to be lower than normal in clients with FMS (Russell, 1989; Russell et al., 1990).

Another neurotransmitter that may be a key to FMS is substance P, a neuropeptide believed to play a role in the transmission of nociceptive information. Elevated levels of substance P have been found in the cerebrospinal fluid of FMS clients, resulting in an exaggerated response to normal stimuli (Vaeroy et al., 1988). Vaeroy has also examined the production of opioids in the cerebrospinal fluid of 37 FMS clients. The concentrations of both prodynorphin and proenkephalin-derived peptides were found to be elevated at the opioid receptors in the central nervous system (Vaeroy et al., 1991).

Vaeroy hypothesized that this apparent opioid hypersecretion could lead to receptor desensitization, which would lessen the capacity for pain modulation. When serotonin levels are low, substance P may exert an amplified effect on pain.

Pain is often associated with inflammation. In the case of FMS, muscle biopsy studies have failed to demonstrate an inflammatory process. Other muscle abnormalities, such as lower-than-normal ATP at the trigger point sites (Bengtsson et al., 1986) and uneven oxygen distribution in the muscles (Lund et al., 1986), have been reported.

The exercising muscle blood flow has been shown to be abnormally low in FMS even when compared with matched sedentary controls. The aerobic capacity of FMS clients is below the norm (Bennett et al., 1989; McCluskey et al., 1990). This is not a surprising finding, because these clients present with fatigue and pain and often report increased muscular pain after exercise, resulting in a downward spiral of deconditioning (Bennett, 1989a).

Researchers are currently determining the role of viruses, yeasts, parasites, and bacteria in the development of FMS. The basis of most viral theories was the discovery that cancer clients temporarily develop FMS (or CFS) while they receive treatment with interleukin-II and alpha-interferon. These two compounds, called cytokines, are chemicals produced by the immune system when the body is fighting an infection. Overproduction of interleukins (the IL-1 beta inhibitory theory) has been documented to cause musculoskeletal pain, fatigue, memory problems, and other symptoms and may be involved in the pathogenesis of CFS/FMS (Wallace, 1989).

Clinical Signs and Symptoms. The core features of FMS include widespread pain lasting more than 3 months and widespread local tenderness in all clients. Fatigue, morning stiffness, and sleep disturbance with nonrefreshed awakening may be present but are not necessary for the diagnosis.

Any or all of these symptoms are found in 75 per cent of the clients. Twenty-five per cent or more of the clients may have irritable bowel syndrome, Raynaud's phenomenon, headache, a subjective sensation of swelling, paresthesias, psychologic dysfunction, and/or functional disability (Hartman, 1993). Symptoms are aggravated by cold, stress, excessive or no exercise, and physical activity ("overdoing it"), including overstretching, and may be improved by warmth or heat, rest, and exercise, including gentle stretching.

Sleep disturbances in stage 4 of nonrapid eye movement sleep (needed for healing of muscle tissues), sleep apnea, difficulty getting to sleep or staying asleep, nocturnal myoclonus (involuntary arm and leg jerks), and bruxism (teeth grinding) cause clients with FMS to wake up feeling unrested and unrefreshed as if they had never gone to sleep (Hamm et al., 1989).

▼ *Clinical Signs and Symptoms of*
Fibromyalgia Syndrome

- Fatigue
- Sleep disturbances
- Tender points on palpation
- Myalgias (generalized aching)
- Tendinitis
- Cold-induced vasospasm (hypersensitivity to cold; Raynaud's phenomenon)
- Dyspnea
- Headache
- Morning stiffness (more than 15 minutes)
- Paresthesia (numbness and tingling)
- Subjective swelling
- Irritable bowel symptoms
- Urinary urgency
- Dry eyes/mouth
- Depression/anxiety
- Hypothermia (mild decrease in core body temperature)
- Premenstrual syndrome (PMS)

Stage 4 sleep disturbances are characterized by an alpha-wave intrusion pattern superimposed on slow-wave delta sleep. It has been hypothesized that this sleep anomaly may interfere with the release of a growth hormone that is also thought to play a role in restorative sleep (Bennett, 1989b). Delta-wave sleep (non-REM) is required for replenishment of the muscles. Deficiency of delta-wave sleep reduces the amount of time that muscles enter a state of resting muscle tone. The alpha-EEG anomaly is not unique to FMS and has been observed in many clients with RA, osteoarthritis, and other painful rheumatic diseases (Moldofsky, 1989).

Diagnosis. In 1990, a multicenter criteria

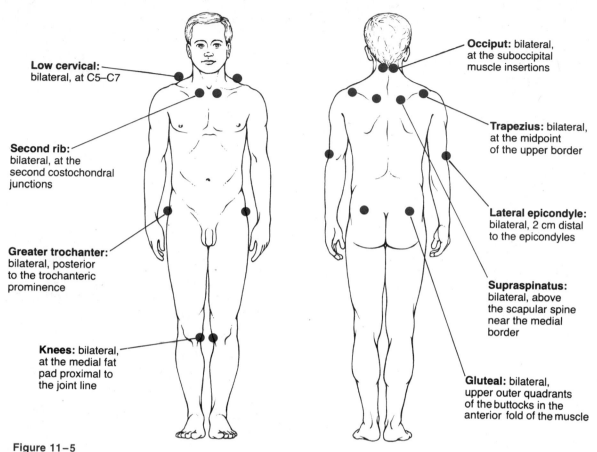

Low cervical: bilateral, at C5–C7

Second rib: bilateral, at the second costochondral junctions

Greater trochanter: bilateral, posterior to the trochanteric prominence

Knees: bilateral, at the medial fat pad proximal to the joint line

Occiput: bilateral, at the suboccipital muscle insertions

Trapezius: bilateral, at the midpoint of the upper border

Lateral epicondyle: bilateral, 2 cm distal to the epicondyles

Supraspinatus: bilateral, above the scapular spine near the medial border

Gluteal: bilateral, upper outer quadrants of the buttocks in the anterior fold of the muscle

Figure 11–5

Anatomic locations of tender points associated with fibromyalgia, according to the American College of Rheumatology 1990 classification for fibromyalgia.

committee of the American College of Rheumatology published the most current criteria for the diagnosis of fibromyalgia (see American College of Rheumatology 1990 Criteria for the Classification of Fibromyalgia; also Fig. 11–5). Although all investigators include generalized body pain and the prescribed number of tender points to palpation as necessary for the diagnosis, some stress the presence of associated symptoms as essential (Campbell et al., 1983; Clark et al., 1985; Wolfe, 1989).

Numerous other diseases and conditions may present with pain, tender points, and some of the symptoms commonly asso-

ciated with fibromyalgia, making this a diagnosis of exclusion. The American College of Rheumatology recommends that the diagnosis be made on the basis of the clinical presentation of the client alone and does not differentiate whether the condition is primary or secondary to another underlying disease (Wolfe et al., 1990).

Other researchers recommend screening laboratory testing for all clients with possible fibromyalgia. These tests include a complete blood count, sedimentation rate, and creatinine phosphokinase and thyroid-stimulating hormone levels. When the chemical presentation warrants it, rheuma-

---

AMERICAN COLLEGE OF RHEUMATOLOGY 1990 CRITERIA FOR THE CLASSIFICATION OF FIBROMYALGIA*

HISTORY OF WIDESPREAD PAIN

DEFINITION: Pain is considered widespread when all the following are present:

■ Pain in the left side of the body

■ Pain in the right side of the body

■ Pain above the waist

■ Pain below the waist

■ Axial skeletal pain (cervical spine, anterior chest, thoracic spine, or low back)

In this definition, shoulder and buttock pain is considered pain for each involved side. "Low back" pain is considered lower segment pain.

PAIN IN 11 OF 18 TENDER POINTS ON DIGITAL PALPATION†

DEFINITION: Pain on digital palpation must be present in at least 11 of the following 18 tender point sites:

■ Occiput: Bilateral, at the suboccipital muscle insertions

■ Low cervical: Bilateral, at the anterior aspects of the intertransverse spaces at C_5-C_7

■ Trapezius: Bilateral, at the midpoint of the upper border

■ Supraspinatus: Bilateral, at origins, above the scapular spine near the medial border

■ Second rib: Bilateral, at the second costochondral junctions, just lateral to the junctions on upper surfaces

■ Lateral epicondyle: Bilateral, 2 cm distal to the epicondyles

■ Gluteal: Bilateral, in upper outer quadrants of buttocks in anterior fold of muscle

■ Greater trochanter: Bilateral, posterior to the trochanteric prominence

■ Knees: Bilateral, at the medial fat pad proximal to the joint line

---

* For classification purposes, clients are said to have fibromyalgia if both criteria are satisfied. Widespread pain must be present for at least 3 months. The presence of a second clinical disorder does not exclude the diagnosis of fibromyalgia.

† Digital palpation should be performed with an approximate force of 4 kg (approximately the pressure to indent a tennis ball.) For a tender point to be considered positive, the subject must state that the palpation was "painful:" a reply of "tender" is not to be considered painful.

From Wolfe, F., et al.: The American College of Rheumatology 1990 criteria for the classification of fibromyalgia. Arthritis and Rheumatism *33:*160–172, 1990.

---

toid factor, antinuclear antibodies, calcium, growth hormone, conventional radiography, or scintigraphy should be checked (Bennett, 1989c; Goldenberg, 1990).

Prognosis and Treatment. The prognosis for recovery from FMS is poor, with most clients experiencing symptoms for their lifetime. Self-management of symptoms is

▼ *Differential Diagnosis of*
Fibromyalgia*

- Hypothyroidism
- Polymyalgia rheumatica/giant cell arteritis
- Rheumatoid arthritis
- Polymyositis/dermatomyositis
- Systemic lupus erythematosus
- Myofascial pain syndrome
- Metabolic myopathy (e.g., alcohol)
- Neurosis (depression/anxiety)
- Metastatic cancer
- Chronic fatigue syndrome
- Temporomandibular joint dysfunction

* Adapted from Harvey, C.K., et al.: Fibromyalgia. Part 1. Review of the literature. Journal of the American Podiatric Medical Association. *83*(7):413, 1993.

the cornerstone of treatment. Approaches to helping clients with FMS must be multidisciplinary and include education and support, stress management and life style training (including psychotherapy, coping strategies, and applying ergonomic principles), medications,* including analgesics and antidepressants as needed, local modalities and techniques for pain and trigger point management, and carefully graded consistent exercise (both aerobic and conditioning) per client tolerance.

Often, the client's condition will not tolerate exercise immediately; exercise at the right time and in the right amount is an essential element of the treatment program. Although it is understandable that these clients may not want to exercise because of fatigue and pain, the prognosis is greatly improved if they do so (McCain et al.,

---

* The use of low-dose tricyclic antidepressants at night in an attempt to modulate the sleep disturbance has been effective (Carette et al., 1986; Goldenberg, 1989b).

1988). The therapist is a key person in educating the client about the importance and difficulty of proceeding with an exercise regimen, encouraging the gradual development of conditioning.

PHYSICIAN REFERRAL

In most immunologic disorders, physicians must rely on the client's history and clinical findings in association with supportive information from diagnostic tests to make a differential diagnosis. Often, there are no definitive diagnostic tests, such as in the case of multiple sclerosis. The physician relies instead on objectively measured central nervous system abnormalities, a history of episodic exacerbations, and remissions of symptoms with progressive worsening of symptoms over time (O'Toole, 1992).

In other situations, such as with dermatomyositis, various tests may be used by the physician in conjunction with the presence of the characteristic skin rash and proximal muscle weakness to determine the diagnosis.

In the early stages of treating disorders like multiple sclerosis, Guillain-Barré syndrome, and myositis, factors such as the effect of fatigue on the client's progress and fragile muscle fibers necessitate that the physical therapist keep close contact with the physician, who will use a physical examination and laboratory tests to determine the most opportune time for an exercise program. While the physician is monitoring serum enzyme levels and the overall medical status of the client, the physical therapist will continue to provide the physician with essential feedback regarding objective findings, such as muscle tenderness, muscle strength, and overall physical endurance.

A careful history and close clinical observations may elicit indications that the client is demonstrating signs and symptoms unrelated to a musculoskeletal disorder. Because the immune system can implicate many of the body systems, the physical therapist should not hesitate to relay to the physician any unusual findings reported or observed.

Clinical Signs and Symptoms Requiring Physician Referral

Anaphylactic reaction

Ataxia

Bowel/bladder dysfunction

Calcinosis

Change in voice

Choking, difficulty in chewing

Chronic diarrhea

Dry eyes/mouth

Dysarthria

Dysphagia

Dyspnea on exertion

Easy bruising

Enlarged lymph nodes

Fatigue

Fever, malaise

Finger ulceration

Headache

Heartburn

Hoarseness

Incoordination

Increased deep tendon reflexes

Joint inflammation

Loss of appetite

Morning stiffness

Muscle fatigue with exertion

Myalgia

Myositis (inflamed muscle)

Nausea, vomiting

Night sweats

Paresthesias

Persistent, dry cough

Polyarthralgia

Positive Babinski/clonus

Progressive dyspnea

Proximal muscle weakness

Ptosis

Raynaud's phenomenon

Recurrent influenza-like symptoms

Skin rash or thickening

Sleep disturbances

Spasticity

Speech impairment

Subcutaneous nodules

Tender points

Thrush in the mouth/tongue

Vertigo

Visual disturbances (diplopia, nystagmus, scotomas)

Weight loss

Wheals

 Key Points to Remember

■ Pain in the knees, hands, wrists, or elbows may indicate an autoimmune disorder; aching in the bones can be caused by expanding bone marrow.

■ Any change in cough, pain, or fever, or any change or new presentation of symptoms, should be reported to the physician.

■ Physical therapists in every clinical setting must be familiar with universal precautions (see Appendix to Chapter 8).

■ Be alert to any warning signs of hypersensitivity response (allergic reaction) during therapy and be prepared to take necessary measures (e.g., graded exercise to client tolerance, control of room temperature, client use of medications).

■ Immediate emergency procedures are required when a client has a severe allergic reaction (anaphylactic shock).

■ For the client with Guillain-Barré syndrome, active exercise must be at a level consistent with the client's muscle strength. Overstretching and overuse of painful muscles may result in prolonged or lack of recovery.

■ For the client with multiple sclerosis, treatment should take place in the coolest (temperature) setting possible.

■ For the client with early stage myositis, muscle fibers are fragile and could be damaged further by exercises and other forms of physical therapy. Maintain close contact with the physician for laboratory test results to determine the most opportune time for each level of the exercise program.

■ For the client with ankylosing spondylitis, the risk of fracture from even minor trauma and the development of atlantoaxial subluxation necessitate the use of extreme caution in treatment procedures. The most common site of fracture is the lower cervical spine.

SUBJECTIVE EXAMINATION *Special Questions to Ask*

Signs and symptoms of immune disorders can appear in any body system. A thorough review of the Family/Personal History form, subjective interview, and appropriate follow-up questions will help the physical therapist identify signs and symptoms that are not part of a musculoskeletal pattern. Special attention should be given to the question on the Family/Personal History form concerning general health. Clients with immune disorders often have poor general health or recurrent infections.

■ Have you ever been told that you had/have an immune disorder, autoimmune disease, or cancer? (Predisposes the person to other diseases)

■ Have you ever received radiation treatment? (Diminishes blood cell production, predisposes to infection)

■ Have you ever had an organ transplant (especially kidney) or removal of your thymus? **(Myasthenia gravis)**

■ Do you have difficulty with combing your hair, raising your arms, getting out of a bathtub, bed, or chair, or climbing stairs? **(Polymyositis, dermatomyositis, myasthenia gravis)**

■ Do you have difficulty when raising your head from the pillow when you are lying down on your back? **(Polymyositis, dermatomyositis, myasthenia gravis)**

■ Do you have difficulty with swallowing or have you noticed any changes in your voice? **(Polymyositis, dermatomyositis, myasthenia gravis)**

■ Do you have any trouble taking a deep breath? **(Weak chest muscles secondary to polymyositis, dermatomyositis, myasthenia gravis)**

■ Have you noticed any changes in your skin texture or pigmentation? Do you have any skin rashes? **(Scleroderma, allergic reactions, SLE, RA, dermatomyositis, psoriatic arthritis, AIDS, Lyme disease)**

  ■ Have you noticed any association between the development of the skin rash and pain or swelling in any of your joints (or other symptoms)?

  ■ Do these other symptoms go away when the skin rash clears up?

  ■ Have you been exposed to ticks? For example, have you been out walking in the woods or in tall grass or in contact with pets? **(Lyme disease)**

■ Have you had any recent vision problems? **(Multiple sclerosis, SLE)**

■ Have you had any difficulties with urination, for example, a change in appearance of urine, accidents, increased frequency? **(Multiple sclerosis, myasthenia gravis)**

For the person with known allergies (check the Family/Personal History form):

■ What are the usual symptoms that you experience in association with your allergies?

■ Describe a typical allergic reaction for you.

■ Do the symptoms relate to physical changes (e.g., cold, heat, or dampness)?

■ Do the symptoms occur in association with activities (e.g., exercise)?

■ Do you take medication for your allergies?

For the client reporting fatigue and weakness:

■ Do you feel tired all the time or only after exertion?

■ Do you get short of breath after mild exercise or at rest?

■ How much sleep do you get at night?

■ Do you take naps during the day?

■ Have you ever been told by a physician that you are anemic?

■ How long have you had this weakness?

■ Does it come and go or is it persistent (there all the time)?

■ Are you able to perform your usual daily activities without stopping to rest or nap?

For the client with fever (fevers recurring every few days, fevers that rise and fall within 24 hours, and fevers that recur frequently should be documented and reported to the physician):

■ When did you first notice this fever?

■ Is it constant or does it come and go?

■ Does your temperature fluctuate?

   If yes, over what period of time does this occur?

Fibromyalgia Syndrome (FMS) Screen

1) Do you have trouble sleeping through the night?	YES	NO
2) Do you feel rested in the morning?	YES	NO
3) Are you stiff and sore in the morning?	YES	NO
4) Do you have daytime fatigue/exhaustion?	YES	NO
5) Do your muscle pain and soreness travel?	YES	NO
6) Do you have tension/migraine headaches?	YES	NO
7) Do you have irritable bowel symptoms (e.g., nausea, diarrhea, stomach cramping)?	YES	NO

Continued on following page

8) Do you have swelling, numbness, or tingling in your arms   YES   NO
   or legs?

9) Are you sensitive to temperature and humidity or changes   YES   NO
   in the weather?

CASE STUDY

REFERRAL

A 28-year-old Hispanic man has come to you for an evaluation without a medical referral. He has seen no medical practitioner for his current symptoms that consist of an unusual gait pattern and weakness of the lower extremities, which he noticed during the last 2 days. He speaks English with a heavy accent, making it difficult to obtain a clear medical history, but the Personal/Family History form indicates no previous or current health or medical problems of any kind. He does note that he has had influenza in the last 3 weeks, but that he is fully recovered now.

PHYSICAL THERAPY INTERVIEW

Using the format outlined in the chapter on *The Physical Therapy Interview*, begin with an open-ended question and follow up with additional appropriate questions incorporating the following:

Current Symptoms

Tell me why you are here (open-ended question) . . . or you may prefer to say, "I notice from your intake form that you have had some weakness in your legs and a change in the way you walk. What can you tell me about this?"

When did you first notice these changes?

What did you notice that made you think that something was happening?

Just before the development of these symptoms, did you injure yourself in any way that you can remember?

Did you have a car accident, fall down, or twist your trunk or hips in any unusual way?

Do you have any pain in your back, hips, or legs? If yes, follow the outline in *The Physical Therapy Interview* to elicit a further description.

Associated Symptoms

Have you had any numbness or tingling in your back, buttocks, or hips or down your legs?

Have you had any other changes in sensation in these areas, such as a burning or prickling feeling?

■ ■ ■ ■ ■ ■ ■ ■ ■ ■ ■ ■

Have you had the "flu," a cold, an upper respiratory infection, or other infection recently?

Have you had a fever or elevated temperature in the last 48 hours?

Do you think that you have a temperature right now?

Have you noticed any other symptoms that I should know about?

> Give the client time to answer the question. Prompt him if you need to with various suggestions (include any others that seem appropriate to the information and responses already given by the client), such as

Nausea or dizziness

Diarrhea or constipation

Unusual fatigue

Recent headaches

Choking, difficulty with chewing

Shortness of breath with mild exertion (e.g., walking to the car or even at rest)

Vomiting

Cold sweats during the day or night

Changes in vision or speech

Skin rashes

Joint pains

Have you noticed any other respiratory, lung, or breathing problems?

Final Question

Is there anything else you think that I should know about your current condition or general health that I have not asked yet?

PROCEDURES TO CARRY OUT DURING THE FIRST SESSION

Given the client's report of lower extremity weakness and antalgic gait of sudden onset without precipitating cause, the following possible problems should be ruled out during the objective assessment:

Neurologic disease or disorder (immunologically based or otherwise), such as:

Discogenic lesion

Tumor

Myasthenia gravis (unlikely due to the man's age)

Guillain-Barré syndrome

Multiple sclerosis

■ ■ ■ ■ ■ ■   ■ ■ ■ ■ ■ ■

Other possible immunologic disorders

AIDS dementia (unlikely from the way the history was presented)

Psychogenic disorder (e.g., hysteria, anxiety, alcoholism, or drug addiction)

Observation/Inspection

- Take the client's vital signs
- Note any obvious changes, such as muscle atrophy, difficulty with breathing or swallowing, facial paralysis, intention tremor
- Describe the gait pattern: Observe for ataxia, incoordination, positive Trendelenburg position, balance, patterns of muscular weakness or imbalance, other gait deviations

Neurologic Screen

- All deep tendon reflexes
- Manual muscle testing of proximal-to-distal large muscle groups looking for a pattern of weakness
- Babinski sign and clonus
- Gross sensory screen looking for any differences in perceived sensation from one side to the other
- Test for dysmetria, balance, and coordination

Orthopedic Assessment

- Lower extremity range of motion (ROM): active and passive
- Back, lower quadrant evaluation protocol (Magee, 1992)

TESTING RESULTS

In the case of this client, the interview revealed very little additional information, because he denied any other associated (systemic) signs or symptoms, denied bowel/bladder dysfunction, precipitating injury or trauma, and neurologic indications such as numbness, tingling, or paresthesias. Although he was difficult to understand, the physical therapist thought that the client had understood the questions and had answered them truthfully. Subjectively, he did not appear to be a malingerer or a hysterical/anxious individual.

His gait pattern could best be described as ataxic. His lower extremities would not support him fully, and he frequently lost his balance and fell down, although he denied any pain or warning that he was about to fall.

Objective findings revealed inconsistent results of muscle testing: The proximal muscles were more involved than the distal muscles (difference of one grade: proximal muscles = fair grade; distal muscles = good grade), but

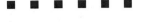

repeated tests elicited alternately strong, weak, or cogwheel responses, as if the muscles were moving in a ratching motion against resistance through the ROM.

The only other positive findings were slightly diminished deep tendon reflexes of the lower extremities compared with the upper extremities, but again these findings were inconsistent when tested over time.

FINAL RESULTS

Because the subjective and objective examinations were so inconsistent and puzzling, the therapist asked another therapist to briefly examine this client. In turn, they decided to ask the client to return either at the end of the day or for the first appointment of the next day to reexamine him for any changes in the pattern of his symptoms. It was more convenient for him to return the next day and he did.

At that time, it became clear that the therapist's difficulty in understanding the client had less to do with his use of English as a second language and more to do with an increasingly slurred speech pattern. His gait remained unchanged, but the muscle strength of the proximal pelvic muscles was consistently weak over several trials spread out during the therapy session, which lasted for 1 hour. This time, the therapist checked the muscles of his upper extremities and found that the scapular muscles were also unable to move against any manual resistance. Deep tendon reflexes of the upper extremities were inconsistently diminished, and reflexes of the lower extremities were now consistently diminished.

The client was referred to a physician for further follow-up and was not treated at the physical therapy clinic that day. He was examined by his family physician, who referred him to a neurologist. A diagnosis of Guillain-Barré syndrome was confirmed when the client's symptoms progressed dramatically, requiring hospitalization.

References

Anderson, J.F.: Mammalian and avian reservoirs for *Borrelia burgdorferi*. Annals of the New York Academy of Science 539:180–191, 1988.

Andreoli, T.E., et al.: Cecil Essentials of Medicine, 3rd ed. Philadelphia, W.B. Saunders, 1993.

Anvari, A., Graninger, W., Schneider, B., et al.: Cardiac involvement in systemic sclerosis. Arthritis and Rheumatism 35:1356–1361, 1992.

Ball, B.V.: Ankylosing spondylitis. In McCarty, D.J.: Arthritis and Allied Conditions. A Textbook of Rheumatology, 11th ed. Philadelphia, Lea & Febiger, 1989, pp. 934–943.

Baum, J.: Laboratory tests in rheumatoid arthritis. Journal of Musculoskeletal Medicine 10(5):55–65, 1993.

Belec, L., Bouquety, J.C., Georges, A.J., et al.: Antibodies to human immunodeficiency virus in the breast milk of healthy, seropositive women. Pediatrics 85:1022–1026, 1990.

Bengtsson, A., et al.: Reduced high-energy phosphate levels in the painful muscles of patients with primary fibromyalgia. Arthritis and Rheumatism 29(7): 817–821, 1986.

Bennett, J.C.: Rheumatoid arthritis: Clinical features. In Schumacher, H.R. (ed.): Primer on the Rheumatic Diseases, 9th ed. Atlanta, Arthritis Foundation, 1988, pp. 87–92.

Bennett, R.M.: Physical fitness and muscle metabolism in the fibromyalgia syndrome: An overview. Journal of Rheumatology 19:28, 1989a.

Bennett, R.M.: Beyond fibromyalgia: Ideas on etiology and treatment. Journal of Rheumatology 19:185, 1989b.

Bennett, R.M.: Confounding features of the fibromyalgia syndrome: A current perspective of differential diagnosis. Journal of Rheumatology 19:58, 1989c.

Bennett, R., et al.: Aerobic fitness in patients with fibrositis. Arthritis and Rheumatism *32*(4):454–460, 1989.

Bennett, R., Clark, S.R., Campbell, S.M., and Burckhardt, C.S.: Low levels of somatomedin-C in patients with FMS: A possible link between sleep and muscle pain. Arthritis and Rheumatism *35*(10):1113–1116, 1992.

Biggar, R.J.: Cancer in acquired immunodeficiency syndrome: An epidemiological assessment. Seminars in Oncology *17*:251–260, 1990.

Bova, C., and Matassarin-Jacobs, E.: Nursing care of clients with altered immune systems. *In* Black, J.M., and Matassarin-Jacobs, E. (eds.): Luckmann and Sorensen's Medical-Surgical Nursing, 4th ed. Philadelphia, W.B. Saunders, 1993, pp. 549-578.

Bucens, M., Armstrong, J., and Stuckey, M.: Virological and microscopic evidence for postnatal HIV transmission via breast milk. Presented at the IVth International Conference on AIDS, Stockholm, Sweden, June 1988.

Calin, A.: Ankylosing spondylitis and the spondyloarthropathies. *In* Schumacher, H.R. (ed.): Primer on the Rheumatic Diseases, 9th ed. Atlanta, Arthritis Foundation, 1988, pp. 142–147.

Calin, A.: Ankylosing spondylitis. *In* Kelley, W.N.: Textbook of Rheumatology, 3rd ed. Philadelphia, W.B. Saunders, 1989, pp. 1021–1037.

Campbell, S.M., Clark, S., Tindall, E.A., et al.: Clinical characteristics of fibrositis: A blinded controlled study of symptoms and tender spots. Part 1. Arthritis and Rheumatism *26*:817, 1983.

Carette, S., McCain, G.A., Bell, D.A., et al.: Evaluation of amitriptyline in primary fibrositis. Arthritis and Rheumatism *29*:655, 1986.

Casabona, J., Melbye, M., and Biggar, R.J.: Kaposi's sarcoma and non-Hodgkin's lymphoma in European AIDS cases. International Journal of Cancer *47*:49–53, 1991.

Centers for Disease Control: Purified protein derivative (PPD)—Tuberculin anergy and HIV infection. Morbidity and Mortality Weekly Report *140*(RR-5):27–33, 1989.

Clark, S., Campbell, S.M., Forehand, M.E., et al.: Clinical characteristics of fibrositis: A blinded controlled study using standard psychological tests. Part 2. Arthritis and Rheumatism *28*:132, 1985.

Curran, J.W.: Epidemiology of HIV infection and AIDS. *In* Wyngaarden, J.B., et al.: Cecil Textbook of Medicine, 19th ed. Philadelphia, W.B. Saunders, 1992, pp. 1918–1925.

Erhardt A.A., and Wasserheit, J.N.: Age, gender, and sexual risk behaviors for sexually transmitted diseases in the United States. *In* Wasserheit, J.N., Aral, S.O., and Holmes, K.K.: Research Issues in the AIDS era. Washington, D.C., American Society for Microbiology, 1991.

Ferraccioli, A.: Neuroendocrinologic findings in FMS. Journal of Rheumatology *17*(7):869–873, 1990.

Fibromyalgia Network: Fibromyalgia syndrome (FMS): Advances in research. April 1992.

Forseth, K., and Gran, J.: The prevalence of FMS among women aged 20–49 years in Adrendal, Norway. Scandinavian Journal of Rheumatology *21*:74–78, 1992.

Fye, K.H., and Sack, K.E.: Rheumatic diseases. *In* Stites, D.P., Stobo, J.D., and Wells, J.V.: Basic and Clinical Immunology, 7th ed. Norwalk, Connecticut, Appleton & Lange, 1991.

Gail, M.H., Pluda, J.M., Rabkin, C.S., et al.: Projections of the incidence of non-Hodgkin's lymphoma related to acquired immunodeficiency syndrome. Journal of the National Cancer Institute *83*:695–701, 1991.

Gall, E.P.: Pathophysiology of rheumatic disease. *In* Banwell, B.F., and Gall, E.P. (eds.): Clinics in Physical Therapy Series: Pathophysiology of Rheumatic Disease. Vol. 16. New York, Churchill Livingstone, 1988, pp. 1–15.

Gladman, D.D.: Psoriatic arthritis. *In* Kahn, M. (ed.): Spine: State of the Art Reviews. Philadelphia, Hanley and Belfus, Inc. *4*:637–656, 1990.

Gladman, D.D.: Psoriatic arthritis. Recent advances in pathogenesis and treatment. Rheumatic Disease Clinics of North America *18*:247–256, 1992.

Gladman, D.D., Shuckett, R., Russell, M.L., et al.: Psoriatic arthritis (PsA): An analysis of 220 patients. Quarterly Journal of Medicine *62*:127–141, 1987.

Gladman, D.D., Blake, R., Brubacher, B., et al.: Chloroquine therapy in psoriatic arthritis. Journal of Rheumatology *19*:1724–1726, 1992.

Goldenberg, D.L.: Fibromyalgia and other chronic fatigue syndromes: Is there evidence for viral disease? Seminars in Arthritis and Rheumatism *18*:111, 1988.

Goldenberg, D.L.: Fibromyalgia and its relation to chronic fatigue syndrome, viral illness and immune abnormalities. Journal of Rheumatology *19*:71, 1989a.

Goldenberg, D.L.: Management of fibromyalgia syndrome. Rheumatic Disease Clinics of North America *15*:499, 1989b.

Goldenberg, D.L.: Fibromyalgia and chronic fatigue syndrome: Are they the same? Journal of Musculoskeletal Medicine, May 19, 1990.

Greenberg, A.: Interactions of HIV and other diseases. *In* Mann, J., Tarantola, D.J.M., and Netter, T.W. (eds.): AIDS in the World: A Global Report. Cambridge, Massachusetts, Harvard University Press, 1992, pp. 133–163.

Guccione, A.A.: Rheumatoid arthritis. *In* O'Sullivan, S.B., and Schmitz, T.J.: Physical Rehabilitation: Assessment and Treatment, 2nd ed. Philadelphia, F.A. Davis, 1988, pp. 435–453.

Guyton, A.: Human Physiology and Mechanisms of Disease, 5th ed., Philadelphia, W.B. Saunders, 1992.

Hadler, N.M.: The patient with low back pain. Hospital Practice, Oct. 30, 1987, pp. 17–22.

Hakala, M., Kontkanen, E., and Koivisto, O.: Simultaneous presentation of upper lobe fibrobullous disease and spinal pseudoarthrosis in a patient with ankylosing spondylitis. Annals of Rheumatic Disease *49*:728–729, 1990.

Hamm, C., Derman, S., and Russell, I.: Sleep parameters in FMS. Arthritis and Rheumatism *32*(4 suppl):S70, 1989.

Hartman, S.S.: Fibrositis, or the fibromyalgia syndrome. *In* Camasta, C.A., Vickers, N.S., and Ruchs, J.A. (eds.): Reconstructive surgery of the Foot and Leg: Update 93. Tucker, Georgia, Podiatry Institute Inc., 1993, pp. 11–14.

Harvey, C.K., Cadena, R., and Dunlap, L.: Fibromyalgia. Part 1. Review of the literature. Journal of the American Podiatric Medicine Association *83*(7):412–417, 1993.

Hollander, H., and Katz, M.H.: HIV infection. *In* Tierney, L.M., et al.: Current Medical Diagnosis and Treatment. Norwalk, Connecticut, Appleton & Lange, 1993, pp. 1008–1028.

Hollister, R.: Collagen vascular disease. *In* Bierman, C.W., and Pearlman, D.S. (eds.): Allergic Diseases from Infancy to Adulthood, 2nd ed. Philadelphia, W.B. Saunders, 1988, pp. 779–787.

Hunder, G.G., Kaye, R.L., and Williams, R.C.: Rheumatology symposium: OA, osteoporosis, fibromyalgia. Journal of Musculoskeletal Medicine *10*(9):16–34, 1993.

Hunter, T.: The spinal complications of ankylosing spondylitis. Seminars in Arthritis and Rheumatism *19*:172–182, 1989.

Istfan, M.A., and LeRoy, E.C.: When systemic sclerosis involves the viscera. Journal of Musculoskeletal Medicine *7*(12):36–50, 1990.

Kidd, B., Mulle, M., Frank, A., et al.: Disease expression of ankylosing spondylitis in males and females. Journal of Rheumatology *15*:1407–1409, 1988.

Koop, C.E.: Surgeon General's Report on Acquired Immune Deficiency Syndrome. Bethesda, Maryland, U.S. Department of Health and Human Services, 1986.

Krown, S.E.: Treatment of AIDS-associated malignancy. Cancer Detection and Prevention *14*:405–409, 1993.

Lab Tech/Med Tech Professional Bulletin: Improving symptoms in M.S. May 1990:5–7.

Lahita, R.G.: What Is Lupus? New York, Lupus Foundation of America, 1992.

Layzer, R.B.: Neuromuscular manifestations of systemic disease. Philadelphia, F.A. Davis, 1985.

Liles, W.C., and Ramsey, P.G.: Infectious diseases. *In* Ramsey, P.G., and Larson, E.B. (eds.): Medical Therapeutics, 2nd ed. Philadelphia, W.B. Saunders, 1993, pp. 62–127.

Long, B., and Wright, R.: Management of persons with problems of the immune system. *In* Phipps, W., Long, B., Woods, N., and Cassmeyer, V. (eds.): Medical-Surgical Nursing: Concepts and Clinical Practice, 4th ed. St. Louis, Mosby Year Book, 1991, pp. 2199–2224.

Lund, N., et al.: Muscle tissue oxygen pressure in FMS. Scandinavian Journal of Rheumatology *15*:165–173,1986.

Lydyard, P., and Grossi, C.: Components of the immune system. *In* Riott, I., Brastoff, J., and Male, D. (eds.): Immunology, 3rd ed. St. Louis, Mosby Year Book, 1993, pp. 2.2–3.11.

Mader, R., and Gladman, D.D.: Psoriatic arthritis: Making the diagnosis and treating early. Journal of Musculoskeletal Medicine *10*(5):18–28, 1993.

Magee, D.J.: Orthopedic Physical Assessment. Philadelphia, W.B. Saunders, 1992, p. 273.

Mann, J., Tarantola, D.J.M., and Netter, T.W. (eds.): AIDS in the World: A Global Report. Cambridge, Massachusetts, Harvard University Press, 1992.

Matassarin-Jacobs, E.: Nursing care of clients with connective tissue disorders. *In* Black, J.M., and Matassarin-Jacobs, E. (eds.): Luckmann and Sorensen's Medical-Surgical Nursing, 4th ed. Philadelphia, W.B. Saunders, 1993, pp. 593–614.

McCain, G.A., Bell, D.A., Mai, F.M., et al.: A controlled study of the effects of a supervised cardiovascular fitness training program on the manifestations of primary fibromyalgia. Arthritis and Rheumatism *31*:1135, 1988.

McCluskey, D., et al.: Aerobic work capacity in patients with CFS. British Medical Journal *301*:953–956, 1990.

McDuffie, F.C.: Pathogenesis of systemic lupus erythematosus. Journal of Musculoskeletal Medicine *7*(1):97–107, 1990.

McEwan, C.: Ankylosing spondylitis and spondylitis accompanying ulcerative colitis, regional enteritis, psoriasis and Reiter's disease: A comparative study. Arthritis and Rheumatism *14*:291, 1971.

Medsger, T.A.: Systemic sclerosis and localized scleroderma. *In* Schumacher, H.R. (ed.): Primer on the Rheumatic Diseases, 9th ed. Atlanta, Arthritis Foundation, 1988, pp. 111–117.

Moldofsky, H.: Nonrestorative sleep and symptoms after a febrile illness in patients with FMS and CFS. Journal of Rheumatology *16*(Suppl 19):150–153, 1989.

Moutsopoulos, H.M., and Youinou, P.: New developments in Sjögren's syndrome. Current Opinions in Rheumatology *3*:815–822, 1991.

Neeck, G., and Riedel, W.: Thyroid function in patients with FMS. Journal of Rheumatology *19*(7):1120–1122, 1992.

Nies, K.M.: Treatment of the fibromyalgia syndrome. Journal of Musculoskeletal Medicine *9*(5):20–26, 1992.

Oddis, C.V., and Medsger, T.A.: Chronic inflammatory myopathies: Polymyositis and dermatomyositis. Journal of Musculoskeletal Medicine *8*(3):26–37, 1991.

O'Toole, M. (ed.): Miller-Keane Encyclopedia and Dictionary of Medicine, Nursing and Allied Health, 5th ed. Philadelphia, W.B. Saunders, 1992.

Ozuna, J.: Nursing care of clients with degenerative neurologic disorders. *In* Black, J.M., and Matassarin-Jacobs, E. (eds.): Luckmann and Sorensen's Medical-Surgical Nursing, 4th ed. Philadelphia, W.B. Saunders, 1993, pp. 773–792.

Pellegrino, M., et al.: Prevalence of mitral valve prolapse in primary fibromyalgia: A pilot investigation. Archives of Physical Medicine Rehabilitation *70*:541–543, 1989.

Phillips, P.E., and Goldberger, E.: Bacterial arthritis: Uncovering the underlying cause. Journal of Musculoskeletal Medicine 7(12):55–64, 1990.

Purtilo, D.T., and Purtilo, R.B.: A Survey of Human Diseases, 2nd ed. Boston, Little, Brown, 1989.

Rabkin, C.S., Biggar, R.J., and Horm, J.W.: Increasing incidence of cancers associated with the human immunodeficiency virus epidemic. International Journal of Cancer 47:692–696, 1991.

Ramanujam, T., and Schumacher, H.R.: Ankylosing spondylitis: Early recognition and management. Journal of Musculoskeletal Medicine 9(1):75–92, 1992.

Robertson, C.R.: Silicone breast implants not proved as cause of musculoskeletal problems. The Journal of Musculoskeletal Medicine 10(9):13–14, 1993.

Ruff, A., Coberly, H., Farzadegan, H., et al.: Detection of HIV-1 by PCR in breast milk. Presented at the VIIth International Conference on AIDS, Florence, Italy, June, 1991.

Russell, I.: Neurohormonal aspects of fibromyalgia syndrome. Rheumatic Disease of North America 15(1):149–168, 1989.

Russell, I., Vaeroy, H., et al.: Cerebrospinal fluid (CSF) biogenic amines in fibromyalgia syndrome. ACR Scientific Abstracts S55, 1990.

Saag, M.S.: Renal, Cardiac, Endocrine, and Rheumatologic Manifestations of HIV Infection. In Wyngaarden, J.B., Smith, L.H., and Bennett, J.C. (eds.): Cecil Textbook of Medicine, 19th ed. Philadelphia, W.B. Saunders, 1992, pp. 1952–1957.

Sattler, F.R.: Pulmonary manifestations of AIDS: Special emphasis on *Pneumocystosis*. In Wyngaarden, J.B., et al.: Cecil Textbook of Medicine, 19th ed. Philadelphia, W.B. Saunders, 1992, pp. 1939–1942.

Schenk, B.. Management of persons with neurologic problems. In Phipps, W., Long, B., Woods, N., and Cassmeyer, V. (eds.): Medical-Surgical Nursing: Concepts and Clinical Practice, 4th ed. St. Louis, Mosby Year Book, 1991, pp. 1817–1896.

Schoen, R.T., and Rahn, D.W.: Lyme disease update: Tips on recognition and treatment. Journal of Musculoskeletal Medicine 8(5):75–90, 1991.

Steere, A.C., Batsford, W.P., Weinburg, M., et al.: Lyme carditis: Cardiac abnormalities of Lyme disease. Annals of Internal Medicine 93:8–16, 1980.

Steere, A.C., Bartenhagen, N.H., Craft, J.E., et al.: The early clinical manifestations of Lyme disease. Annals of Internal Medicine 99:76–82, 1983.

Suarez-Almazor, M.E., and Russell, A.S.: Anterior atlantoaxial subluxation in patients with spondyloarthropathies: Association with peripheral disease. Journal of Rheumatology 15:973–975, 1988.

Talal, N., Carsons, S., Udell, I., and Sciubba, J.J.: Sjögren's Syndrome. Port Washington, New York, Sjögren's Syndrome Foundation, Inc., 1991.

Thiry, L., Sprecher-Goldberger, S., Jonekheer, R., et al.: Isolation of AIDS virus from cell-free breast milk of three healthy virus carriers. Lancet 2:891–892, 1985.

Tullous, M.W., Skerhut, H.E.I., Story, J.L., et al.: Cauda equina syndrome of long-standing ankylosing spondylitis. Case report and review of the literature. Journal of Neurosurgery 73:441–447, 1990.

U.S. Department of Health and Human Services: Lyme Disease: The Facts, the Challenge. National Institutes of Health, Publication No. 92-3193, April 1992.

Vaeroy, H., et al.: Elevated CSF levels of substance P and high incidence of Raynaud phenomenon in patients with fibromyalgia. Pain 32:21–26, 1988.

Vaeroy, H., et al.: No evidence for endorphin deficiency in fibromyalgia. Pain 46:139–143, 1991.

Van de Perre, P., Hitimana, D.G., and Lepage, P.: Human immunodeficiency virus antibodies of IgG, IgA, and IgM subclasses in milk of seropositive mothers. Journal of Pediatrics 113:1039–1041, 1988.

Vonesch, N., Caprilli, F., Castiglione, H.A., et al.: The human colostrum as a route of HIV-1 transmission. Presented at the VIIth International Conference on AIDS, Florence, Italy, June 1991.

Wallace, D.: Cytokine and immune regulation in FMS. Arthritis and Rheumatism 32(10):1334–1335, 1989.

Wasserheit, J.N.: Epidemiological synergy: Inter-relationships between HIV infection and other STDs. In Chen, L., Armor, J.S., and Segal, S. J. (eds.): AIDS and Women's Reproductive Health. New York, Plenum Press, 1992.

Will, R.K.: The changing epidemiology of rheumatic disease. British Journal of Rheumatology 29:299–300, 1990.

Williams, R.C.: Infection and arthritis: How are they related? Journal of Musculoskeletal Medicine 10(6):38–51, 1993.

Wolfe, F., Smythe, H.A., Yunus, M.B., et al.: The American College of Rheumatology 1990 criteria for the classification of fibromyalgia. Arthritis and Rheumatism 33:160, 1990.

Wright, R., and Long, B.: Assessment of the immune system. In Phipps, W., Long, B., Woods, N., and Cassmeyer, V. (eds.): Medical-surgical Nursing: Concepts and Clinical Practice, 4th ed. St. Louis, Mosby Year Book, 1991, pp. 2191–2198.

Wyngaarden, J.B., at al.: Cecil Textbook of Medicine, 19th ed. Philadelphia, W.B. Saunders, 1992.

Yunus, M., Masi, A.T., Calabro, J.J., Miller, K.A., and Feigenbaum, S.L.: Primary fibromyalgia (fibrositis): Clinical study of 50 patients with matched normal controls. Seminars in Arthritis and Rheumatism 11:151–171, 1981.

Yunus, M., Kaylan-Raman, U., and Kaylan-Raman, K.: Primary fibromyalgia syndrome and myofascial pain syndrome: Clinical features and muscle pathology. Archives of Physical Medicine and Rehabilitation 69:451–454, 1988.

Yunus, M., et al.: A controlled study of primary fibromyalgia syndrome: Clinical features and association with other functional syndromes. Journal of Rheumatology 16(Suppl 19):62–71, 1989.

Zvaifler, N.J.: Rheumatoid arthritis. In Schumacher, H.R. (ed.): Primer on Rheumatic Diseases, 9th ed. Atlanta, Arthritis Foundation, 1988, pp. 83–87.

Bibliography

DeVita, V.T., Hellman, S., and Rosenberg, S.A.: AIDS: Etiology, Diagnosis, Treatment and Prevention, 3rd ed., Philadelphia, J.B. Lippincott, 1993.

Friction, J.R., and Awad, E.A. (eds.): Myofascial Pain and Fibromyalgia. Vol. 17. New York, Raven Press, 1990.

Galantino, M.L.: Clinical Assessment and Treatment of HIV. Thorofare, New Jersey, Charles B. Slack, Inc., 1991.

Harris, E.K. (ed.): The Sjögren's Syndrome Handbook. Port Washington, New York, Sjögren's Syndrome Foundation, 1991.

McCain, G.: Toward an integrated understanding of FM syndrome. Pain *45*:227–248, 1991.

Moldofsky, H.: Sleep physiology and psychological aspects of FM. Canadian Journal of Psychology *45*(2):179–184, 1991.

Shafran, S.: The chronic fatigue syndrome. American Journal of Medicine *90*:730–739, 1991.

12

Systemic Origins of Musculoskeletal Pain: Associated Signs and Symptoms

■ ■ ■ ■ ■ ■ ■ ■ ■ ■ ■

Musculoskeletal and Systemic Causes of:

Chest Pain
Back Pain:
    Cervical
    Thoracic
    Scapular
    Lumbar
    Sacroiliac Joint/Sacral

Shoulder Pain
Pelvic Pain
Hip Pain
Groin Pain

The potential for referral of pain from systemic diseases to specific muscles and joints is well documented in the medical literature. These referral patterns most often affect the back and shoulder but may also present in the chest, thorax, hip, groin, or sacroiliac joint. In this chapter, we have attempted to provide an overview of systemic diseases that can refer pain or symptoms to the aforementioned musculoskeletal areas. Unless otherwise stated, in each section of this chapter it is assumed that the text pertains to systemic origins of symptoms for specific joints or areas of the body.

Up to this point, the text has focused on each organ system and the pain or other signs and symptoms referred from organs to musculoskeletal sites. In this chapter, we have turned the focus around so that the reader can quickly refer to the site of presenting pain or other symptoms and determine possible systemic involvement. The physical therapist may then question the client, as suggested, and determine the possible need for a medical referral. For an in-depth discussion of the specific systemic causes of musculoskeletal signs or symptoms, the reader is referred to the individual chapters within this text.

DECISION-MAKING PROCESS

As discussed in Chapter 1, four guiding parameters are used throughout this text to help physical therapists with the decision-making process. These parameters are

- **Client History** (Chapter 2)
- **Pain Patterns/Pain Types** (Chapter 1)
- **Systems Review** (Chapter 12)
- **Signs and Symptoms of Systemic Diseases** (Chapter 12)

It is essential that the physical therapist conduct a thorough interview and correlate the subjective findings with the objective findings in order to recognize presenting conditions that require medical follow-up. Accordingly, the physical therapist will want to obtain the client's history, conduct a systems review, and remain familiar with types of pain, pain patterns, and signs and symptoms that may suggest systemic origins of problems presenting in the musculoskeletal system. A brief review of each of these parameters has been included in this chapter for the clinician who is using this text as a quick reference guide.

These guidelines for collecting and correlating subjective and objective information are suggested for all clients who develop musculoskeletal symptoms insidiously (i.e., without a traumatic origin or known precipitating cause), as well as for the client being treated by a physical therapist for any reason.

Even with a history of trauma or injury, the physical therapist should keep in mind that trauma has been related to symptoms in 10 per cent of people with neoplasm, compared with 10 per cent to 30 per cent or more in people with discogenic pain. In most cases, an injury associated with a neoplasm is precipitated by a neurologic deficit that is caused by cord or root compression due to the tumor (Hadler, 1987a).

Finally, trauma does not solely imply some external force creating injury. Trauma may be intrinsic, resulting from internal derangement of either muscle (e.g., ruptures of the tendinous insertion) or joint (e.g., meniscal injury or joint dysfunction). Intrinsic trauma is associated with an unguarded movement occurring during the performance of a normal functional activity. If the episode producing the pain is the result of extrinsic trauma, the history of onset is usually quite clear. However, extrinsic trauma to one part of the musculoskeletal system may be associated with intrinsic trauma of another part (Zohn, 1988).

For example, a direct injury to the cervical spine during an automobile accident also may result in an intrinsic injury to the lumbar spine that goes unnoticed at the time of the more severe and obvious injury (Zohn, 1988). These cases point out the need to question the client carefully regarding previous trauma, because the client may not realize the potential importance of such information.

CLIENT HISTORY
(Diagnostic Interviewing)

A carefully taken, detailed medical history is the most important single element in the evaluation of a client presenting with musculoskeletal pain of unknown origin or etiology. It is essential for the recognition of systemic disease that may be causing muscle or joint symptoms. Symptoms are likely to appear some time before striking physical signs of disease are evident and before laboratory tests are useful to the physician in detecting disordered physiology. Thus, an accurate and sufficiently detailed history provides historical clues that can be significant in determining when the client should be referred to a physician.

It is important to know the client's age, occupation, and previous illnesses and injuries. The age is important because some musculoskeletal or systemic problems are likely to affect people during specific decades of life (see Table 2–2). Occupation is important because well-defined problems occur in people who engage in different occupational activities such as occupations that involve exposure to gases or chemicals (Zohn, 1988). See Chapter 2 for further explanation.

Other important information may include recent travel (hepatitis, tropical diseases associated with arthralgias), ingestion of raw cow's or goat's milk (tuberculosis), or ingestion of undercooked meat or fish (hepatitis). If the client indicates that illness occurred while traveling abroad, it should be remembered that amebiasis (infections with amebas), fungal infections, and some rare tropical diseases may manifest themselves as joint pain in their chronic course (Mennell, 1964). A remembered accident or childhood disease or illness may contribute important information.

The past history of a client with joint pain must be examined, because there may be a clue to the true nature of the pathologic cause of the pain. A previous history of heart disease in childhood, chorea, or St. Vitus' dance suggests that the cause of pain may be acute rheumatic fever. Migraine or allergic conditions, such as asthma or hay fever, suggest a diagnosis of nonspecific intermittent hydrarthrosis (fluid in a joint). A chronic cough, loss of weight, unexplained fever, undue sweating, and the drinking of raw milk in the past suggest that the underlying cause of the joint symptoms may be tuberculosis or brucellosis, whereas fleeting pains in the small joints of the extremities are suggestive of rheumatoid arthritis. Joint pain after dietary extravagance may suggest gout, and the history of recent injection of antitoxin or the administration of a new drug might suggest an allergic basis for the joint symptoms (Mennell, 1964).

Acute pain in joints may have a sudden onset at rest. In this event, systemic disease should be suspected. It is more often the case that the history will reveal a gradual onset, starting with aching and progressing with time to a state of severe discomfort or even acute pain (Zohn, 1988).

A previous history of cancer, either personal or family, is always a reason to question the client further regarding the onset and the pattern of current symptoms. This is especially true for women with a previous personal or family history of breast cancer or cancer of the reproductive system who now present with shoulder, chest, back, hip, or sacroiliac pain of unknown etiology. Likewise, anyone with back problems should be questioned with regard to both the previous history of cancer and the presence of any other pain or symptoms before the onset of back pain. The client may not realize that pain that begins in one anatomic location and then migrates to the back (e.g., referred pain; metastases) may be caused by the same phenomenon, and thus a good history-taking is important.

If pain has commenced for no apparent reason and is gradually and insidiously increasing, serious pathology should be suspected, particularly if the person feels or looks unwell. A careful evaluation of the client's information regarding the onset of the symptoms is important. The client may think that the pain began for no apparent reason, whereas the alert therapist may recognize a causative factor. Alternatively, the client may wrongfully relate the onset of certain activities in an attempt to identify a cause for pain that really appeared for very different reasons (McKenzie, 1981). When the symptoms seem out of proportion to the injury, or if they persist beyond the expected time for the nature of the injury, the presence of a tumor may be suspected (D'Ambrosia, 1986).

If, during the examination, no position or movement can be found that reduces the presenting pain, the existence of serious pathology should be considered. This is especially true when the client states that there has been no apparent reason for the onset of symptoms or that the symptoms have been present for weeks or months and have been increasing in intensity. There is usually no loss of function or postural deformity (McKenzie, 1981).

Women with back pain who have an unusual menstrual history should be questioned in greater detail regarding gynecologic function to rule out any relationship between the reproductive system and back pain. Any suspicious findings should be reported to the physician for further consideration in making a medical diagnosis.

Corticosteroid use must also be disclosed, because it may be associated with osteoporosis, compression fractures, and infection (Sasso et al., 1991). Both men and women with back pain should be questioned regarding the potential for urologic conditions causing back pain.

It is the associated signs and symptoms that are most often warning signs indicating the possibility of systemic origin of presenting musculoskeletal problems. Because the client may not associate such symptoms with the current joint, muscular, or skeletal pain, the therapist must know the possible systemic causes of musculoskeletal pain and the appropriate questions to ask to elicit the presence of associated symptoms in the client's history.

For example, more obvious examples of related gastrointestinal (GI) complaints include a history of nausea and vomiting of recently ingested food, significant weight loss without effort, a change in the bowel habits or the character of the stool, and increase or decrease of musculoskeletal symptoms with ingestion of food. These are all important associated features of back, thoracic, or scapular pain.

Such a history, even in the presence of objective musculoskeletal findings, requires careful interpretation of subjective and objective results and consultation with the physician. This principle is even more important when the client does not present with significant objective findings to support a primary musculoskeletal lesion.

PAIN PATTERNS/PAIN TYPES

An in-depth discussion of pain patterns and pain types is presented in Chapter 1. In this chapter, pain associated with each anatomic part (e.g., back, chest, shoulder, pelvis, sacrum/sacroiliac, hip, and groin) is discussed and differentiated as systemic from musculoskeletal whenever possible.

Characteristics of pain, such as onset, description, duration, pattern, aggravating and relieving factors, and associated signs and symptoms, are presented. This comparison will assist the therapist in recognizing a systemic presentation from a musculoskeletal presentation of signs and symptoms.

Systemic pain may decrease with a change in position of the hollow organs. For example, esophageal pain may decrease with an upright position, kidney pain may decrease when the client leans toward the uninvolved side, pleural pain may decrease with autosplinting (decreasing respiratory movements by lying on the involved side), gallbladder pain may decrease when the client leans forward, and pancreatic pain may decrease when the client leans forward or sits upright.

Aggravating factors for systemic pain may be organ dependent. For example, any pain pattern associated with the heart can be aggravated by cold, exertion, or stress. Peristalsis caused by eating or drinking may aggravate symptoms associated with the GI tract.

Muscles may be responsible for pain in the areas that may also be focal points for pain of a systemic origin. The muscles most likely to refer pain to a given area are listed in Table 12–1 (Travell and Simons, 1983). For more specific information regarding examination of these muscles, the reader is referred to the Travell and Simons texts listed in the References.

Joint pain can have systemic or musculoskeletal origins. The differences are listed in Table 12–2.

Stiffness. Muscular stiffness and joint stiffness increase as a person ages. Connective tissue changes may occur as fibrinogen produced in the liver is normally converted to fibrin to serve as a clotting factor.

Small amounts of fibrinogen normally leak out of the vasculature into the intracellular spaces, adhering to cellular structures and thus causing microfibrinous ad-

Table 12–1

TRIGGER POINT PAIN GUIDE

Location	Potential Muscles Involved	Location	Potential Muscles Involved
Front of chest pain	Pectoralis major Pectoralis minor Scaleni Sternocleidomastoid (sternal) Sternalis Iliocostalis cervicis Subclavius External abdominal oblique	Lumbar pain	Longissimus thoracis Iliocostalis lumborum Iliocostalis thoracis Multifidi Rectus abdominis
Side of chest pain	Serratus anterior Lattissimus dorsi	Sacral and gluteal pain	Longissimus thoracis Iliocostalis lumborum Multifidi
Low thoracic back pain	Iliocostalis thoracis Multifidi Serratus posterior inferior Rectus abdominis Lattissimus dorsi	Abdominal pain	Rectus abdominis Abdominal obliques Transversus abdominis Iliocostalis thoracis Multifidi Pyramidalis

Adapted from Travell, J.G., and Simons, D.G.: Myofascial Pain and Dysfunction: The Trigger Point Manual. Baltimore, Williams & Wilkins, 1983, p. 574.

hesions among the cells. Activity and movement normally break these adhesions, but with the aging process, with production of fewer and less efficient macrophages, and especially with immobility for any reason, the lysis of these adhesions is reduced. The resultant increase in stiffness occurs as adhesions accumulate in the muscle and fascia (Sinnott, 1993).

Other researchers suggest that increased stiffness may occur as a result of increased collagen fibers, increased cross-links of aged collagen fibers, changes in the mechanical properties of connective tissues, structural and functional changes in the collagen protein, and reduced physical activity (Neumann, 1993; Rauterberg, 1989).

Table 12–2

COMPARISON OF SYSTEMIC AND MUSCULOSKELETAL JOINT PAIN

Systemic	Musculoskeletal

Awakens at night
Deep aching, throbbing
Reduced by pressure
Constant or waves/spasm
Associated signs and symptoms:
  Jaundice
  Migratory arthralgias
  Skin rash
  Fatigue
  Weight loss
  Low-grade fever
  Muscular weakness
  Cyclic, progressive symptoms
  History of infection (hepatitis, streptococcosis, mononucleosis, measles)
	Decreases with rest
	Sharp
	Ceases when stressful action is stopped
	Associated signs and symptoms:
	  Usually none
	  Trigger points may be accompanied by nausea, sweating

Clinical Signs and Symptoms of
Systemic Pain

Onset
- Recent, sudden
- Does not present as chronically observed for several years intermittently

Description
- Knifelike quality stabbing from the inside out, boring, deep aching
- Cutting, gnawing
- Throbbing
- Bone pain
- Unilateral or bilateral

Intensity (related to the degree of noxious stimuli)
- Dull to severe
- Mild to severe

Duration
- Constant, no change, awakens the person at night

Pattern
- Although constant, may come in waves
- Gradually progressive, cyclic
- Night pain, especially night pain relieved by aspirin* (characteristic of osteoid osteoma)
- Symptoms unrelieved by rest or change in position
- Migratory arthralgias: pain/symptoms last for 1 week in one joint, then resolve and appear in another joint

Clinical Signs and Symptoms of
Musculoskeletal Pain (Kirkaldy-Willis, 1983)

Onset (may be sudden or gradual, depending on the history)
- Sudden: Usually associated with acute overload stress, traumatic event, repetitive motion
- Gradual: Secondary to chronic overload of the affected part
    May be present off and on for a period of years

Description
- Local tenderness to pressure is present
- Achy, cramping pain
- May be stiff after prolonged rest, but pain level decreases
- Usually unilateral

Intensity
- May be mild to severe
- May depend on the person's anxiety level—the level of pain may increase in a client fearful of a "serious" condition

Duration
- May be constant but is more likely to be intermittent, depending on the activity or the position

Pattern
- Restriction of active/passive/accessory movement observed
- One or more particular movements "catch" the client and aggravate the pain

Continued on following page

▼ Systemic Pain

Aggravating Factors

- Depends on the organ involved (see specific chapters)

Relieving Factors

- Usually none
- If rest or position change relieves the pain, there is usually a cyclic progression of increasing frequency, intensity, or duration of pain until rest or change in position is no longer a relieving factor

Associated Signs and Symptoms

- Fever, chills
- Night sweats
- Unusual vital signs
- Warning signs of cancer (see Chapter 10)
- GI symptoms: nausea, vomiting, anorexia, unexplained weight loss, diarrhea, constipation
- Early satiety (feeling full after eating)
- Bilateral symptoms (e.g., paresthesias [abnormal sensation], weakness), edema, nail bed changes, skin rash
- Painless weakness of muscles: more often proximal but may occur distally
- Dyspnea (breathlessness at rest or after mild exertion)
- Diaphoresis (excessive perspiration)
- Headaches, dizziness, fainting
- Visual disturbances
- Skin lesions, rashes, or itching that the client may not associate with the musculoskeletal symptoms
- Bowel/bladder symptoms
  - Hematuria (blood in the urine)
  - Nocturia
  - Urgency (sudden need to urinate)
  - Frequency
  - Melena (blood in feces)
  - Fecal or urinary incontinence
  - Bowel smears

---

* Relief with aspirin in these cases demonstrates a greater effect than expected (i.e., the relief is out of proportion to the severity of pain).

▼ Musculoskeletal Pain

Aggravating Factors

- Pain may become worse by movement (some myalgia decreases with movement)

Relieving Factors

- Pain is relieved by *short* periods of rest without resulting stiffness
- Stretching

Associated Signs and Symptoms

- Usually none, although stimulation of trigger points may cause sweating, nausea, blanching

SYSTEMS REVIEW

GENERAL QUESTIONS

- Fever, chills, sweating
- Excessive, unexplained weight gain or loss
- Appetite loss
- Vital signs: blood pressure (BP), temperature, pulse

RHEUMATOLOGIC

- Presence/location of joint swelling
- Muscle pain, weakness
- Skin rashes
- Reaction to sunlight
- Raynaud's phenomenon

NEUROLOGIC

- Headaches
- Vision changes
- Vertigo
- Paresthesias
- Weakness
- Atrophy
- Radicular pain

VASCULAR

- Claudication (limping)
- Coldness of extremities; discoloration; response to cold
- Peripheral edema
- Fatigue, dyspnea, syncope
- Differences in BP from side to side with position change (10 mm Hg or more; increase or decrease/diastolic or systolic; associated symptoms: dizziness, headache, nausea, vomiting, diaphoresis, heart palpitations, increased primary pain or symptoms)

PSYCHOLOGIC

- Sleeping patterns
- Stress levels
- Changes in personal habits

GASTROINTESTINAL

- Abdominal pain
- Indigestion; difficulty in swallowing
- Nausea/vomiting
- Change in bowel habits
- Rectal bleeding

Continued on following page

GENITOURINARY

- Reduced stream
- Burning, bleeding, color
- Incontinence

- Hesitation, urgency
- Nocturia, frequency
- Dysuria (painful or difficult urination)

ENDOCRINE

- Hair and nail changes
- Temperature intolerance
- Cramps

- Edema, polyuria
- Unexplained weakness, fatigue

PULMONARY

- Cough
- Sputum

- Night sweats

GYNECOLOGIC

- Irregular menses, menopause
- Pain with menses, intercourse
- Vaginal discharge

- Surgical procedures
- Birth/abortion histories
- Spotting, bleeding

SYSTEMS REVIEW

Musculoskeletal symptoms accompany many systemic diseases. By using the interview format, a complete review of a client's visceral systems should be undertaken. Cutaneous (skin) manifestations and joint pain may be the presenting feature of systemic disease such as systemic lupus erythematosus (SLE), scleroderma, dermatomyositis, Reiter's disease, progressive systemic sclerosis (PSS), and psoriatic arthritis. Symptoms of joint pain may be associated with and draw attention to acromegaly, pulmonary disease, and kidney diseases (Mennell, 1964).

Arthralgia (joint pain) may be associated with ulcerative colitis and Crohn's disease (regional enteritis). These diseases primarily involving the GI tract may begin with a disturbance of peripheral joints or spine (see Systems Review chart).

General questions about fevers, excessive weight gain or loss, and appetite loss should be followed by questions related to specific organ systems. Questions about *rheumatologic* problems focus on the presence and location of joint swelling, muscle pains and weakness, skin rashes, reaction to sunlight (SLE), and Raynaud's phenomenon.

Appropriate questions about *neurologic* problems deal with headaches, vision changes, vertigo, paresthesias, weakness, atrophy, and radicular pains. *Vascular* problems are identified by questions about claudication (limping), coldness of extremities, discoloration, and the client's response to cold.

Psychologic problems are elicited by questions about sleeping patterns, stress levels, and changes in personal habits. Questions about *GI* problems deal with abdominal pain, indigestion, nausea and vomiting, change in bowel habits, and rectal bleeding.

Genitourinary problems are identified by questions about bleeding, burning, frequency, hesitation, nocturia (excessive urination at night), and dysuria (painful or difficult urination). *Endocrine* disturbances are discovered by questions about hair and nail changes, temperature intolerance, cramps, unexplained weakness, and edema. *Gynecologic* problems are identified by questions about irregularity of menses, pain with menses, vaginal discharge, surgical procedures, birth histories, spotting, or bleeding (Zohn, 1988).

Questions about *pulmonary* problems might center on the presence of cough, sputum, and night sweats.

Vital signs, including blood pressure, temperature, and pulse, must be taken to avoid overlooking a problem of systemic origin. In assessing pulses, a comparison should be made of their force on both sides of the body, as well as in various positions. Differences in the blood pressure between the limbs of each side may be a clue of vascular disease (Zohn, 1988). A difference of 10 mm Hg (increase or decrease) of the diastolic or systolic blood pressure with a position change should be considered a possible indication of systemic problems, especially when accompanied by associated symptoms such as dizziness, headache, nausea, vomiting, diaphoresis (perspiration), heart palpations, and increased primary pain or symptoms.

CHEST PAIN (see also Chapter 3)

Musculoskeletal causes of chest (wall) pain must be differentiated from pain of cardiac, pulmonary, epigastric, and breast origins (Table 12–3) before physical therapy treatment begins. Chest pain also can occur as a result of cervical spine disorders because nerves originating as high as C3 and C4 can extend as far as the nipple line. Pectoral, suprascapular, dorsal scapular, and long thoracic nerves originate in the lower cervical spine, and impingement of these nerves also can cause chest pain.

Tietze's syndrome, costochondritis, the hypersensitive xiphoid, and the syndrome of the slipping rib must be differentiated from problems involving the thoracic viscera, particularly those of the heart, great vessels, and mediastinum, as well as from illness originating in the head, neck, or abdomen.

Because of the potentially confusing nature of chest pain, this is the only section in which musculoskeletal causes of pain are discussed. Whereas the musculoskeletal causes of back, scapula, hip, shoulder, and sacrum/sacroiliac pain are well addressed in other texts, it has been our experience that this information (as it relates to the chest) is not readily available. Understanding both the systemic and musculoskeletal causes of chest pain or symptoms is essential when determining the need for medical referral.

Musculoskeletal Causes

Tietze's Syndrome

Tietze's syndrome (inflammation of a rib and its cartilage; costal chondritis) may be one possible cause of anterior chest wall pain, manifested by painful swelling of one or more costochondral articulations. In most cases, the cause of Tietze's syndrome is unknown. Onset is usually before 40 years of age, with a predilection for the second and third decades, but it also occurs in children.

Approximately 80 per cent of clients have only single sites of involvement, most commonly the second or third costal cartilage (costochondral joint). Anterior chest pain may begin suddenly or gradually and may be associated with increased blood pressure, increased heart rate, and pain radiating down the left arm aggravated by sneezing, coughing, deep inspirations, or twisting motions of the trunk. These symptoms may seem similar to those of a heart

Table 12–3
CAUSES OF CHEST PAIN

Systemic Causes	Neuromusculoskeletal Causes
Pulmonary Pulmonary embolism Spontaneous pneumothorax Pulmonary hypertension Cor pulmonale Pleurisy with pneumonia **Cardiac** Myocardial ischemia 　(angina) Pericarditis Myocardial infarct Dissecting aortic aneurysm **Epigastric/Upper GI** Esophagitis Upper GI ulcer **Breast** Breast tumor Abscess Mastitis Lactation problems Mastodynia Trigger points **Other** Rheumatic diseases Anxiety	Tietze's syndrome Costochondritis Hypersensitive xiphoid Slipping rib syndrome Trigger points Myalgia Rib fracture Cervical spine disorders Neurologic 　Thoracic outlet syndrome 　Neuritis 　Shingles (herpes zoster) 　Dorsal nerve root 　　irritation

attack, but the raised blood pressure and aggravating factors differentiate Tietze's syndrome from myocardial infarction (Zohn, 1988).

Costochondritis

The terms Tietze's syndrome and costochondritis are used interchangeably, although these two conditions are not the same. Costochondritis is more common than Tietze's syndrome and is also known as the anterior chest wall syndrome, the costosternal syndrome, and parasternal chondrodynia (pain in a cartilage).

▼ *Clinical Signs and Symptoms of*
Tietze's Syndrome or Costochondritis

- Sudden or gradual onset of upper anterior chest pain
- Pain/tenderness of costochondral joint(s)
- Bulbous swelling of the involved costal cartilage (Tietze's syndrome)
- Mild-to-severe chest pain that may radiate to the left shoulder and arm
- Pain is aggravated by sneezing, coughing, inspiration, bending, recumbency, or exertion

Although both disorders are characterized by inflammation of one or more costal cartilages, costochondritis refers to pain in the costochondral articulations without swelling. This disorder is observed in people over age 40 years, tends to affect the third, fourth, and fifth costochondral joints, and occurs more often in women.

Costochondritis is characterized by pain of the anterior chest wall that may radiate widely, stimulating intrathoracic (including cardiac) or intraabdominal disease. Costochondritis can be similar to muscular pain and is elicited by pressure over the costochondral junctions. It may follow trauma or may be associated with systemic rheumatic disease. Inflammation of upper costal cartilages may cause annoying chest pain, whereas inflammation of lower costal cartilages is more likely to cause abdominal discomfort.

Other Causes

The *hypersensitive xiphoid* (xiphodynia) is tender to palpation, and local pressure may cause nausea and vomiting. This syndrome is manifested as

- Epigastric pain
- Nausea
- Vomiting

In the syndrome of the *slipping rib* (usually the tenth), the involved cartilage moves upward and overrides the cartilage above it, thus causing pain.

Trigger Points

Trigger points (hypersensitivity) in the thoracic paravertebral muscles refer pain to the chest, as do trigger points in the pectoralis major, pectoralis minor, and scalenus anterior muscles (see Table 12–1). Posterior chest wall pain may also be caused by irritable trigger points.

One of the most extensive patterns of pain from irritable trigger points is the complex pattern from the anterior scalene muscle. This may produce ipsilateral sternal pain, anterior chest wall pain, or breast pain; also, vertebral border of the scapula, shoulder, shawl, and arm pain radiating to the thumb and index finger (Zohn, 1988). Trigger points in the pectoral muscles can also cause anterior chest wall pain.

On examination, the physical therapist should palpate for tender points and taut bands of muscle tissue, squeeze the involved muscle, observe for increased pain with palpation, test for increased pain with resisted motion, and correlate symptoms with respiratory movements. The client should be questioned about a possible history of upper respiratory infection with repeated, forceful coughing, prolonged vigorous activity requiring repetitive motion(s), bending, lifting, or forceful abdominal breathing such as accompanies long-distance running.

Myalgia

Myalgia (muscular pain) in the respiratory muscles is well localized, reproducible by palpation, and exacerbated by manipulations of the chest wall. The discomfort of myalgia is almost always described as aching and may range from mild to intense. Diaphragmatic irritation may be referred to the ipsilateral neck and shoulder, lower thorax, lumbar region, or upper abdomen (see Fig. 3–7).

Neurologic Causes (see also Chapter 3)

Thoracic outlet syndrome (TOS) refers to a compression of the neural and vascular structures that leave or pass over the superior rim of the thoracic cage. The compressive forces associated with this neurovascular problem can be caused by musculoskeletal forces and can result in chest pain. TOS usually affects the upper extremity in the distribution of the ulnar nerve, with possible radiation to the neck, shoulder, scapula, or axilla, but the pain may occur primarily in the anterior chest wall, mimicking coronary heart disease. Usually, associated changes in sensation and neurologic findings will point to chest pain with an underlying neurologic cause.

Intercostal neuritis, such as herpes zoster or shingles produced by a viral infection of a dorsal nerve root, can cause neuritic chest wall pain, which can be differentiated from coronary pain. Neuritic pain occurs unrelated to effort or only with use of the upper extremities; it lasts longer (hours) than angina; and it may be associated with chills, fever, headache, malaise, and skin rash. Symptoms are confined to the somatic distribution of one of the spinal nerves.

Dorsal nerve root irritation of the thoracic spine is another neuritic condition that can refer pain to any point along the peripheral nerve. This condition can be caused by infectious processes (e.g., radiculitis or inflammation of the spinal nerve root dural sheath) and mechanical irritation caused by spinal deformities (e.g., bone spur or cervical rib).

Symptoms of lateral or anterior chest wall pain also may be referred to one or both arms through the brachial plexus, and there is often a history of associated back pain. The pain of dorsal nerve root irritation is more superficial than that of cardiac pain, but it can be aggravated by exertion of just the upper extremities. It is usually accompanied by other neurologic signs, such as muscle atrophy and numbness or tingling.

Rib Fractures

Periosteal (bone) pain is usually described as being intense and can be well localized, whereas chronic disease, often affecting the bone marrow and endosteum, may result in poorly localized pain of varying degrees of severity. Occult (hidden) rib fractures may occur, especially in a client with a chronic cough or someone who has had an explosive sneeze. Fractures may also occur as a result of trauma, but painful symptoms may not be perceived at first if other injuries are more significant. Rib fractures must be confirmed by x-ray diagnosis. Rib pain without fracture may indicate bone tumor or disease affecting bone, such as multiple myeloma (Zohn, 1988).

Systemic Causes

Pulmonary Causes

Parietal (somatic) pain refers to pain generating from the wall of any cavity, such as the chest or pelvic cavity. Whereas the visceral pleura is insensitive to pain, the parietal pleura is well supplied with pain nerve endings. Parietal pain may present as unilateral chest pain (rather than midline only) because at any given point, the parietal peritoneum obtains innervation from only one side of the nervous system. Parietal chest pain is usually more precisely localized to the site of the lesion than is visceral pain. When pain is referred, the pattern is usually along the costal margins or into the upper abdominal quadrants.

Pleural Pain

This type of pain is a common chest discomfort usually associated with infectious diseases, but it is also seen in spontaneous pneumothorax, rib fractures, and pulmonary embolism (blood clot) with infarction (death of tissue owing to occlusion of the blood supply). The pleural pain is characteristically close to the chest wall, sharp in character, and exacerbated by inspiration, coughing, and movement. In contrast to chest wall pain, it is usually not localized by palpation.

Spontaneous pneumothorax occasionally affects the exercising individual and occurs without obvious preceding trauma or infection. Peak incidence is in adults 20 to 40 years of age. Clients frequently present with the acute onset of pleuritic chest pain localized to the side of the pneumothorax. The pain may be referred to the shoulder or scapula (see Fig. 4–5). Any chest pain accompanied by a persistent cough (whether dry or productive) or other constitutional symptoms, such as vomiting, fever, hemoptysis, dizziness, dyspnea (with or without exertion), or night sweats, must be medically diagnosed.

Cardiac Causes

There are many causes of chest pain, both cardiac and noncardiac in origin. Cardiac-related pain may arise secondary to angina, myocardial infarction, pericarditis, or dissecting aortic aneurysm.

Cardiac-related chest pain also can occur when there is normal coronary circulation, as in the case of clients with pernicious anemia (chronic, progressive reduction of erythrocytes and subsequent loss of oxygen). These clients may have chest pain (angina) on physical exertion because of the lack of nutrition to the myocardium. (For more detailed information on cardiac causes of chest pain, see Chapter 3.)

Noncardiac causes of chest pain include pleuropulmonary disorders, musculoskeletal disorders, neurologic disorders, GI disorders, breast pain, and anxiety states. Cardiac- and noncardiac-related causes of chest pain are discussed in detail in Chapter 3 and are not repeated here.

Epigastric Causes

Epigastric pain is typically characterized by substernal or upper abdominal (just below the xiphoid process) discomfort (see Fig. 3–13). This may occur with radiation posteriorly to the back secondary to longstanding ulcers. Lesions of the upper esophagus may cause pain in the (anterior) neck, whereas lesions of the lower esophagus are more likely to be characterized by pain originating from the xiphoid process, radiating around the thorax to the middle of the back. Epigastric pain or discomfort may occur in association with disorders of the liver, gallbladder, common bile duct, and pancreas, with referral of pain to the interscapular, subscapular, or middle/low back regions.

Breast Pain (see also Chapter 3)

Although it is more typical in women, both men and women can have chest, back, scapular, and shoulder pain referred by pathology of the breast. The typical referral pattern for breast pain is around the chest into the axilla, to the back at the level of the breast, and occasionally into the neck and posterior aspect of the shoulder girdle (see Fig. 3–14).

The pain may continue along the medial aspect of the ipsilateral arm to the fourth and fifth digits. Pain in the upper inner arm may arise from outer quadrant breast tumors, but pain in the local chest wall may point to any breast pathology, such as abscess, mastitis (inflammation of the breast), or lactation (breast feeding) problems.

Mastodynia (irritation of the upper dorsal intercostal nerve) causing chest pain is almost always associated with ovulatory cycles, especially premenstrually.

Any recently discovered or changing tumors (lumps or nodules) must be examined by a physician. Any suspicious finding reported, observed, or palpated should be checked by a physician, especially in the case of a woman with a previous personal or family history of breast cancer.

A previous history of cancer is always cause to question the client further regarding the onset and pattern of current symptoms. This is especially true for women with a previous history of breast cancer or cancer of the reproductive system now presenting with shoulder, chest, hip, or SI pain of unknown etiology.

Jarring or movement of the breasts and

movement of the arms may aggravate the pain, with radiation to the inner aspect of the arm(s). This pattern occurs when the tumor is attached to surrounding tissues, thus preventing normal movement of skin, fascia, and muscle. Look for changes (e.g., prominent vein, skin redness, or dimpling) in the skin surface over the breast and chest.

Removal of a breast due to primary cancer may seem so far remote from symptoms of these body locations that the client may not volunteer this essential information (Cyriax, 1982; Wedge, 1983).

Trigger points of the pectoral muscles can mimic cardiac chest pain, but trigger point pain shows a wider variation in daily activities than does the more consistent limit imposed by angina (Travell and Simons, 1983). Chest pain caused by repetitive overuse can result in pectoral myalgia. This condition may occur separately from trigger points, and painful chest symptoms will be reproduced by squeezing the muscle belly.

As mentioned, the trigger point pattern from the anterior scalene muscle may produce ipsilateral sternal pain, anterior chest wall pain, or breast pain (Travell and Simons, 1983; Zohn, 1988).

BACK PAIN

Back pain is a symptom, not a diagnosis, but many times a specific diagnosis is impossible or unavailable. Back pain may arise in the spine from mechanical, inflammatory, metabolic, or neoplastic disorders, or it can be referred from abdominal or pelvic disease (Jayson, 1984).

The therapist must be aware that many different diseases can present as low back pain. The clues about the quality of pain, the age of the client, and the presence of systemic complaints or associated signs and symptoms indicate the need to investigate further. The history and physical therapy examination provide essential clues in determining the need for referral to a physician (Hadler, 1987a).

Effect of Position

Systemic back pain is not relieved by recumbency. The bone pain of metastasis or myeloma tends to be more continuous, progressive, and prominent when the client is recumbent. A history of fever and chills with or without previous infection anywhere in the body may indicate a low-grade infection (Nelson, 1993).

Beware of the client with acute backache who is unable to lie still, because almost all clients with regional or nonspecific backache seek the most comfortable position (usually recumbency) and stay in that position. In contrast, people with systemic backache move. In particular, visceral diseases, such as pancreatic neoplasm, pancreatitis, and posterior penetrating ulcers, often present with a systemic backache that causes the client to curl up, sleep in a chair, or pace the floor at night.

Primary tumors of the spinal cord or its roots (notably cauda equina tumor) may also present as low back pain. People with the lesions try to sleep in a chair and often pace the floor at night. Some clients with systemic backache writhe; they may have had a vascular catastrophe, such as an abdominal aortic dissection or rupture of an abdominal aortic aneurysm (sac formed by dilatation of blood vessel) (Hadler, 1987b).

Back pain that is unrelieved by rest or change in position, or pain that does not fit the expected mechanical or neuromusculoskeletal pattern, should serve as a red flag. When the symptoms cannot be reproduced, aggravated, or altered in any way during the examination, additional questions to screen for medical disease are indicated.

Night Pain

Long-standing night pain unaltered by positional change suggests a space-occupying lesion, such as a tumor. Systemic back pain may get worse at night with any of the following problems (Hadler, 1987b):

- Vertebral osteomyelitis
- Septic discitis
- Cushing's disease
- Osteomalacia
- Primary and metastatic cancer
- Paget's disease
- Ankylosing spondylitis
- Tuberculosis (of the spine)

Age

The risk of certain diseases associated with back pain increases with advancing age; these include systemic diseases and neoplastic disorders. If a client has had a low backache for years, progressive, serious disease is unlikely. However, a month or two of increasing backache, often in an elderly client, may be a signal of lumbar metastases.

Associated Signs and Symptoms

When back pain is accompanied by severe or chronic pain and fever, referral to a physician is necessary. Other possible associated symptoms may include fatigue, dyspnea, sweating after only minor exertion, and GI symptoms (Cyriax, 1982). See Clues Suggesting Systemic Back Pain.

Back pain accompanied by sustained morning stiffness may be caused by a spondyloarthropathy (disease of the joints of the spine). Extraarticular involvement of the eyes, skin, and GI system often accompanies spondyloarthropathy. Such symptoms present a red flag identifying clients who should be referred to a physician.

Referred pain originates in organs outside the spine that share pain innervation with areas of the lumbosacral spine. Colicky pain is associated with spasm in a hollow viscus. Severe, tearing pain with sweating and dizziness may originate from an

---

CLUES SUGGESTING SYSTEMIC BACK PAIN

- Age over 45 years
- Nocturnal back pain
- Back pain that causes writhing, prompts the client to move about, or curl up in the sitting position
- Back pain with constitutional symptoms: nausea, fatigue, vomiting, diarrhea, fever
- Back pain that is insidious in onset and progression
- Previous history of cancer
- Back and abdominal pain at the same level (may occur simultaneously or alternately)
- Sacral pain in the absence of history of trauma or overuse
- Elevated body temperature, night sweats, febrile chills
- Back pain that is unrelieved by recumbency
- Back pain that does not vary with exertion or activity
- Severe, persistent back pain with full and painless movement of the spine
- Severe back and lower extremity weakness without pain
- Back pain associated with meals (increase or decrease in symptoms)

expanding abdominal aortic aneurysm. Burning pain may originate from a duodenal ulcer (see Clues Suggesting Systemic Back Pain).

Classifications

There are many ways to examine and classify back pain. We have divided back pain into six categories:

■ Visceral

■ Neurogenic

■ Vasculogenic

■ Psychogenic

■ Spondylogenic

■ Primary or secondary cancer

Visceral

Visceral back pain is more likely to result from visceral disease in the abdomen and pelvis than from intrathoracic disease, which refers pain to the neck and shoulder. Visceral back pain is not very often confused with pain originating in the spine, because sufficient specific symptoms and signs are usually present to localize the problem correctly. For example, pancreatic carcinoma can cause severe and persistent back pain. However, this lesion causes other problems that turn attention away from the spine. When pain is referred to the back from an intra-abdominal or pelvic viscus (organs in the pelvis and abdomen), the outstanding finding is a full and painless range of movement at the lumbar spine. This finding focuses attention on the nonmoving parts of the body: the kidney, colon, ovary, uterus, and rectum.

Referred Pain (McCowin et al., 1991). Disorders of the vascular, genitourinary, and GI systems can cause stimulation of sensory nerves that results in the perception of pain both at the damaged area and at superficial tissues supplied by the same segments of the spinal cord. This is called referred pain.

Visceral sensory input travels to the brain by the same pathways as somatic sensory input, but higher perceptive centers may selectively diminish or enhance either form of sensory input. Sensory stimulation may cross over in the dorsal horn of the spinal cord to result in pain felt only in somatic locations, or it may stimulate anterior horn cells to produce muscle spasm.

True visceral pain is felt at the site of primary stimulation and is dull, aching, diffuse, and deep. Deep somatic abdominal pain from the parietal peritoneum is localized, sharp, intense, and often associated with reflex abdominal wall muscle spasm. Referred pain to the lumbrosacral spine is sharp and well localized and may be associated with reflex muscle contraction and hyperalgesia.

Back pain associated with perforation of organs, gynecologic conditions, or gastroenterologic disease seldom mimics "typical back pain" because of the history, associated symptoms, and lack of accompanying objective findings to support a musculoskeletal origin of pain. For example, low back pain of mechanical spondylitic origin is normally relieved by rest, whereas lesions in solid or hollow viscera may be relieved by change in position, but over time, even a change in position does not provide relief (Cyriax, 1982; Wedge, 1983).

Neurogenic

Neurogenic back pain is not easily differentiated. A serious delay in diagnosis can result from failure to appreciate the fact that neoplasms of the cord and cauda equina can mimic spondylogenic pain.

Diabetic neuropathy can cause nerve root irritation. A clinical picture that is indistinguishable from sciatica can result, and this similarity may lead to long and serious delays in diagnosis (Wedge, 1983). Such a situation may require persistence on the part of the therapist and client in requesting further medical follow-up.

The small vertebral canal also increases the risk of development of *sciatica* from a prolapsed intervertebral disc without any suggestion of claudication (Porter et al., 1978). Sciatica develops not only because of the disc prolapse but also because the person was already at risk for compression of the sciatic nerve owing to alteration in the shape and use of the vertebral canal.

Confusion with spinal stenosis syndromes may occur owing to ischemia of the sciatic nerve. Atheromatous change in the internal iliac artery may lead to sciatic pain with claudication-like symptoms.

Spinal stenosis is caused by a narrowing of the spinal canal, nerve root canals, or intervertebral foramina. The canal tends to be narrow at the lumbrosacral junction, and the nerve roots in the cauda equina are tightly packed. The emerging nerve root exits through a shallow lateral recess and may be compressed easily (Jayson, 1984). Any combination of degenerative changes, such as disc protrusion, osteophyte formation, and ligamentous thickening, reduces the space needed for the spinal cord and its nerve roots.

Clinical Signs and Symptoms. The client with spinal stenosis may develop a characteristic pattern of symptoms, with back pain, numbness, and paresthesia in the leg developing after the person walks a few hundred yards. The person may be forced to stop walking and obtains relief after resting for 4 or 5 minutes. The pattern of symptoms is similar to that of intermittent claudication (Table 12–4).

The vertebral canal is wider when the spine is flexed, so symptoms vary; when walking, some people will squat as if to tie their shoe laces to avoid the embarrassment of appearing to flex their spines forward.

Table 12–4
SYMPTOMS AND DIFFERENTIATION OF CLAUDICATION

Vascular Claudication	Neurogenic Claudication	Spinal Stenosis
Pain* is usually bilateral	Pain is usually bilateral, but may be unilateral	Usually bilateral pain
Occurs in the calf (foot, thigh, hip, or buttocks)	Occurs in back, buttocks, thighs, calves, feet	Occurs in back, buttocks, thighs, calves, feet
Pain consistent in all spinal positions	Pain decreased in spinal flexion	Pain decreased in spinal flexion
	Pain increased in spinal extension	Pain increased in spinal extension
Pain brought on by physical exertion (e.g., walking)	Pain increased with walking	Pain increased with walking
Pain relieved promptly by rest (1–5 min)	Pain decreased by recumbency	Pain relieved with prolonged rest (may persist hours after resting)
Pain increased by walking uphill		Pain decreased when walking uphill
No burning or dysesthesia	Burning and dysesthesia from the back to the buttocks and leg(s)	Burning and numbness present in lower extremities
Decreased or absent pulses in lower extremities	Normal pulses	Normal pulses
Color and skin changes in feet Cold, numb, dry, or scaly skin Poor nail and hair growth	Good skin nutrition	Good skin nutrition
Affects ages from 40 to over 60 years	Affects ages from 40 to over 60 years	Peaks in seventh decade Affects men primarily

* "Pain" associated with vascular claudication may also be described as an "aching," "cramping," or "tired" feeling.

Vasculogenic

The symptoms of vasculogenic back pain may be mistaken for those of a wide variety of musculoskeletal, neurologic, and arthritic disorders. Conversely, the diagnosed presence of vascular impairment of a minor degree may direct attention away from a primary disorder that originates elsewhere. Such disorders include low back pain of musculoskeletal origin, nerve root compression, spinal cord tumor, arthritis of the hip, or peripheral neuritis (Zohn and Mennell, 1988).

Peripheral arterial disease (PAD) is a medical problem that affects millions of Americans and can ultimately lead to amputation if not caught by screening. The most common cause of PAD is atherosclerosis, the hardening of fatty substances in the arteries (see Chapter 3).

Risk factors include smoking, hypertension, elevated serum cholesterol, diabetes, and age. PAD most often affects men older than 50 years, although more and more women are being affected because of an increase in smoking among women.

PAD with claudication can be confused with neurogenic claudication and spinal stenosis. Intermittent claudication is distinguished from other leg pain by its characteristic occurrence while walking or exercising, prompt relief upon rest, and position of the spine (see Table 12–4).

The medical diagnosis is difficult to make, because vascular and neurogenic claudication occur in approximately the same age group and can coexist in the same individual. Vascular studies and myelography may be required to help determine which problem dominates (Zohn, 1988).

Clinical Signs and Symptoms. Symptoms of occlusive disease occur as arteries become narrowed or blocked, limiting regional blood flow. The most common symptom is intermittent claudication, which occurs because blood flow to the legs is diminished and exercise increases the demands for oxygen.

The location of vasculogenic pain depends on the location of the vascular pathology (Zohn and Mennell, 1988). Gradual *obstruction of the aortic bifurcation* produces

■ Bilateral buttock and leg pain

■ Weakness and fatigue of the lower extremities

■ Atrophy of the leg musculature

■ Absent femoral pulses

■ Color and temperature changes in the lower extremities

When the pathology is in the *iliac artery,* symptoms may include

■ Pain in the low back, buttock, and leg of the affected side

■ Numbness

Involvement of the *femoral artery,* along its course or at the femoropopliteal junction, produces

■ Thigh and calf pain

■ Pulses absent below femoral pulse

Obstruction of the *popliteal artery* or its branches produces

■ Pain in the calf, ankle, or foot

Case Example. A 68-year-old woman with a long history of degenerative arthritis of the spine was referred to physical therapy for conservative treatment toward a goal of improving function despite her painful symptoms. Her symptoms were diffuse bilateral lumbosacral back pain into the buttocks and thighs, which increased with walking or any activity and did not subside substantially with rest (except for prolonged rest and immobility).

On examination, this client moved slowly and with effort, complaining of the painful symptoms described. There was no tenderness of the sacroiliac joint or sciatic notch but a subjective report of tenderness over L4–L5 and L5–S1. There was no palpable step-off or dip of the spinous processes for spondylolisthesis and no paraspinal spasm, but a marked right lumbar scoliosis with a lateral shift to the left was noted. She reported knowledge of scoliosis since she was a child.

A neurologic screening examination revealed normal straight leg raise and normal sensation and reflexes in both lower extremities. Motor examination was unremarkable for an inactive 68-year-old woman. Dorsalis pedis and posterior tibialis pulses were palpable but weak, bilaterally.

Despite physical therapy treatment and compliance on the part of the client with a home program, her symptoms persisted and progressively worsened. She returned to her physician with a report of these findings. Further testing showed that in addition to degenerative arthritis of the lumbrosacral spine, there was secondary stenosis and marked aortic calcification, indicating a vascular component to her symptoms.

Surgery was scheduled: an L4–L5 laminectomy with fusion, iliac crest bone graft, and decompression foraminotomies. Postoperatively, she subjectively reported 80 per cent improvement in her symptoms with an improvement in function, although she was still unable to return to work.

Spondylogenic

Spondylogenic back pain (or the symptoms produced by bone lesions) is relatively limited in nature and quality, although the conditions producing these symptoms are numerous. The age of the person, character of the pain, weight loss, fever, deformity, and bone tenderness are most helpful to the physician in making the correct diagnosis.

Osteoporosis (see also Chapter 9). Osteoporosis has many different causes and is associated with a loss of bone mass per unit volume, with a normal ratio of bone mineral to matrix. Loss of bone mass predisposes a person to vertebral body fracture, back pain, and deformity. Senile osteoporosis is found in aging men, whereas postmenopausal osteoporosis occurs in women (McCowin et al., 1991).

The acute pain of a compression fracture superimposed on chronic discomfort, often in the absence of a history of trauma, may be the only presenting symptom. The client may recall a "snap" associated with mild pain, or there may have been no pain at all after the "snap." More intense pain may not develop for hours or until the next day.

Back pain over the thoracic or lumbar spine that is intensified by prolonged sitting, standing, and the Valsalva maneuver may resolve after 3 or 4 months as the fractures of the vertebral bodies heal. The pain may persist owing to microfractures or biomechanical effects from deformity.

Other symptoms include pain on percussion over the fractured vertebral bodies, paraspinal muscle spasms, loss of height, and kyphoscoliosis.

Osteomalacia (see also Chapter 9). Osteomalacia is a metabolic bone disease in which the ratio of bone mineral content to bone matrix is decreased. The bone is weakened and vulnerable to fractures, which may produce back pain and progressive kyphoscoliosis. Osteomalacia may be caused by vitamin D deficiency, intestinal disorders, drugs, metabolic acidosis, phosphate deficiencies, and primary and secondary mineralization defects.

Symptoms may include back pain, fractures, bone tenderness on palpation, muscle weakness, kyphoscoliosis, bowing of the lower extremities, and enlargement of the costochondral junctions.

Fractures. Fractures occurring after trauma, in the osteoporotic spine, or in the spine affected by osteomalacia are usually easily diagnosed by the physician based on both the history and the radiographs. Acute, localized bone pain occurs secondary to a vertebral fracture. Vertebral body fracture without a history of trauma suggests a pathologic process affecting the bone (McCowin et al., 1991).

Small fractures, however, may occur in the apophyseal processes and in the trabeculae (Simms-Williams et al., 1978), particularly around the vertebral end-plates (Vernon-Roberts and Pirie, 1973), and may cause sudden severe episodes of back pain that resolve with a few days' rest. These fractures are difficult if not impossible to recognize in conventional radiographs.

Vertebral Osteomyelitis. Vertebral osteomyelitis is a bone infection most often affecting the first and second lumbar vertebrae, causing low back pain. There are many causative factors. Osteomyelitis may occur in diabetics, injection drug users (IDUs), alcoholics, clients on corticosteroid drugs, and otherwise debilitated or immune-suppressed clients.

Osteomyelitis also can occur after surgery, open fractures, penetrating wounds, and systemic infections; *Staphylococcus aureus* is the most common causative organism (Dirschl and Almekinders, 1993). It may result from a hematogenous spread through arterial and venous routes secondary to pelvic inflammatory disease or genitourinary tract infection.

Acute hematogenous osteomyelitis is seen most commonly in children, usually originating in the metaphysis of a long bone. Precipitating trauma is often present in the history, and well-localized, acute bone pain of 1 to several days' duration is the primary symptom. The pain is most commonly severe enough to limit or restrict the use of the involved extremity, and fever and malaise consistent with sepsis are usual (Green, 1988).

In the adult, usually two adjacent vertebrae and their intervening disc are involved, and the verebral body(ies) may undergo destruction and collapse. Abscess formation may result, with possible neurologic involvement.

The most consistent clinical finding is marked tenderness over the spinous process of the involved vertebrae with "nonspecific backache." Movement is painful, and there is marked muscular guarding of the paravertebral muscles and the hamstrings. The involved vertebrae are usually exquisitely sensitive to percussion, and pain is more severe at night. There may be no rise in temperature or abnormality in white blood cell count because generalized sepsis is not present, but an elevated erythrocyte sedimentation rate is likely.

Disc Space Infection. Disc space infection is a form of subacute osteomyelitis involving the vertebral end-plates and the disc in both children and adults. Symptoms associated with postoperative disc space infection occur 2 to 8 weeks after discectomy. Discitis of an infectious type occurs following bacteremia secondary to urinary tract infection, with or without instrumentation (e.g., catheterization or cystoscopy).

Adults with disc space infection often complain of low back pain localized around the disc area. The pain can range from mild to "excruciating;" excruciating pain is accompanied by restricted movement and constant pain, present both day and night. The pain is usually made worse by activity, but unlike most other causes of back pain, it is *not* relieved by rest. If the condition becomes chronic, pain may radiate into the abdomen, pelvis, and lower extremities.

Physical examination may reveal localized tenderness over the involved disc space, paraspinal muscle spasm, and restricted lumbar motion. A straight leg raise (SLR) may be positive, and fever is common (Morgenlander, 1991).

Rheumatic Diseases. Rheumatic diseases such as ankylosing spondylitis, Reiter's syndrome, psoriatic arthritis, and arthritis associated with chronic inflammatory bowel (enteropathic) disease may present with back and sacroiliac joint pain. Clients with these diseases have a genetic predisposition to these arthropathies, which are triggered by a number of environmental factors such as trauma and infection (McCowin et al., 1991). Each of these clinical entities has been discussed in detail in Chapter 11.

Spondyloarthropathy is characterized by

morning pain that improves with activity. There is limitation of motion in all directions and tenderness over the spine and sacroiliac joints. The most significant finding in ankylosing spondylitis is that the client presents with night (back) pain and morning stiffness as the two major complaints, but asymmetric sacroiliac involvement with radiation into the buttock and thigh can occur.

In addition to back pain, these rheumatic diseases usually include a constellation of associated signs and symptoms, such as fever, skin lesions, anorexia, and weight loss, that alert the physical therapist to the presence of systemic disease.

Polymyalgia rheumatica and fibromyalgia syndrome (formerly called fibrositis) are muscle syndromes associated with lumbosacral pain. Fibromyalgia syndrome refers to a syndrome of pain and stiffness that can occur in the back with localized tender areas. Both these disorders are also discussed in Chapter 11.

Hypercortisolism. Cushing's syndrome, or hypercortisolism, results from overactivity of the adrenal gland, with consequent hypersecretion of glucocorticoids. Iatrogenic Cushing's syndrome, another form of this disorder, results from exogenous administration of synthetic glucocorticoids in supraphysiologic amounts (Loriaux, 1993).

Although it is a relatively rare condition, it can cause demineralization of bone; in severe cases this may lead to pathologic fractures. More commonly, wedging of the vertebrae, kyphosis, bone pain, and back pain secondary to bone loss occur.

Psychogenic (see also Psychologic Factors in Pain Assessment, Chapter 1)

Psychogenic back pain is observed in the hysterical client or in the client who has extreme anxiety that increases the person's perception of pain. The hysterical client has severe pain as a product of inadequate defense mechanisms or severe anxiety. The anxiety leads to muscle tension, more anxiety, and then to muscle spasm. In either situation, look for bizarre signs, such as

- Paraplegia with only stocking-glove anesthesia
- Reflexes inconsistent with the presenting problem or other symptoms present
- Cogwheel motion of muscles for weakness
- Straight leg raising (SLR) in the sitting versus the supine position (person is unable to complete SLR in supine but can easily perform an SLR in a sitting position)
- SLR supine with plantar flexion instead of dorsiflexion reproduces symptoms

Primary or Secondary Cancer

It is essential to review the client's medical history regarding previous cancer when assessing back pain, especially back pain of insidious onset (whether gradual or sudden). For example, removal of a breast owing to primary cancer or a previous history of prostate cancer may seem so remote from the present back pain that the client may not volunteer this essential information (Cyriax, 1982; Wedge, 1983).

Neoplasm (whether primary or secondary) may interfere with the sympathetic nerves; if so, the foot on the affected side is warmer than the foot on the unaffected side. Paresis of the gross muscles of one or both feet in the absence of nerve root pain suggests a tumor. The client often looks anxious and fatigued and is often desperate for relief.

Primary Neoplasm. *Multiple myeloma* is the most common malignant primary bone tumor, and early in its course it can easily be overlooked as the cause of back pain, which is present in 35 per cent of clients with multiple myeloma. The symptoms may be nonspecific, but the general lack of well-being is an indicator of the need for medical referral. When pain is present, it is mild, aching, and intermittent, relieved by rest, and aggravated by weight bearing. There may be neurologic symptoms secondary to vertebral body collapse or extradural extension of the tumor.

Osteoid osteoma (benign, blood-filled tumor of cortical bone; osteoblastoma) of the spine may not present with the characteristic history of night pain relieved by aspirin. Some of these tumors are painless. When present, the pain is intermittent and vague initially but becomes constant, with a boring quality (McCowin et al., 1991). Hamstring spasm with marked limitation of SLR is often found with osteoid osteoma of the lumbar spine, causing further confusion.

Skeletal Metastases. Secondary cancer causing back pain is usually metastatic from the breast, thyroid, lung, kidney, or prostate and is much more common than primary bone cancer. The first suggestion of malignant disease lies in the history, which is not of pain varying with exertion but of pain of steady aggravation irrespective of activity. This distinguishing pain is unrelenting, intense, and progressive. In comparison, back pain owing to degenerative joint disease is seldom, if ever, unrelenting and usually responds to bed rest.

A short period of increasing central backache in an elderly person is always a red flag symptom. The pain spreads down both lower limbs in a distribution that does not correspond with any one nerve root level. Bilateral sciatica then develops, and the back pain becomes worse. Severe weakness without pain is very suggestive of spinal metastases. Gross muscle weakness with a full range of SLR and without a history of recent acute sciatica at the upper two lumbar levels is also suggestive of spinal metastases (Cyriax, 1982).

It is more difficult to detect sacral neoplasm than lower lumbar metastasis, because the spinal joints retain a full and painless range of movement. The client reports sacral pain, sometimes coccygodynia (pain in the coccyx) only.

Cervical Pain (Table 12–5)

Pain in the neck, shoulder, and arm may be secondary to a local abnormality or to a

Table 12–5

VISCEROGENIC CAUSES OF NECK AND BACK PAIN

Cervical	Thoracic/Scapular	Lumbar	Sacroiliac (SI)/Sacral
Tracheobronchial irritation	Pleuropulmonary disorders	Metastatic lesions	Prostatitis/cancer
Cervical bone tumors (benign or malignant)	Peptic ulcer	Kidney disorders	Gynecologic disorders
Cervical cord tumors	Pancreatic cancer	Pyelonephritis	Enteropathic disorders
Pancoast tumors	Pancreatitis	Perinephric abscess	Ulcerative colitis
Vertebral osteomyelitis	Cholecystitis	Nephrolithiasis	Crohn's disease
	Biliary colic	Ureteral colic	Colon cancer
	Pyelonephritis	UTI	Irritable bowel syndrome
	Kidney disease	Prostatitis/cancer	Endocarditis
	Mediastinal tumors	Testicular cancer	Spondyloarthropathies
	Aortic aneurysm	Abdominal aortic aneurysm	Ankylosing spondylitis
	Esophagitis (severe)	Endocarditis	Reiter's syndrome
	Myocardial infarct	Acute pancreatitis	Psoriatic arthritis
	Gallbladder	Small intestine	Inflammatory bowel disease arthritis
	Acromegaly	Obstruction (neoplasm)	Paget's disease
		Irritable bowel syndrome	
		Crohn's disease (regional enteritis)	
		Gynecologic disorders	
		Tuberculosis	

systemic disorder. Although referred neck pain and disability resulting from cervical spine disorders are most commonly caused by intervertebral disc degeneration, referred pain also may be caused by an inflammatory process such as rheumatoid arthritis; infectious disease (e.g., vertebral osteomyelitis); cancer; or cardiac, pulmonary (Pancoast's tumor), or abdominal disorders (Cyriax, 1982; Pedowitz et al., 1988).

Tracheobronchial Irritation. Tracheobronchial irritation can cause pain to be referred to sites in the neck or anterior chest at the same levels as the points of irritation in the air passages (see Fig. 4–6). This irritation may be caused by inflammatory lesions, irritating foreign materials, or cancerous tumors (Bauwens and Paine, 1983).

Cervical Bone Tumors. These may be benign or malignant primary (arising from bone), secondary (i.e., metastatic from a distant primary site), extramedullary, or intramedullary neoplasms. Primary neoplastic tumors of the cervical spine are rare in adults. They are much more common in younger people and more likely to be benign in this age group (Pedowitz et al., 1988).

The most common benign tumors in adults are osteochondromas, osteoblastomas, aneurysmal bone cysts, chondromas, osteoid osteomas, and hemangiomas (blood-filled tumor). The most common malignant tumors are osteogenic sarcoma, giant cell tumor, and chordoma.

The primary first symptom is persistent, local neck pain of insidious onset, with or without neurologic signs and symptoms (e.g., upper extremity pain, weakness, and sensory loss). The pain may be severe and constant (i.e., through the night) and is not usually relieved by rest. Occipital headache may accompany the neck pain (Phillips and Levine, 1989).

There may be a palpable external mass and pain on motion of the cervical spine. With progressive vertebral body collapse, bone may protrude into the spinal canal, compressing the anterior spinal cord surface and producing paralysis.

Cervical (Spinal) Cord Tumors. These account for 15 per cent of primary central nervous system tumors. Metastatic lesions are much more common than primary lesions, with 15 per cent of spine metastases localized in the cervical region.

Pancoast's Tumors. Pancoast's tumors of the lung may invade the roots of the brachial plexus as they enlarge, so that the client with Pancoast's tumor may present with pain in the C8 to T1 region, wasting of the muscles of the hand, and/or Horner's syndrome (unilateral constricted pupil, ptosis, loss of facial sweating).

Vertebral Osteomyelitis. This occurs infrequently, with approximately 8 per cent of the cases localized to the cervical spine. Epidural extension may cause radicular pain or neurologic deficit. Previous infection can be identified in 30 per cent to 40 per cent of cases, including tuberculosis as a potential source of cervical spine infections (Pedowitz et al., 1988).

Thoracic Pain (D'Ambrosia, 1986)
(Table 12–6)

Systemic origins of musculoskeletal pain in the thoracic spine (see Tables 12–5 and 12–6) are usually accompanied by constitutional symptoms (affecting the whole body, systemic) and other associated symptoms that the client may not relate to the back pain and, therefore, may fail to mention to the physical therapist. Such additional symptoms should be discovered during the subjective examination by the careful interviewer. When the client (or the objective examination) indicates the presence of a fever (or night sweats), a referral to a physician is indicated.

The close proximity of the thoracic spine to the chest and respiratory organs may result in a correlation between respiratory movements and increased thoracic symptoms. This situation requires careful screening of *pleuropulmonary* (involving the pleura and the lungs) symptoms.

Table 12-6

SYSTEMIC CAUSES OF THORACIC/SCAPULAR PAIN

Systemic Origin	Location
Pleuropulmonary disorders	
Basilar pneumonia	Right upper back
Empyema	Scapula
Pleurisy	Scapula
Spontaneous pneumothorax	Ipsilateral scapula
Peptic ulcer: stomach/duodenal ulcers	6th–10th thoracic vertebrae
Pancreatic carcinoma	Midthoracic or lumbar spine
Gallbladder disease	Midback between scapulae; right upper scapula
Acute cholecystitis	Right subscapular area; between scapulae
Biliary colic	Right upper back; midback between scapulae; right interscapular or subscapular areas
Acute pyelonephritis	Costovertebral angle (posteriorly)
Esophagitis	Midback between scapulae
Myocardial infarct	Midthoracic spine
Acromegaly	Midthoracic or lumbar spine

When screening the client by means of the physical therapy interview, the physical therapist should remember that symptoms of pleural, intercostal, muscular, costal, and dural origin all increase on coughing or deep inspiration; thus, only pain of a cardiac origin is ruled out when symptoms increase in association with respiratory movements (Cyriax, 1982).

Clients with acute deterioration of neurologic status frequently have thoracic lesions. The ratio of canal diameter to cord size is small, resulting in early neural compression. Collateral circulation to the midthoracic region is limited, and tumor involvement may produce ischemic damage to the cord with resultant rapid worsening of neurologic status (O'Connor and Currier, 1992).

Peptic Ulcer

The pain of peptic ulcer (see Fig. 6–6) occasionally occurs only in the back between the eighth and tenth thoracic vertebrae. Duodenal ulcers may refer pain from the fifth to tenth thoracic vertebrae, either at the midline or just to one side of the spine (may be either side). This localization accompanies posterior penetration through the duodenum. The client usually describes a typical history of ulcers, with periodic symptoms, relief with antacids, and the relationship of pain to certain foods and the timing of meals. For example, the client may have relief from pain after eating initially, but the pain then returns and increases 1 to 2 hours after eating when the stomach is emptied. When questioned further, the client may indicate that blood is present in the feces.

Pancreatic Carcinoma

In pancreatic carcinoma (see Figs. 6–13 and 8–5), the most frequent symptom is pain. It can be first noted as a paroxysmal or steady, dull pain radiating from the epigastrium into the back. The pain is usually slowly progressive, is worse at night, and is unrelated to digestive activities. Other signs and symptoms may include jaundice, anorexia, severe weight loss, and GI difficulties that are unrelated to meals. This disease is predominantly found in men (3:1) and occurs in the sixth and seventh decades.

Acute Cholecystitis

Acute cholecystitis (gallbladder infection) (see Fig. 8–5) may refer intense, sudden, paroxysmal (sudden, recurrent or intensifying) pain to the right upper quadrant of the back, especially the tip of the right scapula, with muscle guarding. This muscle guarding causes tenderness, pain, and biomechanical disturbances that further increase the client's pain. Fever and chills are common associated symptoms.

Biliary Colic

The pain of biliary colic (see Fig. 8–5) (bile duct obstruction that may be caused by various disorders, including stones, stricture, pancreatic carcinoma, and primary biliary cirrhosis) refers to the right upper quadrant posteriorly, with pain in the right shoulder. There may be back pain between the scapulae, with referred pain to the right side in the interscapular or subscapular area. Occasionally, the pain beneath the right costal margin may be confused with the shoulder girdle pain secondary to intracostal nerve compression.

Acute Pyelonephritis

Acute pyelonephritis (see Fig. 7–3) (inflammation of the kidney and renal pelvis) and other kidney conditions present with aching pain at one or several costovertebral areas, posteriorly, just lateral to the muscles at T12–L1, from acute distention of the capsule of the kidney. The pain is usually dull and constant, with possible radiation to the pelvic crest or groin. The client may describe febrile chills, frequent urination, hematuria, and shoulder pain (if the diaphragm is irritated). Percussion to the flank areas reveals tenderness.

Mediastinal Lesions

Mediastinal tumors or an aortic aneurysm (see Fig. 3–11) may refer pain to the thoracic spine, but the pain is agonizing and is disproportionate to any musculoskeletal problem. In the case of neoplasm, the client may report symptoms typical of cancer (see Chapter 10). Tumors occur most often in the thoracic spine because of its length, the proximity to the mediastinum, and the proximity to direct metastatic extension from lymph nodes involved with lymphoma, breast, or lung cancer.

With *aortic aneurysm,* there may be a history of cardiac involvement. Vascular pain from abdominal aortic aneurysm is secondary to compression of surrounding structures or extension or rupture of the aneurysm. Most clients experience dull, steady abdominal pain that is unrelated to activity. Back pain is usually associated with epigastric discomfort and may radiate to the lumbar spine, hips, or thighs. Rupture of an abdominal aneurysm is associated with excruciating pain, circulatory shock, and an expanding mass (McCowin et al., 1991).

Severe Esophagitis

Severe esophagitis (see Fig. 6–10) may refer pain to the thoracic spine. This referred pain is always accompanied by epigastric pain and heartburn. The client may be an alcoholic and have esophageal varices (distention of veins in lower esophagus) in association with the esophagitis.

Myocardial Infarction

The pain of an acute myocardial infarction (see Fig. 3–9) ("heart attack") may radiate into the thoracic spine area. It is accompanied usually by a crushing, compressing pain or a sensation across the chest with an associated cold sweat, weak blood pressure, and thready pulse.

Scapular Pain (see Table 12–6)

Most causes of scapular pain occur along the vertebral border and result from various primary musculoskeletal lesions. However, respiratory viral infections or pulmonary disorders, such as empyema (pus in the pleural cavity), pleurisy (inflammation of the pleura), or spontaneous pneumothorax (air in the pleural cavity), can cause scapular pain.

Clients with these pulmonary or respiratory origins of pain usually also show signs of general malaise and associated symptoms related to the pulmonary system. Gallbladder disease and biliary colic from other causes may also refer pain to the interscapular or right subscapular area. Specific questions should be asked to rule out potential pulmonary or GI problems, because the client may not associate such signs and symptoms with scapular pain.

Clients presenting with a pneumothorax develop acute pleuritic chest pain localized to the side of the pneumothorax. This pain may be referred to the ipsilateral scapula or shoulder, across the chest, or over the abdomen (see Fig. 4–5); associated symptoms may include dyspnea, cough, hemoptysis (blood in sputum), tachycardia (increased heart rate), tachypnea (rapid respirations), and cyanosis (blue lips and skin due to a lack of oxygen).

The client may have severe pain in the upper and lateral thoracic wall, which is aggravated by any movement and by the cough and dyspnea that accompany it (Bauwens and Paine, 1983). The client may be most comfortable sitting in an upright position.

Lumbar Pain (Low Back Pain)
(see Table 12–5; Table 12–7)

Metastatic Lesions

Metastatic lesions affecting the lumbar spine occur most commonly from breast, lung, prostate, kidney, and GI cancer and myelomas and lymphomas (McClain and Weinstein, 1990). Cancer of the prostate is the second most common site of cancer among men and is often diagnosed when the man seeks medical assistance because of symptoms of urinary obstruction or sciatica. The sciatic (low back, hip, and leg)

pain is caused by metastasis of the cancer to the bones of the pelvis, lumbar spine, or femur.

The high frequency of metastatic involvement of the spine may be due to tumor spread via the paravertebral venous plexus. This thin-walled and valveless venous system probably accounts for the higher incidence of metastases in the thoracic spine from breast carcinoma and in the lumbar region from prostatic carcinoma (Harrington, 1986).

As discussed earlier, pain due to neoplasm is typically progressive, is more pronounced at night, and may not have a clear association with activity level, as is characteristic of mechanical back pain. The usual progression of symptoms in clients with cord compression is back pain followed by radicular pain, lower extremity weakness, sensory loss, and, finally, loss of sphincter (bowel and bladder) control (O'Connor and Currier, 1992).

When there is a delay of less than 24 hours between the onset of symptoms and the appearance of full-blown neurologic involvement, the prognosis for recovery is poor no matter what treatment is offered (Harrington, 1986).

Kidney Disorders

Kidney disorders (see Figs. 7–4, 7–6, and 7–7), such as acute pyelonephritis and perinephric abscess of the kidney, may be confused with a back condition. Most renal and urologic conditions present with a combination of systemic signs and symptoms accompanied by pelvic, flank, or low back pain. The client may have a history of recent trauma or a past medical history of urinary tract infections to alert the clinician to a possible systemic origin of symptoms. In *pyelonephritis,* an aching pain is noted in one or both costovertebral areas (see Fig. 7–5). The client usually has a fever and shaking chills. The flank areas are tender to percussion.

Nephrolithiasis (kidney stones) may present as back pain radiating to the flank

Table 12–7

LOW BACK PAIN: SYMPTOMS AND CAUSES

Symptom	Possible Cause
Night pain unrelieved by rest or position change	Tumor
Fever, chills, sweats	Infection
Unremitting, throbbing lumbar pain	Aortic aneurysm
Abdominal pain radiating to midback	Pancreatitis, gastrointestinal disease, peptic ulcer
Morning stiffness that improves as day goes on	Inflammatory arthritis
Leg pain increased by walking and relieved by standing	Vascular claudication
Leg pain increased by walking, unaffected by standing, but relieved by sitting	Neurogenic claudication
"Stocking-glove" numbness	Referred pain, nonorganic pain
Global pain	Nonorganic pain
Long-standing back pain aggravated by activity	Deconditioning
Pain increased by sitting	Discogenic disease
Sharp, narrow band of pain radiating below the knee	Herniated disc
Chronic spinal pain (unsatisfying job/home life)	Stress
Back pain dating to specific injury	Strain or sprain
Back pain in athletic teenager	Epiphysitis, juvenile discogenic disease, spondylolysis, or spondylolisthesis

Adapted from Nelson, B.W.: A rational approach to the treatment of low back pain. Journal of Musculoskeletal Medicine *10*(5):75, 1993.

or the iliac crest. These stones are subsequently passed through the ureters to the bladder and then through the urethra. They are usually due to the precipitation of calcium salts but can be urate salts, cystine (amino acid), or rarely xanthine (purine compound).

The calcium-containing variety most often occurs with diseases associated with hypercalcemia (excess calcium in the blood), such as hyperparathyroidism, metastatic carcinoma, multiple myeloma, senile osteoporosis, specific renal tubular disease, hyperthyroidism, and Cushing's disease.

Other conditions associated with calcu-lus formation are infection, urinary stasis, dehydration, and excessive ingestion or absorption of calcium. Urate crystals are associated with gouty conditions and hyperuricemia (excess uric acid in blood) (D'Ambrosia, 1986). The focal symptoms of nephrolithiasis are characterized by back pain radiating to the flank or iliac crest (see Fig. 7–4).

Ureteral colic, caused by passage of a calculus (kidney stone), presents as an excruciating pain that radiates down the course of the ureter into the urethra or groin area. These attacks are intermittent and can be accompanied by nausea, vomiting, sweating, and tachycardia. The urine usually contains erythrocytes or is grossly bloody (D'Ambrosia, 1986).

Urinary tract infection affecting the lower urinary tract is related directly to irritation of the bladder and urethra. The intensity of symptoms depends on the severity of the infection, and although low back pain may be the client's chief complaint, further questioning usually elicits additional urologic symptoms, such as urinary frequency, urinary urgency, dysuria, or hematuria. Clients can be asymptomatic with regard to urologic symptoms, and a medical work-up will be necessary for making the diagnosis.

Prostatitis

Prostatitis or prostate cancer can cause low back, pelvic, and leg pain. In addition, metastases from prostate cancer to the pelvis, femur, and/or lumbar spine can produce sciatica. Associated symptoms include melena (blood in stool), sudden moderate-to-high fever, chills, and changes in bowel function. Men from the fifth decade on are most commonly affected.

Testicular Cancer (Richie, 1993)

Testicular cancer is a relatively uncommon disease with an incidence of only about 3 cases per 100,000 men per year. Nonetheless, testicular cancer represents the most common malignancy in men from ages 15 to 35 and is the second most common malignancy from ages 35 to 39.

Involvement of the epididymis or spermatic cord may lead to pelvic or inguinal lymph node metastases, although most tumors confined to the testis proper will spread primarily to the retroperitoneal lymph nodes. Subsequent cephalad drainage may be to the thoracic duct and supraclavicular nodes. Hematogenous spread to the lungs, bone, or liver may occur as a result of direct tumor invasion. In about 10 per cent of clients, dissemination along

these pathways may result in thoracic, lumbar, supraclavicular, neck, or shoulder pain or mass as the first symptom. Other symptoms related to this pathway of dissemination may include respiratory symptoms or GI disturbance.

The usual presentation of testicular cancer is a painless swelling nodule in one gonad, noted incidentally by the client or his sexual partner. This is described as a lump or hardness of the testis, with occasional heaviness or a dull aching sensation in the lower abdomen or scrotum. Acute pain is the presenting symptom in about 10 per cent of clients.

Abdominal Aortic Aneurysm

On occasion, an abdominal aortic aneurysm (see Fig. 3–11) can cause severe back pain. Prompt medical attention is imperative because rupture can result in death. The clients are usually men in the sixth or seventh decade of life who present with a deep, boring pain in the midlumbar region. Other historical clues of coronary disease or intermittent claudication of the lower extremities may be present. An objective examination may reveal a pulsing abdominal mass. Peripheral pulses may be diminished or absent (D'Ambrosia, 1986).

Endocarditis

A significant number of clients (up to 45 per cent) with bacterial endocarditis present initially with musculoskeletal symptoms, including arthralgia, arthritis, low back pain, and myalgias. Half of these clients will have only musculoskeletal symptoms, without other signs of endocarditis. The early onset of joint pain and myalgia is more likely if the client is older and has had a previously diagnosed heart murmur.

Almost one third of clients with bacterial endocarditis have low back pain; in many clients, it is the principal musculoskeletal symptom reported. Back pain is accompanied by decreased range of motion and spinal tenderness. Pain may affect only one side, and it may be limited to the paraspinal muscles. Endocarditis-induced low back pain may be very similar to that associated with a herniated lumbar disc: it radiates to the leg and may be accentuated by raising the leg, coughing, or sneezing. The key difference is that neurologic deficits are usually absent in clients with bacterial endocarditis.

The cause of back pain and leg myalgia associated with bacterial endocarditis has not been determined. Some authors suggest that concurrent aseptic meningitis may contribute to both leg and pack pain. Others suggest that leg pain is related to emboli that break off from the infected cardiac valves. The latter theory is supported by biopsy evidence of muscle necrosis or vasculitis in clients with bacterial endocarditis.

Acute Pancreatitis

The pain of acute pancreatitis (see Fig. 6–13) originates in the epigastrium and may radiate into the midback to low back in the region of L1 (referred). Pain from the head of the pancreas is felt to the right of the spine, whereas pain from the body and tail is felt to the left of the spine (McCowin et al., 1991). It is sudden, severe, and widespread. Associated symptoms, including diarrhea, pain after a meal, anorexia, and unexplained weight loss, are related primarily to the GI system. The pain is relieved initially by heat, which decreases muscular tension, and may be relieved by leaning forward, sitting up, or lying motionless (D'Ambrosia, 1986).

Diseases of the Small Intestine

Diseases of the small intestine (see Fig. 6–11), such as Crohn's disease (regional enteritis), irritable bowel syndrome, or obstruction (neoplasm), usually produce abdominal pain, but the pain may be referred to the back if the stimulus is sufficiently intense or if the individual's pain threshold is low. There will almost always be accompanying GI symptoms to alert the careful examiner.

Gynecologic Disorders

Gynecologic disorders can cause midpelvic or low back discomfort (see also Pelvic Pain in this chapter). These conditions can include

- Retroversion (tipping back) of the uterus
- Ovarian cysts
- Uterine fibroids (fibrous connective tissue)
- Endometriosis (uterine lining attaches to pelvic cavity and organs therein)
- Pelvic inflammatory disease (PID)
- Cystocele (herniation of the urinary bladder into the vagina)
- Rectocele (hernial protrusion of part of the rectum into the vagina)
- Ectopic or normal pregnancy

The woman may have sharp, bilateral, and cramping pain in the lower quadrants. These conditions are most common in women aged 20 to 45 years. A diagnosis of pelvic disorders as the cause of low back pain in the woman is made by careful pelvic examination by the physician. A gynecologic/obstetric screen should be included in all complete back work-ups, because these conditions can be confused with ruptured appendix, ectopic pregnancy (fertilized ovum implants outside the uterus), or perforation of GI abscesses.

Low back pain associated with pregnancy may occur as a result of a variety of causes, including changes that occur with ligamentous relaxation of the pelvic girdle (Golightly, 1982; Grieve, 1976; Magee, 1992), rotation of the pelvis at the sacroiliac joint (Spankus, 1965), faulty body mechanics and poor posture leading to increased musculoskeletal stress and strain (Spankus, 1965), and stretch placed on the dorsolumbar fascia through its attachment to the abdominal muscles (Sullivan, 1989).

Pain of vascular origin is usually throbbing or pulsatile. Although vascular accidents are rare during pregnancy, in a few cases vascular anomalies of spinal vessels first appear during pregnancy. Presenting symptoms are sudden onset of back pain, followed by rapidly progressive motor loss (Collins et al., 1986).

In addition, it should be remembered that pain from hip pathology can be referred to the groin, ankle, knee, thigh, low back, or sacroiliac areas. The client may reveal rectal and lower sacral or coccygeal pain that can be referred menstrual pain. There may be a history of sexually transmitted disease, ectopic pregnancy, use of an intrauterine contraceptive device, dysuria, or a recent abortion. With a cystocele or a rectocele, there may be a history of multiparity (two or more pregnancies resulting in viable offspring), prolonged

▼ *Associated Signs and Symptoms of* **Gynecologic Disorders**

- Missed menses, irregular menses, history of menstrual disturbances
- Tender breasts
- Nausea, vomiting
- Chronic constipation (with laxative and enema dependency)
- Pain on defecation
- Fever, night sweats, chills
- History of vaginal discharge
- Abnormal uterine bleeding
  - Late menstrual periods with persistent bleeding
  - Irregular, longer, heavier menstrual periods, no specific pattern
  - Any postmenopausal bleeding

labor, instrument (e.g., forceps) delivery, chronic cough, or lifting heavy objects.

Tumors, masses, and even endometriosis may involve the sacral plexus or its branches, causing severe, burning pain that is sciatic in nature. Multiple roots are usually involved, and the pain is severe and burning (D'Ambrosia, 1986).

Current efforts to identify the pathogenesis of obstetric low back pain are devoted to the study of normal and abnormal biomechanics of the spine and the influence of physiologic changes of pregnancy on the musculoskeletal system (Hummel-Berry, 1990).

The physical therapist is encouraged to ask appropriate questions to determine the need for a gynecologic evaluation (see *Special Questions for Women* in this chapter), especially in the absence of objective musculoskeletal findings.

Tuberculosis (see also Chapter 4)

Tuberculous spondylitis (Pott's disease) most commonly affects the lower thoracic vertebrae at the level of the kidney, producing nagging local back pain referred to the anterior abdominal wall (mistaken for appendicitis). A tender, prominent spinal process may develop because of anterior wedging of two vertebral bodies. A paraspinal abscess may extend and present as a mass in the groin or supraclavicular space. A paraspinal abscess that compresses the spinal cord or granulation tissue that intrudes on the anterior aspects of the cord may cause symptoms ranging from minor loss of bowel and urinary sphincter control to abrupt and irreversible paraplegia (Berkow and Fletcher, 1992). Immobilization and avoidance of weight bearing may be required to relieve pain, with attention to maintaining strength and range of motion.

There may be a history of previous lymph or pulmonary infection or a positive family history for tuberculosis. The tuberculosis bacilli spread through the bloodstream with the following musculoskeletal findings:

- Kyphosis secondary to the destruction of vertebral bodies (especially the thoracolumbar junction)
- Spasticity or paraplegia if abscess or bone impingement puts pressure on the cord
- Low-grade fever, pallor
- Local back pain aggravated by movement
- Listlessness, muscle atrophy
- Night pain

Sacroiliac Joint/Sacral Pain
(see Table 12–5)

The most common clinical presentation of sacroiliac pain is in a person who has had a memorable *physical event* that initiated the pain, such as a misstep off a curb, lifting of a heavy object in a twisted position, or childbirth, possibly due to the relationship of birthing positions to pelvic/low back/sacral pain (Mens et al., 1992; Mooney, 1993). The person usually experiences severe pain over the posterior sacroiliac joint and medial buttock, with some distal referral.

The most typical pain referral patterns of *systemic disease* to the sacrum and sacroiliac joint include prostatitis, prostate cancer, and gynecologic disorders. These specific disorders also refer pain to the lumbar spine and have already been discussed in that section.

Disorders of the large intestine and colon, such as ulcerative colitis, Crohn's disease (regional enteritis), carcinoma of the colon, and the irritable bowel syndrome, can refer pain to the sacrum when the rectum is stimulated.

Most commonly, unless pain causes muscle spasm, splinting, and subsequent biomechanical changes, these clients demonstrate a remarkable lack of objective findings to implicate the sacroiliac joint or sacrum as the causative factor in the symptoms presented.

Mennell (1964) suggests that sacral pain in the absence of history of trauma or overuse is a clue to the presentation of systemic backache. Pain elicited by pressing on the sacrum with the client in a prone position suggests sacroiliitis (inflammation of the sacroiliac joint) (Hadler, 1987a).

Endocarditis

Endocarditis may produce destructive changes in the sacroiliac joint, probably as a result of seeding of the joint by septic emboli. The pain will be localized over the sacroiliac joint, and the physician will use x-ray studies and bone scans to verify this diagnosis. See Chapter 3 for an in-depth discussion of endocarditis.

Spondyloarthropathies

Spondyloarthropathies, representing a group of noninfected, inflammatory, erosive rheumatic diseases, target the sacroiliac joints. Sacroiliac and back pain are present in clients who have ankylosing spondylitis, Reiter's syndrome, psoriatic arthritis, or arthritis associated with chronic inflammatory bowel disease. Each of these disorders is characterized by additional systemic signs and symptoms that should be discovered by the careful interviewer (see individual chapters for an in-depth discussion of each disease). Such findings will assist the physical therapist in determining the need for further medical follow-up.

Paget's Disease (see also Chapter 9)

Paget's disease (osteitis deformans) is a metabolic bone disorder characterized by slowly progressive enlargement and deformity of multiple bones associated with unexplained acceleration of both deposition and resorption of bone that causes the bones to become spongelike, weakened,

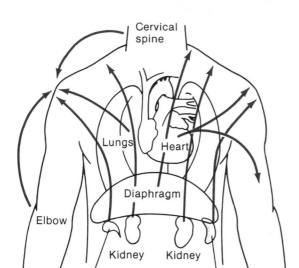

Figure 12-1

Musculoskeletal and systemic structures referring pain to the shoulder. (Adapted from Magee, D.J.: Orthopedic Physical Assessment, 2nd ed. Philadelphia, W.B. Saunders, 1992, p. 125.)

and deformed. The bones most commonly involved are the pelvis, lumbar spine, and sacrum. Although this disorder is often asymptomatic, when symptoms do occur, they occur insidiously and may include deep, aching bone pain, nocturnal pain, joint stiffness, fatigue, headaches, dizziness, increased temperature over the long bones, and periosteal tenderness.

SHOULDER PAIN (Fig. 12-1)

Systemic disease may also present itself clinically as shoulder pain. Pain is commonly referred to one of the shoulder joints (Table 12-8) from diseased viscera in the chest and in the upper abdomen. Other pathologic conditions in the neck, cervical spine, axilla, thorax, thoracic spine, and chest wall (Table 12-9) also can refer pain to the shoulder.

Differential diagnosis of shoulder pain is sometimes especially difficult, because any pain that is felt in the shoulder will affect

Table 12-8
SHOULDER PAIN

Right Shoulder		Left Shoulder	
Systemic Origin	*Location*	*Systemic Origin*	*Location*
Peptic ulcer	Lateral border, R scapula	Ruptured spleen	L shoulder (Kehr's sign)
Myocardial ischemia	R shoulder, down arm	Myocardial ischemia	L pectoral/L shoulder
Hepatic/biliary:		Pancreas	L shoulder
Acute cholecystitis	R shoulder; between scapulae; R subscapular area	Ectopic pregnancy (rupture)	L shoulder (Kehr's sign)
Liver abscess	R shoulder		
Gallbladder	R upper trapezius		
Liver disease (hepatitis, cirrhosis, metastatic tumors)	R shoulder, R subscapula		
Pulmonary:	Ipsilateral shoulder; upper trapezius	Pulmonary:	Ipsilateral shoulder; upper trapezius
Pleurisy		Pleurisy	
Spontaneous pneumothorax		Spontaneous pneumothorax	
Pancoast's tumor		Pancoast's tumor	
Kidney	Ipsilateral shoulder	Kidney	Ipsilateral shoulder
		Postoperative laparoscopy	L shoulder (Kehr's sign)

Table 12-9

SYSTEMIC CAUSES OF SHOULDER PAIN

Shoulder pain may be referred from the neck, chest (thorax or thoracic spine), and abdomen, and from systemic diseases. The following have been diagnosed as having the onset or origin of presenting symptoms in the shoulder.

Neck	Chest	Abdomen	Systemic Disease
Bone tumors	Angina/myocardial infarct	Liver disease	Collagen vascular disease
Metastases	Pericarditis	Ruptured spleen	Gout
Tuberculosis	Aortic aneurysm	Spinal metastases	Syphilis/gonorrhea
Nodes in neck (from	Empyema and lung abscess	Dissecting aortic aneurysm	Sickle cell anemia
metastases, leukemia,	Pulmonary tuberculosis	Diaphragmatic irritation	Hemophilia
and Hodgkin's disease)	Pancoast's tumor	Peptic ulcer	Rheumatic disease
Cervical cord tumors	Lung cancer (bronchogenic	Gallbladder disease	Metastatic cancer
	carcinoma)	Subphrenic abscess	Breast
	Spontaneous pneumothorax	Hiatal hernia	Prostate
	Nodes in mediastinum/axilla	Pyelonephritis	Kidney
	Metastases in thoracic spine	Diaphragmatic hernia	Lung
	Breast disease	Ectopic pregnancy	Thyroid
	Primary or secondary	(rupture)	Testicle
	cancer	Upper urinary tract	
	Mastodynia		
	Hiatal hernia		

Adapted from Zohn, D.A.: Musculoskeletal Pain: Diagnosis and Physical Treatment, 2nd ed. Boston, Little, Brown, 1988, p. 178.

the joint as though the pain were originating in the joint (Mennell, 1964).

Many visceral diseases are notorious for presenting as unilateral shoulder pain. Esophageal, pericardial, or myocardial diseases, aortic dissection, and diaphragmatic irritation from thoracic or abdominal diseases can all present as unilateral shoulder pain.

For example, distention of the renal cap from kidney disorders can refer pain to the ipsilateral shoulder via pressure on the diaphragm. Usually with referred pain from the thoracic or abdominal viscera, the history will present sufficient symptoms in the chest or abdomen to indicate a systemic problem (Riggins, 1986).

Left shoulder pain lasting several days after diagnostic laparoscopy results from free air in the peritoneum from gas used to expand the area during the procedure (Haicken, 1991; Narchi et al., 1991).

Shoulder pain with any of the following features should be approached as a manifestation of systemic visceral illness, even if the pain is exacerbated by shoulder movement or if there are objective findings at the shoulder (Hadler, 1987a):

- Pleuritic component
  - Persistent dry, hacking, or productive cough
  - Blood-tinged sputum
  - Musculoskeletal symptoms aggravated by respiratory movements, such as coughing, laughing, deep breathing
  - Chest pain
- Exacerbation by recumbency
- Coincident diaphoresis
- Coincident nausea, vomiting, dysphagia
- Other GI complaints:
  - Anorexia
  - Early satiety
  - Epigastric pain or discomfort and fullness
- Exacerbation by exertion unrelated to shoulder movement (cardiac)
- Urologic complaints (see Fig. 7-4)
- Jaundice (see Fig. 8-5)

Pulmonary Diseases and Shoulder Pain

Extensive disease may occur in the periphery of the lung without pain until the process extends to the parietal pleura. Pleural irritation then results in sharp, localized pain that is aggravated by any respiratory movement. Clients usually note that the pain is alleviated by lying on the affected side, which diminishes the movement of that side of the chest ("autosplinting") (Scharf, 1989). Shoulder pain of musculoskeletal origin is usually aggravated by lying on the symptomatic shoulder.

Cardiac Diseases and Shoulder Pain

Pain of cardiac and diaphragmatic origin is often experienced in the shoulder, because the heart and diaphragm are supplied by the C5–C6 spinal segment, and the visceral pain is referred to the corresponding somatic area (Scharf, 1989).

The most frequent musculoskeletal symptom in clients with *bacterial endocarditis* is arthralgia, generally in the proximal joints. The shoulder is the most commonly affected site, followed (in declining incidence) by the knee, hip, wrist, ankle, metatarsophalangeal, and metacarpophalangeal joints and by acromioclavicular involvement.

Most endocarditis clients with arthralgias have only one or two painful joints, although some may have pain in several joints. Painful symptoms begin suddenly in one or two joints, accompanied by warmth, tenderness, and redness. One helpful clue: as a rule, morning stiffness is not as prevalent in clients with endocarditis as in those with rheumatoid arthritis or polymyalgia rheumatica.

The inflammatory process accompanying *pericarditis* may result in an accumulation of fluid in the pericardial sac, preventing the heart from expanding fully. The subsequent chest pain of pericarditis (see Fig. 3–10) closely mimics that of a myocardial infarction because it is substernal, is associated with cough, and may radiate to the shoulder. It can be differentiated from myocardial infarction by the pattern of relieving and aggravating factors.

For example, the pain of a myocardial infarction is unaffected by position, breathing, or movement, whereas the pain associated with pericarditis may be relieved by kneeling with hands on the floor, leaning forward, or sitting upright. Pericardial pain is often worse with breathing, swallowing, or belching.

Aortic aneurysm presents as sudden, severe chest pain with a tearing sensation (see Fig. 3–11), and the pain may extend to the neck, shoulders, lower back, or abdomen but rarely to the joints and arms, which distinguishes it from a myocardial infarction. Isolated shoulder pain is not associated with aortic aneurysm. Shoulder pain associated with *angina* and *myocardial infarct* is presented in Chapter 3. See also Figures 3–8 and 3–9.

Painful Shoulder-Hand Syndrome
(see also Chapter 3)

The shoulder-hand syndrome is uncommon and remains a poorly understood condition of the upper extremity, believed to be caused by a malfunction of the autonomic nervous system. In fact, the term shoulder-hand syndrome represents outdated, though still used, nomenclature. Reflex sympathetic dystrophy (RSD) is a more descriptive term that better reflects the underlying sympathetic dysfunction.

The client has severe and bizarre pains in the extremity associated with excessive sweating and coolness. There is glossiness of the skin with a loss of normal skin texture and associated joint stiffness. This syndrome occurs more commonly in people who are emotionally unstable and who have extremely low pain thresholds (Riggins, 1986).

The initiating factor may be trauma, often quite minor, or it may result from

Table 12–10
STAGES OF SHOULDER-HAND SYNDROME (REFLEX SYMPATHETIC DYSTROPHY–RSD)

Stage 1	Stage 2	Stage 3
Limited shoulder range of motion with or without pain	Shoulder pain subsides, and shoulder range may even increase	Progressive atrophy of the bones, skin, and muscles
Swelling of the dorsum of the hand	Edema of the hand may subside, but fingers will become even stiffer	Limitation of hands, wrists, and fingers increases, leaving the hand painless but in a useless, atrophied, clawed position
Full flexion of the fingers and joints	Sensitivity decreases	
Wrist assumes a flexed posture	No change in skin appearance—pale, atrophic	
Skin is usually moist with small bubbles of perspiration, and the hand may be pale and cool or assume a pink hue		

From Cailliet, R.: Shoulder Pain. Philadelphia, F.A. Davis, 1981.

remote disease of the thoracic or abdominal viscera that causes referred pain to the shoulder and arm (Riggins, 1986). A painful shoulder-hand presentation may follow a myocardial infarction or cerebral vascular accident (stroke). RSD can occur from 1 to 3 months after the infarction or cerebral vascular accident. It was a more common complication of myocardial infarctions when clients were treated with strict, prolonged bed rest and immobilization. The change from prolonged bed rest to early ambulation has almost eliminated this problem (Morris et al., 1990).

This syndrome occurs with equal frequency in either or both shoulders and, except when caused by coronary occlusion, is most frequent in women. The shoulder is generally involved first, but the painful hand may precede the shoulder. Regardless of the site or source of the pain sensation, the syndrome follows a specific pattern.

Pain Pattern

Three stages of the complex are recognized (Table 12–10). First the shoulder becomes "stiff," is limited in range of motion, and may proceed to a "frozen shoulder." Even after a myocardial infarction, the shoulder initially resembles the pericapsulitis from other causes. Tenderness about the shoulder is diffuse and not localized to a specific tendon or bursal area. The duration of the initial shoulder stage, before the hand component begins, is extremely variable.

The shoulder may be "stiff" for several months before the hand becomes involved, or both may become stiff simultaneously. The hand and fingers become diffusely swollen. At first, the edema is pitting and may be relieved by prolonged elevation of the arm. This edema is noted predominantly on the dorsum of the hand and is usually observed over the metacarpophalangeal and proximal interphalangeal joints. The skin over the knuckles becomes puffy and loses the normal creases. The hand becomes boggy and painful. As the edema forms under the extensor tendons, flexion becomes increasingly limited. The collateral ligaments, which must elongate to permit flexion of the metacarpophalangeal joints, become shortened and thus prevent or limit full flexion.

Limited shoulder action prevents elevation of the arm above shoulder level so that lymphatic and vascular pumping actions are restricted. The skin gradually becomes shiny, hairless, and atrophic. The edema containing protein converts into a diffuse, cobweb-like tissue that adheres to the tendons and joint capsules and prevents further movement. The joints undergo disuse atrophy of the cartilage, and the capsule thickens. The bones become osteoporotic (Cailliet, 1981).

Hepatic and Biliary Diseases and Shoulder Pain

As with many of the organ systems in the human body, the hepatic and biliary organs (liver, gallbladder, and common bile duct) can develop diseases that mimic primary musculoskeletal lesions.

The musculoskeletal symptoms associated with hepatic and biliary pathology are generally confined to the midback, scapular, and right shoulder regions. These musculoskeletal symptoms can occur alone (as the only presenting symptom) or in combination with other systemic signs and symptoms. Fortunately, in most cases of shoulder pain referred from visceral processes, shoulder motion is not compromised and local tenderness is not a prominent feature.

Diagnostic interviewing is especially helpful when clients have avoided medical treatment for so long that shoulder pain caused by hepatic and biliary diseases may in turn create biomechanical changes in muscular contractions and shoulder movement. These changes eventually create pain of a biomechanical nature (Rose and Rothstein, 1982).

Referred shoulder pain may be the only presenting symptom of hepatic or biliary disease. Sympathetic fibers from the biliary system are connected through the celiac and splanchnic plexuses to the hepatic fibers in the region of the dorsal spine. These connections account for the intercostal and radiating interscapular pain that accompanies gallbladder disease (see Fig. 8–5). Although the innervation is bilateral, most of the biliary fibers reach the cord through the right splanchnic nerves, producing pain in the right shoulder (Given and Simmons, 1979; Ridge and Way, 1993).

Rheumatic Diseases and Shoulder Pain

A number of systemic rheumatic diseases can present as shoulder pain, even as unilateral shoulder pain. The HLA-B27–associated spondyloarthropathies (diseases of the joints of the spine), such as ankylosing spondylitis, most frequently involve the sacroiliac joints and spine. Involvement of large central joints, such as the hip and shoulder, is common, however.

Rheumatoid arthritis and its variants likewise frequently involve the shoulder girdle. These systemic rheumatic diseases are suggested by the details of the shoulder examination, by coincident systemic complaints of malaise and easy fatigability, and by complaints of discomfort in other joints either coincidental with the presenting shoulder complaint or in the past (Hadler, 1987a).

Other systemic rheumatic diseases with major shoulder involvement include polymyalgia rheumatica and polymyositis (inflammatory disease of the muscles). Both may be somewhat asymmetric but almost always present with bilateral involvement and impressive systemic symptoms (Hadler, 1987a).

Neoplasm (Cyriax, 1982)

Questions about visceral function are relevant when the pattern for malignant invasion at the shoulder emerges. Invasion of the upper humerus and glenoid area by secondary malignant deposits affects the joint and the adjacent muscles.

Muscle wasting is greatly in excess of any attributable to arthritis and follows a bizarre pattern that does not conform to any one neurologic lesion or to any one

Clinical Signs and Symptoms of
Neoplasm

- Marked limitation of movement at the shoulder joint
- Severe muscular weakness and pain with resisted movements

muscle. Localized warmth felt at any part of the scapular area may prove to be the first sign of a malignant deposit eroding bone. Within 1 or 2 weeks after this observation, a palpable tumor will have appeared, and erosion of bone will be visible on x-ray.

Primary Neoplasm

This neoplasm occurs chiefly in young people, in whom a causeless limitation of movement of the shoulder leads the physician to a study of the radiographic appearances. If the tumor originates from the shaft of the humerus, the first symptoms may be a feeling of "pins and needles" in the hand, associated with fixation of the biceps and triceps muscles and leading to limitation of movement at the elbow.

Pulmonary (Secondary) Neoplasm

Occasionally the client requires medical referral because shoulder pain is referred from metastatic lung cancer. When the shoulder is examined, the client is unable to lift the arm beyond the horizontal position. Muscles respond with spasm that limits joint movement.

If the neoplasm interferes with the diaphragm, diaphragmatic pain (C3, C4, C5) is often felt at the shoulder at each breath (at the fourth cervical dermatome [i.e., at the deltoid area]), in correspondence with the main embryologic derivation of the diaphragm. Pain arising from the part of the pleura that is not in contact with the diaphragm is also brought on by respiration but is felt in the chest.

Although the lung is insensitive, large tumors invading the chest wall set up local pain and cause spasm of the pectoralis major muscle, with consequent limitation of elevation of the arm. If the neoplasm encroaches on the ribs, stretching the muscle attached to the ribs leads to sympathetic spasm of the pectoralis major.

By contrast, the scapula is mobile, and a full range of passive movement is present at the shoulder joint. The same signs are found in contracture of the pectoral scar after radical mastectomy, but there may be no pain.

Pancoast's tumors of the lung apex usually do not cause symptoms while confined to the pulmonary parenchyma. They can extend into the surrounding structures, infiltrating the chest wall into the axilla, presenting with shoulder pain and occasionally with brachial plexus (eighth cervical and first thoracic nerve) involvement.

This nerve involvement produces sharp neuritic pain in the axilla, shoulder, and subscapular area on the affected side, with eventual atrophy of the upper extremity muscles. Bone pain is aching, is exacerbated at night, and is a cause of restlessness and musculoskeletal movement. Usually associated general systemic signs and symptoms are present (Cailliet, 1991). These features are not found in any regional musculoskeletal disorder, including such disorders of the shoulder (Hadler, 1987a).

For example, a similar pain pattern caused by trigger points of the serratus anterior can be differentiated from neoplasm by the lack of true neurologic findings (indicating trigger point) or by lack of improvement after treatment to eliminate the trigger point (indicating neoplasm).

PELVIC PAIN (Hughes et al., 1990)

Female pelvic pain is a common medical problem that is usually evaluated and diagnosed by a physician. However, because pelvic diseases can refer pain to the low back, groin, and thigh, the physical therapist may be the first health care professional responsible for adequate medical screening. In the case of chronic, medically evaluated but undiagnosed pelvic pain, the therapist may see the need for further medical follow-up, necessitating physician referral.

The pelvic cavity is in direct communication with the abdominal cavity. Its anterior wall is part of the musculature of the abdominal cavity. The lateral walls of the pelvic cavity are covered by the iliopsoas, iliacus, and obturator muscles, and inferiorly the outlet is guarded by the levator ani and pubococcygeus muscles, which, with the corresponding muscles of the opposite side, form the pelvic diaphragm. Any organ disease or systemic condition altering the normal anatomic relationships can cause musculoskeletal pelvic pain, described in this section.

Types

On the basis of innervation of the pelvic organs, two types of pelvic pain are recognized: *visceral pain* caused by stimulation of autonomic nerves (T11, T12, L1, L2, S2, S3) and *somatic pain* caused by stimulation of sensory nerve endings in the pudendal nerve (S2, S3). Pain in the female pelvis and perineum may be visceral or somatic or, rarely, a mixture of both. Pain in the pelvis may be acute, chronic, or referred from the hip, sacroiliac/sacrum, or low back regions.

Visceral pelvic peritoneum, which covers the upper third of the bladder, the body of the uterus, and the upper third of the rectum and the rectosigmoid junction, is an integral part of these organs and is innervated by autonomic nerves supplying these viscera. It is insensitive to touch but responds with pain on traction, distention, spasm, or ischemia of the viscus.

Parietal pelvic peritoneum, which covers the upper half of the lateral wall of the pelvis and the upper two thirds of the sacral hollow, is supplied by somatic nerves. These somatic nerves also supply corresponding segmental areas of skin and muscles of the trunk and anterior abdominal wall. Painful stimulation of the parietal pelvic peritoneum may cause referred segmental pain and spasm of the iliopsoas muscle and muscles of the anterior abdominal wall.

The *viscera* are innervated by the autonomic nervous system, which has sympathetic and parasympathetic components. The efferent fibers of the sympathetic system emerge through the thoracic and upper lumbar spinal nerves, and the parasympathetic efferent fibers emerge through certain cranial and sacral spinal nerves.

As mentioned previously in this text, viscera are insensitive to cutting, crushing, or bruising. Excessive distention, contraction, and pulling, however, together with some pathologic conditions, excite nociceptive afferents and may result in pain. The sensation aroused by stimulation of these afferents is usually a poorly localized ache, or colic when caused by excessive contractions.

Occasionally, the pain may be referred to the same dermatome as that innervated by somatic sensory nerves that share the same vertebral inlet. The segmental inlet levels of sympathetic pelvic afferents are listed below.

- Sigmoid colon and rectum   L1–L2
- Ureter   T11–L2
- Ovary   T10–T11
- Urinary bladder   T11–L2
- Uterus   T12–L1
- Fallopian tube   T10–L1

Children under 14 years of age rarely present with pelvic pain of gynecologic origin. Those who do will be suffering from one of a comparatively small group of diseases. Infection is the most likely cause and is limited to the vulva and vagina. Theoretically, infection can ascend to involve the peritoneal cavity, causing iliopsoas abscess and pelvic, hip, or groin pain, but this rarely happens in this age group (Rocker, 1990a).

Causes (Table 12–11)

Gynecologic causes of pain are related to the classic pathologic subdivision of congenital anomaly, inflammatory process (in-

Table 12–11
CAUSES OF PELVIC PAIN

Uterus
   Prolapse
   Dysmenorrhea
   Endometriosis
   Tumors
Neoplasm
Surgical
Vascular disorders
"Gynecalgia" (see text)
Pregnancy
Infectious/inflammatory
   Septic arthritis
   Ileal Crohn's disease
   Acute appendicitis
   Osteomyelitis
   Vaginal infection
   Pelvic inflammatory disease (PID)
Enteropathic disease
   Crohn's disease
   Diverticular disease
   Irritable bowel syndrome (IBS)
Urologic
Ovarian cysts
Trauma
Dyspareunia
Premenstrual tension
Sexually transmitted disease (STD)
Sexual assault/incest
Psychogenic
Musculoskeletal

cluding infection), neoplasia, or trauma. In addition, there are anomalies associated with pregnancy and endometriosis. The most common tumors are those arising in the ovaries and uterus (Rocker, 1990b).

Uterus

Uterovaginal prolapse can cause low-grade and persistent pain. This type of prolapse is a combination of basic anatomic structure, the effects of pregnancy and labor, postmenopausal hormone deficiency, and poor general muscular fitness. The addition of obesity, chronic cough, and constipation makes permanent correction of this disorder difficult.

Secondary prolapse may occur with large intrapelvic tumors, with sacral nerve disor-

ders, or following surgical resection. Pain is due primarily to stretching of the ligamentous supports and secondarily to the excoriation (scratch or abrasion) that can occur to the prolapsed cervical or vaginal tissue. The pain of prolapse is central, suprapubic, and dragging in the groin, and there is a sensation of a lump at the vulva. Symptoms are relieved by rest and lying down and may be aggravated by sitting, walking, coughing, intercourse, or straining. There are no significant associated systemic signs and symptoms (Rocker, 1990b).

Dysmenorrhea, defined as painful menstruation, is divided into two types: primary and secondary. *Primary dysmenorrhea* occurs in the absence of identifiable pathology and develops at the onset of menses, continuing into the third decade. *Secondary dysmenorrhea* occurs after the age of 20 years and is the result of pelvic pathology related to endometriosis, intrauterine myomas (tumors or polyps containing muscle tissue), uterine prolapse, pelvic inflammatory disease, cervical stenosis, and adenomyosis (benign invasive growths of the endometrium into the muscular layers of the uterus).

Dysmenorrhea is characterized by spasmodic, cramplike pain that comes and goes in waves and radiates over the lower abdomen and pelvis, thighs, and low back, sometimes accompanied by headache, irritability, mental depression, fatigue, and GI symptoms (O'Toole, 1992).

Endometriosis is a pathologic condition in which tissue resembling the mucous membrane lining the uterus occurs aberrantly in various locations of the pelvic cavity and elsewhere (O'Toole, 1992). It is related mainly to the reproductive years and is seen rarely in women younger than 20 years; the mean age at diagnosis is 35 years.

The symptoms closely reflect the physical signs, and the severity of pain is related more to the site than to the extent of disease. Untreated, endometriosis spreads progressively, and natural remission takes place only with menopause. Damage owing to fibrosis and adhesion resolves slowly, but stenosis is likely to produce partial or complete obstruction of organs within the pelvic cavity (Rocker, 1990b).

Pelvic pain referred to the rectum and lower sacral or coccygeal regions, starting before or after the onset of menstruation and improving after cessation of menstrual flow, with cyclic recurrence, is the classic symptom of endometriosis. As the condition extends, pain remains throughout the cycle, with exacerbation at menstruation and finally, constant severity at all times.

Other pelvic organ dysfunctions causing clinical pelvic pain (and sometimes low back with pelvic pain) include uterine fibroids, nonmalignant tumors that attach to the uterine wall and can grow to a very large size; vulvar or vaginal infection associated with yellow, odorous vaginal discharge; pelvic congestion; and varicosities.

Neoplasm (Sturdy, 1990)

The female pelvis is a depository for malignant tissue after incomplete removal of a primary carcinoma within the pelvis, for recurrence of cancer after surgical resection or radiotherapy of a pelvic neoplasm, or for metastatic deposits from a primary lesion elsewhere in the abdominal cavity.

Primary colonic and rectal tumors spread locally, by the lymphatics or by the bloodsteam. Extension through the bowel wall may fix the tumor to the musculoskeletal walls of the pelvic cavity or to surrounding organs and may produce fistulas into the small intestine, bladder, or vagina. Advanced rectal tumors are frequently "fixed" to the sacral hollow. Deep pain within the pelvis is a poor prognostic sign, because it may indicate spread of neoplasm into the sacral nerve plexuses.

Surgery

Hysterectomy is the most common major surgical procedure in America and Europe. Up to 15 per cent of women between the ages of 40 and 70 years undergo this operation. The immediate postoperative phase in the hospital is associated with varying amounts of pain from problems such as hematoma formation with infection, which causes backache and pelvic pain. The second phase of convalescence takes place at home and may be accompanied by varying degrees of lower abdominal discomfort, backache, vaginal discharge, and fatigue (Rocker, 1990b).

Vascular Disorders (Sturdy, 1990)

The iliac arteries may be gradually occluded by atherosclerosis or obstructed by an embolus. The resultant ischemia produces pain in the affected limb but may also give rise to pelvic pain. Whether the occlusion is thrombotic or embolic, the client will complain of pain in the affected limb and probably pain in the buttocks. The pain characteristically is aggravated by exercise (claudication). The affected limb becomes colder and paler, and in sudden occlusion, diminished sensation to pinprick may be observed on examination. Femoral and distal arteries should be palpated for pulsation.

Thrombosis of the large iliac veins may occur spontaneously, following injury to the lower limb and pelvis, or it may appear after pelvic surgical procedures. An estimated 30 per cent of clients have asymptomatic deep vein thrombosis after major surgery. Thrombosis occluding the iliac vein produces an enlarged, warm, and painful leg and only occasionally discomfort in the pelvis.

Gynecalgia

Although a pathologic cause can be identified for most cases of chronic pelvic pain, a small percentage remains for which no physical cause can be found, and the term "gynecalgia" is used. Women with gynecalgia syndrome are usually 25 to 40 years of age and have at least one child. The symptoms are of at least 2 (and often many more) years' duration, infrequently with acute exacerbation.

Pain is vague and poorly localized, although it is usually confined to the lower abdomen and pelvis, radiating to the groin and upper and inner thighs. Other symptoms include dyspareunia, menstrual change, low back pain, urinary and bowel changes, fatigue, and obvious anxiety and depression (Rocker, 1990b).

Pregnancy

Pelvic pain associated with normal pregnancy is similar to low back pain as discussed earlier in this chapter. About 1 per cent of all pregnancies are outside the endometrium, or ectopic, with the majority of ectopic implantations being in the fallopian tube. Symptoms of an ectopic pregnancy are usually spotting and sudden lower abdominal and pelvic cramping pain shortly after the first missed menstrual period. Gradual hemorrhage causes pelvic (and sometimes low back) pain and pressure, but rapid hemorrhage results in hypotension or shock (Berkow and Fletcher, 1992). Tubal rupture is common, bringing about medical attention and diagnosis.

Infection/Inflammation

Acute appendicitis, sigmoid diverticulitis, ileal Crohn's disease, and salpingitis (inflammation of the fallopian tube) are acute inflammatory disorders within the pelvis that produce both visceral and somatic pain because of involvement of the parietal peritoneum. All these disorders in the acute phase have the following signs and symptoms (Sturdy, 1990):

■ Lower abdominal pelvic pain (right sided = appendicitis; left sided = diverticulitis)

■ Pain aggravated by increased abdominal pressure (e.g., coughing, walking)

■ Nausea and vomiting

■ Tachycardia

■ Pelvic abscess (iliopsoas abscess)

The bones of the pelvis as well as the joints can be affected by generalized diseases, including infection such as osteomyelitis and septic arthritis of the sacroiliac joint.

Pelvic inflammatory disease is an infectious process caused by gonococci, staphylococci, streptococci, and other pus-producing (pyogenic) organisms; rarely, tuberculosis travels through the blood, causing pelvic inflammatory disease. Pelvic inflammatory disease refers to ascending pelvic infections, i.e., those involving the upper genital tract beyond the cervix, including the fallopian tubes, uterus, pelvic connective tissue, pelvic peritoneum veins, and rarely, ovaries. It has a wide spectrum of presentation (Matassarin-Jacobs and Clark, 1993).

Pelvic inflammatory disease may be asymptomatic and discovered incidentally, or it may be symptomatic of major pelvic peritonitis. The first attack of primary infection is characterized by fever, general malaise, bilateral lower abdominal pain with secondary nausea and vomiting, and disturbance in urination with associated heavy, odorous vaginal discharge (Rocker, 1990c). Low back and pelvic symptoms may be minimal and reported as "discomfort" rather than actual pain, or the woman experiences acute, sharp, severe aching on both sides of the pelvis.

Secondary pelvic infection may follow surgery, septic abortion, or pregnancy, owing to the entry of endogenous bacteria into the damaged pelvic tissues. Other factors associated with the increase in pelvic inflammatory disease include sexually transmitted diseases and the fitting of an intrauterine contraceptive device (IUCD). Infection associated with an IUCD seems less likely if the device contains copper, which is probably bactericidal (Glencross, 1990).

Chronic pelvic inflammatory disease is associated with lower abdominal pain and groin discomfort that persists and may radiate to the inner aspects of the thigh. Backache and dyspareunia (difficult or painful intercourse) are also noted.

Enteropathy

The small bowel, sigmoid, and rectum (as well as the bladder, a nonenteropathic organ) may be affected by gynecologic disease, and the response will be in relation to the pressure or displacement of these organs by direct swelling or by reaction to an adjacent infection or to the spilling of blood, menstrual fluid, or infected material. Bowel function may be altered, or alternating bowel symptoms with normal bowel function, rather than persistent symptoms, may occur (Rocker, 1990b).

Crohn's disease may affect the terminal ileum and cecum or the rectum and sigmoid colon in the pelvis. Crohn's disease is a chronic inflammation of all layers of the bowel wall, with an unknown etiology, possibly autoimmune (see Chapter 6). In addition to pelvic and low back pain, the systemic manifestations of Crohn's disease include fever, malaise, anemia, arthralgias, and bowel symptoms.

Diverticular disease of the colon (diverticulosis) is an acquired condition that appears in the fifth to seventh decades with equal frequency in the two sexes. Symptoms, when present, are intermittent, moderate-to-severe pain in the left lower abdomen and left side of the pelvis and a feeling of bowel distention. Accompanying bowel symptoms, including hard stools, alternating diarrhea and constipation, mucus in the stools, and rectal bleeding, may be present (Sturdy, 1990).

Irritable bowel syndrome (IBS) produces persistent, colicky lower abdominal and pelvic pain associated with anorexia, belching, abdominal distention, and bowel changes. The symptoms are produced by excessive colonic motility and spasm of the bowel (spastic colon), and in many cases, the disorder has a large psychogenic component (Sturdy, 1990).

Psychogenic (See also Psychologic Factors in Pain Assessment in Chapter 1)

Psychogenic pain is often ill-defined, and its anatomic distribution depends more on the person's concepts than on clinical disease processes. Such pain does not radiate; commonly, the client presents with multiple unrelated symptoms, and the fluctuations in the course of symptoms are determined more by crises in the person's psychosocial life than by physical changes.

Musculoskeletal Causes (Jones, 1990)

In general, orthopedic causes of pelvic pain in women are easily recognized by the physical therapist. They are usually made worse by exercise and weight bearing and are relieved by rest. *Posterior pelvic pain* originating in the lumbosacral, sacroiliac, coccydynial, and sacrococcygeal regions usually presents as localized pain in the lower lumbar spine and over the sacrum, often radiating over the sacroiliac ligaments and referred into the posterior thigh and buttock.

Pain radiating from the sacroiliac joint can commonly be felt in both the buttock and the posterior thigh and is often aggravated by rotation of the lumbar spine on the pelvis. Coccydynial and sacrococcygeal pain is a very common presentation in women, often associated with a fall on the buttocks, and presents with the person's having difficulty sitting on firm surfaces and with pain in the coccygeal region on defecation or straining.

In the physically active client, proximal hamstring injury, including avulsion of the ischial epiphysis in the adolescent, can cause posterior pelvic and buttock pain.

Anterior pelvic pain commonly occurs as a result of any disorder affecting the hip joint, including inflammatory arthritis; pregnancy with separation of the symphysis pubis; local injury to the insertion of the rectus abdominis, rectus femoris, or adductor muscles; femoral neuralgia; and psoas abscess. (See Hip Pain in this chapter.)

Referred pain in the true *sciatic* distribution and in the L5 or S1 nerve roots is felt below the knee joint. This may be accompanied by signs of nerve root disorder, such as dermatome sensory deficit or myotome weakness. In elderly clients, neurogenic claudication is not uncommon.

The *myofascial component* of pelvic floor pain has been a focus of recent attention in the field of physical therapy. The pelvic floor is a muscular floor providing support for the abdominal contents and sphincter control for the perineal openings. When this muscular floor sags or sustains a muscle tear during childbirth or sexual abuse, weakness results in pelvic laxity and disrupts the positioning and functioning of the pelvic organs; it can also affect the function of the lumbosacral spine (Dunbar, 1991).

Chronic back, leg, and pelvic pain or discomfort, persistent groin pressure, urinary incontinence, and organ prolapse may accompany pelvic floor weakness. Severe pain in the pelvic region of women with fibromyalgia syndrome is not uncommon.

Excess pelvic tension can cause levator ani syndrome and tension myalgia, with symptoms of pain, pressure, and discomfort in the rectum, vagina, perirectal area, or low back. The spasm and tenderness in the levator ani may occur in men and women and can be caused by birthing trauma, neurologic abnormalities in the lumbosacral spine, sexual assault or abuse, or anal fissures. Tension myalgia refers to symptoms of pain in the pelvic floor muscles, rectum, low back, and pelvis. This disorder may be accompanied by constipation, impaired bowel and bladder function, and pain during sexual intercourse.

Stress fractures of the pubis are common in osteomalacia and Paget's disease. Paget's disease frequently affects the pelvis but is usually painless until it secondarily affects the joints by causing osteoarthrosis or stress fractures. Traumatic stress fractures also can occur in joggers, military recruits, athletes, and pregnant women during delivery, with symptoms of pain in the involved area, aggravated by active motion of the limb or deep pressure and weight bearing during ambulation (Moran, 1988).

Femoral hernia accounts for 20 per cent of female hernias. Diagnosis is rarely possible until the hernia strangulates, causing lateral wall pelvic pain that may be referred down the medial side of the thigh to the knee along the geniculate branch of the obturator nerve (L2–L4). Immediate surgical repair is indicated (Sturdy, 1990).

HIP PAIN

Regional pain referred from disorders affecting the low back, abdomen, or retroperitoneal region (with irritation of the psoas muscle); nerve roots; peripheral nerves; or overlying soft tissue structures (e.g., femoral hernia, bursitis, fasciitis) may present as "hip pain." These disorders may include primary musculoskeletal lesions as well as disorders affecting the organs within the pelvic cavity and other diseases.

Additionally, pain from hip pathology can be referred to the groin, ankle, knee, anterior thigh, low back, or sacroiliac area, radiating as far as the knee via the obturator nerve. Postoperatively, orthopedic pins may migrate, referring pain from the hip to the back, tibia, or ankle. Referred pain originating from hip pathology potentially can be confused with pain referred from ligamentous structures of the lumbar spine or

Table 12–12
CAUSES OF HIP PAIN

Spinal metastases
Bone tumors
   Osteoid osteoma
   Chrondroblastomas
   Chondrosarcoma
   Giant cell tumor
   Ewing's sarcoma
Osteoporosis
Iliopsoas abscess
Appendicitis
Pelvic inflammatory disease
Crohn's disease (regional enteritis)
Femoral hernia
Ureteral colic
Reiter's syndrome
Ankylosing spondylitis
Tuberculosis
Sickle cell anemia
Hemophilia
Arterial insufficiency

---

sacroiliac joints (Hummel-Berry, 1990; Two-mey and Taylor, 1987).

A careful history and physical examination usually differentiate these entities from true hip disease (Hadler, 1987a).

Causes

Normal rotations in extension in the reproduction of hip pain should alert one to consider an extraarticular cause. Pain in the lumbosacral region of any etiology may be referred to the hip. The classic example of this is referred pain along the course of T12 to L1 secondary to prolapsed intervertebral disc. However, pain originating from such diverse causes as simple low back strain or metastatic carcinoma to the vertebrae may also cause referred pain to the hip. Hip pain referred from the lower lumbar vertebrae and sacrum is usually felt in the gluteal region, with radiation down the back or outer aspect of the thigh. Lesions in the upper lumbar vertebrae often refer pain into the anterior aspect of the thigh (Hadler, 1987a).

Systemic Causes (Table 12–12)

SPINAL METASTASES

Spinal metastases to the femur or lower pelvis may present as hip pain. Although it may be said that any metastatic tumor may appear in bone, this is true for many tumors only when they have existed long enough and are in the terminal stage. Tumors have usually been recognized much earlier and no longer present a diagnostic problem. With the exception of myeloma and a rare lymphoma, metastasis to the synovium is unusual, so that joint motion is not compromised by these bone lesions. Although any tumor of the bone, cartilage, or soft tissue may present at the hip, some benign and malignant neoplasms have a propensity to occur in this location (Hadler, 1987a).

OSTEOID OSTEOMA

Osteoid osteoma, a small, benign but painful tumor, is relatively common, with 20 per cent of lesions occurring in the proximal femur. Ten per cent of the lesions occur in the pelvis. The client usually presents in the second decade of life complaining of chronic dull hip, knee, or thigh pain that is worse at night and alleviated by activity and aspirin. A physical examination usually reveals an antalgic gait and may demonstrate point tenderness over the lesion and restriction of hip motion. The physician's diagnosis takes into consideration the typical pain pattern, the person's age, the pain's response to aspirin, and radiographic findings (Hadler, 1987a).

OTHER BONE TUMORS

A great many varieties of benign and malignant tumors may present differently, depending on the age of the client, the site, and the duration of the lesion. Other bone tumors, such as chondroblastoma, chondrosarcoma, giant cell tumors, and Ewing's sarcoma causing hip pain, are discussed in greater detail in Chapter 10. In each case, the client's age and the location of symptoms are used by the physician in conjunction with radiographs to make a positive diagnosis.

OSTEOPOROSIS

Hip fracture associated with osteoporosis is a common cause of hip pain, especially in women over 65 years of age. Osteoporosis accompanying the postmenopausal period, combined with a circulatory impairment, postural hypotension, or some medications, can increase a client's risk of falling and incurring hip fracture.

Transient osteoporosis of the hip occurs infrequently during pregnancy but presents a particularly challenging disorder for the treating physical therapist. Although the actual incidence is unknown, reports in the literature indicate that it may be under-diagnosed (Lose and Lindholm, 1986).

Symptoms include progressive hip pain, sometimes referred to the lateral thigh. The pain develops shortly before or during the last trimester and is aggravated by weight bearing. The pain subsides and the x-ray appearance returns to normal within several months following delivery.

Any evaluation procedures performed by the physical therapist that produce significant shear through the femoral head of a pregnant woman must be performed with extreme caution. The transient osteoporosis of pregnancy is not limited to the hip, and vertebral compression may also occur (Hummel-Berry, 1990).

Treatment. Treatment for pregnancy-induced osteoporosis is bed rest, pain relief, and gentle mobility exercise until delivery, after which gradual weight bearing is reinstated (Lose and Lindholm, 1986).

INFLAMMATORY DISEASES

Abdominal or intraperitoneal inflammation, which leads to irritation of the psoas muscle and psoas abscess, may present as hip pain.

Psoas abscess, a localized collection of pus, most commonly affects the right hip and can be caused by any peritoneal inflammatory process such as Crohn's disease, appendicitis, or pelvic inflammatory disease. Pain in the hip may also involve the medial aspect of the thigh and femoral triangle area. Once the abscess is formed, a muscular spasm may be provoked, producing hip flexion and even flexion contracture of the hip.

Hemarthrosis associated with *hemophilia* may affect the hip and result in a GI bleed, causing hemorrhage within the psoas muscle. The subsequent bleeding-spasm cycle produces increased hip pain and hip flexion spasm/contracture. These systemic causes of hip pain are usually associated with loss of appetite, fever, and night sweats.

Psoas abscess must be differentiated from trigger points of the psoas muscle causing the psoas minor syndrome, which is easily mistaken for appendicitis. Hemorrhage within the psoas muscle, either spontaneous or associated with anticoagulation therapy, can cause a painful compression syndrome of the femoral nerve. Symptoms from the iliopsoas trigger point are aggravated by weight-bearing activities and relieved by recumbency or rest. Relief is greater when the hip is flexed (Travell and Simons, 1992).

Other Causes

Referred symptoms from *femoral hernia* or *ureteral coli* can be distinguished from musculoskeletal hip pain by the history, presence of systemic symptoms, and pattern of pain. There have been reports of Reiter's syndrome or ankylosing spondylitis presenting as referred pain to the hip (Hadler, 1987a).

Although *ankylosing spondylitis* is primarily an arthritis of the spine, one fifth of the clients notice the first symptoms in the peripheral joints, and approximately one third of these clients ultimately develop hip disease. Late in the disease, marked hip flexion contractures are present, and bony ankylosis of the hip may occur.

Tubercular disease of the hip is rare in developed countries but can occur. The client usually presents with a chronic limp and pain in the hip that persists at rest. Approximately 60 per cent of clients do not have constitutional symptoms, although the tuberculin skin test is usually positive, and radiographs are similar to those for septic arthritis (Hadler, 1987a).

Sickle cell anemia resulting in avascular necrosis (death of cells due to lack of

blood supply) of the hip and hemarthrosis (blood in the joint) associated with *hemophilia* are two of the most common hematologic diseases to cause pain in the hip.

GROIN PAIN

The physical therapist is not likely to be faced with a client complaining of just groin pain or symptoms. It is more typical to see a person who has low back, hip, or sacroiliac problems and who has a secondary complaint of groin pain. However, on examination, the physical therapist may palpate enlarged lymph nodes in the groin area, or the client may indicate these nodes to the examiner.

Painless, progressive enlargements of lymph nodes that persist for more than 4 weeks or that involve more than one area are an indication of a need for a medical referral.

Hodgkin's disease arises in the lymph glands most commonly on one side of the neck or groin, but lymph nodes also enlarge in response to infections throughout the body, so the client must seek medical diagnosis to be certain of the cause of enlarged lymph nodes.

As always, the physical therapist must question the client further regarding the onset of symptoms and the presence of any associated symptoms, such as fever, weight loss, bleeding, and skin lesions.

▼ *Clinical Signs and Symptoms of*

Hip Avascular Necrosis

- Pain in the groin or thigh
- Tenderness to palpation over the hip joint
- Antalgic gait with a limp
- Hip motion decreased in flexion, internal rotation, and abduction

▼ *Clinical Signs and Symptoms of*

Hip Hemarthrosis

- Pain in the groin and thigh
- Fullness in the hip joint, both anterior in the groin and over the greater trochanter
- Limited motion in hip flexion, abduction, and external rotation (allows most room for the blood in the joint capsule)

Causes (Table 12–13)

Musculoskeletal Causes
(Garrett, 1992)

The most common musculoskeletal cause of groin pain is strain of the adductor muscles, most often involving the adductor longus. The history includes a specific trauma or injury, which occurs primarily at the junction of the muscle fibers with the extended tendon of origin. Acutely, this injury causes pain with passive stretch or

Table 12–13

CAUSES OF GROIN PAIN

Systemic Causes of Groin Pain	Musculoskeletal Causes of Groin Pain
Spinal cord tumors	Adductor muscle strain
Ureteral pain	Pubalgia
Ascites	Osteitis pubis
Hemophilia gastrointestinal bleeding	Trauma (including sexual assault)
Abdominal aortic aneurysm	Inguinal hernia
	Hip joint pathology
	Trigger points

active contraction; eccentric activation may be even more painful. Acute injury may be followed in several days by ecchymosis.

Other musculoskeletal causes of groin pain may include trauma (including sexual assault), inguinal hernia (fairly common in young athletes), pubalgia, osteitis pubis, and hip joint disease such as slipped capital femoral epiphysis, intraarticular disease, and avulsion of the rectus femoris from the anterior inferior iliac spine and the sartorius from the anterior superior iliac spine.

Pubalgia is characterized by pain in the inguinal area, most often near the middle of the inguinal ligament. The pain results from an abdominal wall muscular injury. Active abdominal flexion (e.g., sit-ups) and passive stretching of abdominal muscles (e.g., prone extension) cause pain. This problem occurs most frequently in soccer players.

Osteitis pubis, which may be mistaken for adductor strain, is located at the symphysis pubis and is characterized by tenderness to direct pressure about the symphysis. This is also most likely to occur in participants of any active sport.

Underlying hip joint pathology can also mimic an adductor strain. Pain associated with this entity is described as being directly in the inguinal area and limits hip rotation.

Active trigger points along the upper rim of the pubis and the lateral half of the inguinal ligament may lie in the lower internal oblique muscle and possibly in the lower rectus abdominis. These trigger points can cause increased irritability and spasm of the detrusor and urinary sphincter muscles, producing urinary frequency, retention of urine, and groin pain (Travell and Simons, 1983).

Systemic Causes

Primary and secondary *spinal cord tumors* may initially present with discomfort in the thoracolumbar area in a beltlike distribution. The pain may extend to the groin or legs and may be constant or intermittent; a dull ache; or a sharp, knifelike sensation (Andreoli et al., 1993).

The pain can be primarily at the site of the lesion or may refer to the ipsilateral groin and down the ipsilateral extremity with radicular involvement (nerve root compression or irritation).

Ureteral pain is felt in the groin and genital area (see Fig. 7–6) with radiation forward around the flank into the lower abdominal quadrant. Abdominal muscle spasm with rebound tenderness can occur on the same side as the source of pain. The pain also can be generalized throughout the abdomen and associated with nausea, vomiting, and impaired intestinal motility. Abdominal rebound tenderness results when the adjacent peritoneum becomes inflamed (Wilson and Klahr, 1993).

Ascites, an abnormal accumulation of serous (edematous) fluid within the peritoneal cavity, also can cause low back pain or groin pain. This condition is associated with liver disease and alcoholism. The person presents with a distended abdomen, lumbar lordosis, and possible edema bilaterally in the ankles.

Hemophilia may involve GI bleeding accompanied by low abdominal and groin pain owing to bleeding into the wall of the large intestine or iliopsoas muscle. This retroperitoneal hemorrhage produces a muscle spasm of the iliopsoas muscle with a subsequent hip flexion contracture. Other symptoms may include melena, hematemesis, and fever.

Abdominal aortic aneurysm may be asymptomatic, and discovery occurs on physical or x-ray examination of the abdomen or lower spine for some other reason. The most common symptom is awareness of a pulsating mass in the abdomen, with or without pain, followed by abdominal and back pain. Groin pain and flank pain may be experienced because of increasing pressure on other structures. For detailed information, see Chapter 3.

PHYSICIAN REFERRAL

A careful history and close observation of the client are important in determining whether a person may need a medical referral for possible systemic origin of pain or symptoms masquerading as musculoskeletal involvement. Anyone presenting with chest, back (cervical, thoracic, scapular, lumbar, sacroiliac), hip, or shoulder pain without a history of trauma (including forceful movement of the spine, repetitive movements of the shoulder or back, or easy lifting) should be screened for a possible systemic origin of symptoms.

It is not the physical therapist's responsibility to differentiate diagnostically among the various causes of systemic signs and symptoms, but rather to identify when the client's history, subjective report, and objective findings do not support the presence of a musculoskeletal problem, thus requiring a medical follow-up.

Each of the visceral systems reviewed in this text has specific patterns of pain referral with accompanying signs and symptoms or history to assist the physical therapist in making a thorough investigation of the presenting problem. Familiarity with these patterns and the appropriate follow-up questions is essential when considering medical referral for possible visceral involvement.

Physical therapists are often the health care representatives to whom clients describe problems or concerns that are more appropriately reported to the physician. Conversations of this nature are not unusual when considering the consistent daily or weekly contact that physical therapists may have with clients. The knowledgeable physical therapist who can recognize this information may also be able to guide the client effectively in seeking the necessary medical attention.

Additionally, exercise may be the precipitating or aggravating factor for the onset of some conditions, such as angina, asthma, vascular or migraine headaches, spontaneous pneumothorax, or dehydration secondary to the use of diuretic medications, requiring that the physical therapist communicate and collaborate with the physician. Knowledge of the correct information to give the physician can facilitate the communication process.

Systemic Signs and Symptoms Requiring Physician Referral

Systemic signs and symptoms generally follow patterns characteristic of the organ or system involved. Constitutional (i.e., systemic) symptoms that are characteristic of multisystems should serve as red flags to alert the physical therapist to the possibility that a client's complaints are more than just musculoskeletal in nature. The following signs and symptoms are the most common.

Abdominal pain	Dysphagia
Anorexia	Dyspnea
Bilateral symptoms	Early satiety
Bowel/bladder changes	Fatigue
Chills	Fever
Constipation	Headaches
Diaphoresis	Heartburn
Diarrhea	Hemoptysis
Dizziness	Hoarseness
Dysesthesia	Indigestion
	Jaundice

Nausea	Palpitations	Skin rash	Weakness
Night pain	Paresthesia	Vision changes	Weight loss/gain
Night sweats	Persistent cough	Vomiting	

Key Points To Remember

- Clients may inaccurately attribute symptoms to a particular incident or activity, or they may fail to recognize causative factors.

- Any person presenting with musculoskeletal pain of unknown cause and/or a past medical history of cancer should be screened for medical disease. *Special Questions for Men and Women* may be helpful in this screening process.

- When symptoms seem out of proportion to the injury, or if they persist beyond the expected time for the nature of the injury, medical referral may be indicated.

- Pain that is unrelieved by rest or change in position or pain/symptoms that do not fit the expected mechanical or neuromusculoskeletal pattern should serve as red flag warnings.

- When symptoms cannot be reproduced, aggravated, or altered in any way during the examination, additional questions to screen for medical disease are indicated.

- Shoulder pain aggravated by the supine position may be an indication of mediastinal or pleural involvement. Shoulder or back pain alleviated by lying on the painful side may indicate autosplinting (pleural). See Figure 12–1.

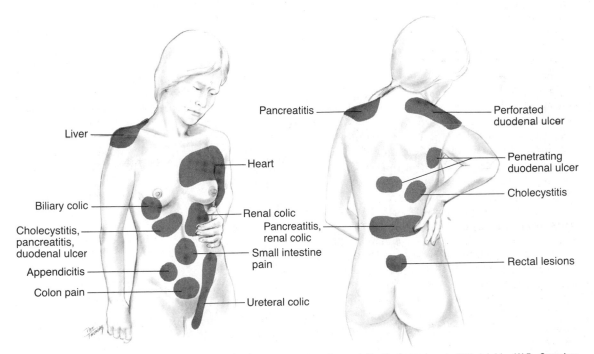

Common sites of referred pain. (From Jarvis, C.: Physical Examination and Health Assessment. Philadelphia, W.B. Saunders, 1992.)

- Trigger points should always be considered as a possible cause of a presentation like systemic symptoms.

- Chest pain can occur as a result of cervical spine disorders because nerves originating as high as C3, C4 can extend as far as the nipple line.

- Postoperative infection of any kind may not present with any clinical signs/symptoms for weeks or months.

- Muscle weakness without pain, without history of sciatica, and without a positive straight leg raising (SLR) is suggestive of spinal metastases.

- Sciatica may be the first symptom of prostate cancer metastasized to the bones of the pelvis, lumbar spine, or femur.

- Sacral pain, in the absence of a history of trauma or overuse, that is not reproduced with pressure on the sacrum (client is prone) is a red flag presentation indicating a possible systemic cause of symptoms.

SUMMARY

Throughout this text, the physical therapist has been encouraged to assess musculoskeletal complaints of unknown origin affecting the back, shoulder, chest, thorax, hip, groin, or sacroiliac joint with the idea that a systemic origin of symptoms must be considered.

A carefully taken medical history, review of systems, evaluation of pain patterns/pain types, and appropriate questions asked during the physical therapy interview must be correlated with the objective findings. These tools will help the physical therapist in making a physical therapy diagnosis or

in making the decision to refer the client to another health care practitioner.

This chapter has compared specifically the possible systemic versus musculoskeletal causes of pain associated with the chest/thorax, back, shoulder, hip, groin, or sacroiliac joint. Special questions to ask are provided to assist the physical therapist in identifying the potential presence of signs and symptoms associated with systemic disease. Additionally, special questions appropriate for women and men are outlined, depending on the presenting musculoskeletal complaints.

In discussing musculoskeletal versus systemic symptoms, we have attempted to provide the physical therapist with important information needed when making an assessment of the client, including

- Client's history and systems review
- Characteristics of pain
  - Signs and symptoms of systemic pain
  - Signs and symptoms of musculoskeletal pain
- Chest pain
  - Musculoskeletal causes
- Back pain
  - Classifications
  - Cervical
  - Thoracic
  - Scapular
  - Lumbar (LBP)
  - Sacroiliac joint/sacral
- Shoulder pain
- Pelvic pain
  - Types
  - Causes
- Hip pain
- Groin pain
- Special questions to ask by anatomic location

SUBJECTIVE EXAMINATION	*Special Questions to Ask: Chest/Thorax*

Musculoskeletal

- Have you strained a muscle from coughing?

- Have you ever injured your chest?

- Does it hurt to touch your chest or to take a deep breath (e.g., coughing, sneezing, sighing, or laughing)? **(Myalgia, fractured rib, costochondritis, myofascial trigger point)**

- Do you have frequent attacks of heartburn, or do you take antacids to relieve heartburn or acid indigestion? **(Noncardiac cause of chest pain, abdominal muscle trigger point, GI disorder)**

Neurologic

- Do you have any trouble taking a deep breath? **(Weak chest muscles secondary to polymyositis, dermatomyositis, myasthenia gravis)**

- Does your chest pain ever travel into your armpit, arm, neck, or wing bone (scapula)? **(Thoracic outlet syndrome)**

  - If yes, do you ever feel burning, pricking, numbness, or any other unusual sensation in any of these areas?

Pulmonary

- Have you ever been treated for a lung problem?

  - If yes, please describe what this problem was, when it occurred, and how it was treated.

- Do you think your chest or thoracic (upper back) pain is caused by a lung problem?

- Have you ever had trouble with breathing?

- Are you having difficulty with breathing now?

- Do you ever have shortness of breath, breathlessness, or can't quite catch your breath?

  - If yes, does this happen when you rest; lie flat; walk on level ground; walk up stairs; or when you are under stress or tension?

  - How long does it last?

  - What do you do to get your breathing back to normal?

- How far can you walk before you feel breathless?

- What symptom stops your walking (e.g., shortness of breath, heart pounding, or weak legs)?

- Do you have any breathing aids (e.g., oxygen, nebulizer, humidifier, or intermittent positive pressure breathing [IPPB] machine)?

- Do you have a cough? (Note whether the person smokes, for how long and how much.) Do you have a smoker's hack?

  - If yes to having a cough, distinguish it from a smoker's cough. Ask when it started.

  - Does coughing increase or bring on your symptoms?

  - Do you cough anything up? If yes, please describe the color, amount, and frequency.

  - Are you taking anything for this cough? If yes, does it seem to help?

- Do you have periods when you can't seem to stop coughing?

- Do you ever cough up blood?

  - If yes, what color is it? (Bright red = fresh; brown or black = older)

  - If yes, has this been treated?

- Have you ever had a blood clot in your lungs? If yes, when and how was it treated?

- Have you had a chest x-ray film taken during the last 5 years? If yes, when and where did it occur? What were the results?

- Do you work around asbestos, coal, dust, chemicals, or fumes? If yes, please describe.

  - Do you wear a mask at work? If yes, approximately how much of the time do you wear a mask?

- If the person is a farmer, ask what kind of farming, because some agricultural products may cause respiratory irritation.

- Have you ever had tuberculosis or a positive skin test for tuberculosis?

  - If yes, when did it occur and how was it treated? What is your current status?

- When was your last test for tuberculosis? Was the result normal?

Cardiac

- Has a physician ever told you that you have heart trouble?

- Have you ever had a heart attack? If yes, when? Please describe.

  - If yes to either question: Do you think your current symptoms are related to your heart problems?

- Do you have angina (pectoris)?

  - If yes, please describe the symptoms and tell me when it occurs.

  - If no, pursue further with the following questions.

- Do you ever have discomfort or tightness in your chest? **(Angina)**

- Have you ever had a crushing sensation in your chest with or without pain down your left arm?
- Do you have pain in your jaw, either alone or in combination with chest pain?
- If you climb a few flights of stairs fairly rapidly, do you have tightness or pressing pain in your chest?
- Do you get pressure or pain or tightness in the chest if you walk in the cold wind or face a cold blast of air?
- Have you ever had pain or pressure or a squeezing feeling in the chest that occurred during exercise, walking, or any other physical or sexual activity?
- Do you ever have bouts of rapid heart action, irregular heart beats, or palpitations of your heart?

Epigastric

- Have you ever been told that you have an ulcer?
- Does the pain under your breast bone radiate (travel) around to your back or do you ever have back pain at the same time that your chest hurts?
- Have you ever had heartburn or acid indigestion?
  - If yes, how is this pain different?
  - If no, have you noticed any association between when you eat and when this pain comes on?

Breast

- Do you have any discharge from your breasts or nipples?
  - If yes, do you know what is causing this discharge?
  - Have you received medical treatment for this problem?
- Are you lactating (nursing a baby)?
- Have you examined yourself for any lumps or nodules and found any thickening or lump?
  - If yes, where was it and how long was it present?
  - Has your physician examined this lump?
  - If no (for women), do you examine your own breasts?
  - If yes, when was the last time that you did a breast self-examination?
- Have you been involved in any activities of a repetitive nature that could cause sore muscles (e.g., painting, washing walls, push-ups or other calisthenics, heavy lifting or pushing, overhead movements, prolonged running, or fast walking)?
- Have you recently been coughing excessively?

SUBJECTIVE EXAMINATION	*Special Questions to Ask: Back*

When did the pain or symptoms start?

- Did it (they) start gradually or suddenly? **(Vascular versus trauma problem)**

- Was there an illness or injury before the onset of pain?

- Have you noticed any changes in your symptoms since they first started up to the present time?

- Is the pain aggravated or relieved by coughing or sneezing? **(Nerve root involvement, muscular)**

- Is the pain aggravated or relieved by activity?

- Are there any particular positions (sitting, lying, standing) that aggravate or relieve the pain?

- Does the pain radiate down the leg? If so, where?

- Have you noticed any muscular weakness?

- Have you had a fever, chills, or burning with urination during the last 3 to 4 weeks?

- Have you been treated previously for back disorders?

- How has your general health been both before the beginning of your back problem and now today?

- How does rest affect the pain or symptoms?

- Do you feel worse in the morning or evening . . . **OR** . . . what difference do you notice in your symptoms from the morning when you first wake up, until the evening when you go to bed?

- Do you ever have swollen feet or ankles? If yes, are they swollen when you get up in the morning? **(Edema/congestive heart failure)**

- Do you ever get cramps in your legs if you walk for several blocks? **(Intermittent claudication)**

General Systemic

Most of these questions may be asked of clients with pain or symptoms anywhere in the musculoskeletal system.

- Have you ever been told that you have osteoporosis or brittle bones, fractures, back problems? **(Wasting of bone matrix in Cushing's syndrome)**

- Have you ever been diagnosed or treated for cancer in any part of your body?

- Do you ever notice sweating, nausea, or chest pains when your current symptoms occur?

■ What other symptoms have you had with this problem? For example, state whether you have had any:

    Numbness

    Burning, tingling

    Nausea, vomiting

    Loss of appetite

    Unexpected or significant (10 or 15 lb) weight gain or loss

    Diarrhea, constipation, blood in your stool or urine

    Difficulty in starting or continuing the flow of urine or incontinence (inability to hold your urine)

    Hoarseness or difficulty in swallowing

    Heart palpitations or fluttering

    Difficulty in breathing while just sitting or resting or with mild effort (e.g., when walking from the car to the house)

    Unexplained sweating or perspiration

    Night sweats, fever, chills

    Changes in vision: blurred vision, black spots, double vision, temporary blindness

    Fatigue, weakness, sudden paralysis of one side of your body, arm, or leg **(TIA)**

    Headaches

    Dizziness or fainting spells

Gastrointestinal

■ Have you noticed any association between when you eat and when your symptoms increase or decrease?

  ■ Do you notice any change in your symptoms 1 to 3 hours after you eat?

  ■ Do you notice any pain beneath the breastbone (epigastric) or just beneath the wing bone (subscapular) 1 to 2 hours after eating?

■ Do you have a feeling of fullness after only one or two bites of food?

■ Is your back pain relieved after having a bowel movement? **(GI obstruction)**

■ Do you have rectal, low back, or sacroiliac pain when passing stool or having a bowel movement?

■ Do you have frequent heartburn or take antacids to relieve heartburn or acid indigestion?

Urology

■ Have you noticed any changes in your bowel movement or the flow of urine since your back/groin pain started?

- If no, it may be necessary to provide prompts or examples of what changes you are referring to (e.g., difficulty in starting or continuing the flow of urine, numbness or tingling in the groin or pelvis)
- Have you had burning with urination during the last 3 to 4 weeks?
- Do you ever have blood in your stool or notice blood in the toilet after having a bowel movement? **(Hemorrhoids, prostate problems, cancer)**
- Do you have any problems with your kidneys or bladder? If so, please describe.
- Have you ever had kidney or bladder stones? If so, how were these stones treated?
- Have you ever had an injury to your bladder or to your kidneys? If so, how was this treated?
- Have you had any infections of the bladder, and how were these infections treated?
  - Were they related to any specific circumstances (e.g., pregnancy, intercourse)?
- Have you had any kidney infections, and how were these treated?
  - Were they related to any specific circumstances (e.g., pregnancy, after bladder infections, a strep throat, or strep skin infections)?
- Do you ever have pain, discomfort, or a burning sensation when you urinate? **(Lower urinary tract irritation)**
- Have you noticed any blood in your urine?

SUBJECTIVE EXAMINATION	*Special Questions to Ask: Sacroiliac/Sacrum*

Follow the same format as for *Special Questions to Ask: Back,* with particular emphasis on gynecologic (for women) and urologic questions for both men and women.

SUBJECTIVE EXAMINATION	*Special Questions for Women: Screening For Medical Disease*

General Health

- Date of last Pap smear:
- Date of last breast examination:
- Do you perform a monthly breast self-examination?
- Where are you in your menstrual cycle (pre/mid/postmenopausal)?
- Are you taking birth control pills?

- For the menopausal woman: Are you taking estrogen replacement therapy (ERT)?
- Have you experienced any of the following (constitutional) symptoms associated with your current problem(s):

    (Night) sweats

    Low-grade fever

    Nausea

    Diarrhea/constipation

    Dizziness

    Fainting

    Fatigue

Past Medical History

- Have you had vaginal surgery or a hysterectomy? **(Hysterectomy: joint pain and myalgias may occur. Vaginal surgery: incontinence)**
- Have you ever had (or do you now have) pelvic inflammatory disease or any sexually transmitted disease (STD)?
- How many pregnancies have you had?
- How many live births have you had?
- Have you had any spontaneous or induced (therapeutic) abortions?
- Do you have "brittle bones" (osteoporosis)?
- Have you ever had a compression fracture of your back?

SUBJECTIVE EXAMINATION	*Special Questions for Women Experiencing Back, Groin, Pelvic, Hip, or Sacroiliac (SI) Pain*

Since your back/SI (or other type) of pain/symptoms started, have you seen a gynecologist to rule out any gynecologic cause of this problem?

- Have you ever been told that you have

    Retroversion of the uterus (tipped back)

    Ovarian cysts

    Fibroids or tumors

    Endometriosis

    Cystocele (sagging bladder)

    Rectocele (sagging rectum)

- Have you ever had pelvic inflammatory disease (PID)?

- Do you have any known sexually transmitted diseases? **(Cause of PID)**

- Do you have any premenstrual symptoms (e.g., water retention, mood changes including depression, headaches, food cravings, painful or tender breasts)? Have you noticed any pattern between your back/SI (or other) symptoms and PMS?

- Do you have an intrauterine coil or loop (IUCD)? **(PID and ectopic pregnancy can occur)**

- Have you (recently) had a baby? **(Birth trauma)**

  - If yes, did you have an epidural (anesthesia)? **(Postpartum back pain)**

  - Did you have any significant medical problems during your pregnancy or delivery?

- Have you ever had a tubal or ectopic pregnancy? Is it possible you may be pregnant now?

- Have you had any spontaneous or induced abortions? **(Weakness secondary to blood loss, infection, scarring; blood in peritoneum irritating diaphragm)** If yes, how many, when, onset of symptoms in relation to incident?

- Do you ever leak urine with coughing, laughing, lifting, exercising, or sneezing? **(Stress incontinence; tension myalgia of pelvic floor)**

- Do you ever have a "falling-out" feeling or pelvic heaviness after standing for a long time? **(Incontinence; prolapse; pelvic floor weakness)**

  - If yes to incontinence, ask several additional questions to determine the frequency, the amount of protection needed as measured by the number and type of pads used daily, and how much this problem interferes with daily activities and lifestyle.

- Recent history of bladder or kidney infections? **(Referred back pain)**

- Presence of vaginal discharge? **(Referred back pain)**

  - If yes, do you know what is causing this discharge?

  - How long have you had this problem? Is there any connection between when the discharge started and when you first noticed your back/sacroiliac (or other) symptoms?

- Is there any connection between your (back, hip, sacroiliac) pain/symptoms and your menstrual cycle (related to ovulation, midcycle, or menses)?

- Where were you in your menstrual cycle when your injury or illness occurred?

- Have you ever been told you have endometriosis?

SUBJECTIVE EXAMINATION	*Special Questions for Men Experiencing Back, Hip, Groin, or SI Pain/Symptoms*

- Do you ever have difficulty with urination (e.g., difficulty starting or continuing flow or a very slow flow of urination)?
- Do you ever have blood in your urine?
- Do you ever have pain, burning, or discomfort on urination?
- Have you ever been treated for prostate problems (prostate cancer, prostatitis)?
- Have you recently had kidney stones or bladder or kidney infections?
- Have you ever been told you have a hernia, or do you think you have a hernia now?

SUBJECTIVE EXAMINATION	*Special Questions to Ask: Shoulder*

General Systemic

- Does your pain ever wake you at night from a sound sleep? **(Cancer)** Can you find any way to relieve the pain and get back to sleep?
  - If yes, how? **(Cancer: nothing relieves it)**
- Have you sustained any injuries in the last week during a sports activity, car accident, etc? **(Ruptured spleen associated with pain in the left shoulder: positive Kehr's sign)**
- Since the beginning of your shoulder problem, have you had any unusual perspiration for no apparent reason, night sweats, or fever?
- Have you had any unusual fatigue (more than usual with no change in life style), joint pain in other joints, or general malaise? **(Rheumatic disease)**

Pulmonary

- Do you currently have a cough?
  - If yes, is this a smoker's cough?
  - If no, how long has this been present?
  - Is this a productive cough (can you bring up sputum) and is the sputum tinged with blood?
- Does your shoulder pain increase when you cough, laugh, or take a deep breath?
- Do you have any chest pain?
- What effect does lying down or resting have on your shoulder pain?

(A pulmonary problem may be made worse, whereas a musculoskeletal problem may be relieved; on the other hand, pain may be relieved when the client lies on the affected side, which diminishes the movement of that side of the chest.)

Cardiac

■ Do you ever notice sweating, nausea, or chest pain when the pain in your shoulder occurs?

■ Have you noticed your shoulder pain increasing with exertion that does not necessarily cause you to use your shoulder (e.g., climbing stairs)?

Gastrointestinal

■ Have you ever had an ulcer?

  ■ If yes, when? Do you still have any pain from your ulcer?

  ■ Have you noticed any association between when you eat and when your symptoms increase or decrease?

■ Does eating relieve your pain? **(Duodenal or pyloric ulcer)**

  ■ How soon is the pain relieved after eating?

■ Does eating aggravate your pain? **(Gastric ulcer, gallbladder inflammation)**

■ Does your pain occur 1 to 3 hours after eating or between meals? **(Duodenal or pyloric ulcers, gallstones)**

■ Have you ever had gallstones?

■ Do you have a feeling of fullness after only one or two bites of food? **(Early satiety: stomach and duodenum or gallbladder)**

■ Have you had any nausea, vomiting, difficulty in swallowing, loss of appetite, or heartburn since the shoulder started bothering you?

| SUBJECTIVE EXAMINATION | *Special Questions for Women Experiencing Shoulder Pain/Dysfunction* |

Have you had any recent kidney infections, tumors, or kidney stones? **(Pressure from kidney on diaphragm referred to shoulder)**

■ Have you ever had a breast implant or mastectomy? **(Altered lymph drainage, scar tissue)**

■ Have you ever had a tubal or ectopic pregnancy?

- Have you had any spontaneous or induced abortions recently? **(Blood in peritoneum irritating diaphragm)**
- Have you recently had a baby? **(Excessive muscle tension during birth)**
  - If yes: Are you breast feeding with the infant supported on pillows?
  - Do you have a breast discharge or have you had mastitis?

SUBJECTIVE EXAMINATION | *Special Questions to Ask: Hip*

Because hip pain can be caused by referred pain from disorders of the low back, abdomen, and reproductive and urologic structures, special questions should include consideration of the following:

Special questions for women

Special questions for men

Special questions for back patients:

   General systemic questions

   GI questions

   Urologic questions

These questions are fully outlined elsewhere in this chapter and are not repeated here.

SUBJECTIVE EXAMINATION | *Special Questions to Ask: Groin*

Refer to the *Special Questions to Ask: Sacroiliac/Sacrum* section.

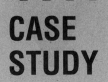

CASE STUDY

REFERRAL

   A 65-year-old retired railroad engineer has come to you with a left "frozen shoulder." During the course of the subjective examination, he also tells you that he is taking two cardiac medications.

   What questions should you ask that might help you relate these two problems (shoulder/cardiac) or to rule out any relationship?

■ ■ ■ ■ ■ ■ ■ ■ ■ ■ ■

PHYSICAL THERAPY INTERVIEW

Onset/History

What do you think is the cause of your shoulder problem?

When did it occur or how long have you had this problem (sudden or gradual onset)?

Can you recall any specific incident when you injured your shoulder, for example, by falling, being hit by someone or something, automobile accident?

Did you ever have a snapping or popping sensation just before your shoulder started to hurt? **(Ligamentous or cartilagenous lesion)**

Did you injure your neck in any way before your shoulder developed these problems?

Have you had a recent heart attack? Have you had nausea, fatigue, sweating, chest pain, or pressure with or without pain in your neck, jaw, left shoulder, or down your left arm?

Has your left hand ever been stiff or swollen? **(Shoulder-hand syndrome [reflex sympathetic dystrophy] after myocardial infarction)**

Do you associate the symptom relating to your shoulder with your heart problems?

Shortly before you first noticed difficulty with your shoulder, were you involved in any kind of activities that would require repetitive movements, such as painting, gardening, playing tennis or golf?

MEDICAL HISTORY

Have you had any surgery during the past year?

How has your general health been? **(Shoulder pain is a frequent site of referred pain from other internal medical problems; see Figure 12-1.)**

Did you ever have rheumatic fever when you were a child?

What is your typical pattern of chest pain or angina?

Has this pattern changed in any way since your shoulder started to hurt? For example, does the chest pain last longer, come on with less exertion, and feel more intense?

Do your heart medications relieve your shoulder symptoms, even briefly?

If so, how long after you take the medications do you notice a difference?

Does this occur every time that you take your medications?

MEDICAL TESTING

Have you had any recent x-rays taken of the shoulder or your neck?

Have you received medical or physical therapy treatment for shoulder problems before?

If so, where, when, why, who, and what (see The Core Interview in Chapter 2 for specific questions)?

Have you had any (extensive) medical testing during the past year?

PAIN/SYMPTOMS

Is your shoulder painful?

If yes, how long has the shoulder been painful?

Follow the usual line of questioning regarding the pattern, frequency, intensity, and duration outlined in The Core Interview to establish necessary information regarding pain.

Aggravating/relieving activities

How does rest affect your shoulder symptoms? **(True muscular lesions are relieved with prolonged rest [i.e., more than 1 hour], whereas angina is usually relieved more immediately by cessation of activity or rest [i.e., usually within 2 to 5 minutes, up to 15 minutes]**

Does your shoulder pain occur during exercise (e.g., walking, climbing stairs, mowing the law) or any other physical or sexual activity? (Evaluate the difference between total body exertion causing shoulder symptoms versus movements of the upper extremities only reproducing symptoms. Total body exertion causing shoulder pain may be secondary to angina or myocardial infarction; whereas movements of just the upper extremities causing shoulder pain are indicative of a primary musculoskeletal lesion.)

Subacute/acute/chronic musculoskeletal lesion versus systemic pain pattern (see The Core Interview for specific meaning to the client's answers to these questions):

Can you lie on that side?

Does the shoulder pain awaken you at night?

If so, is this because you have rolled onto that side?

Do you notice any chest pain, night sweats, fever, or heart palpitations when you wake up at night?

Have you ever noticed these symptoms (e.g., chest pain, heart palpitations) with your shoulder pain during the day?

Do these symptoms wake you up separately from your shoulder pain or does your shoulder pain wake you up and you have these additional symptoms? (As always when asking questions about sleep patterns, the person may be unsure of the answers to the questions. In such cases, the physical therapist is advised to ask the client to pay attention to what happens related to sleep during the next few days up to 1 week and report back with more definitive information.)

References

Andreoli, T.E., Bennett, J.C., Carpenter, C.C.J., Plum, F., Smith, L.H. (eds.): Cecil Essentials of Medicine, 3rd ed. Philadelphia, W.B. Saunders, 1993, pp. 799–805.

Bauwens, D.B., and Paine, R.: Thoracic pain. In Blacklow, R.S. (ed.): MacBryde's Signs and Symptoms, 6th ed. Philadelphia, J.B. Lippincott, 1983, pp. 139–164.

Berkow, R., and Fletcher, A.J. (eds.): The Merck Manual of Diagnosis and Therapy, 16th ed. Rahway, New Jersey, Merck Sharp & Dohme Research Laboratory, 1992.

Cailliet, R.: Shoulder Pain. Philadelphia, F.A. Davis, 1981.

Cailliet, R.: Shoulder Pain, 3rd ed. Philadelphia, F.A. Davis, 1991.

Collins, J.H., Oser, F., Garcia, C.A., and Robertson, H.J.: Sudden paralysis in pregnancy due to spinal cord vascular accidents. Journal of Louisiana State Medical Society 138:44–48, 1986.

Cyriax, J.: Textbook of Orthopaedic Medicine, 8th ed. Vol. 1. London, Bailliere Tindall, 1982.

D'Ambrosia, R.: Musculoskeletal Disorders: Regional Examination and Differential Diagnosis, 2nd ed. Philadelphia, J.B. Lippincott, 1986.

Dirschl, D.R., and Almekinders, L.C.: Osteomyelitis: Common causes and treatment recommendations. Drugs 45(1):29–43, 1993.

Dunbar, A.: The silent problem: Taking the patient history one step further. Journal of Obstetric and Gynecologic Physical Therapy 15(2):4–5, 1991.

Garrett, W.E.: Strain, hernia, joint disease: Cause of youth's groin pain? Journal of Musculoskeletal Medicine 9(1):17–18, 1992.

Given, B.A., and Simmons, S.J.: Gastroenterology in Clinical Nursing. Baltimore: C.V. Mosby, 1979.

Glencross, E.J.G.: Bacteriological investigation of genitourinary infections. In Rocker, I. (ed.): Pelvic Pain in Women: Diagnosis and Management. New York, Springer-Verlag, 1990, pp. 31–40.

Golightly, R.: Pelvic arthropathy in pregnancy and the puerperium. Physiotherapy 68:216–220, 1982.

Green, N.E.: What to do when you suspect acute hematogenous osteomyelitis in children. Journal of Musculoskeletal Medicine 5(8):62–74, 1988.

Grieve, G.P.: The sacroiliac joint. Physiotherapy 62:384–399, 1976.

Hadler, N.M.: Medical management of regional musculoskeletal diseases: Backache, neck pain, disorders of the upper and lower extremities. Orlando, Florida, Grune and Stratton, 1984.

Hadler, N.M. (ed.): Clinical Concepts in Regional Musculoskeletal Illness. Orlando, Florida, Grune and Stratton, 1987a.

Hadler, N.M.: The patient with low back pain. Hospital Practice, Oct. 30, 1987b, pp. 17–22.

Haicken, B.N.: Laser laparoscopic cholecystectomy in the ambulatory setting. Journal of Post-Anesthesia Nursing 6(1):33–39, 1991.

Harrington, K.D.: Metastatic disease of the spine. Journal of Bone and Joint Surgery 68A:1110–1115, 1986.

Hollander, H., and Katz, M.H.: HIV infection. In Current Medical Diagnosis and Treatment. Norwalk, Connecticut, Appleton and Lange, 1993, p. 1008.

Hughes, J.M., Sturdy, D.E., and Thomas, G.D.: General aspects. In Rocker, I. (ed.): Pelvic Pain in Women: Diagnosis and Management. New York, Springer-Verlag, 1990, pp. 1–20.

Hummel-Berry, K.: Obstetric low back pain: A comprehensive review. Part One. Journal of Obstetric and Gynecologic Physical Therapy 14(1):10–13, 1990.

Jayson, M.I.V.: Difficult diagnoses in back pain. British Medical Journal 288:740–741, 1984.

Jones, D.G.: Orthopedic causes of pelvic pain. In Rocker, I. (ed.): Pelvic Pain in Women: Diagnosis and Management. New York, Springer-Verlag, 1990, pp. 150–156.

Kirkaldy-Willis, W.H. (ed.): Managing Low Back Pain. New York, Churchill Livingstone, 1983.

Loriaux, T.C.: Nursing care of clients with adrenal, pituitary, and gonadal disorders. In Black, J.M., and Matassarin-Jacobs, E.: Luckmann and Sorensen's Medical-Surgical Nursing, 4th ed. Philadelphia, W.B. Saunders, 1993, pp. 1837–1862.

Lose, G., and Lindholm, P.: Transient painful osteoporosis of the hip in pregnancy. International Journal of Gynecology and Obstetrics 24:13–16, 1986.

Magee, D.J.: Orthopedic Physical Assessment. Philadelphia, W.B. Saunders, 1992.

Matassarin-Jacobs, E., and Clark, A.J.: Nursing care of women with gynecologic disorders. In Black, J.M., and Matassarin-Jacobs, E.: Luckmann and Sorensen's Medical-Surgical Nursing, 4th ed. Philadelphia, W.B. Saunders, 1993, pp. 2119–2156.

McClain, R.F., and Weinstein, J.N.: Tumors of the spine. Seminar in Spine Surgery 2:157–180, 1990.

McCowin, P.R., Borenstein, D., and Wiesel, S.W.: The current approach to the medical diagnosis of low back pain. Orthopedic Clinics of North America 22(2):315–325, 1991.

McKenzie, R.A.: The Lumbar Spine: Mechanical Diagnosis and Therapy. Waikanae, New Zealand, Spinal Publications, 1981.

Mennell, J.M.: Joint Pain: Diagnosis and Treatment Using Manipulative Techniques. Boston, Little, Brown, 1964.

Mens, J.M.A., Stam, H.J., Stoeckhart, R., et al.: Peripartum pelvic pain: A report of the analysis of an inquiry among patients of the Dutch Patients Society. In Vleeming, A., Mooney, V., Snijjders, C., et al. (eds.): The First Interdisciplinary World Congress on Low Back Pain and Its Relation to the Sacroiliac Joint. Rotterdam, The Netherlands, ECO, 1992, pp. 521–533.

Mooney, V.: Understanding, examining for, and treating sacroiliac pain. Journal of Musculoskeletal Medicine 10(7):37–49, 1993.

Moran, J.: Stress fractures in pregnancy. American Journal of Obstetrics and Gynecology 158(6):1274–1277, 1988.

Morgenlander, J.C.: Disc space infection. The Black Letter 5(3):3, January 1991.

Morris, D.C., Hurst, J.W., and Walter, P.F.: The recognition and treatment of myocardial infarction and its complications. In Hurst, J.W. (ed.): The Heart, 7th ed. New York, McGraw-Hill, 1990, pp. 1054–1078.

Narchi, P., Benhamou, D., and Fernandez, H.: Intraperitoneal local anesthetic for shoulder pain after day-case laparoscopy. Lancet 338(8782–8783):1569–1570, 1991.

Nelson, B.W.: A rational approach to the treatment of low back pain. Journal of Musculoskeletal Medicine 10(5):67–82, 1993.

Neumann, D.A.: Arthrokinesiologic considerations in the aged adult. In Guccione, A.A. (ed.): Geriatric Physical Therapy. St Louis, Mosby, 1993, pp. 47–70.

O'Connor, M.I., and Currier, B.L.: Metastatic bone disease: Metastatic disease of the spine. Orthopedics 15(5):611–620, 1992.

O'Toole, M. (ed.): Encyclopedia and Dictionary of Medicine, Nursing and Allied Health, 5th ed. Philadelphia, W.B. Saunders, 1992.

Pedowitz, R.A., Garfin, S.R., Roberts, W.A., and White, A.A.: Evaluating the causes of neck, shoulder, and arm pain. Journal of Musculoskeletal Medicine 5(6):61–74, 1988.

Phillips, E., and Levine, A.M.: Metastatic lesions of the upper cervical spine. Spine 14:1071–1077, 1989.

Porter, R.W., Hibbert, C.S., and Wicks, M.: The spinal canal in symptomatic lumbar disc lesions. Journal of Bone and Joint Surgery (Br) 60B:485–487, 1978.

Rauterberg, J.: Age-dependent changes in structure, properties, and biosynthesis of collagen. In Platt, D. (ed.): Gerontology: 4th International Symposium. New York, Springer-Verlag, 1989.

Richie, J.P.: Detection and treatment of testicular cancer. Ca—A Journal for Clinicians 43(3):151–175, 1993.

Ridge, J.R., and Way, L.W.: Abdominal pain. In Sleisenger, M.H., and Fordtran, J.S. (eds.): Gastrointestinal Disease, 5th ed. Philadelphia, W.B. Saunders, 1993, pp. 150–161.

Riggins, R.S.: The shoulder. In D'Ambrosia, R.: Musculoskeletal Disorder: Regional Examination and Differential Diagnosis, 2nd. ed. Philadelphia, J.B. Lippincott, 1986, pp. 367–393.

Rocker, I.: Reproduction and pain. In Rocker, I. (ed.): Pelvic Pain in Women: Diagnosis and Management. New York, Springer-Verlag, 1990a, pp. 59–61.

Rocker, I.: Gynecological examination and investigation. In Rocker, I. (ed.): Pelvic Pain in Women: Diagnosis and Management. New York, Springer-Verlag, 1990b, pp. 26–28.

Rocker, I.: Gynecological pain. In Rocker, I. (ed.): Pelvic Pain in Women: Diagnosis and Management. New York, Springer-Verlag, 1990c, pp. 103–132.

Rose, S.J., and Rothstein, J.M.: Muscle mutability: General concepts and adaptations to altered patterns of use. Physical Therapy 62:1773, 1982.

Sasso, R.C., Cotler, H.B., and Guyer, R.D.: Evaluating low back pain: The role of diagnostic imaging. Journal of Musculoskeletal Medicine 8(5):21–37, 1991.

Scharf, S.M.: History and physical examination. In Baum, G.L., and Wolinsky, E. (eds.): Textbook of Pulmonary Diseases, 4th ed. Boston, Little, Brown, 1989, pp. 213–226.

Simms-Williams, H., Jayson, M.I.V., and Baddeley, H.: Small spinal fractures in back pain patients. Annals of Rheumatic Disease 37:262–265, 1978.

Sinnott, M.: Assessing musculoskeletal changes in the geriatric population. American Physical Therapy Association Combined Sections Meeting, February 3–7, 1993.

Spankus, J.D.: Cause and treatment of low back pain during pregnancy. Wisconsin Medical Journal 64: 303–304, 1965.

Sturdy, D.E.: Surgical causes of pelvic pain. In Rocker, I. (ed.): Pelvic Pain in Women: Diagnosis and Management. New York, Springer-Verlag, 1990, pp. 133–150.

Sullivan, M.S.: Back support mechanisms during manual lifting. Physical Therapy 69:38–45, 1989.

Travell, J.G., and Simons, D.G.: Myofascial Pain and Dysfunction: The Trigger Point Manual. Vol. 1. Baltimore, Williams and Wilkins, 1983.

Travell, J.G., and Simons, D.G.: Myofascial Pain and Dysfunction: The Trigger Point Manual. Vol. 2. Baltimore, Williams and Wilkins, 1992.

Twomey, L.T., and Taylor, J.R. (eds.): Physical Therapy of the Low Back. Edinburgh, Churchill Livingstone, 1987.

Vernon-Roberts, B., and Pirie, C.J.: Healing trabecular microfractures in the bodies of lumbar vertebrae. Annals of Rheumatic Disease, 32:406–412, 1973.

Wedge, J.H.: Differential diagnosis of low back pain. In Kirkaldy-Willis, W.H. (ed.): Managing Low Back Pain. New York, Churchill Livingstone, 1983, pp. 129–143.

Wilson, D.L., and Klahr, S.: Urinary tract obstruction. In Schrier, R.W., and Gottschalk, C.W. (eds.): Diseases of the Kidney, 5th ed. Vol. 1. Boston, Little, Brown, 1993.

Zohn, D.A.: Musculoskeletal Pain: Diagnosis and Physical Treatment, 2nd ed. Boston, Little, Brown, 1988.

Zohn, D.A., and Mennell, J.: Musculoskeletal Pain: Principles of Physical Diagnosis and Physical Treatment, 2nd ed. Boston, Little, Brown, 1988.

Bibliography

Benson, J.T. (ed.): Female Pelvic Floor Disorders; Investigation and Management. New York, W.W. Norton, 1992.

Cyriax, J., and Cyriax, P.: Illustrated Manual of Orthopaedic Medicine. London, Butterworths, 1983.

King, P.M., et al.: Musculoskeletal factors in chronic pelvic pain. Journal of Psychosomatic Obstetrics and Gynaecology 12(Suppl.):87–98, 1991.

Layzer, R.B.: Neuromuscular Manifestations of Systemic Disease. Philadelphia, F.A. Davis, 1985.

Lile, A., and Hagar, T.: Survey of current physical therapy treatment for the pregnant client with lumbo-pelvic dysfunction. Journal of Obstetrics and Gynecology 15(4):10–12, 1991.

Nachemson, A.L.: Newest knowledge of low back pain. A critical look. Clinical Orthopedics 279:8–20, 1992.

Reiter, R.: Chronic pelvic pain. Clinics in Obstetrics and Gynecology 33(1):117–211, 1990.

Urinary Incontinence in Adults: Clinical Practice Guideline. AHCPR Pub. No. 92-0038. Rockville, Maryland, Agency for Health Care Policy and Research, Public Health Service, U.S. Department of Human and Health Services, March 1992.

Wall, L., and Davidson, T.: The role of muscular re-education by physical therapy in the treatment of genuine stress urinary incontinence. Obstetrical and Gynecological Survey 47(5):322–331, 1992.

Acetylcholine: An acetic acid ester of choline, normally present in many parts of the body, having important physiologic functions; it is a neurotransmitter at cholinergic synapses

Achalasia: Failure to relax the smooth muscle fibers of the gastrointestinal tract at any junction of one part with another; especially failure of the lower esophagus to relax with swallowing

Acidosis: A pathologic condition resulting from accumulation of acid or depletion of the alkaline reserve (bicarbonate content) in the blood and body tissues and characterized by an increase in hydrogen ion concentration (decrease in pH); the opposite of alkalosis

Acquired immunodeficiency syndrome (AIDS): Suppression or deficiency of the cellular immune response, acquired by exposure to the human T-cell lymphotrophic virus (HIV); infection by the virus and the consequent suppression of the immune response predisposes the infected person to opportunistic infections and malignancies

Acromegaly: Abnormal enlargement of the extremities of the skeleton (nose, jaw, hands, feet) resulting from hypersecretion of growth hormone (GH) from the pituitary gland

Acroparesthesia: An abnormal sensation, such as tingling, numbness, "pins and needles" in the digits

Adenoma: A benign epithelial tumor in which the cells form recognizable glandular structures or in which the cells are derived from glandular epithelium

Agglutination: Aggregation of separate particles into clumps or masses, especially the clumping together of bacteria by the action of a specific antibody directed against a surface antigen

Agoraphobia: An anxiety disorder characterized by intense, irrational fear of open places, especially a marked fear of being alone or of being in public places where escape would be difficult or help might be unavailable

Albumin: A plasma protein formed principally in the liver and responsible for much of the colloidal osmotic pressure of the blood

Alkalosis: A pathologic condition resulting from an accumulation of base or from a loss of acid without comparable loss of base in the body fluids, characterized by a decrease in hydrogen ion concentration (increase in pH)

Allergen: A substance, protein or nonprotein, capable of inducing allergy or specific hypersensitivity

Allergy: A state of abnormal and individual hypersensitivity acquired through exposure to a particular allergen; reexposure reveals a heightened capacity to react

Alopecia: Loss of hair, baldness

Alveoli: Air sac or thin-walled chamber in the lungs, surrounded by networks of capillaries through whose walls exchange of carbon dioxide and oxygen takes place

Amebiasis: Infection with amebas, especially *Entamoeba histolytica;* amebic dysentery

Amenorrhea: Absence of the menses

Amyloidosis: The deposition in various tissues of amyloid, a protein resembling starch, that causes tissues to become waxy and nonfunctioning

Anabolism: The constructive phase of metabolism in which the body cells synthesize protoplasm for growth and repair; the opposite of catabolism

Anaplasia: Loss of differentiation of cells; a characteristic of tumor cells

Anastomoses: Connecting channels between blood vessels

Androgens: Any steroid hormone that promotes male characteristics; the two main androgens are androsterone and testosterone

Anemia: A reduction below normal in the number of erythrocytes (red blood cells or RBCs) or in the quantity of hemoglobin in the blood

Aneurysm: A sac formed by the dilatation of the wall of an artery, a vein, or the heart

Angina (pectoris): Spasmodic, choking, suffocating chest pain usually due to a lack of adequate blood supply (oxygen) to the heart muscle

Angiodysplasia: Small vascular abnormalities, especially of the intestinal tract

Angiogenesis: The development of blood vessels in the embryo
tumor a., the induction of the growth of blood vessels from surrounding tissue into a solid tumor by a diffusible chemical factor released by the tumor cells

Angioma (spider): Branched dilatation of the superficial capillaries, resembling a spider

Angiotensin: A vasoconstrictive principle formed in the blood when renin is released from the juxtaglomerular apparatus in the kidney

Anicteric: Without jaundice

Anisocytosis: The presence in the blood of erythrocytes showing abnormal variations in size

Ankylosis: Immobility and consolidation or fusion of a joint due to disease, injury, or surgical procedure; ankylosis may be caused by destruction of the membranes that line the joint or by faulty bone structure

Anorexia: Loss of appetite due to emotional state

Antibody: An immunoglobulin molecule having a specific amino acid sequence that gives each antibody the ability to adhere to and interact with only the antigen that induced its synthesis; this antigen-specific property of the antibody is the basis of the antigen-antibody reaction that is essential to an immune response

Antigen: Any substance that is capable, under appropriate conditions, of inducing a specific immune response and of reacting with the products of that response; that is, with specific antibody or specifically sensitized T lymphocytes, or both; antigens may be soluble substances, such as toxins and foreign proteins, or particulates, such as bacteria and tissue cells

Anuria: Complete suppression of urine formation by the kidney

Aplastic anemia: A deficiency of circulating erythrocytes because of the arrested development of erythrocytes within the bone marrow

Arrhythmia: Any irregularity of the heartbeat; any variation from the normal regular rhythm of the heart

Arteriosclerosis: A group of diseases characterized by the thickening and hardening of the usually supple arterial walls; it comprises three distinct forms: atherosclerosis, Mönckeberg's arteriosclerosis, and arteriolosclerosis

Arteriosclerosis obliterans: Atheroscleromas (plaques) of the intima (innermost structure) of small vessels has caused complete obliteration of the lumen (cavity or channel within a tube) of the artery; affects the aorta and its branches to the extremities

Arteritis: Inflammation of an artery

Arthralgia: Pain in a joint

Ascites: Effusion and accumulation of serous (clear liquid) fluid that accumulates in the peritoneal (abdominal) cavity

Aspirate: To inhale vomitus, mucus, or food into the respiratory tract

Asterixis: A motor disturbance marked by intermittent lapses of an assumed posture as a result of intermittency of sustained contraction of groups of muscles; called liver flap because of its occurrence in liver disease

Atheroma: Slow deterioration of arteries in which fatty deposits called plaque (lipids such as triglycerides and cholesterol) are laid down in the (intima) inner lining of the arteries; occurring in atherosclerosis, a form of arteriosclerosis

Atherosclerosis: An extremely common form of arteriosclerosis in which deposits of yellow plaques (atheromas) containing cholesterol, lipoid material, and lipophages are formed within the intima and inner media of large and medium-sized arteries

Atopy: A clinical hypersensitivity state or allergy with a hereditary predisposition

Atrial septal defect: Hole between the atria of the heart

Autoantibody: An antibody formed in response to, and reacting against, an antigenic constituent of the individual's own tissues

Autoimmune disease: Disease due to immunologic action of one's own cells or antibodies on components of the body

Autonomic: Not subject to voluntary control; the branch of the nervous system that works without conscious control

Autosplinting: Lying down on the painful side to relieve pleuritic or pulmonary pain by reducing respiratory excursion or movements

Avascular necrosis: Death of cells due to a lack of blood supply

B cells: B lymphocytes, white blood cells of the immune system derived from bone marrow and involved in the production of antibodies; associated with humoral-mediated immunity

Bacteriuria: Bacteria in the urine

Basophil: A granular leukocyte with an irregularly shaped, relatively pale-staining nucleus that is partially constricted into two lobes, and with cytoplasm containing coarse blue-black granules of variable size; basophils contain vasoactive amines, for example, histamine and serotonin, that are released on appropriate stimulation

Basophilia: Abnormal increase of basophilic leukocytes in the blood

Bile: A clear yellow or orange fluid produced by the liver; it is concentrated and stored in the gallbladder and is poured into the small intestine via the bile ducts when needed for digestion; bile helps in alkalinizing the intestinal contents and plays a role in the emulsification, absorption, and digestion of fat

Bilirubin: A bile pigment produced by the breakdown of heme and reduction of biliverdin; failure of the liver cells to excrete

bile (or obstruction of the bile ducts) can cause an increased amount of bilirubin in the body fluids and lead to obstructive jaundice

Biliverdin: A green bile pigment formed by catabolism of hemoglobin and converted to bilirubin in the blood

Bradycardia: Slowness of the heart beat, which is shown by slowing of the pulse rate to less than 60 beats/min

Bradykinin: A nonpeptide kinin formed from a plasma protein, high-molecular-weight (HMW) kininogen by the action of kallikrein (enzyme that release kinins); it is a very powerful vasodilator that increases capillary permeability and, in addition, constricts smooth muscle and stimulates pain receptors

Bronchiectasis: Chronic dilatation of the bronchi and bronchioles with secondary infection, usually involving the lower lobes of the lung

Bronchus (pl. bronchi): Any of the larger passages conveying air to and within the lungs

Buerger's disease: See Thromboangiitis obliterans

Bulimia: Eating disorder characterized by episodic binge eating followed by purging behavior, such as self-induced vomiting and laxative abuse

CAL: Chronic airflow limitation, a term used by pulmonary medicine specialists to describe more accurately the condition otherwise called chronic obstructive pulmonary disease (COPD)

Calcinosis: A condition characterized by abnormal deposition of calcium salts in the tissues

Calculus (pl. calculi): Stones either in the kidney or gallbladder, composed of mineral salts

Caliculus (pl. caliculi): Small cup or cup-shaped structure

Canaliculus (pl. canaliculi): An extremely narrow tubular passage or channel

Cancellous: Of a lattice or spongelike structure; referring to bone

Cancer: Any malignant cellular tumor; this word encompasses a group of neoplastic diseases in which there is a transformation of normal body cells into malignant ones

Carcinoma: A malignant new growth made up of epithelial cells tending to infiltrate surrounding tissues and give rise to metastases

Carcinoma in situ: A neoplastic entity in which the tumor cells have not invaded the basement membrane but are still confined to the epithelium of origin

Carcinomatous neuromyopathy: There are many types of carcinomatous neuromyopathy; however, pertinent to the physical therapist, presentation may be as idiopathic weakness of the proximal muscles that may be accompanied by the diminution of two or more deep tendon reflexes

Catabolism: Any destructive process by which complex substances are converted by living cells into simpler compounds, with release of energy; the opposite of anabolism

Celiac plexus: A network of ganglia and nerves supplying the abdominal viscera; also called solar plexus

Cheirarthritis: Inflammation of the joints of the hands and fingers

Chemotaxis: Force or movement in response to the influence of chemical stimulation; for example, the attraction of neutrophils to the immune complex

Cholangiocarcinoma: A primary (fatal) cancer of the liver that develops in the bile ducts

Cholecystectomy: Excision of the gallbladder

Cholecystitis: Inflammation of the gallbladder, acute or chronic

Cholecystokinin: A polypeptide hormone secreted in the small intestine that stimulates gallbladder contraction and secretion of pancreatic enzymes

Choledocholithiasis: Calculi in the common duct

Cholelith: Gallstone

Cholelithiasis: The presence or formation of gallstones

Chondrocalcinosis: Deposition of calcium salts in the cartilage of joints; when accompanied by attacks of goutlike symptoms, it is called pseudogout

Chondrodynia: Pain in a cartilage

Chondroma: A tumor or tumor-like growth of cartilage cells; it may remain in the interior or substance of a cartilage or bone (true chondroma or enchondroma), or it may develop on the surface of a cartilage and project under the periosteum of bone (ecchondroma or ecchondrosis)

Chondrosarcoma: A malignant tumor derived from cartilage cells or their precursors

Chondrosternal: Pertaining to the costal cartilages and sternum

Chordoma: A malignant tumor arising from embryonic remains of the notochord (cylindrical cord of cells on the dorsal aspect of an embryo, marking its longitudinal axis; it is the center of development of the axial skeleton)

Chyme: The semifluid material produced by action of the gastric juice on ingested food and discharged through the pylorus into the duodenum

Cirrhosis: A liver disease characterized by the loss of the normal microscopic lobular architecture and regenerative replacement of necrotic parenchymal tissue with fibrous bands of connective tissue that eventually constrict and partition the organ into irregular nodules

Claudication: Limping or lameness caused by ischemia or insufficient blood flow in occlusive arterial disease of the limbs; if claudication is intermittent, this represents a complex of symptoms characterized by the absence of pain or discomfort in a limb when at rest and the commencement of pain, tension, and weakness after walking is begun with intensification of the condition until walking is impossible, requiring rest until the symptoms have disappeared

Clearance: Complete removal by the kidneys of a solute or substance from a specific volume of blood per unit of time

Closed-ended question: Question that requires only a "yes" or "no" answer

Clotting factors: Factors essential to normal blood clotting whose absence, diminution, or excess may lead to abnormality of the clotting; there are 12 factors, commonly designated by Roman numerals

Clubbing: Bulbous swelling of the terminal phalanges of the fingers and toes, giving them a "club" appearance

Coagulation: Formation of a clot

Coccygodynia: Pain in the coccyx and neighboring region

COLD: Chronic obstructive lung disease; also called chronic obstructive pulmonary disease (COPD)

Collagen: A fibrous structural protein that constitutes the protein of the white fibers (collagenous fibers) of skin, tendon, bone, cartilage, and all other connective tissues

Colloid osmotic pressure (oncotic): Pressure exerted by proteins in the blood to pull fluid from the interstitial space back into the vascular area

Colposcopy: Procedure that visualizes the cervical canal by use of a speculum with a magnifying lens

Complement: A term originally used to refer to the heat-labile factor in serum that causes immune cytolysis, the lysis of antibody-coated cells, and now refers to the entire functionally related system, consisting of at least 20 distinct serum proteins, which is the effector of immune cytolysis and other biologic functions

Congestive heart failure: The heart's inability to pump enough blood for the body to function well; the heart muscles gradually fail to contract vigorously enough to cycle adequately the total volume of circulating blood

Conization: Removal of a cone of tissue, as in partial excision of the cervix uteri

Conjugate: In biochemistry, the joining of a toxic substance with some natural substance of the body to form a detoxified product for elimination from the body

Constipation: A condition in which waste matter in the bowel is too hard to pass easily or in which bowel movements are so infrequent that discomfort and other symptoms interfere with one's usual daily activities and sense of well-being; constipation can be said to exist when a person reports a frequency of bowel elimination that is less than the usual pattern or when defecation occurs less than three times a week, with stools that are hard and well-formed and possibly less than the usual amount; straining at stool occurs regularly and the person experiences headache, abdominal pain, a feeling of fullness in the abdomen or rectum, and either diminished appetite or nausea

Constitutional symptoms: Affecting the whole constitution of the body; not local; systemic

Conversion symptoms: A mental disorder in which a person "converts" the anxiety caused by a psychologic conflict into physical symptoms

COPD: Chronic obstructive pulmonary disease; also called chronic obstructive lung disease (COLD)

Cor pulmonale: Heart disease (enlargement of the right ventricle) secondary to pulmonary disease

Coronary thrombosis: Sudden blockage of the coronary artery

Costochondral: Pertaining to a rib and its cartilage

Costochondritis: Inflammation of the costal cartilage or rib and rib cartilage

Cretinism: Arrested physical and mental development with dystrophy of bones and soft tissues, due to congenital lack of thyroid gland secretion from hypofunctioning or absence of the gland

Crohn's disease: Inflammation of the terminal portion of the ileum; also called regional enteritis and regional ileitis; it can affect any segment of the intestinal tract, although it is more commonly located in the terminal ileum

Cutaneous: Pertaining to the skin

Cyanosis: Blue discoloration of the skin and mucous membranes due to excessive concentration of reduced hemoglobin in the blood

Cystine: A naturally occurring amino acid, the chief sulfur-containing component of the protein molecule; it is sometimes found in the urine and in the kidneys in the form of minute hexagonal crystals that frequently form cystine calculus (stones) in the bladder.

Cystitis: Inflammation of the bladder

Cystocele: Herniation of the urinary bladder into the vagina

Cystoscopy: Examination of the bladder by means of a scope especially designed for passing through the urethra into the bladder to permit visual inspection of the interior of that organ

Cytology (cytologic): The study of cells, their origin, structure, function, and pathology

Cytolysis: Cell lysis produced by antibody with the participation of complement

Cytotoxic: Adjectival form of cytotoxicity, the degree to which an agent possesses a specific destructive action on certain cells; used particularly in referring to the lysis of cells by immune phenomena and to antineoplastic drugs that selectively kill dividing cells

Dactylitis: Inflammation of a finger or toe

Demyelinization (or demyelination): Destruction, removal, or loss of the myelin sheath of a nerve or nerves

Dependent edema: Edema (abnormal accumulation of fluid in the intercellular spaces of the body) affecting most severely the lowermost parts of the body that are maintained in a dependent (unsupported) position.

Depolarization: The rapid reversal of the resting membrane potential that results from a sequence of events in which the cell membrane permeability to sodium increases spontaneously (e.g., in pacemaking cells) or in response to a stimulus, then a rapid influx of sodium occurs and potassium moves out of the cell; this movement of ions across the membrane creates an electrical current or impulse that spreads as a wave of depolarization to adjacent cells

Diaphoresis: Perspiration, especially excessive or profuse perspiration

Diarrhea: Rapid movement of fecal matter through the intestine, resulting in poor absorption of water, nutritive elements, and electrolytes and producing abnormally frequent evacuation of watery stools

Diastole: The phase of the cardiac cycle in which the heart relaxes between contractions; specifically, the period when the two ventricles are dilated by the blood flowing into them

Differentiation: The process of acquiring completely individual characteristics, such as occurs in the progressive diversification of cells and tissues

Diffuse lymphoma: A malignant lymphoma in which the neoplastic cells infiltrate the entire lymph node without any organized pattern; this unorganized infiltration is called effacement

Diffusion: Movement of solutes of particles from an area of greater concentration to an area of lesser concentration through a semipermeable membrane

Diplopia: Double vision; the perception of two images of a single object

Disseminated: Scattered; distributed over a considerable area

Disseminated intravascular coagulation: Widespread formation of thromboses in the microcirculation, mainly within the capillaries; it is a secondary complication of a diverse group of obstetric, surgical, infectious, hemolytic, and neoplastic disorders, all of which intrinsically affect the coagulation sequence

Diuresis: Increased excretion of the urine

Dysesthesias: Impairment of any sense, especially the sense of touch; a painful, persistent sensation induced by a gentle touch of the skin

Dyspareunia: Difficult or painful coitus

Dysphagia: Difficulty in swallowing

Dysplasia (dysplastic): Alteration in size, shape, and organization of adult cells

Dyspnea: Labored or difficult breathing; it is a symptom of a variety of disorders and is primarily an indication of inadequate ventilation or insufficient amounts of oxygen in the circulating blood

Dysuria: Painful or difficult urination

Ecchymosis: Hemorrhagic spot, larger than a petechia, in the skin or mucous membrane, forming a nonelevated, rounded or irregular, blue or purple patch; a bruise

Ectopic: Pertaining to or characterized by displacement or malposition, especially if congenital

Ectopic pregnancy: Pregnancy in which the fertilized ovum becomes implanted outside the uterus instead of in the wall of the uterus; also called extrauterine pregnancy

Effusion: Escape of fluid into a body part

Embolism: The sudden blocking of an artery by a clot of foreign material (embolus) that has been brought to its site of lodgment by the blood current; may also be a fat globule, air bubble, piece of tissue, or clump of bacteria

Embolus (pl. emboli): Part or all of a clot that breaks away and circulates through the bloodstream

Emphysema: A pathologic accumulation of air in tissues or organs; the term is generally used to designate chronic pulmonary emphysema, a lung disorder in which the terminal bronchioles become plugged with mucus; eventually, there is a loss of elasticity in the lung tissue so that inspired air becomes trapped in the lungs, making breathing difficult, especially during the expiratory phase

Empyema: Accumulation of pus in a body cavity

Endemic: Present in a community at all times

Endocarditis: Inflammation of the endocardium (lining covering the heart and valves)

Endocardium: The endothelial lining membrane of the cavities of the heart and the connective tissue bed on which it lies; the innermost layer lining the heart

Endometriosis: A condition in which tissue more or less perfectly resembling the endometrium (the mucous membrane lining the uterus) occurs aberrantly in various locations in the pelvic cavity and elsewhere

Endothelium (cardiac): Layer of cells lining the cavities of the heart and blood vessels

Enthesitis: Inflammation at the site of attachment of a muscle or ligament to bone

Enuresis: Involuntary discharge of urine, usually referring to involuntary discharge of urine during sleep at night; bed-wetting beyond the age when bladder control should have been achieved

Eosinophil: A granular leukocyte with a nucleus that usually has two lobes connected by a thread of chromatin, and cytoplasm containing coarse, round granules of uniform size

Eosinophilia: The formation and accumulation of an abnormally large number of eosinophils in the blood

Epicardium: The serous pericardium (visceral pleura) or layer on the surface of the heart that immediately envelops the heart

Epigastric: Describes the upper middle region of the abdomen and lower sternum

Epigastrium: The upper and middle region of the abdomen, located within the sternal angle

Epistaxis: Hemorrhage from the nose; nosebleed

Epitope: A characteristic shape or marker on an antigen's surface

Eructation: Belching

Erythema: Redness of the skin caused by congestion of the capillaries in the lower layers of the skin; it occurs with any skin injury, infection, or inflammation

Erythema nodosum: Red bumps/purple knots over the ankles and shins

Erythrocytes: A red blood cell or corpuscle; one of the formed elements of the peripheral blood; the functions of erythrocytes include transportation of oxygen and carbon dioxide; they are important in the maintenance of a normal acid-base balance, and because they help determine the viscosity of the blood, they also influence its specific gravity

Erythropoiesis: The formation of erythrocytes

Erythropoietin: A glycoprotein hormone secreted by the kidney in the adult and by the liver in the fetus, which acts on stem cells of the bone marrow to stimulate red blood cell production

Esophageal varices: Varicosities (distentions) of branches of the azygos vein that anastomose (connection between two normally distinct structures) with tributaries of the portal vein in the lower esophagus; caused by portal hypertension in cirrhosis of the liver

Esophagitis: Inflammation of the esophagus

Exogenous: Developed or originating outside the organism

Exophthalmos, exophthalmia: Abnormal protrusion of the eye

Extracellular fluid (ECF): Body fluid found outside body cells

Extramedullary: Outside the spinal cord but still within the spinal canal

Fiberoptic endoscopy: Visual examination of the interior structures of the body with an instrument (endoscope); used for direct visual inspection of the hollow organs or body cavities

Fibrillations: Involuntary twitching or contraction of the heart muscle fibrils, but not the muscle as a whole

Fibrin: An insoluble protein that is essential to clotting of blood, formed from fibrinogen by action of thrombin

Fibrinogen: A high-molecular-weight protein in the blood plasma that, by the action of thrombin, is converted into fibrin; also called clotting factor I; in the clotting mechanism, fibrin threads form a meshwork for the basis of a blood clot; most of the fibrinogen in the circulating blood is formed in the liver

Fibroids: Having a fibrous structure, fibroma; tumor consisting mainly of fibrous or fully developed connective tissue

Fibrosis: Formation of fibrous tissue

Flatulence: Excessive formation of gases in the intestine or stomach

Frequency: Referring to urinary or bowel frequency: increased number of times urination or defecation occurs without an increase in the daily volume or output, due to reduced bladder or colon capacity

Fulminate: To occur suddenly with great intensity

Funnel technique: Moving from an open-ended line of questions to the closed-ended questions

Giant cell tumor: A bone tumor, ranging from benign to malignant, consisting of cellular spindle cell stroma (tissue containing the ground substance, framework, or matrix of an organ) containing multinucleated giant cells resembling osteoclasts

Gliosis: Fibrous cells (astrocytes) in damaged areas of the central nervous system

Glomerular filtration rate (GFR): The amount of fluid filtered by the glomerular capillaries in 1 minute (approximately 125 ml/min)

Glomerulonephritis: A variety of nephritis (inflammation of the kidney) characterized by inflammation of the capillary loops in the glomeruli of the kidney; it occurs in acute, subacute, and chronic forms and is usually secondary to an infection

Glucagon: A polypeptide hormone secreted by the alpha cells of the islets of Langerhans in response to hypoglycemia or to stimulation by growth hormone; it increases blood glucose concentration by stimulating glycogenolysis in the liver and is administered to relieve hypoglycemic coma from any cause, especially hyperinsulinism

Glucocorticoids: Any corticoid substance that increases gluconeogenesis, raising the concentration of liver glycogen and blood sugar (i.e., cortisol [hydrocortisone], cortisone, and corticosterone)

Glycosuria: The presence of glucose in the urine

Goiter: Enlargement of the thyroid gland, causing a swelling in the front of the neck

Gout: The manifestation of an inherited inborn error of purine metabolism, characterized by an elevated serum uric acid (hyperuricemia); may cause gouty arthritis or renal disease because of the deposition of urate crystals in tissues

Granulocyte: Any cell containing granules, especially a granular leukocyte; a cell of the immune system filled with granules of toxic chemicals that enable the cell to digest microorganisms; basophils, neutrophils, eosinophils, and mast cells are examples of granulocytes

Gynecomastia: Excessive development of mammary glands in men, even to the functional state

Helper T cells (T$_h$): A subset of T cells that initiates antibody production

Hemangioma: Benign tumor composed of newly formed blood vessels clustered together

Hemarthrosis: Blood in the cavity of the joint

Hematemesis: Vomiting of blood

Hematochromatosis, hemochromatosis: A disorder of iron metabolism with excess deposition of iron in the tissues, bronze skin pigmentation, cirrhosis of the liver, and diabetes mellitus; also called bronze diabetes and iron storage disease

Hematogenous: Disseminated by the bloodstream or by the circulation

Hematoma: A localized collection of extravasated (escaped) blood, usually clotted, in an organ, space, or tissue

Hematopoiesis: The formation and development of blood cells, usually taking place in the bone marrow

Hematopoietic: Pertaining to or affecting the formation of blood cells; an agent that promotes the formation of blood cells

Hematuria: The discharge of blood in the urine; the urine may be slightly blood-tinged, grossly bloody, or a smoky brown color

Heme: The nonprotein, insoluble, iron protoporphyrin (a porphyrin, which in combination with iron, forms hemes) constituent of hemoglobin; it is responsible for oxygen-carrying properties of hemoglobin

Hemoglobin: A protein found in the erythrocytes (red blood cells), which transports molecular oxygen (O_2) in the blood; symbol Hb

Hemolysis: Rupture of erythrocytes (red blood cells) with the release of hemoglobin into the plasma

Hemoptysis: Coughing and spitting of blood as a result of bleeding from any part of the respiratory tract

Hemorrhoids: Enlarged (varicose) veins in the mucous membrane inside or just outside of the rectum; also called "piles"

Hemostasis: The arrest of the escape of blood by either natural (clot formation or vessel spasm) or artificial (compression or ligation) methods, or the interruption of blood flow to a part

Hepatic encephalopathy: A condition, usually occurring secondarily to advanced liver disease, marked by disturbances of consciousness that may progress to deep coma (hepatic coma), psychiatric changes of varying degree, flapping tremor, and fetor hepaticus (characteristic breath odor)

Hepatomegaly: Enlargement of the liver

HLA-B27: A genetic marker: human leukocyte antigen

Homans' sign: Slight pain or discomfort at the back of the knee or calf when the ankle is forcibly dorsiflexed, indicative of thrombus in the veins of the leg

Homocystinuria: An inborn error of sulfur amino acid metabolism caused by lack of the enzyme cystathionine synthase

Hormone: A chemical transmitter substance produced by cells of the body and transported by the bloodstream to the cells and organs on which it has a specific regulatory effect

Hyalinization: Conversion into a substance resembling glass

Hydrarthrosis: Accumulation of watery fluid in the cavity of a joint

Hydrostatic pressure: Pressure exerted by a stationary fluid

Hyperalgesia: Excessive sensitivity to pain

Hyperalimentation: A program of parenteral administration of all nutrients for people with gastrointestinal dysfunction; also called total parenteral alimentation (TPA) and total parenteral nutrition (TPN)

Hyperbilirubinemia: An excess of bilirubin in the blood as a result of liver or biliary tract dysfunction, or with excessive destruction of erythrocytes

Hypercalcemia: An excess of calcium in the blood

Hypercholesteremia: An excess of cholesterol in the blood

Hyperesthesia: Increased sensitivity to touch or other sensory stimulation

Hyperfunction: Excessive functioning of a part or a gland

Hyperglycemia: An excess of glucose in the blood

Hyperkalemia: Abnormally high potassium concentration in the blood, most often due to defective renal excretion, such as in kidney disease, severe and extensive burns, intestinal obstruction, and Addison's disease

Hyperkeratosis: Hypertrophy of the horny layer of the skin (e.g., nails, soles, or any disease characterized by it

Hyperkinesis: Abnormal increase in motor function or activity

Hyperlipidemia: A general term for elevated concentrations of any or all of the lipids in the plasma

Hyperosmolar: A solution that consists of a large amount of solute and a small amount of water

Hyperplasia: Abnormal increase in the volume of tissue or organ caused by the formation and growth of new normal cells

Hypersplenism: A condition characterized by exaggeration of the hemolytic function (rupture of the erythrocytes with the release of hemoglobin into the plasma) of the spleen, resulting in deficiency of peripheral blood elements

Hypertension: Persistent elevation of blood pressure

Hypertonic: Same as hyperosmolar

Hypertrophy: Increase in volume of a tissue or organ produced entirely by enlargement of existing cells

Hyperuricemia: An excess of uric acid or urates in the blood

Hyperuricosuria: An excess of uric acid excreted in the urine

Hypesthesia (hypoesthesia): Abnormal decrease in sensitivity to sensory stimulation

Hypochromia: Decrease of hemoglobin in the erythrocytes so that the erythrocytes are abnormally pale

Hypofunction: Diminished functioning of a part or gland

Hyponatremia: Deficiency of sodium in the blood

Hypoosmolar: Describes a solution that consists of a large amount of water and a small amount of solute

Hypophosphatemia: Deficiency of phosphates in the blood

Hypotonic: Same as hypoosmolar

Hypovolemic shock: Abnormally decreased volume of circulating fluid (plasma) in the body

Hypoxia: A broad term meaning diminished availability of oxygen to the body tissues

Icteric: Pertaining to or affected by jaundice, yellowed

IgE: Immunoglobulin E, a protein of animal origin with known antibody activity

Ileum: The distal portion of the small intestine, extending from the jejunum to the cecum

Immune complex: Large molecules formed when antigen and antibody bind together

Immunocompetence: The capacity to develop an immune response after exposure to antigen

Immunodeficient: Describes a deficiency of immune response or a disorder characterized by deficient immune response

Immunoglobulin: There are five classes of immunoglobulins: IgM, IgG, IgA, IgE, and IgD; each immunoglobulin is a protein of animal origin with known antibody activity; immunoglobulins are major components of what is called the humoral immune response system; they are synthesized by lymphocytes and plasma cells and are found in the serum and in other body fluids and tissues, including the urine, spinal fluid, lymph nodes, and spleen

Incontinence: Inability to control excretory functions (may be bowel or urinary)

Induration: The quality of being hard

Infarction: Irreversible tissue damage (necrosis) due to lack of oxygen resulting from obstruction of an artery, most commonly by a thrombus or embolus

Insulin: A double-chain protein hormone formed in the beta cells of the pancreatic islets of Langerhans; the major fuel-regulating hormone, it is secreted into the blood in response to a rise in concentration of blood glucose or amino acids

Interferon: A natural glycoprotein released by cells invaded by viruses; it is not itself an antiviral agent, but acts instead as a stimulant to noninfected cells causing them to synthesize another protein with antiviral characteristics

Internuncial: Neurons connecting other neurons

Interstitial compartment: Space between cells

Intracellular fluid (ICF): Body fluid found inside body cells

Intradural: Within or beneath the dura mater, the outermost, toughest, and most fibrous of the three membranes (meninges) covering the brain and spinal cord

Intramedullary: Within the spinal cord

Intravascular compartment: Vascular spaces; spaces within the blood vessels

Iridocyclitis: Inflammation of the iris and ciliary body of the eye

Iritis: Inflammation of the iris, the circular pigmented membrane behind the cornea of the eye

Ischemia: Loss of blood supply in an area, usually caused by a functional constriction or mechanical obstruction of a blood vessel

Isotonic: Describes a solution that contains both water and solutes in the same concentration as that of the fluid in the body

Jaundice: Yellowness of the skin, sclerae, mucous membranes, and excretions due to hyperbilirubinemia and deposition of bile pigments; also called icteric

Kernicterus: A condition in the newborn infant marked by severe neural symptoms associated with high levels of bilirubin in the blood

Ketonuria: An excess of ketone bodies (normal metabolic products of lipid and pyruvate within the liver) in the urine

Kussmaul's respiration: A distressing dyspnea characterized by increased respiratory rate (above 20/min), increased depth of respiration, panting, and labored respiration typical of air hunger; seen in metabolic acidosis, especially diabetic ketoacidosis and renal failure

Lactation: The secretion of milk by the breast; also describes the period of weeks or months during which a child is nursed at the breast

Laparoscopy: Examination of the peritoneal cavity by means of an endoscope called a laparoscope

Leukocyte: A colorless blood corpuscle capable of ameboid movement, whose chief function is to protect the body against microorganisms causing disease, classified into two main groups: granular (basophils, neutrophils, eosinophils) and nongranular (lymphocytes, monocytes)

Leukocytosis: A transient increase in the number of leukocytes in the blood, due to various causes

Leukopenia: Also known as leukocytopenia; a reduction in the number of leukocytes in the blood, the count being 5000 or less

Leukopoiesis: Production of leukocytes

Leukopoietin: Any factor or agent promoting leukopoiesis

Lithotomy: Incision of a duct or organ for removal of calculi

Lithotomy position: The person lies on the back, legs flexed on the thighs, thighs flexed on the abdomen and abducted

Lumen: The cavity or channel within a tube or tubular organ, such as a blood vessel or the intestine

Lymph: A transparent, usually slightly yellow liquid found within the lymphatic vessels and collected from tissues in all parts of the body and returned to the blood via the lymphatic system

Lymph nodes: Any of the accumulations of lymphoid tissue organized as definite lymphoid organs along the course of lymphatic vessels; they are the main source of lymphocytes in the peripheral blood and act as a defense mechanism by removing noxious agents (e.g., bacteria, toxins)

Lymphadenopathy: Disease of the lymph nodes

Lymphedema: An excessive accumulation of fluid in tissue spaces

Lymphocytes: Any of the mononuclear, nonphagocytic leukocytes found in the blood, lymph, and lymphoid tissues that comprise the body's immunologically competent cells and their precursors; they are divided into two classes of B lymphocytes, responsible for humoral and cellular immunity, respectively

Lymphoid cells: Cells pertaining to lymph or to tissue of the lymphatic system, specifically lymphocytes and plasma cells

Lymphokines: A general term for soluble protein mediators released by sensitized lymphocytes on contact with antigen; believed to play a role in macrophage activation, lymphocyte transformation, and cell-mediated immunity

Lymphomas: Any neoplastic disorder of lymphoid tissue, including Hodgkin's disease; often used to denote malignant lymphoma, classifications of which are based on predominant cell type and degree of differentiation; various categories may be subdivided into nodular and diffuse types, depending on the predominant pattern of cell arrangement

Lysis: Destruction or decomposition, especially by enzymatic digestion

Macrophage: Any of the large, mononuclear, highly phagocytic cells derived from monocytes that occur in the walls of blood vessels and in loose connective tissue; they function in phagocytosis, presentation of antigens or T lymphocytes and B lymphocytes, and secretion of a variety of products, including enzymes, several complement components and coagulation factors, some prostaglandins, and several regulatory molecules

Mast cells: A connective tissue cell capable of releasing basophilic granules that contain histamine, heparin, hyaluronic acid, and slow-reacting substance of anaphylaxis (SRS-A); in some species, capable of releasing serotonin

Mastitis: Inflammation of the breast occurring in a variety of forms and in various degrees of severity

Mastodynia: Mammary neuralgia of the intercostal nerves of the upper dorsal branches on one side

Mediastinum: The mass of tissues and organs separating the sternum in front and the vertebral column behind, containing the heart and its large vessels, trachea, esophagus, thymus, and lymph nodes

Megaloureter: Congenital ureteral dilatation without demonstrable cause

Melanoma: A tumor arising from the skin; refers to malignant melanoma

Melena: Blood in stool characterized by a dark, tarry color

Menarche: Establishment of beginning of the menstrual function

Menorrhagia: Excessive menstruation

Metaplasia: The change in the type of adult cells in a tissue to a form abnormal for that tissue

Metastases: The transfer of cancer cells from one organ or part to another not directly connected with the original organ

Microangiopathy: A disorder involving the small blood vessels
   thrombotic m., formation of thrombi in the arterioles and capillaries

Micturition: Urination

Mineralocorticoids: Any of a group of hormones elaborated by the cortex of the adrenal gland, so called because of their effects on sodium, chloride, and potassium concentrations in the extracellular fluid to regulate fluid and electrolyte balance; the primary mineralocorticoid is aldosterone

Monoarthritis: Asymmetric presentation of arthritis, affecting one joint at a time

Monocytes: A mononuclear, phagocytic leukocyte derived from promonocytes in the bone marrow; they circulate in the blood for about 24 hours before migrating to the tissues, such as in the lung and liver, where they develop into macrophages

Monokines: A general term for soluble mediators of immune responses that are not antibodies nor complement components and that are produced by mononuclear phagocytes (monocytes or macrophages)

Morbidity: A condition of being diseased (sickness or illness)

Morphea: A condition in which there is a connective tissue replacement of the skin and sometimes of the subcutaneous tissue, marked by the formation of ivory white or pink patches, bands, or lines that are sometimes bordered by a purple areola; the lesions are firm but not hard and are usually depressed; they may remain localized or may involute, leaving atrophy and scarring; also called localized scleroderma

Multiparity: Two or more pregnancies, in one woman, resulting in viable offspring

Multiple myeloma: A malignant neoplasm of plasma cells in which the plasma cells proliferate and invade the bone marrow, causing destruction of the bone and resulting in pathologic fracture and bone pain

Myalgia: Muscular pain

Myelin: Lipid substance forming a sheath around the axons of certain nerve fibers

Myelofibrosis: Replacement of bone marrow by fibrous tissue

Myocardial infarct: Necrosis of the cells of an area of the heart muscle (myocardium) occurring as a result of oxygen deprivation, which in turn is caused by obstruction of the blood supply; commonly referred to as a "heart attack"

Myocardium: The middle and thickest layer of the heart wall consisting of cardiac muscle

Myoedema: Localized knot or edema of contracting muscle induced by direct percussion or by some other form of mechanical irritation of the muscle

Myokymia: A benign condition in which there is persistent quivering of the muscles

Myopathy: Any disease of a muscle

Myositis: Inflammation of a voluntary muscle

Myxedema: A condition resulting from advanced hypothyroidism or a deficiency of thyroxine

Necrosis: Morphologic changes indicative of cell death caused by enzymatic degradation; death of tissue

Neoplasm: Tumor; any new and abnormal growth, specifically one in which cell multiplication is uncontrolled and progressive. Neoplasms may be benign or malignant

Nephrolithiasis: A condition marked by the presence of renal calculi or kidney stones

Neuraxis: Axon; central nervous system

Neuritis: Constant irritation of nerve endings; inflammation of a nerve

Neurogenic: Forming nervous tissue or originating in the nervous system

Neurohormones: A hormone stimulating the neural mechanism

Neutrophil: A granular leukocyte that has a nucleus with three to five lobes connected by threads of chromatin and cytoplasm containing very fine granules; neutrophils have the property of chemotaxis, adherence to immune complexes, and phagocytosis; also called polymorphonuclear, polynuclear, or neutrophilic leukocyte

Night sweats: Gradual increase in body temperature above normal, followed by a sudden drop in temperature that usually occurs during sleep; the person affected may awaken when the sudden reduction of body temperature results in profuse sweating

Nitroglycerin: Medication used as a coronary artery vasodilator

Nocturia: Excessive urination at night

Nodular lymphoma: Malignant lymphoma in which the lymphomatous cells are clustered into identifiable nodules within the lymph nodes that somewhat resemble the germinal centers of lymph node follicles

Nystagmus: Involuntary, rapid, rhythmic movement (horizontal, vertical, rotatory, or mixed) of the eyeball

Obstipation: Intractable (not easily relieved) constipation

Occult: Hidden from view, obscure

Odynophagia: Painful swallowing of food

Oliguria: Diminished urine secretion in relation to fluid intake

Oncogene: A gene found in the chromosomes of tumor cells whose activation is associated with the initial and continuing conversion of normal cells into cancer cells

Oncogenesis: The production or causation of tumors

Onycholysis: Loosening or separation of a nail from its bed

Oophorectomy: Removal of one or both ovaries; also called ovariectomy

Open-ended question: Question that elicits more than a one-word response

Orthopnea: Difficult breathing except in the upright position; the person must sit or stand to breathe

Orthostatic hypotension: Excessive fall (20 or more mm Hg) in blood pressure on assuming the erect position

Osmolality: The concentration of a solution in terms of osmoles of solutes per kilogram of solvent

Osmosis: Movement of water from an area of high concentration of water to an area of low concentration of water through a semipermeable membrane

Osmotic diuresis: Rapid loss of sodium and water through the inhibition of their reabsorption in the kidney tubules and the loop of Henle

Osteoblastomas: A benign, painful, vascular tumor of bone marked by the formation of osteoid tissue and primitive bone

Osteochondromas: A benign bone tumor consisting of projection adult bone capped by cartilage

Osteodystrophy (renal): Demineralization of bones related to decreased calcium absorption and resultant calcium/phosphorus imbalance

Osteogenic sarcoma (osteosarcoma): A malignant primary tumor of bone consisting of a malignant connective tissue stroma (tissue forming the framework, ground substance of matrix of an organ)

Osteoid osteoma: A benign hemarthromatous (blood-filled) lesion of cortical bone in young individuals

Osteolytic lesions: Dissolution of bone; removal or loss of calcium from the bone

Osteomalacia: Softening of the bones, resulting from impaired mineralization with excess accumulation of osteoid (bone that has not calcified), caused by vitamin D deficiency in adults

Osteomyelitis: Inflammation of bone, localized or generalized, due to a pyogenic (producing pus) infection; it may result in bone destruction and in stiffening of joints if the infection spreads to the joints

Osteopenia: Reduced bone mass due to a decrease in the rate of osteoid synthesis to a level insufficient to compensate for normal bone lysis; any bone mass below the normal

Osteoporosis: Decreased mass per unit volume of normally mineralized bone compared with age-and sex-matched controls

Palpitations: Subjective sensation of throbbing, fluttering, skipping, rapid, or forcible pulsation of the heart; may be regular or irregular

Pannus: An inflammatory exudate overlying synovial cells on the inside of a joint capsule, usually occurring in rheumatoid arthritis; fatty, bloody, edematous mass within the synovial membrane

Papilledema: Edema and hyperemia (excess blood) of the optic disc usually associated with increased intracranial pressure

Papilloma: A benign tumor derived from epithelium; papillomas may arise from skin, mucous membranes, or glandular ducts

Paracentesis: Surgical puncture of a cavity for the aspiration of fluid

Paraneoplastic syndrome: A collective term for disorders arising from metabolic effects of cancer on tissues remote from the tumor; such syndromes may appear as primary endocrine, hematologic, or neuromuscular disorders

Paraphrasing technique: Repeating information presented by the client for clarification

Parenchyma: The essential or functional elements of an organ; for example, the kidney itself

Parenteral: Not through the alimentary canal, but by subcutaneous, intramuscular, intrasternal, or intravenous injection

Paresthesias: Abnormal sensation, such as burning or prickling without a loss of objective neurologic findings

Parietal: Of or pertaining to the walls of an organ or cavity

Parietal pericardium: The serous membrane between the (fibrous) pericardium and the epicardium (or visceral surface) of the heart

Parietal pleura: The serous membrane lining the walls of the thoracic cavity

Paroxysmal: A sudden, recurrent intensification of symptoms; a spasm

Paroxysmal nocturnal dyspnea: Acute dyspnea occurring suddenly at night, usually waking the person after a few hours of sleep; caused by pulmonary congestion and edema that result from left-sided heart failure; varies in severity from nocturnal restlessness or anxiety to extreme respiratory distress

Patent ductus arteriosus: Shunt caused by an opening between the aorta and the pulmonary artery

Pericardial: Related to the pericardium; the fibroserous sac enclosing the heart and the roots of the great vessels

Pericardium: The fibrous sac enveloping the entire heart, consisting of two layers: the epicardium (visceral layer immediately surrounding the heart) and the serous parietal pericardium

Peristalsis: The wormlike movement by which the alimentary canal or other tubular organs with both longitudinal and circular muscle fibers propel their contents, consisting of a wave of contraction passing along the tube

Petechiae: Minute, pinpoint, nonraised, perfectly round, purple-red spots caused by intradermal or submucous hemorrhage; later turns blue or yellow

Peyer's patches: White, oval, elevated patches of closely packed lymph follicles in mucous and submucous layers of the small intestine

pH: The negative logarithm of the hydrogen ion concentration $[H^+]$, a measure of the degree to which a solution is acidic or alkaline

Phagocyte: Any cell capable of ingesting particulate matter; the term refers to two types of phagocytes: polymorphonuclear leukocytes and mononuclear phagocytes (macrophages and monocytes); these cells ingest microorganisms and other particulate antigens that are coated with antibody or complement, a process that is mediated by specific cell-surface receptors

Phagocytosing: The process of ingesting particulate matter by phagocytes

Phagocytosis: The engulfing of microorganisms or other cells and foreign material

Phimosis: Constriction of the orifice or opening of the prepuce or foreskin so that it cannot be drawn back over the glans

Phlebitis: Inflammation of a vein

Phlebotomy: Incision of a vein and removal of blood

Phrenic nerve: A major branch of the cervical plexus that extends through the thorax to provide innervation of the diaphragm; nerve impulses from the inspiratory center in the brain travel down the phrenic nerve, causing contraction of the diaphragm and inspiration occurs

Piloerection: Erection of the hair

Pitting edema: Edema in which pressure leaves a persistent depression in the tissues

Platelet: A small disc or platelike structure, the smallest of the formed elements in blood; also called thrombocytes; these disc-shaped, nonnucleated blood elements are very fragile and tend to adhere to uneven or damaged surfaces; their rate of formation is governed by the amount of oxygen in the blood and the presence of nucleic acid derivatives from injured tissue; the functions of platelets are related to coagulation and the clotting of blood; because of their adhesion and aggregation capabilities, platelets can occlude small breaks in blood vessels and prevent blood from escaping;

platelets are also able to take up, store, transport, and release serotonin and platelet factor III

Pleura: A thin, transparent, moist serous membrane enveloping the lungs (pulmonary pleura) and lining the thoracic cavity (parietal pleura), completely enclosing a potential space known as the pleural cavity

Pleural space: The potential space between the parietal pleura and the pulmonary pleura (visceral pleura of the lungs)

Pleurisy: Inflammation of the pleura; it may be caused by infection, injury, or tumor; it may be a complication of lung diseases, particularly of pneumonia or sometimes tuberculosis, lung abscess, or influenza

Pleuropulmonary: Pertaining to the pleura (serous membrane around the lungs and lining the thoracic cavity enclosing the pleural cavity) and the lungs

Pneumatocele: Hernia of lung tissue; a benign, thin-walled, air-containing cyst of the lung

Pneumothorax: Accumulation of gas or air in the pleural cavity resulting in the collapse of the lung on the affected side

Poikilocytosis: The presence of abnormally shaped red blood cells in the blood

Polyarthritis: Inflammation of several joints

Polycythemia: An increase in the total red cell mass of the blood

Polydypsia: Excessive thirst

Polymyositis: A chronic, progressive inflammatory disease of skeletal muscle, occurring in both children and adults

Polyp: Any growth or mass protruding from a mucous membrane

Polyphagia: Excessive ingestion of food

Polyuria: Excessive excretion of urine

Portal hypertension: Abnormally increased pressure in the portal circulation (i.e., circulation from the gastrointestinal tract and spleen through the portal vein to the liver) due to narrowing of the capillary branches of the portal vessels; the result is impairment of the liver's ability to detoxify wastes and transport nutrients, resulting in hepatic encephalopathy, anorexia, and metabolic acidosis; the increased pressure can lead to escape of fluid through the liver capsule and into the abdominal cavity (ascites)

Precordia(ium): The region over the heart and lower part of the thorax; sometimes the diaphragm is referred to as the precordium

Prolapse: The falling down or downward displacement of a part or organ

Prostaglandins: A group of naturally occurring, chemically related, long-chain hydroxy fatty acids that stimulate contractility of the uterine and other smooth muscles and have the ability to lower blood pressure, regulate acid secretion of the stomach, regulate body temperature and platelet aggregation, and control inflammation and vascular permeability; they also affect the action of certain hormones

Proteinuria: An excess of serum proteins in the urine; may cause foamy urine

Pruritus: Itching common in many skin disorders, especially allergic inflammation and parasitic infestation; systemic diseases that may cause pruritus include diabetes mellitus and liver disorders with jaundice

Ptosis: Drooping of the upper eyelid (caused by extraocular muscle weakness)

Pulmonary infarct: Localized necrosis of lung tissue due to obstruction of the arterial blood supply

Pulmonary pleura: Membrane enveloping the lungs

Purkinje's fibers: Modified cardiac muscle fibers in the subendothelial tissue, concerned with conducting impulses to the heart

Purpura: A hemorrhagic disease characterized by extravasation of blood into the tissues, under the skin, and through the mucous membranes, and producing spontaneous ecchymoses (bruises) and petechiae (small red patches) on the skin

Pyelonephritis: Inflammation of the kidney and renal pelvis (funnel-shaped expansion of the upper end of the ureter into which the renal cavities open, usually the renal sinus); also called nephropyelitis

Pyoderma: Any purulent (containing or forming pus) skin disease; deep ulcers or canker sores

Raynaud's disease: Vasospasm of digital arteries with blanching and numbness of fingers

Raynaud's phenomenon: Intermittent spasm of the digital arteries, with blanching and numbness of the fingers or toes bilaterally

Rectocele: Hernial protrusion of part of the rectum into the vagina

Referred: Related to a remote origin

Reflux: A backward or return flow

Regional enteritis: See Crohn's disease

Relaxin: A hormone that produces relaxation of the symphysis pubis and dilation of the uterine cervix

Renin: A proteolytic enzyme synthesized, stored, and secreted by the juxtaglomerular cells of the kidney; it plays a role in the regulation of blood pressure by catalyzing the conversion of the plasma glycoprotein angiotensinogen to angiotensin I

Reticuloendothelial: Pertaining to the reticuloendothelium or to the reticuloendothelial system that is a network of cells and tissues found throughout the body, especially in the blood, general connective tissue, spleen, liver, lungs, bone marrow, and lymph nodes; reticuloendothelial cells are involved in blood cell formation and destruction, storage of fatty materials, and metabolism of iron and pigment; they play a role in inflammation and immunity; some of the cells are motile (capable of motion) and phagocytic, ingesting and destroying unwanted foreign material; the reticuloendothelial cells of the spleen possess the ability to dispose of disintegrated erythrocytes, but they do not destroy hemoglobin that is liberated in the process

Retinopathy: Noninflammatory disease of the retina

Retrosternum: Behind the sternum

Retroversion: Tipping backward of an entire organ, specifically the uterus

Retrovirus: A large group of RNA viruses that includes the leukoviruses and lentiviruses; so called because they carry reverse transcriptase

Sacroiliitis: Inflammation of the sacroiliac joint

Salpingitis: Inflammation of a fallopian tube

Sarcoma: A tumor, often highly malignant, consisting of cells derived from connective tissue, such as bone and cartilage, muscle, blood vessel, or lymphoid tissue; these tumors usually develop rapidly and metastasize through the lymph channels

Satiety: State or condition of satisfaction, as full gratification of appetite or thirst with abolition of the desire to ingest further food or liquids

Sclerae: The tough, white outer coat of the eyeballs

Sclerodactyly: Chronic hardening and shrinking of the fingers and toes

Scotomas: An area of lost or depressed vision within the visual field; perceived as black spots before the eyes

Septic (sepsis): Characterized by the presence of blood or other tissues of pathogenic microorganisms or their toxins

Septicemia: Blood poisoning

Signs: Any objective evidence of disease or dysfunction; an observable physical phenomenon

Sinoatrial node: The cardiac pacemaker located in the right atrium of the heart

Sinusitis: Inflammation of one or more of the paranasal sinuses, often occurring during an upper respiratory infection when the infection in the nose spreads to the sinuses

Sinusoids: Resembling a sinus; a form of terminal blood channel consisting of large, irregular, anastomosing vessels with a lining of reticuloendothelium

Somatic: Pertaining to or characteristic of the body (soma); the body as distinguished from the mind; the body tissue as distinguished from the germ cells

Spider angiomas: Branched dilatation of the superficial capillaries, resembling a spider

Splenectomy: Excision of the spleen

Splenomegaly: Enlargement of the spleen

Spondylitis: Inflammation of the vertebrae

Spondyloarthropathy: Disease of the joints of the spine

Spondylotic bars: A union of the bones of a joint by proliferation of bone cells in the shape of a bar extending between two bones (or vertebrae)

Spontaneous pneumothorax: Accumulation of air or gas in the pleural cavity, resulting in collapse of the lung on the affected side

Stem cells: Any precursor cell; a mother cell with the capacity for replication and differentiation

Stenosis: Narrowing or stricture of a duct, canal, body passage, or opening

Stress incontinence: Involuntary escape of urine due to strain on the orifice of the bladder, such as in coughing or sneezing

Stricture: An abnormal narrowing of a duct or passage

Suppressor T cells (T_s): Subset of T cells that "turn off" antibody production

Surfactant: A mixture of phospholipids secreted by the alveolar cells into the alveoli and respiratory passages that reduce the surface tension of pulmonary fluids and thus contribute to the elastic properties of pulmonary disease

Symptoms: Any indication of disease as perceived by the client

Syncope: Episodes of fainting or loss of consciousness due to generalized cerebral ischemia

Syndesmophyte: Ossification of connective tissue other than bone, such as ligaments, tendons, or outer margins of the intervertebral disc

Systole: The contraction, or period of contraction, of the heart, especially of the ventricles, during which blood is forced into the aorta and pulmonary artery

T cells: White blood cells that are processed in the thymus and then produce lymphokines; responsible in part for carrying out the immune response; also called T lymphocytes

Tachycardia: Rapid beating of the heart; the term is usually applied to a heart rate above 100 beats/min

Tachypnea: Very rapid, shallow breathing; respiratory rate greater than 20 breaths/min

Target gland: Glands in the body that are specifically affected by pituitary hormones

Telangiectasia: Vascular lesion formed by dilation of a group of small blood vessels

Tenesmus: Ineffective and painful straining at stool or in urinating

Tetralogy of Fallot: A combination of congenital cardiac defects, consisting of pulmonary stenosis, interventricular septal defect, displacement of the aorta so that it overrides the interventricular septum and receives venous as well as arterial blood, and right ventricular hypertrophy

Thrombin: An enzyme resulting from the activation of prothrombin, which catalyzes the conversion of fibrinogen to fibrin

Thromboangiitis obliterans (Buerger's disease): An intense inflammatory and obliterative disease of the blood vessels of primarily the lower extremities

Thrombocyte: A blood platelet

Thrombocytopenia: Decrease in the number of platelets in circulating blood, resulting from decreased or defective platelet production or from accelerated platelet destruction.

Thrombocytosis: Increase in the number of platelets in the circulating blood

Thrombophlebitis: Inflammation of a vein, accompanied by thrombus formation

Thrombopoiesis: Thrombogenesis; clot formation

Thrombopoietin: Any agent or factor involved in thrombopoiesis (clot formation)

Thromboxanes: An intermediate in the metabolic pathway of arachidonic acid, formed from prostaglandin endoperoxides and released from suitably stimulated platelets; the unstable form, thromboxane A_2, is a potent inducer of platelet aggregation and constrictor of arterial smooth muscle

Thrombus (pl. thrombi): A blood clot formed within a blood vessel or cavity of the heart that remains attached to the site at which it formed; an aggregation of blood factors, primarily platelets and fibrin, with entrapment of cellular elements, frequently causing vascular obstruction at the point of its formation. Some experts differentiate a thrombus from a blood clot

Thymectomy: Excision of the thymus

Thymus: A ductless, glandlike body lying in the upper mediastinum beneath the sternum, which plays an immunologic role throughout life; a lymphoid organ

Tophus (pl. tophi): A chalky deposit of sodium urate occurring in gout; tophi form most often around the joints in cartilage, bone, bursae, and subcutaneous tissue, producing a chronic, foreign body inflammatory response

Total parenteral nutrition (TPN): See Hyperalimentation

Transient ischemic attacks (TIAs): Temporary disruption of blood supply to part of the brain, lasting 5 to 20 minutes; an early warning signal of possible impending CVA or stroke

Trigger point: Hypersensitive spot in the skeletal musculature that produces pain that can be referred to other parts of the body

Ulcerative colitis: A recurrent acute and chronic disorder characterized by extensive inflammatory ulceration in the colon, chiefly of the mucosa and submucosa

Urate salts: Salts of uric acid

Uremia: An excess in the blood of urea, creatinine, and other nitrogenous end-products of protein and amino acid metabolism; referred to more correctly as azotemia and, in current medical usage, the entire complex of signs and symptoms of chronic renal failure

Uremic breath: Characteristic urine-like odor of breath secondary to a build-up and release of uremic toxins

Urethritis: Inflammation of the urethra, a tubular passage through which urine is discharged from the bladder to the exterior of the body

Urgency: Referring to bowel and bladder urgency: the sudden compelling desire to urinate or defecate

Urgency incontinence: Inability to hold back urination when feeling the urge to void; a major complaint of people with urinary tract infections

Urinary urgency: The sudden compelling desire to urinate

Urticaria: A vascular reaction of the skin marked by the transient appearance of slightly elevated patches (wheals) that are redder or paler than the surrounding skin and are often attended by severe itching; also called hives

Uveitis: Inflammation of part or all of the middle (vascular) tunic of the eye (uvea)

Varicose: Dilated or distended

Vasodilatory: Capable of opening up the blood vessels

Ventricular septal defect: Hole between the ventricles of the heart

Vertical transmission: Method of transmission by which an infant is infected with hepatitis by its mother either during pregnancy or after birth

Vertigo: An illusion of movement; a sensation as if the external world were revolving around the client; the term is sometimes erroneously used to mean any form of dizziness, but the client will usually use the word "dizzy" to describe the symptom

Viscera (pl. of viscus): Any large interior organs in any of the great body cavities, especially organs in the abdomen

Visceral: Pertaining to a viscus or any large interior organ in any of the great body cavities, especially organs in the abdomen

Visceral peritoneum: The serous membrane lining the organs

Visceral pleura: The membrane enveloping an organ

Viscus (pl. viscera): Any large interior organ in any of the great body cavities, especially organs in the abdomen

Xanthine: A purine compound found in most body tissues and fluids; it is a precursor of uric acid

Index

Page numbers in **boldface** indicate lists of clinical signs and symptoms.
Page numbers in *italics* indicate illustrations.
Page numbers followed by t indicate tables.

609